A Clinician's Guide to Neurodegenerative Disorders

A Clinician's Guide to Neurodegenerative Disorders

Edited by Anna Roberts

STATES
ACADEMIC PRESS
www.statesacademicpress.com

States Academic Press,
109 South 5th Street,
Brooklyn, NY 11249, USA

Visit us on the World Wide Web at:
www.statesacademicpress.com

ISBN: 978-1-63989-001-9

Cataloging-in-Publication Data

A clinician's guide to neurodegenerative disorders / edited by Anna Roberts.
p. cm.
Includes bibliographical references and index.
ISBN 978-1-63989-001-9
1. Nervous system--Degeneration. 2. Degeneration (Pathology). 3. Molecular neurobiology.
4. Neurology. I. Roberts, Anna.
RC365 .C55 2022
616.804 7--dc23

Table of Contents

Preface ... IX

Chapter 1 **Alzheimer's disease, neuroprotection, and CNS immunosenescence** ... 1
Wolfgang J. Streit and Qing-Shan Xue

Chapter 2 **Scale and pattern of atrophy in the chronic stages of moderate-severe TBI** ... 8
Robin E. A. Green, Brenda Colella, Jerome J. Maller, Mark Bayley, Joanna Glazer and David J. Mikulis

Chapter 3 **Current understanding of the glial response to disorders of the aging CNS** ... 17
Roger A Barker and Francesca Cicchetti

Chapter 4 **Is there evidence for neurodegenerative change following traumatic brain injury in children and youth?** ... 22
Michelle L. Keightley, Katia J. Sinopoli, Karen D. Davis, David J. Mikulis, Richard Wennber, Maria C. Tartaglia, Jen-Kai Chen and Charles H. Tator

Chapter 5 **Cerebrospinal fluid biomarkers for differentiation of frontotemporal lobar degeneration from Alzheimer's disease** ... 28
David J. Irwin, John Q. Trojanowski and Murray Grossman

Chapter 6 **Traumatic brain injury and post-acute decline: what role does environmental enrichment play?** ... 39
Diana Frasca, Jennifer Tomaszczyk, Bradford J. McFadyen and Robin E. Green

Chapter 7 **Aspects of innate immunity and Parkinson's disease** ... 61
Yue Huang and Glenda M. Halliday

Chapter 8 **Chronic traumatic encephalopathy and other neurodegenerative proteinopathies** ... 71
Maria Carmela Tartaglia, Lili-Naz Hazrati, Karen D. Davis, Robin E. A. Green, Richard Wennberg, David Mikulis, Leo J. Ezerins, Michelle Keightley and Charles Tator

Chapter 9 **Microglia function in Alzheimer's disease** ... 77
Egle Solito and Magdalena Sastre

Chapter 10 **Absence of chronic traumatic encephalopathy in retired football players with multiple concussions and neurological symptomatology** ... 87
Lili-Naz Hazrati, Maria C. Tartaglia, Phedias Diamandis, Karen D. Davis, Robin E. Green, Richard Wennberg, Janice C. Wong, Leo Ezerins and Charles H. Tator

Chapter 11 **The utility of age-specific cut-offs for visual rating of medial temporal atrophy in classifying Alzheimer's disease, MCI and cognitively normal elderly subjects** ... 96
Ranjan Duara, David A. Loewenstein, Qian Shen, Warren Barker, Daniel Varon, Maria T. Greig, Rosie Curiel, Joscelyn Agron, Isael Santos and Huntington Potter

Chapter 12 **Methodological considerations in longitudinal morphometry of traumatic brain injury** 104
Junghoon Kim, Brian Avants, John Whyte and James C. Gee

Chapter 13 **Evaluation of annexin A5 as a biomarker for Alzheimer's disease and dementia with lewy bodies** 110
Hitoshi Sohma, Shin-ichi Imai, Norio Takei, Hirohito Honda, Kyoichi Matsumoto, Kumiko Utsumi, Kayo Matsuki, Eri Hashimoto, Toshikazu Saito and Yasuo Kokai

Chapter 14 **Traumatic brain injury, neuroimaging, and neurodegeneration** 117
Erin D. Bigler

Chapter 15 **MTA index: a simple 2D-method for assessing atrophy of the medial temporal lobe using clinically available neuroimaging** 132
Manuel Menéndez-González, Alfonso López-Muñiz, José A. Vega, José M. Salas-Pacheco and Oscar Arias-Carrión

Chapter 16 **History of innate immunity in neurodegenerative disorders** 138
Patrick L. McGeer and Edith G. McGeer

Chapter 17 **Biomarker-based prediction of progression in MCI: comparison of AD signature and hippocampal volume with spinal fluid amyloid-β and tau** 143
Bradford C. Dickerson and David A. Wolk

Chapter 18 **Imaging of microglia in patients with neurodegenerative disorders** 152
Marios Politis, Paul Su and Paola Piccini

Chapter 19 **Is the subcallosal medial prefrontal cortex a common site of atrophy in Alzheimer's disease and frontotemporal lobar degeneration?** 162
Olof Lindberg, Eric Westman, Sari Karlsson, Per Östberg, Leif A. Svensson, Andrew Simmons and Lars-Olof Wahlund

Chapter 20 **Microglial activation – tuning and pruning adult neurogenesis** 170
Christine T. Ekdahl

Chapter 21 **Longitudinal diffusion tensor imaging and neuropsychological correlates in traumatic brain injury patients** 179
Kimberly D. Farbota, Barbara B. Bendlin, Andrew L. Alexander, Howard A. Rowley, Robert J. Dempsey and Sterling C. Johnson

Chapter 22 **The role of apolipoprotein E (*APOE*) genotype in early mild cognitive impairment (E-MCI)** 193
Shannon L. Risacher, Sungeun Kim, Li Shen, Kwangsik Nho, Tatiana Foroud, Robert C. Green, Ronald C. Petersen, Clifford R. Jack Jr, Paul S. Aisen, Robert A. Koeppe, William J. Jagust, Leslie M. Shaw, John Q. Trojanowski, Michael W. Weiner and Andrew J. Saykin

Chapter 23 **Primary phagocytosis of neurons by inflamed microglia: potential roles in neurodegeneration** 205
Jonas J. Neher, Urte Neniskyte and Guy C. Brown

Chapter 24 **VBM with viscous fluid registration of gray matter segments in SPM** 214
Joao M. S. Pereira, Julio Acosta-Cabronero, George Pengas, Li Xiong, Peter J. Nestor and Guy B. Williams

Chapter 25 **The role of the innate immune system in ALS** ... **223**
Sudarshan Phani, Diane Berengere Re and Serge Przedborski

Chapter 26 **Environmental enrichment may protect against hippocampal atrophy in the chronic stages of traumatic brain injury** ... **229**
Lesley S. Miller, Brenda Colella, David Mikulis, Jerome Maller and Robin E. A. Green

Chapter 27 **Is abeta a sufficient biomarker for monitoring anti-abeta clinical studies?** ... **237**
Jens Moreth, Chrystelle Mavoungou and Katharina Schindowski

Chapter 28 **PREDICT-HD study** ... **244**
Kevin M. Biglan, Ying Zhang, Jeffrey D. Long, Michael Geschwind, Gail A. Kang, Annie Killoran, Wenjing Lu, Elizabeth McCusker, James A. Mills, Lynn A. Raymond, Claudia Testa, Joanne Wojcieszek and Jane S. Paulsen

Permissions

List of Contributors

Index

Preface

The main aim of this book is to educate learners and enhance their research focus by presenting diverse topics covering this vast field. This is an advanced book which compiles significant studies by distinguished experts in the area of analysis. This book addresses successive solutions to the challenges arising in the area of application, along with it; the book provides scope for future developments.

The diseases which are caused by the loss of function and eventual death of nerve cells in the brain or the peripheral nervous system are termed as neurodegenerative disorders. There are various mechanisms due to which neurodegenerative diseases can occur, such as genetic mutation, accumulation of misfolded proteins, mitochondrial dysfunction and aggregation of proteins. A few of the neurodegenerative diseases are Alzheimer's, Huntington's and Parkinson's disease. Alzheimer's disease causes the patients to lose their memory over a period of time. Huntington's disease causes the degeneration of nerve cells in the brain. It can result in disorders related to movement, cognition and mental abilities. Most of the topics introduced in this book cover new techniques in the diagnosis and management of neurodegenerative disorders. Different approaches, evaluations, methodologies and advanced studies on these medical conditions have been included in it. This book will provide comprehensive knowledge to the readers.

It was a great honour to edit this book, though there were challenges, as it involved a lot of communication and networking between me and the editorial team. However, the end result was this all-inclusive book covering diverse themes in the field.

Finally, it is important to acknowledge the efforts of the contributors for their excellent chapters, through which a wide variety of issues have been addressed. I would also like to thank my colleagues for their valuable feedback during the making of this book.

Editor

1

Alzheimer's disease, neuroprotection, and CNS immunosenescence

Wolfgang J. Streit* and Qing-Shan Xue

Department of Neuroscience, University of Florida College of Medicine and McKnight Brain Institute, Gainesville, FL, USA

Edited by:
Roger A. Barker, University of Cambridge and Addenbrooke's Hospital, UK

Reviewed by:
Francesca Cicchetti, Université Laval, Canada
Hans Lassmann, Center for Brain Research, Austria

****Correspondence:***
Wolfgang J. Streit, Department of Neuroscience, University of Florida, PO Box 100244, Gainesville, FL 32610-0244, USA.
e-mail: streit@mbi.ufl.edu

This review is focused on discussing in some detail possible neuroprotective functions of microglial cells. We strive to explain how loss of these essential microglial functions might contribute toward the development of characteristic neuropathological features that characterize Alzheimer's disease. The conceptual framework guiding our thinking is provided by the hypothesis that microglial senescence accounts for impaired neuronal protection and consequent neurodegeneration.

Keywords: Alzheimer's disease, CNS immunosenescence, impaired neuronal protection, microglial cells, microglial senescence, neurodegeneration, neuropathological features, neuroprotection

INTRODUCTION

The role of CNS microglial cells in the development of Alzheimer's disease(AD) has been the subject of considerable interest since McGeer's initial description of reactive microglia in human AD brain in 1987 (McGeer et al., 1987). Most of the numerous studies that followed corroborated McGeer's findings and collectively over the years they coalesced into the amyloid cascade-neuroinflammation hypothesis, which claims that neurodegenerative changes in AD (neurofibrillary degeneration) are the result of an uncontrolled, chronic intracerebral inflammatory reaction triggered by the accumulation/aggregation of amyloid-beta (Aβ) protein in plaques. Today, the neuroinflammation hypothesis is difficult to uphold given that clinical trials with anti-inflammatory drugs and strategies to remove Aβ from the brain have met with disappointing results and have yielded little in the way of effective treatments for humans. In this paper, we briefly describe our own vision of what may be the role of microglia in AD pathogenesis, which is different in that our primary focus is not on a single protein (Aβ) as the cause of AD, but instead relies on the incontrovertible fact that the incidence of sporadic AD is strongly correlated with aging. Our theory, which we call the microglial dysfunction hypothesis, states that neurodegeneration in AD is the result of an aging-related, gradually progressive breakdown of innate CNS immunity and loss of neuroprotection, i.e., microglial cell senescence. In contrast to normal aging this deterioration of innate CNS immunity appears to be accelerated in AD. The difference in perspective between the dysfunction hypothesis and the neuroinflammation theory is due in large part to our conviction that microglia are entirely beneficial cells, whose single-most important function is to provide neuronal protection at all times in the normal and injured CNS. In the following, we shall discuss succinctly several microglial neuroprotective functions and how senescent deterioration of these could contribute to development of neurodegenerative changes.

THE BRAIN'S INNATE IMMUNE SYSTEM IS NEUROPROTECTIVE

Even though doubts about the very existence of microglia were expressed in textbooks until the early 1990s (Graeber, 2010), the notion that microglia are the key cellular elements comprising the brain's innate immune system (Graeber and Streit, 1990; Streit and Kincaid-Colton, 1995) is now widely recognized. A common view that has been expressed many times is that together with peripheral macrophages, such as Kupffer cells of the liver, Langerhans cells of the epidermis, or alveolar macrophages in the lung, microglia are another member of the mononuclear phagocyte system, i.e., a tissue-specific macrophage. While there is little doubt regarding validity of a mononuclear lineage relationship, microglia in the CNS do not maintain a macrophage state constitutively or continuously. In the normal adult brain, microglia display a well-differentiated, dendritic morphology similar to that of other brain cells. They exhibit multiple, finely branched cytoplasmic processes with which they constantly explore the CNS microenvironment searching for disturbances that may require their quick response (Nimmerjahn et al., 2005; Tremblay et al., 2010). These ramified microglia are sensors of pathology (Kreutzberg, 1996; Stence et al., 2001; Petersen and Dailey, 2004; Davalos et al., 2005) and they do not exhibit macrophage morphology, nor do they express the typical macrophage marker, CD68 (recognized by ED1 antibody in the rat). Even activated microglia with hypertrophic morphology express the CD68 antigen only after having engaged in phagocytic activity (Graeber et al., 1998). It is therefore only under conditions of tissue/cell necrosis when debris must be phagocytized that microglia show expression of CD68 and can therefore be considered brain macrophages. The currently popular idea of differentiating functionally distinct macrophage phenotypes classified as M1 (cytotoxic), M2 (reparative), and a third, "deactivated" form might thus apply merely to those few microglial cells that at any given time are in a macrophage state during CNS injury or disease. To generalize and assume that the M1/M2 classification applies to the microglial population at large represents a rather indiscriminate extrapolation of *in vitro* studies performed with peripheral macrophages (Colton, 2009; Michelucci et al., 2009; Moon et al., 2011), and it could be misleading to assume that resting and activated microglia within the brain microenvironment function in the same manner as peripheral (professional) macrophages that have been cultured and manipulated *in vitro* with cytokines. There is currently no way of reliably identifying functionally distinct microglial phenotypes in brain tissue *in situ* and without this capability no real progress on functional involvement of putative M1 or M2 microglial subtypes in the cellular pathogenesis of AD can be made. In part because of this we are assuming that all microglia are potentially beneficial cells and our view of microglial involvement in AD is rooted firmly in that assumption. It is known that the CNS parenchyma represents a unique compartment that is segregated to a large extent from the rest of the body by the blood brain barrier (BBB), and that it represents an immunologically subdued environment (Ford et al., 1995; Perry et al., 1995; Carson et al., 1998; Hoek et al., 2000; Cardona et al., 2006), although not necessarily an "immunologically privileged site" (Galea et al., 2007). There are no constitutively active (professional) macrophages in the brain parenchyma under normal conditions. Our definition of a microglial cell is that of a cell type of the mononuclear cell lineage that has evolved to be highly adapted and specialized for residing within the unique CNS microenvironment. As such its immunological potential is limited largely to phagocytosis while its neuroprotective capabilities are maximized, and one might thus view microglia as a hybrid between a moderately immunocompetent mononuclear cell and a powerful neuroprotective glial cell.

We view the neuroprotective capabilities of microglia in the broadest possible meaning of the term, namely, anything that microglia do that is beneficial for and/or conducive toward proper neuronal functioning. One obvious beneficial function of microglia is simply their ability to transform into macrophages that can clear out debris and process waste when/if the need arises. These microglia-derived macrophages are not necessarily cytotoxic because much of the debris generated within the brain, for example after trauma or is chemia, is sterile (Chen and Nunez, 2010) and would thus not require elaboration of cytotoxins to kill microorganisms. Direct infection of the CNS with microorganisms is largely prevented by the natural barriers of skull, meninges, and BBB, but if these fail and when microorganisms do gain access to the parenchyma, they are likely to be eliminated quickly and efficiently by microglial cells and probably without too much collateral damage, as there are multiple mechanisms involved in post-infection neuropathology other than microglial neurotoxicity (Nau and Bruck, 2002; Mariani and Kielian, 2009; Ribes et al., 2011). One condition that deserves special mention is infection with the human immunodeficiency virus-1 (HIV-1), where microglial cells themselves are the target of the infectious agent (Michaels et al., 1988). It is therefore reasonable to assume that the functionality of HIV-infected microglia is compromised, although in ways that are not yet entirely understood. From our perspective, compromised microglial function includes primarily an impaired ability to provide neuroprotection, and it is perhaps because of this that patients with HIV/AIDS frequently suffer from the consequences of neurodegeneration, a.k.a. HIV-associated dementia (Anthony and Bell, 2008). It seems obvious that compromised innate immunity within the CNS due to HIV infection is what accounts at least in part for the high incidence of opportunistic CNS infections in HIV/AIDS patients, notably toxoplasmosis (Mariani and Kielian, 2009).

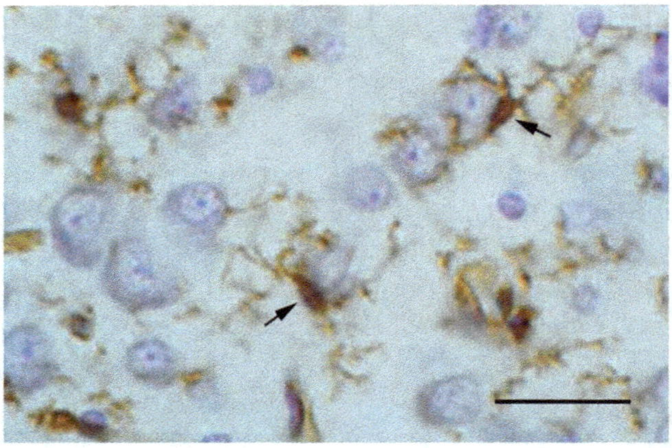

FIGURE 1 | Lectin staining of microglia (brown) in the normal cerebral cortex of a rabbit shows two microglial cells (arrows) extending their processes around cortical neurons. This close spatial relationship suggests ongoing interactions between resting microglia and neurons. Neurons are stained with cresyl violet. Scale bar: 50 μm.

A second and very direct neuroprotective function provided by microglia is the production and secretion of neurotrophic factors, notably BDNF (Elkabes et al., 1996; Batchelor et al., 1999; Suzuki et al., 2001; Nakajima et al., 2002; Coull et al., 2005) and NGF (Mallat et al., 1989; Heese et al., 1997; Frade and Barde, 1998), but also others like TGF-β (Kiefer et al., 1993; Lehrmann et al., 1998), bFGF (Araujo and Cotman, 1992), and GDNF (Batchelor et al., 1999; Suzuki et al., 2001). Production of neurotrophins by microglia is usually increased after injury/during recovery when the cells become activated and neurons require more neurotrophic support than under normal conditions. However, even under normal conditions microglia are likely to sustain neuronal functioning during periods of high activity or sub-pathological stress when smaller doses of neurotrophic factors may be required. Although it is difficult to demonstrate directly that this type of specific microglial-neuronal interaction actually occurs, histological images showing some neurons covered tightly by microglial processes suggests that this could be the case (**Figure 1**). Different neuronal populations require different neurotrophic factors and quite possibly microglia have the ability to sense which factors and how much of them may be needed in any particular circumstance. Their ability to migrate and home in on neurons in need is essential for facilitating such targeted neuroprotection.

A third way in which microglia can be neuroprotective is by diverting noxious and potentially harmful substances away from neurons. It has long been known that astrocytes take up excess glutamate from the extracellular space under conditions of heightened neuronal activity in an effort to minimize glutamate-mediated excitotoxicity. During the past 10 years it has become clear that astrocytes are not alone in this effort and that activated microglial cells also participate in the removal of glutamate by upregulating primarily glutamate transporter-1 (GLT-1) *in vivo* following traumatic lesions as well as *in vitro* after stimulation with LPS, TNF-α, or neuronal conditioned medium (Lopez-Redondo et al., 2000; Nakajima et al., 2001, 2008; van Landeghem et al., 2001). Interestingly, glutamate uptake by microglia is coupled to enhanced glutathione synthesis by microglia, perhaps reflecting an effort by the cells to protect themselves from damage (Persson et al., 2006). These studies underscore the extensive crosstalk that takes place continuously between microglia and neurons. In addition to glutamate, a second substance with considerable and non-specific damage potential is free, redox-active iron, which may be present either as ferric (Fe^{+3}) or ferrous (Fe^{+2}) ions. We propose that the sequestration of free iron in the CNS by ferritin in microglia constitutes an important neuroprotective mechanism that becomes most relevant when there is a breach in the BBB and the possibility exists of free iron entering the brain parenchyma. The evidence for this mechanism of microglial neuroprotection is as follows: we and others have previously reported that many of the dystrophic (senescent) microglia in human brain are positive for the iron storage protein, ferritin (Simmons et al., 2007; Lopes et al., 2008), suggesting that the sequestration and concomitant accidental escape of free iron atoms can contribute to microglial senescence by increasing oxidative stress within these cells. This has raised the interesting and novel possibility that microglia rather than neurons may be primary victims of oxidative damage (Dringen, 2005; Lopes et al., 2008; Nakanishi and Wu, 2009), representing somewhat of a paradigm shift since in the past microglia have been seen primarily as a source of free radicals that endanger neuronal survival (Colton and Gilbert, 1987; Boje and Arora, 1992; Chao et al., 1992). It seems plausible then to think that microglia can protect neurons by taking the brunt of at least some oxidative stress and deflecting it away, which makes sense since microglia are relatively expendable and possess renewal capacity from within the CNS (mitosis) or from bone-marrow derived precursor cells. One might draw the analogy to the game of chess where pawns are sacrificed to save the more valuable pieces. Compatible with this idea of microglial self-sacrifice is evidence from animal experiments showing that activated microglia in the axotomized facial nucleus are negative for ferritin (unpublished) and that therefore ferritin expression in microglia is not necessarily linked to microglial activation. Importantly, transection of the facial nerve leaves the BBB undisturbed, but conversely, when a brain lesion does result in a breach of the BBB some microglia do become ferritin-positive and even dystrophic (Xue et al., 2010). Thus, neuroprotective microglia are like the HazMat Team in the CNS which will put itself in harm's way to protect neurons.

A final aspect of microglial neuroprotection within the scope of this discussion concerns their emerging role in the regulation of the plasticity of neuronal circuits, that is, their involvement in the pruning/elimination and maintenance of synaptic connections. This aspect of the microglial functional repertoire was recognized for the first time more than 40 years ago by Blinzinger and Kreutzberg (1968), yet it remained largely unexplored until quite recently when a number of laboratories started to reexamine and delve deeper into this phenomenon. It now appears that microglial regulation of neuronal connectivity is important during development, as well as in the normal and injured adult brain (Wake et al., 2009; Tremblay et al., 2010; Paolicelli et al., 2011). The stripping of synapses from axotomized motoneurons (Blinzinger and Kreutzberg, 1968) perhaps best illustrates a direct neuroprotective effect of such cellular action in that displacement of synapses from the surface of injured motoneurons may prevent afferent excitation, which is hardly needed at a time when motoneurons are working to regenerate their severed axons (Streit, 1993). In fact, tight microglial ensheathment of injured motoneurons instantaneously fulfills multiple goals of neuroprotection: while preventing unnecessary excitation through synaptic displacement, it also puts microglia into very close proximity to the neuronal cell soma to facilitate targeted delivery of neurotrophic factors and, in addition, it perfectly prepositions microglia for rapid phagocytosis should a neuron fail to survive as a result of having been axotomized. Elimination of synapses during development (Paolicelli et al., 2011) or during altered sensory processing (Tremblay et al., 2010) is neuroprotective insofar as it facilitates the proper formation and rearrangement of synaptic connections and thus optimizes neuronal functioning.

NEUROINFLAMMATION AND THE SIGNIFICANCE OF MICROGLIAL ACTIVATION IN AD

Countless studies in laboratory animals involving experimental CNS lesions have shown that microglia become activated rapidly in response to neuronal injury (Kreutzberg, 1996; Kettenmann et al., 2011). This prompt cellular reaction to CNS tissue injury (glial activation), which can occur within seconds after injury (Nimmerjahn et al., 2005), constitutes acute neuroinflammation. The primary purpose of such acute inflammation, being limited in its range to the immediate vicinity of the lesion, is to initiate wound healing and to restore homeostasis as soon as possible, and microglial activation subsides as healing occurs. Excess microglia generated during the activation response *via* mitosis of resident cells undergo programmed cell death which reduces cell numbers back to baseline (Gehrmann and Banati, 1995; Jones et al., 1997; Conde and Streit, 2006), constituting a form of physiological cell death perhaps similar to what happens in normal ontogenetic development. One seemingly trivial insight to be gained from these lesion studies is that they clearly establish the cause-and-effect relationship between injury and subsequent microglial activation underscoring the fundamental definition of inflammation, i.e., the cellular response to injury. In the context of AD and the amyloid cascade-neuroinflammation theory a cause-and-effect relationship is anything but trivial. Although deposition of the Aβ protein is seen by many as a trigger for microglial activation in AD and has thus given rise to a large body of literature resulting from sundry experimental approaches, there is no consensus to date whether or not Aβ actually stimulates microglial activation. Case in point, we and others have observed that some human brains with substantial Aβ loads reveal a notable lack of microglial activation (Itagaki et al., 1989; Ohgami et al., 1991; Streit et al., 2009; **Figure 2**). Similarly, the supposition that microglial cells are involved in the clearance of Aβ has not been proven. Generally speaking, studies performed *in vitro* with cultured microglia

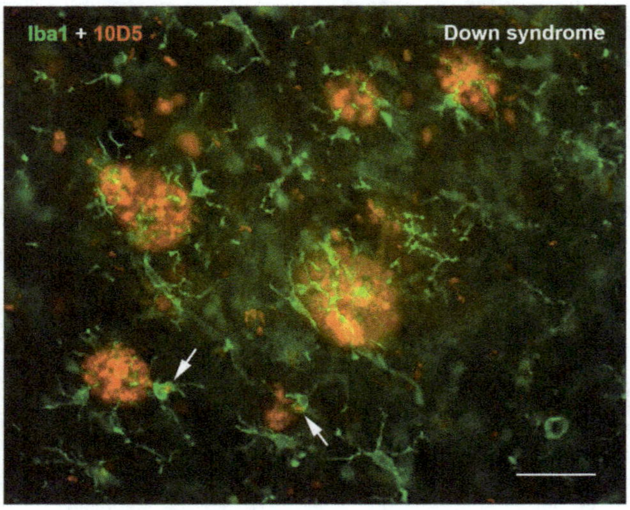

FIGURE 2 | Double immunofluorescent staining for microglia (Iba1) and Aβ protein (10D5) in the cerebral cortex of a human with Down syndrome reveals apparently normal, non-activated microglia in and around Aβ deposits. Microglia are ramified and show no evidence of having internalized any Aβ protein. Two microglial cells show presence of intracellular, autofluorescent lipofuscin (arrows). Scale bar: 50 μm.

provide the only convincing evidence that microglia can phagocytize Aβ protein, but these stand in stark contrast to most studies in Aβ-overexpressing animal models (which do not) and certainly to studies in human brain which reveal a lack of Aβ phagocytosis by microglia. Thus, the relationship between Aβ, microglial activation, and/or neuroinflammation remains enigmatic and perplexing even after more than 20 years of intense research. If one also considers the alleged causal connection between amyloid deposits and neurofibrillary degeneration the picture gets blurred even more as this connection seems to grow weaker and evidence is mounting against rather than in favor of it.

Yet another issue that complicates our understanding of neuroinflammation in AD is found in the fact that primary infections outside of the CNS influence the state of microglial cells. In particular, sepsis, which is more commonly found in elderly patients due to compromised immune function, will induce microglial activation within the brain (Lemstra et al., 2007; Streit et al., 2009). It is likely that there are other types of systemic pathology that may do so as well (Mattiace et al., 1990). Nearly all prior studies that have reported microglial activation and/or upregulation of inflammatory cytokines in the CNS of AD subjects have not made a distinction between cases that were free of peripheral infectious disease and those that were not, and it is therefore quite possible that neuroinflammatory changes reported could have been the result of peripheral diseases. Studies are underway in our laboratory to further investigate this possibility.

MICROGLIAL SENESCENCE AND NEURODEGENERATION – CONNECTING THE DOTS

The discovery of dystrophic microglia in human brain represents a critical step in conceiving the microglial dysfunction hypothesis because it raises the possibility that microglia are subject to senescence and degeneration (Streit et al., 2004). Dystrophic microglia were first identified in the aged human brain as cells displaying abnormal morphological features, such as shortened, gnarled, beaded, or fragmented cytoplasmic processes, as well as loss of fine ramifications and formation of spheroidal swellings. Because they are present in greater numbers in aged vs. young humans microglial dystrophy is thought to reflect degenerative changes related to cell senescence. Our subsequent demonstration of a close spatial and temporal relationship between neurofibrillary degeneration (tau pathology) and microglial dystrophy in subjects with either AD or Down syndrome has provided another crucial piece in the puzzle consolidating the dysfunction theory by linking microglial senescence and neurodegeneration (Streit et al., 2009; Xue and Streit, 2011). Additional support for this link is derived also from the well-known fact that aged rodents typically do not develop neurofibrillary degeneration, and that microglial degeneration has been undetectable in uninjured rodent brain (Streit and Xue, 2010). Clearly, the next major step in advancing this line of thinking would be to induce microglial dystrophy experimentally and determine if it is accompanied by neurodegenerative changes. Current efforts in our laboratory are directed toward that goal.

The morphological abnormalities that characterize dystrophic microglia have been described in detail before (Streit et al., 2004, 2009; Xue and Streit, 2011), suffice it to say here that the most advanced and striking change involves fragmentation of the cells' cytoplasm, which is termed cytorrhexis (**Figure 3**). Cytorrhexis reflects obvious degeneration of cell structure and it appears to be the end result of a progression from beading of processes to subsequent fragmentation not unlike what has been observed during axonal degeneration (Kerschensteiner et al., 2005; Coleman and Freeman, 2010). We view microglial cytorrhexis as a form of accidental cell death with as of yet unknown causes, although much points toward undue oxidative stress as a likely etiologic factor. Our prior work has shown that cytorrhexis does not involve detectable nuclear fragmentation further supporting the idea of an accidental rather than an apoptotic mechanism (Fendrick et al., 2007).

With regard to the aforementioned neuroprotective roles of microglia, there are a number of interesting points to consider in terms of how deterioration of these neuroprotective functions could be critically important in the development of aging-related neurodegenerative diseases. Phagocytosis of debris by microglia is an essential cellular activity that ensures maintenance of a clean, debris-free brain parenchyma, and is conducive toward facilitating optimal interneuronal electrochemical signaling. A substantial decline in microglial phagocytosis due to cell senescence and/or degeneration would almost certainly contribute to NDD development (Neumann et al., 2009). In addition, impaired phagocytosis could be a factor contributing to reduced clearance of amyloid deposits, a possibility that has been raised in previous reports (Fiala et al., 2005; Streit et al., 2008; Njie et al., 2012). Areas of the human brain showing advanced tau pathology are characterized by widespread presence of cytorrhectic microglia but also reveal a conspicuous absence of phagocytic activity. This very likely reflects the fact that fragmented microglia cells no longer are capable of performing phagocytosis, which explains why areas of tau pathology are littered with uncleared microglial debris. Although not yet shown, it would hardly come as a surprise to find out that the ability

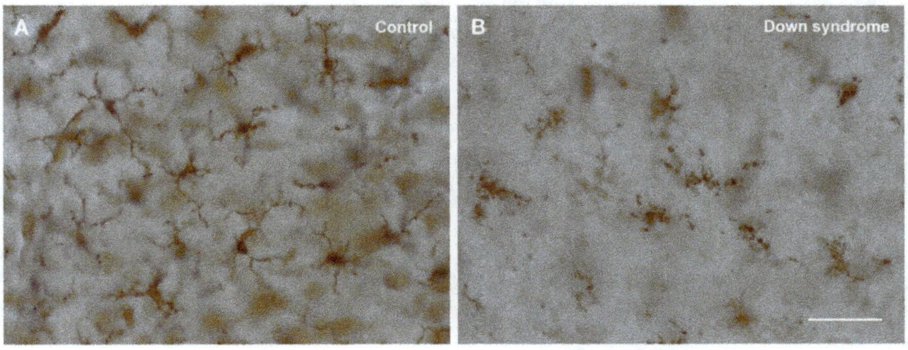

FIGURE 3 | Comparison of normal (ramified) and degenerating (dystrophic) microglia using Iba1 immunostaining in human cerebral cortex. (A) 22-year-old male non-demented subject reveals cells with normal morphology; **(B)** 48-year-old female subject with Down syndrome shows cells displaying obvious cytoplasmic fragmentation. Scale bar: 50 μm.

of cytorrhectic microglia to produce sufficient amounts of neurotrophic factors is much reduced. The possibility also exists that dying microglial cells could elaborate toxic factors, which might be a way to reconcile the dysfunction and neuroinflammation ideas.

For quite some time now the presence of increased brain iron and/or a disturbance in iron metabolism has been seen as a major factor contributing directly to free radical mediated neuronal degeneration (Jellinger et al., 1990; Dexter et al., 1991; Youdim and Riederer, 1993; Lynch et al., 2000; Berg et al., 2001; Zecca et al., 2004; Smith et al., 2010). Here again, microglial degeneration offers an opportunity to deepen our understanding of the importance of brain iron in the pathogenesis of neurodegenerative diseases. As levels of brain iron increase with aging, perhaps due in part to presence of microbleeds, the burden for resident microglial cells in sequestering free iron through ferritin expression becomes progressively higher. At the same time the risk for microglia to develop degenerative changes through iron-mediated oxidative stress is heightened, thus resulting in an ever increasing number of dystrophic and dysfunctional microglial cells with impaired ability to provide neuroprotection. Observations in humans showing that a large proportion of ferritin-positive microglia are dystrophic and that these dystrophic cells accumulate in advanced lesions (senile plaques) substantiate this line of thinking (Kaneko et al., 1989; Lopes et al., 2008; Xue and Streit, 2011).

As mentioned, there is an increasing number of recent studies that suggest significant involvement of microglia in synaptic plasticity (Tremblay et al., 2011). If microglia are indeed the electricians of the brain and important for maintaining synaptic integrity of neuronal circuits (Graeber, 2010), then their deterioration in the AD brain could certainly play a direct role in the loss of synapses which represents a hallmark feature of the disease (DeKosky and Scheff, 1990; Terry et al., 1991; Lassmann et al., 1993). Naturally, if the dysfunction hypothesis is correct and microglial degeneration contributes to neurodegeneration, the loss of synapses secondary to neuronal degeneration would also fit into this scenario. Some studies have suggested a role for microglia in synapse elimination as well as in synaptogenesis during CNS development (Bessis et al., 2007), and these functions are likely to be performed much more effectively by young microglial cells in the developing brain than by senescent ones in the aged CNS.

CONCLUSION

As the brain's innate immune system one might be inclined to think of microglia primarily as immunological defenders that fight invading microorganisms. However, in so doing one underestimates their importance as supportive and neuroprotective glial cells essential for helping to maintain neuronal functioning in the normal CNS and especially their crucial involvement in CNS repair and regeneration during injury and disease. We believe that microglial neuroprotection constitutes a most important aspect of the cells' biological significance because it defines a single common denominator that contributes to improved understanding of CNS development, normal adult brain function, as well mechanisms of injury, disease, and repair. Specifically, with regard to aging-related neurodegenerative diseases, which represent one of the greatest challenges for biomedical science in this day and age, we think that the concept of CNS immunosenescence has considerable potential for advancing progress in terms of new and improved approaches toward treatment and prevention.

REFERENCES

Anthony, I. C., and Bell, J. E. (2008). The neuropathology of HIV/AIDS. *Int. Rev. Psychiatry* 20, 15–24.

Araujo, D. M., and Cotman, C. W. (1992). Beta-amyloid stimulates glial cells in vitro to produce growth factors that accumulate in senile plaques in Alzheimer's disease. *Brain Res.* 569, 141–145.

Batchelor, P. E., Liberatore, G. T., Wong, J. Y., Porritt, M. J., Frerichs, F., Donnan, G. A., and Howells, D. W. (1999). Activated macrophages and microglia induce dopaminergic sprouting in the injured striatum and express brain-derived neurotrophic factor and glial cell line-derived neurotrophic factor. *J. Neurosci.* 19, 1708–1716.

Berg, D., Gerlach, M., Youdim, M. B., Double, K. L., Zecca, L., Riederer, P., and Becker, G. (2001). Brain iron pathways and their relevance to Parkinson's disease. *J. Neurochem.* 79, 225–236.

Bessis, A., Bechade, C., Bernard, D., and Roumier, A. (2007). Microglial control of neuronal death and synaptic properties. *Glia* 55, 233–238.

Blinzinger, K., and Kreutzberg, G. (1968). Displacement of synaptic terminals from regenerating motoneurons by microglial celss. *Z. Zellforsch.* 85, 145–157.

Boje, K. M., and Arora, P. K. (1992). Microglial-produced nitric oxide and reactive nitrogen oxides mediate neuronal cell death. *Brain Res.* 587, 250–256.

Cardona, A. E., Pioro, E. P., Sasse, M. E., Kostenko, V., Cardona, S. M., Dijkstra, I. M., Huang, D., Kidd, G., Dombrowski, S., Dutta, R., Lee, J.-C., Cook, D. N., Jung, S., Lira, S. A., Littman, D. R., and Ransohoff, R. M. (2006). Control of microglial neurotoxicity by the fractalkine receptor. *Nat. Neurosci.* 9, 917–924.

Carson, M. J., Reilly, C. R., Sutcliffe, J. G., and Lo, D. (1998). Mature microglia resemble immature antigen-presenting cells. *Glia* 22, 72–85.

Chao, C. C., Hu, S., Molitor, T. W., Shaskan, E. G., and Peterson, P. K. (1992). Activated microglia mediate neuronal cell injury via a nitric oxide mechanism. *J. Immunol.* 149, 2736–2741.

Chen, G. Y., and Nunez, G. (2010). Sterile inflammation: sensing and reacting to damage. *Nat. Rev. Immunol.* 10, 826–837.

Coleman, M. P., and Freeman, M. R. (2010). Wallerian degeneration, wld(s), and nmnat. *Annu. Rev. Neurosci.* 33, 245–267.

Colton, C. A. (2009). Heterogeneity of microglial activation in the innate immune response in the brain. *J. Neuroimmune Pharmacol.* 4, 399–418.

Colton, C. A., and Gilbert, D. L. (1987). Production of superoxide anions by a CNS macrophage, the microglia. *FEBS Lett.* 223, 284–288.

Conde, J. R., and Streit, W. J. (2006). Effect of aging on the microglial response to peripheral nerve injury. *Neurobiol. Aging* 27, 1451–1461.

Coull, J. A., Beggs, S., Boudreau, D., Boivin, D., Tsuda, M., Inoue, K., Gravel, C., Salter, M. W., and De Koninck, Y. (2005). BDNF from microglia causes the shift in neuronal anion gradient underlying neuropathic pain. *Nature* 438, 1017–1021.

Davalos, D., Grutzendler, J., Yang, G., Kim, J. V., Zuo, Y., Jung, S., Littman, D. R., Dustin, M. L., and Gan, W. B. (2005). ATP mediates rapid microglial response to local brain injury in vivo. *Nat. Neurosci.* 8, 752–758.

DeKosky, S. T., and Scheff, S. W. (1990). Synapse loss in frontal cortex biopsies in Alzheimer's disease: correlation with cognitive severity. *Ann. Neurol.* 27, 457–464.

Dexter, D. T., Carayon, A., Javoy-Agid, F., Wells, F. R., Daniel, S. E., Lees, A., Jenner, P., and Marsden, C. D. (1991). Alterations in levels of iron, ferritin and other trace metals in Parkinson's disease and other neurodegenerative diseases affecting the basal ganglia. *Brain* 114, 1953–1975.

Dringen, R. (2005). Oxidative and antioxidative potential of brain microglial cells. *Antioxid. Redox Signal.* 7, 1223–1233.

Elkabes, S., DiCicco-Bloom, E. M., and Black, I. B. (1996). Brain microglia/macrophages express neurotrophins that selectively regulate microglial proliferation and function. *J. Neurosci.* 16, 2508–2521.

Fendrick, S. E., Xue, Q. S., and Streit, W. J. (2007). Formation of multinucleated giant cells and microglial degeneration in rats expressing a mutant Cu/Zn superoxide dismutase gene. *J. Neuroinflammation* 4, 9.

Fiala, M., Lin, J., Ringman, J., Kermani-Arab, V., Tsao, G., Patel, A., Lossinsky, A. S., Graves, M. C., Gustavson, A., Sayre, J., Sofroni, E., Suarez, T., Chiappelli, F., and Bernard, G. (2005). Ineffective phagocytosis of amyloid-beta by macrophages of Alzheimer's disease patients. *J. Alzheimers Dis.* 7, 221–232.

Ford, A. L., Goodsall, A. L., Hickey, W. F., and Sedgwick, J. D. (1995). Normal adult ramified microglia separated from other central nervous system macrophages by flow cytometric sorting. Phenotypic differences defined and direct ex vivo antigen presentation to myelin basic protein-reactive CD4+ T cells compared. *J. Immunol.* 154, 4309–4321.

Frade, J. M., and Barde, Y. A. (1998). Microglia-derived nerve growth factor causes cell death in the developing retina. *Neuron* 20, 35–41.

Galea, I., Bechmann, I., and Perry, V. H. (2007). What is immune privilege (not)? *Trends Immunol.* 28, 12–18.

Gehrmann, J., and Banati, R. B. (1995). Microglial turnover in the injured CNS: activated microglia undergo delayed DNA fragmentation following peripheral nerve injury. *J. Neuropathol. Exp. Neurol.* 54, 680–688.

Graeber, M. B. (2010). Changing face of microglia. *Science* 330, 783–788.

Graeber, M. B., Lopez-Redondo, F., Ikoma, E., Ishikawa, M., Imai, Y., Nakajima, K., Kreutzberg, G. W., and Kohsaka, S. (1998). The microglia/macrophage response in the neonatal rat facial nucleus following axotomy. *Brain Res.* 813, 241–253.

Graeber, M. B., and Streit, W. J. (1990). Microglia: immune network in the CNS. *Brain Pathol.* 1, 2–5.

Heese, K., Fiebich, B. L., Bauer, J., and Otten, U. (1997). Nerve growth factor (NGF) expression in rat microglia is induced by adenosine A2a-receptors. *Neurosci. Lett.* 231, 83–86.

Hoek, R. M., Ruuls, S. R., Murphy, C. A., Wright, G. J., Goddard, R., Zurawski, S. M., Blom, B., Homola, M. E., Streit, W. J., Brown, M. H., Barclay, A. N., and Sedgwick, J. D. (2000). Down-regulation of the macrophage lineage through interaction with OX2 (CD200). *Science* 290, 1768–1771.

Itagaki, S., McGeer, P. L., Akiyama, H., Zhu, S., and Selkoe, D. (1989). Relationship of microglia and astrocytes to amyloid deposits of Alzheimer disease. *J. Neuroimmunol.* 24, 173–182.

Jellinger, K., Paulus, W., Grundke-Iqbal, I., Riederer, P., and Youdim, M. B. (1990). Brain iron and ferritin in Parkinson's and Alzheimer's diseases. *J. Neural Transm. Park. Dis. Dement. Sect.* 2, 327–340.

Jones, L. L., Banati, R. B., Graeber, M. B., Bonfanti, L., Raivich, G., and Kreutzberg, G. W. (1997). Population control of microglia: does apoptosis play a role? *J. Neurocytol.* 26, 755–770.

Kaneko, Y., Kitamoto, T., Tateishi, J., and Yamaguchi, K. (1989). Ferritin immunohistochemistry as a marker for microglia. *Acta Neuropathol.* 79, 129–136.

Kerschensteiner, M., Schwab, M. E., Lichtman, J. W., and Misgeld, T. (2005). In vivo imaging of axonal degeneration and regeneration in the injured spinal cord. *Nat. Med.* 11, 572–577.

Kettenmann, H., Hanisch, U. K., Noda, M., and Verkhratsky, A. (2011). Physiology of microglia. *Physiol. Rev.* 91, 461–553.

Kiefer, R., Gold, R., Gehrmann, J., Lindholm, D., Wekerle, H., and Kreutzberg, G. W. (1993). Transforming growth factor beta expression in reactive spinal cord microglia and meningeal inflammatory cells during experimental allergic neuritis. *J. Neurosci. Res.* 36, 391–398.

Kreutzberg, G. W. (1996). Microglia: a sensor for pathological events in the CNS. *Trends Neurosci.* 19, 312–318.

Lassmann, H., Fischer, P., and Jellinger, K. (1993). Synaptic pathology of Alzheimer's disease. *Ann. N. Y. Acad. Sci.* 695, 59–64.

Lehrmann, E., Kiefer, R., Christensen, T., Toyka, K. V., Zimmer, J., Diemer, N. H., Hartung, H. P., and Finsen, B. (1998). Microglia and macrophages are major sources of locally produced transforming growth factor-beta1 after transient middle cerebral artery occlusion in rats. *Glia* 24, 437–448.

Lemstra, A. W., Groen in't Woud, J. C., Hoozemans, J. J., van Haastert, E. S., Rozemuller, A. J., Eikelenboom, P., and van Gool, W. A. (2007). Microglia activation in sepsis: a case-control study. *J. Neuroinflammation* 4, 4.

Lopes, K. O., Sparks, D. L., and Streit, W. J. (2008). Microglial dystrophy in the aged and Alzheimer's disease brain is associated with ferritin immunoreactivity. *Glia* 56, 1048–1060.

Lopez-Redondo, F., Nakajima, K., Honda, S., and Kohsaka, S. (2000). Glutamate transporter GLT-1 is highly expressed in activated microglia following facial nerve axotomy. *Brain Res. Mol. Brain Res.* 76, 429–435.

Lynch, T., Cherny, R. A., and Bush, A. I. (2000). Oxidative processes in Alzheimer's disease: the role of a beta-metal interactions. *Exp. Gerontol.* 35, 445–451.

Mallat, M., Houlgatte, R., Brachet, P., and Prochiantz, A. (1989). Lipopolysaccharide-stimulated rat brain macrophages release NGF in vitro. *Dev. Biol.* 133, 309–311.

Mariani, M. M., and Kielian, T. (2009). Microglia in infectious diseases of the central nervous system. *J. Neuroimmune Pharmacol.* 4, 448–461.

Mattiace, L. A., Davies, P., and Dickson, D. W. (1990). Detection of HLA-DR on microglia in the human brain is a function of both clinical and technical factors. *Am. J. Pathol.* 136, 1101–1114.

McGeer, P. L., Itagaki, S., Tago, H., and McGeer, E. G. (1987). Reactive microglia in patients with senile dementia of the Alzheimer type are positive for the histocompatibility glycoprotein HLA-DR. *Neurosci. Lett.* 79, 195–200.

Michaels, J., Price, R. W., and Rosenblum, M. K. (1988). Microglia in the giant cell encephalitis of acquired immune deficiency syndrome: proliferation, infection and fusion. *Acta Neuropathol.* 76, 373–379.

Michelucci, A., Heurtaux, T., Grandbarbe, L., Morga, E., and Heuschling, P. (2009). Characterization of the microglial phenotype under specific pro-inflammatory and anti-inflammatory conditions: effects of oligomeric and fibrillar amyloid-beta. *J. Neuroimmunol.* 210, 3–12.

Moon, M. L., McNeil, L. K., and Freund, G. G. (2011). Macrophages make me sick: how macrophage activation states influence sickness behavior. *Psychoneuroendocrinology* 36, 1431–1440.

Nakajima, K., Tohyama, Y., Kohsaka, S., and Kurihara, T. (2001). Ability of rat microglia to uptake extracellular glutamate. *Neurosci. Lett.* 307, 171–174.

Nakajima, K., Tohyama, Y., Kohsaka, S., and Kurihara, T. (2002). Ceramide activates microglia to enhance the production/secretion of brain-derived neurotrophic factor (BDNF) without induction of deleterious factors in vitro. *J. Neurochem.* 80, 697–705.

Nakajima, K., Yamamoto, S., Kohsaka, S., and Kurihara, T. (2008). Neuronal stimulation leading to upregulation of glutamate transporter-1 (GLT-1) in rat microglia in vitro. *Neurosci. Lett.* 436, 331–334.

Nakanishi, H., and Wu, Z. (2009). Microglia-aging: roles of microglial lysosome- and mitochondria-derived reactive oxygen species in brain aging. *Behav. Brain Res.* 201, 1–7.

Nau, R., and Bruck, W. (2002). Neuronal injury in bacterial meningitis: mechanisms and implications for therapy. *Trends Neurosci.* 25, 38–45.

Neumann, H., Kotter, M. R., and Franklin, R. J. (2009). Debris clearance by microglia: an essential link between degeneration and regeneration. *Brain* 132, 288–295.

Nimmerjahn, A., Kirchhoff, F., and Helmchen, F. (2005). Resting microglial cells are highly dynamic surveillants of brain parenchyma in vivo. *Science* 308, 1314–1318.

Njie, E. G., Boelen, E., Stassen, F. R., Steinbusch, H. W., Borchelt, D. R., and Streit, W. J. (2012). Ex vivo cultures of microglia from young and aged rodent brain reveal age-related changes in microglial function. *Neurobiol. Aging* 33, 195.e1–195.e12.

Ohgami, T., Kitamoto, T., Shin, R. W., Kaneko, Y., Ogomori, K., and Tateishi, J. (1991). Increased senile plaques without microglia in Alzheimer's disease. *Acta Neuropathol.* 81, 242–247.

Paolicelli, R. C., Bolasco, G., Pagani, F., Maggi, L., Scianni, M., Panzanelli, P., Giustetto, M., Ferreira, T. A., Guiducci, E., Dumas, L., Ragozzino, D., and Gross, C. T. (2011). Synaptic pruning by microglia is necessary for normal brain development. *Science* 333, 1456–1458.

Perry, V. H., Bell, M. D., Brown, H. C., and Matyszak, M. K. (1995). Inflammation in the nervous system. *Curr. Opin. Neurobiol.* 5, 636–641.

Persson, M., Sandberg, M., Hansson, E., and Ronnback, L. (2006). Microglial glutamate uptake is coupled to glutathione synthesis and glutamate release. *Eur. J. Neurosci.* 24, 1063–1070.

Petersen, M. A., and Dailey, M. E. (2004). Diverse microglial motility behaviors during clearance of dead cells in hippocampal slices. *Glia* 46, 195–206.

Ribes, S., Ebert, S., Regen, T., Agarwal, A., Tauber, S. C., Czesnik, D., Spreer, A., Bunkowski, S., Eiffert, H., Hanisch, U. K., Hammerschmidt, S., and Nauet, R. (2011). Toll-like receptor stimulation enhances phagocytosis and intracellular killing of nonencapsulated and encapsulated Streptococcus pneumoniae by murine microglia. *Infect. Immun.* 78, 865–871.

Simmons, D. A., Casale, M., Alcon, B., Pham, N., Narayan, N., and Lynch, G. (2007). Ferritin accumulation in dystrophic microglia is an early event in the development of Huntington's disease. *Glia* 55, 1074–1084.

Smith, M. A., Zhu, X., Tabaton, M., Liu, G., McKeel, D. W. Jr., Cohen, M. L., Wang, X., Siedlak, S. L., Dwyer, B. E., Hayashi, T., Nakamura, M., Nunomura, A., and Perry, G. (2010). Increased iron and free radical generation in preclinical Alzheimer disease and mild cognitive impairment. *J. Alzheimers Dis.* 19, 363–372.

Stence, N., Waite, M., and Dailey, M. E. (2001). Dynamics of microglial activation: a confocal time-lapse analysis in hippocampal slices. *Glia* 33, 256–266.

Streit, W. J. (1993). Microglial-neuronal interactions. *J. Chem. Neuroanat.* 6, 261–266.

Streit, W. J., Braak, H., Xue, Q. S., and Bechmann, I. (2009). Dystrophic (senescent) rather than activated microglial cells are associated with tau pathology and likely precede neurodegeneration in Alzheimer's disease. *Acta Neuropathol.* 118, 475–485.

Streit, W. J., and Kincaid-Colton, C. A. (1995). The brain's immune system. *Sci. Am.* 273, 54–55, 58–61.

Streit, W. J., Miller, K. R., Lopes, K. O., and Njie, E. (2008). Microglial degeneration in the aging brain – bad news for neurons? *Front. Biosci.* 13, 3423–3438.

Streit, W. J., Sammons, N. W., Kuhns, A. J., and Sparks, D. L. (2004). Dystrophic microglia in the aging human brain. *Glia* 45, 208–212.

Streit, W. J., and Xue, Q. S. (2010). The Brain's aging immune system. *Aging Dis.* 1, 254–261.

Suzuki, H., Imai, F., Kanno, T., and Sawada, M. (2001). Preservation of neurotrophin expression in microglia that migrate into the gerbil's brain across the blood-brain barrier. *Neurosci. Lett.* 312, 95–98.

Terry, R. D., Masliah, E., Salmon, D. P., Butters, N., DeTeresa, R., Hill, R., Hansen, L. A., and Katzman, R. (1991). Physical basis of cognitive alterations in Alzheimer's disease: synapse loss is the major correlate of cognitive impairment. *Ann. Neurol.* 30, 572–580.

Tremblay, M. E., Lowery, R. L., and Majewska, A. K. (2010). Microglial interactions with synapses are modulated by visual experience. *PLoS Biol.* 8, e1000527. doi:10.1371/journal.pbio.1000527

Tremblay, M. E., Stevens, B., Sierra, A., Wake, H., Bessis, A., and Nimmerjahn, A. (2011). The role of microglia in the healthy brain. *J. Neurosci.* 31, 16064–16069.

van Landeghem, F. K., Stover, J. F., Bechmann, I., Bruck, W., Unterberg, A., Buhrer, C., and von Deimling, A. (2001). Early expression of glutamate transporter proteins in ramified microglia after controlled cortical impact injury in the rat. *Glia* 35, 167–179.

Wake, H., Moorhouse, A. J., Jinno, S., Kohsaka, S., and Nabekura, J. (2009) Resting microglia directly monitor the functional state of synapses in vivo and determine the fate of ischemic terminals. *J. Neurosci.* 29, 3974–3980.

Xue, Q. S., and Streit, W. J. (2011). Microglial pathology in Down syndrome. *Acta Neuropathol.* 122, 455–466.

Xue, Q. S., Yang, C., Hoffman, P. M., and Streit, W. J. (2010). Microglial response to murine leukemia virus-induced encephalopathy is a good indicator of neuronal perturbations. *Brain Res.* 1319, 131–141.

Youdim, M. B., and Riederer, P. (1993). The role of iron in senescence of dopaminergic neurons in Parkinson's disease. *J. Neural Transm. Suppl.* 40, 57–67.

Zecca, L., Youdim, M. B., Riederer, P., Connor, J. R., and Crichton, R. R. (2004). Iron, brain ageing and neurodegenerative disorders. *Nat. Rev. Neurosci.* 5, 863–873.

2

Scale and pattern of atrophy in the chronic stages of moderate-severe TBI

Robin E. A. Green[1,2]*, Brenda Colella[1], Jerome J. Maller[3], Mark Bayley[1], Joanna Glazer[1] and David J. Mikulis[4,5]

[1] Cognitive Neurorehabilitation Sciences Laboratory, Research Department, Toronto Rehabilitation Institute, Toronto, ON, Canada
[2] Department of Psychiatry, Faculty of Medicine, University of Toronto, Toronto, ON, Canada
[3] Brain Stimulation and Neuroimaging Laboratory, Monash Alfred Psychiatry Research Centre, Alfred Hospital, Melbourne, VIC, Australia
[4] fMRI Laboratory, Division of Applied and Interventional Research, Toronto Western Research Institute, Toronto, ON, Canada
[5] Department of Medical Imaging, Faculty of Medicine, University of Toronto, Toronto, ON, Canada

Edited by:
Hauke R. Heekeren, Freie Universität Berlin, Germany

Reviewed by:
Ruthger Righart, Institute for Stroke and Dementia Research, Germany
Erin D. Bigler, Brigham Young University, USA

****Correspondence:***
Robin E. A. Green, Toronto Rehabilitation Institute, 550 University Avenue, Rm. 11-207, Toronto, ON M5G 2A2, Canada
e-mail: robin.green@uhn.ca

Background: Moderate-severe traumatic brain injury (TBI) is increasingly being understood as a progressive disorder, with growing evidence of reduced brain volume and white matter (WM) integrity as well as lesion expansion in the chronic phases of injury. The scale of these losses has yet to be investigated, and pattern of change across structures has received limited attention.

Objectives: (1) To measure the percentage of patients in our TBI sample showing atrophy from 5 to 20 months post-injury in the whole brain and in structures with known vulnerability to acute TBI, and (2) To examine relative vulnerability and patterns of volume loss across structures.

Methods: Fifty-six TBI patients [complicated mild to severe, with mean Glasgow Coma Scale (GCS) in severe range] underwent MRI at, on average, 5 and 20 months post-injury; 12 healthy controls underwent MRI twice, with a mean gap between scans of 25.4 months. Mean monthly percent volume change was computed for whole brain (ventricle-to-brain ratio; VBR), corpus callosum (CC), and right and left hippocampi (HPC).

Results: (1) Using a threshold of 2 z-scores below controls, 96% of patients showed atrophy across time points in at least one region; 75% showed atrophy in at least 3 of the 4 regions measured. (2) There were no significant differences in the proportion of patients who showed atrophy across structures. For those showing decline in VBR, there was a significant association with both the CC and the right HPC ($P < 0.05$ for both comparisons). There were also significant associations between those showing decline in (i) right and left HPC ($P < 0.05$); (ii) all combinations of genu, body and splenium of the CC ($P < 0.05$), and (iii) head and tail of the right HPC ($P < 0.05$ all sub-structure comparisons).

Conclusions: Atrophy in chronic TBI is robust, and the CC, right HPC and left HPC appear equally vulnerable. Significant associations between the right and left HPC, and within substructures of the CC and right HPC, raise the possibility of common mechanisms for these regions, including transneuronal degeneration. Given the 96% incidence rate of atrophy, a genetic explanation is unlikely to explain all findings. Multiple and possibly synergistic mechanisms may explain findings. Atrophy has been associated with poorer functional outcomes, but recent findings suggest there is potential to offset this. A better, understanding of the underlying mechanisms could permit targeted therapy enabling better long-term outcomes.

Keywords: atrophy, chronic, degeneration, traumatic brain injury, progression, MRI

INTRODUCTION

Traumatic brain injury (TBI) is increasingly being understood as a chronic and possibly progressive disease, rather than an injury with a circumscribed period of recovery and a static course thereafter (Ng et al., 2008; Masel and Dewitt, 2010; Bigler, 2013a). Evidence is accumulating from several laboratories including our own that following early cognitive recovery, many patients show statistically and clinically significant cognitive decline in the ensuing months (Ruff et al., 1991) and years (Millis et al., 2001; Till et al., 2008). We and others have also demonstrated that the brain's structure is not static after resolution of acute injuries, with TBI patients showing volume loss and reduced white matter (WM) integrity during the sub-acute and chronic stages of injury (Bendlin et al., 2008; Greenberg et al., 2008; Ng et al., 2008; Sidaros et al., 2009; Farbota et al., 2012; Adnan et al., 2013). Given that such atrophy is observed in some studies well after the resolution of acute events (Greenberg et al., 2008; Ng et al., 2008; Ross et al., 2012), and that sub-acute structural deterioration has been correlated with functional and behavioral outcomes (Bendlin et al., 2008; Sidaros et al., 2009), these changes cannot be attributed simply to encephalomalacia (i.e., scar formation associated with gliosis) or to resolution of edema. The evidence is thus supportive of a progressive neuropathology, possible mechanisms of which have been recently reviewed (Smith et al., 2013).

This very different course of TBI than has been traditionally assumed has clinical and scientific implications for how we understand and treat TBI patients, in both the short and longer term. Therefore, it is important to gain an understanding of the scale of atrophy: What proportion of TBI patients demonstrates progressive loss of brain volume? Previous studies have demonstrated group differences in atrophy and/or WM integrity loss between TBI patients and controls. What has yet to be investigated is the actual prevalence of patients who show decline, and moreover, who do so at what might be considered a clinically significant degree. Such information is needed to understand whether it is a subset of TBI patients who are at risk of degeneration or the majority. While atrophy in a subset would direct researchers (and clinicians) to evaluate risk factors for degeneration; ubiquitous atrophy would suggest that TBI itself is a degenerative disorder. The central aim of this study, therefore, was to begin to shed light on this question of scale.

To address the question, we undertook volumetric MRI measurements in TBI patients at approximately 5 and 20 months post-injury and compared the extent of volume loss across time for each patient to a normative control sample, also measured at two time points. We called patients showing significant volume loss "decliners." In both samples, we examined the whole brain using ventricle-to-brain ratio (VBR), as well as the hippocampi and corpus callosum (CC) and their sub-structures, areas with demonstrated vulnerability to the acute mechanical and neurochemical effects of injury (e.g., axonal deformation, hypoxia, excitotoxic cascades Povlishock and Katz, 2005). Our cohort ranged in severity from complicated mild to severe, but was overall a severely injured group of patients.

With regard to prediction of the scale of atrophy, in a previous study in which we examined lesion expansion, we found that in our sample of 14 patients, 10 showed lesion expansion across time within the chronic stages of injury (Ng et al., 2008). We therefore predicted that at least half of our sample in the current study would show significant volume loss on at least one measure.

We were also interested in the relative vulnerability of the individual structures and sub-structures, and in their pattern of deterioration. With regard to relative vulnerability, we measured the number of decliners (i.e., people who showed atrophy across time points as compared to normative controls) for each structure in order to ascertain whether one structure showed a greater frequency of decliners than another structure.

We speculated that those regions most vulnerable to *acute* injury would show the greatest chronic atrophy. This is because of growing evidence that while "use" increases brain (and in particular hippocampal) volume (Draganski et al., 2006; Maguire et al., 2006), "disuse" mediates volume loss (Underwood and Coulson, 2008; Miller et al., 2013). Therefore, we reasoned that regions most susceptible to initial damage, should sustain greater disuse, and therefore greater later atrophy. Both the CC and the hippocampi are commonly affected in TBI, especially when rotational forces are involved. In one study in children, the hippocampus was identified as the most vulnerable structure to TBI (Wilde et al., 2006), and it is vulnerable to acute phase damage from a variety of mechanisms, (e.g., mechanical deformation, hypoxic/excitotoxic injury, afferent and efferent disconnection of projections, and compromised neurogenesis Greer et al., 2012). The hippocampal head has been shown to be disproportionately vulnerable, as compared to the body and tail (Ariza et al., 2006). We therefore predicted that more individuals would show chronic degeneration in the hippocampal head than any other structure/sub-structure examined.

With regard to the pattern of deterioration, we asked whether the volumes of those regions measured in the study shrink commensurately with one another, and whether their sub-regions would shrink commensurately. In other words, did individuals who showed atrophy on one structure, also necessarily show atrophy on another?

In our previous research into sub-acute cognitive decline (Till et al., 2008), we observed marked variability in the cognitive and psychomotor functions that showed decline from 12 to 24 months post-injury, both within and between subjects. This suggested that atrophy might not have a predictable pattern. On this basis, we predicted that decline in one region would *not* be associated with decline in another, although we expected VBR—as an index that subsumes all other structures—to be associated with the hippocampi and CC.

MATERIALS AND METHODS

All participants gave their informed consent, except where participants were clinically judged as unable to provide informed consent; here, a substitute decision maker provided informed consent. In such cases, all patients gave their assent to participate. The study was approved by the Research Ethics Board of the Toronto Rehabiltation Institute where the research took place

PARTICIPANTS

TBI Patient group

Patient participants were 56 males and females with clinically confirmed TBI. See **Table 1** for injury and demographic characteristics of the sample, which were ascertained through medical records, clinical interview and direct testing. Overall, this was a typical group of adult TBI patients with more males than females, more motor-vehicle accidents than other causes of injury, estimated pre-morbid IQ (as measured by the Wechsler Test of Adult Reading (WTAR) Weschler, 2001; Green et al., 2008) in the average range, and just over high-school education. TBI severity for participants was based on the lowest Glasgow Coma Scale (GCS) score obtained from the acute care medical chart, where GCS was available and valid, or from length of post-traumatic amnesia (PTA), which was obtained from medical records and/or from clinical interview with the patient and family members at approximately 2 months post-injury. PTA classifications were based on

Table 1 | Injury and demographic characteristics of TBI sample ($N = 56$).

Variable	Proportion/mean	*SD* (range)
Age (years)	$M = 40.16$	15.63 (17–73)
Education (years)	$M = 13.63$	3.36 (6–21)
Estimated pre-morbid IQ (WTAR) ($N = 51$)	$M = 98.45$	18.26 (67–125)
Sex	73% = male 27% = female	
SOCIO-ECONOMIC STATUS (BASED ON HOLLINGSHEAD CLASSIFICATION Hollingshead and Redlich, 1958)		
1. Major business/professional	3.8%	
2. Medium business/minor professional, technical	41.5%	
3. Skilled craftsperson, clerical, sales worker	17%	
4. Machine operator, semiskilled worker	18.9%	
5. Unskilled laborer, menial service worker	18.9%	
TYPE OF INJURY		
Motor vehicle accident	57.1%	
Fall	37.5%	
Assault	3.6%	
Sports injury	1.8%	
SEVERITY OF INJURY VARIABLES		
Acute care length of stay (days)	$M = 37.44$days	20.01 (5–98)
GCS (lowest of recorded scores)	$M = 6.19$	3.42(3–13)
Mild (13–15)	10.7	
Moderate (9–12)	5.4%	
Severe (≤8)	69.6%	
Missing data	14.3%	
LENGTH OF POST-TRAUMATIC AMNESIA		
Less then 5 min, very mild	3.6%	
1–24 h, moderate	1.8%	
1–7 days, severe	21.4%	
1–4 weeks, very severe	44.6%	
>4 weeks, extremely severe	23.2%	
Missing data	5.4%	

Lezak (2004). As indicated in **Table 1**, patients ranged in severity from complicated mild to severe or greater, with mean TBI severity based on GCS in the severe range ($M = 6.2$).

All patient participants were recruited at a large, urban rehabilitation teaching hospital in Toronto from the in-patient Acquired Brain Injury service. The patients were part of an ongoing, prospective study on recovery from TBI (*The Toronto Rehab Traumatic Brain Injury Recovery Study*), which includes cognitive, motor, and neuro-imaging assessments at multiple time points. Inclusion criteria for the larger study comprise: clinically confirmed TBI with central (as opposed to orthopedic) injuries severe enough to warrant in-patient neurorehabilitation; out of PTA by 3 months post-injury; aged between 17 and 75; able to use at least one upper extremity; and, functional command of English. An additional inclusion criterion for the present study was completion of two or more MRIs. Exclusion criteria for the larger study include: past history of TBI; history of psychotic or neurological illness; and, TBI sustained secondary to another neurological event (e.g., a stroke). An additional exclusion criterion for the current study was an intervening neurological event between the first and follow-up MRI with the potential to influence the structural status of the brain (e.g., another TBI or intra-cranial infection).

Healthy control group

Twelve healthy adult control participants were recruited to the current study. These individuals were students and staff members at the rehabilitation hospital or friends or family members of students and staff members. Controls were excluded if they had a previous history of TBI, including concussion, or any other disease affecting the central nervous system. The control group was 50% male, with a mean age of 36.3 years ($SD = 12.5$, range 18–60), and a mean education of 17.5 years ($SD = 2.2$, range 11–21).

DESIGN AND PROCEDURES

The study was a prospective, repeated measures design. The normative control group was used to establish the level of decline in each patient for each structure. This was computed for each subject for each structure, as described below. MRIs were administered at two time points. The first was completed for all patients at a mean of 5.2 months post-injury, ($SD = 1.15$; range: 3.7–10.4). The second scan was at a mean of 20 months post-injury ($SD = 4.7$; range = 10.5–56.1), with a mean gap between scans of 14.8 months ($SD = 10.9$; range = 4.4–52.2). For control participants, the mean gap between scans was 25.4 months ($SD = 10.0$; range = 10.4–39.4). The relatively greater gap in the controls biased hypotheses against Type I errors. The longer gap between control scans allowed for greater non-specific decline to transpire, thereby increasing the threshold for reaching decline in the patients.

The MRI outcome measures were as follows: computed monthly percent change for ventricle to brain ratio (VBR), volumes of the left hippocampus (HPC-L; i.e., HPC-L total, HPC-L head, HPC-L body, HPC-L tail), volumes of the right hippocampus (HPC-R; i.e., HPC-R total, HPC-R head, HPC-R body, HPC-R tail), and CC volumes (i.e., CC total, CC genu, CC body, CC splenium).

All participants were required to pass a rigorous, clinical screening procedure prior to the first MRI assessment. All MRIs were conducted at a separate site (Toronto Western Hospital), which is part of the same center. All equipment and acquisition parameters were identical for the initial and follow-up assessments. One of two MRI technologists performed all MRIs.

Acquisition protocol

MRI scans were acquired on a General Electric (GE) Signa-Echospeed 1.5 Tesla HD scanner (SIGNA EXCITE, GE Healthcare, Milwaukee WI), using an eight channel head coil. Sequences included sagittal T1 ($TR/TE = 300/13$ ms), slice thickness = 5 mm, space 2.5 mm, matrix 256 × 128 axial gradient recalled echo (GRE) $TR/TE = 450/20$, flip angle = 20°, slice thickness = 3 mm no gap, matrix 256 × 192 axial fluid-attenuated-inversion-recovery (FLAIR) TR/TE = 9000/45 ms, TI (inversion time) = 2200 ms, slice thickness = 5 mm no gap, matrix 256 × 192 axial fast spin echo (FSE) proton density (PD)/T2 TR/TE 5500/30,90 ms, slice thickness = 3 mm no gap, matrix 256 × 192. All above mentioned sequences were obtained with a 22 cm field of view (FOV). The high-resolution isotropic T1 weighted, three-dimensional IR prepped radio-frequency spoiled-gradient recalled-echo (3D IRSPGR) images $TI/TR/TE$ = 12/300/5,TI, FA = 20, slice thickness = 1 mm no gap, matrix = 256 × 256 were acquired in the axial plane utilizing a 25 cm FOV. The entire scanning session lasted approximately 55 min.

Image processing and analysis

The MR images were transferred to a workstation for image processing. The scans were received in the Digital Imaging and Communications in Medicine (DICOM) file format and were subsequently converted into (Medical Imaging Network Common Data Form; MINC) file format that was created at McConnell Brain maging Centre of the Montreal Neurological Institute. Following this procedure, the files were anonymized.

A number of image processing steps were performed in order to make MRI data usable for image analysis. The first step was the intensity non-uniformity correction (Sled et al., 1998). These images were then linearly registered (aligned) into stereotaxic coordinates (Collins et al., 1994) based on the Talairach atlas (Talairach and Tournoux, 1988). The linear registration to Talairach coordinates was accomplished through 3D cross-correlation between a given volume and an average MR brain image previously converted into the Talairach coordinate system (Collins et al., 1994). After the registration the images had the same size and orientation, allowing for direct anatomical comparisons between subjects. A second non-uniformity correction was performed after the registration, which helped to remove any residual non-uniformity artifacts.

Every voxel in a non-uniformity corrected and registered image was then classified into one of the three classes: cerebrospinal fluid (CSF), gray matter (GM), and WM using an automated tissue classification algorithm (Zijdenbos et al., 1998). Subsequently, cortical surface extraction from the tissue-classified images was performed, resulting in a 3D reconstruction of the cortical surface. Next, the skull and scalp were removed in the tissue-classified images using the 3D surface extraction as a mask in order to obtain the tissue volumes of the whole brain. Thus, the volumes of CSF, GM, and WM reported in this study were calculated using the tissue-classified images, which excluded the skull, scalp, cerebellum, and brainstem. The combination of the GM and WM was used as the whole brain volume in the VBR analysis.

The hippocampi were manually outlined using Analyze TM 8.1 (Brain Imaging Resource, Mayo Clinic, MN) by an experienced tracer (JM) from coronally orientated MR images in the anterior-posterior direction. Calculations of volumes were computed automatically by multiplying the number of voxels traced in each slice, by their depth (i.e., slice thickness). As described by Watson et al. (1992, 1997), the anterior tip of the HPC until the slice before the opening of the crux of the fornix was measured as the HPC head and body and included the subiculum, CA1-areas, and dentate gyrus. The HPC tail was measured from the slice immediately posterior to that which represented the last slice according to the Watson protocol (see Maller et al., 2007 for a more detailed description of this procedure) (Maller et al., 2007).

The CC was manually traced on the midline sagittal slice of the T1 images using anatomical landmarks in an hierarchical order on a Windows XP Professional workstation (Core2Duo CPU, 2GIG RAM) using the Region of Interest module within analyzetm 8.1 (Brain Imaging Resource, Mayo Clinic, MN, USA). The landmarks based on the midline sagittal slice were, first, no WM or only minimal WM in the cortical mantle surrounding the CC, second, the interthalamic adhesion, and third, the transparent septum and the visibility of the aqueduct of Sylvius. To adjust for total brain volume, total midsagittal CC area and every subregional area in the analyses data were normalized by dividing by each individual's total intracranial volume (ICV). ICV was calculated from the total of GM, WM, and cerebrospinal fluid volumes which were estimated from processing the T1-weighted scans through FSL 4.0 (Analysisgroup, 2012), using the FAST module.

Analyses

Percentage of people showing significant decline in volume. As noted above, patients were classified as "decliners" if they showed atrophy in parenchymal tissue at a threshold of at least 2 z-scores below that of controls. (Note that we use the term "below" here rather than "greater than" for clarity of exposition.) We calculated a z-score for each patient participant using the following method: First, for each structure and substructure, percent change from time 1 to time 2 was calculated for patients and controls using the following formula: $[t2 - t1/(t1 + t2)] * 100$. Second, *monthly* percent change was then calculated in order to compare subjects with differing temporal gaps between scans. Third, a z-score was calculated for each patient using his/her *observed* score (i.e., percent change per month), the *expected* score (i.e., mean monthly percent change for controls), and the standard deviation for monthly percent change in the control group. We used a conservative z-score cut-off to classify decliners. Only if the patient was at least 2 z-scores below that of controls was he/she classified as a decliner. This enabled us to compute the percentage of decliners in our sample, in order to address the primary objective of our study.

Relative vulnerability of decline of structures/sub-structures and pattern of deterioration. To examine whether structures were equally vulnerable to decline or whether the number of decliners varied across structures, we calculated 95% confidence intervals for each proportion of decliners across structures, and substructures. To examine whether decline in one structure was associated with decline in another, we calculated PHI coefficients and their 95% confidence intervals between structures and between substructures. This enabled us to measure the degree of overlap within subjects in decliner classification across the structures (i.e., is there a correlation between those classified as decliners and non-decliners in one structure and those in another?). The PHI coefficient is a measure of association for two binary variables, interpreted similarly to the Pearson Correlation Coefficient.

Presentation of findings. Results are presented by each of the three research questions: (1) the overall percentage of people showing decline on at least one structure, and the number of structures on which subjects declined; (2) the relative vulnerability of structures (i.e., respective number of decliners in each structure), and (3) the pattern of atrophy (i.e., whether decline in one structure was associated with decline in another).

RESULTS

DEMOGRAPHIC COMPARISONS BETWEEN CONTROLS AND PATIENTS

There was no significant difference between the patients and controls for age, $t = 0.897$ ($df = 72$), $p = 0.373$, Cohen's $d = 0.211$. The controls had significantly more education than the patients, $t = -4.25$ ($df = 72$), $p < 0.001$, Cohen's $d = -1.00$.

DECLINERS: PERCENTAGE OF PATIENTS WHO SHOW ATROPHY THAT IS AT LEAST 2 z-SCORES BELOW THAT OF CONTROLS

Table 2 shows the monthly percent atrophy in the control group. The control group monthly percent changes were extremely small, with all scores close to 0, consistent with stability over time. [Note that while the primary aim of the study was to ascertain the *percentage* of decliners in our sample, we have included patient means with unpaired t-test results (all assuming unequal variances based on Levene's tests) to permit group mean comparisons]. These illustrate highly significant group differences.

Table 3 shows that compared to the normative group, over 96% of patients showed decline in at least one region. The majority (75%) showed decline in at least three of the four regions measured.

In **Table 4** the absolute number and percentage of decliners by structure are presented. Over 70% of patients showed atrophy within each of the right and left HPC, the CC and the whole brain; moreover, the lower bounds of the confidence intervals for each of these values was greater than 50%. Therefore, the results strongly support our hypothesis that more than 50% of patients would show atrophy of the brain.

RELATIVE VULNERABILITY TO DECLINE OF STRUCTURES AND SUB-STRUCTURES

Examining similarities and differences across structures in the number of decliners, **Table 4** shows that, the highest absolute number of decliners is in VBR; this is not surprising as VBR is an index of total brain volume loss that subsumes all structures. However, none of the structures (including VBR) differed significantly from one another with respect to the number of decliners, with confidence intervals overlapping substantially. Within the substructures, it is interesting to note that only the genu of the CC was different from its respective sub-structures, with significantly fewer decliners than in either the body or the splenium. These results did not support our hypothesis that the hippocampus, and particularly the hippocampal head would show greatest vulnerability.

PATTERN OF ATROPHY ACROSS STRUCTURES

Examining whether atrophy across structures and sub-structures was related, we examined the association between decliners. If a patient showed atrophy across time on one structure, were they likely to also show atrophy on another structure? **Table 5A** shows the PHI coefficients and their 95% confidence intervals between regions measured. There was an overarching relationship, that

Table 2 | Percent decline (by group) across structures and substructures.

Structure	Percent atrophy per month in healthy control participants ($N = 12$)	Percent atrophy per month in patients ($N = 56$)
VBR[a]	0.18 (0.21)	1.32 (1.21)*****
HPC-L head	−0.008 (0.03)	−0.300 (0.63)**
HPC-L body	−0.004 (0.04)	−0.364 (0.59)*****
HPC-L tail	0.054 (0.08)	−0.676 (1.44)*****
HPC-L total	−0.002 (0.02)	−0.348 (0.48)*****
HPC-R head	0.004 (0.03)	−0.248 (0.60)**
HPC-R body	0.005 (0.03)	−0.331 (0.83)**
HPC-R tail	−0.023 (0.05)	−0.662 (1.05)*****
HPC-R total	0.002 (0.03)	−0.324 (0.53)*****
CC genu	−0.14 (0.11)	−0.855 (1.24)*****
CC body	0.09 (0.09)	−0.765 (1.33)*****
CC splenium	0.08 (0.09)	−0.805 (0.81)*****
CC total	−0.02 (0.04)	−0.812 (0.88)*****

[a] *Positive change for VBR denotes atrophy.*
$^{**}P < 0.005$; $^{*****}P < 0.00001$.

Table 3 | The number of patients who show atrophy.

	Number/(percentage) of decliners
Decline in at least 1 structure	**54/56 (96.4%)**
Decline in 4/4 structures	22/56 (39.3%)
Decline in 3/4 structures	20/56 (35.7%)
Decline in 2/4 structures	8/56 (9%)
Decline in 1/4 structures	4/56 (7%)
Decline in 0/4 structures	2/56 (3.6%)

Table 4 | The number of patients who show decline in each structure and substructure.

Structure/ substructure	Number/(percentage) of decliners by structure	Lower and upper 95% CI at 2 z-score < controls
VBR	**45** (80.4)	67.6–89.9
HPC-L head	31 (55.4)	41.5–68.7
HPC-L body	24 (42.9)	29.7–56.8
HPC-L tail	32 (57.1)	43.2–70.3
HPC-L total	**40** (71.4)	57.8–82.7
HPC-R head	38 (67.9)	54.0–79.7
HPC-R body	39 (69.6)	55.9–81.2
HPC-R tail	36 (64.3)	50.4–76.6
HPC-R total	**41** (73.2)	59.7–84.2
CC genu	26 (46.4)*	33.0–60.3
CC body	42 (75.0)	61.6–85.6
CC splenium	42 (75.0)	61.6–85.6
CC total	**43 (76.8)**	63.6–87.0

Table 5A | PHI coefficients across the structures measured.

	PHI coefficients (95% CI)			
	VBR	**HPC-L total**	**HPC-R total**	**CC total**
VBR	–	$r = -0.01$ ($CI = -0.28$–0.25)	$r = 0.31^*$ ($CI = 0.05$–0.53)	$r = 0.37^*$ ($CI = 0.12$–0.57)
HPC-L total	–	–	$r = 0.33^*$ ($CI = 0.08$–0.55)	$r = 0.03$ ($CI = -0.24$–0.29)
HPC-R total	–	–	–	$r = 0.15$ ($CI = -0.12$–0.39)

is, significant overlap, between VBR with both the CC and the right (but not left) HPC. The right and left hippocampus also overlapped significantly. There was no relationship between the CC and the hippocampi. These results partially supported our hypotheses, namely a relationship between VBR and individual structures, and the absence of relationship between some (though not all) of the structures measured.

Table 5B presents the PHI coefficients and their 95% confidence intervals between substructures. Here, significant overlap was observed between the right hippocampus head and tail, and between the genu and body and the genu and splenium of the CC, findings which overall did not support our hypothesis.

Table 5B | PHI coefficients for sub-structures of the left and right hippocampus and the corpus callosum.

	PHI coefficients (95% CI)		
	HPC-L head	**HPC-L body**	**HPC-L tail**
HPC-L head	–	$r = -0.02$ ($CI = -0.28$–0.24)	$r = 0.02$ ($CI = -0.24$–0.28)
HPC-L body	–	–	$r = -0.05$ ($CI = -0.31$–0.21)
	HPC-R head	**HPC-R body**	**HPC-R tail**
HPC-R head	–	$r = 0.13$ ($CI = -0.14$–0.38)	$r = 0.29^*$ ($CI = 0.02$–0.51)
HPC-R body	–	–	$r = 0.16$ ($CI = -0.11$–0.40)
	CC genu	**CC body**	**CC splenium**
CC genu	–	$r = 0.29^*$ ($CI = 0.03$–0.51)	$r = 0.37^*$ ($CI = 0.12$–0.58)
CC body	–	–	$r = 0.14$ ($CI = -0.13$–0.39)

DISCUSSION

The primary purpose of the current study was to gain a better understanding of the scale of atrophy in the chronic phase of TBI. Our cohort was a Canadian sample of patients with brain injuries ranging from complicated mild to severe. More than 96% of our sample showed atrophy over time in at least one region and the large majority showed atrophy in at least three of the four regions measured. Therefore, these findings indicate substantive atrophy—we employed a threshold of at least two z-scores below that of controls—across several structures. Given the relationship between sub-acute atrophy and behavioral and functional outcomes (Sidaros et al., 2008, 2009; Farbota et al., 2012), and between total brain volume loss and clinical impairment (Tate et al., 2011), these findings are clinically concerning, especially as brain atrophy is a known predictor of Alzheimer's Disease (Frisoni et al., 2010).

A secondary purpose of the study was to begin to characterize this chronic atrophy by examining two related features of the data: (i) the extent to which the number of decliners in each structure and sub-structure differed, allowing us to evaluate preliminarily the relative vulnerability of structures examined, and (ii) the extent to which decline in one structure was associated with decline in another. With regard to the first question, we found few differences in the number of decliners across structures and sub-structures, with only the genu differing significantly from the other sub-structures of the CC. Thus, contrary to our hypothesis, the findings in the small number of regions examined in our study do not suggest that one region is more vulnerable to chronic volume loss than another, with the exception of the genu. However, it is possible that limited power may have elevated Type II errors; given the rather large confidence intervals secondary to sample size, the results may under-represent differences between structures.

Regarding the second question, we found more associations across structures than we had predicted. Subjects showing atrophy in the whole brain also showed atrophy in other structures measured (i.e., CC and right HPC) as expected, which likely does not speak to underlying mechanisms, but rather to VBR's inclusive relationship with the other structures measured. However, we also found that those who declined in one HPC were more likely to also decline in the other. Within the sub-structures, those who declined in the right HPC head were more likely to decline in the tail, and those who declined in genu of the CC were more likely to decline in the body and the splenium. It is important to note that wide confidence intervals secondary to sample size bias the findings in favor of Type II errors, and that these findings may actually *underestimate* the degree of association between the structures.

These findings offer some direction for future research into mechanisms. A great deal of research has examined the *acute* primary and secondary mechanical, chemical, and electrophysiological changes in the brain following TBI, which in more serious injuries are ultimately associated with necrotic or apoptotic death (Povlishock and Katz, 2005; Griesbach et al., 2007). In contrast, there has been relatively limited research directly investigating mechanisms of later atrophy of the brain (but see Johnson et al., 2013; Smith et al., 2013).

MECHANISMS OF ATROPHY IN THE CHRONIC STAGE OF TBI

In broad strokes, atrophy in the chronic stages of injury may reflect volume loss, neuronal death or a reduction in neuronal proliferation and/or survival. Cell death may occur due to delayed apoptotic mechanisms (Colicos et al., 1996; Bramlett et al., 1997a,b; Dixon et al., 1999; Williams et al., 2001; Coulson et al., 2008) secondary to trans-neuronal degeneration (Gennarelli and Graham, 1998; Tate and Bigler, 2000) arising from disconnections within or between functionally related structures (Tate and Bigler, 2000; Duering et al., 2012; Bigler, 2013b). Volume loss may reflect decreased complexity of the neuropil, with decreased spines, synapses and arborization or reduced fluid as a result of diminished protein production. Vascular changes might also contribute to volumetric changes over time. For example, reduced functional hyperemia (because of reduced neuronal demand) would reduce blood volume as would disrupted neurovascular coupling. A mechanism receiving increasing scientific attention for chronic stage losses in TBI is persisting inflammation, associated with cytokine release and microglial activation (Gentleman et al., 2004; Rodriguez-Paez et al., 2005; Johnson et al., 2013; Smith et al., 2013). Genetic causes of poorer clinical outcomes have been advanced for a number of years (Ponsford et al., 2011). A highly probable cause of volume losses are the synergistic effects of aging and TBI, as described in detail by Bigler (2013b); such effects may exacerbate the burden of normal and pathological aging, and thereby account for observed volume losses, with such losses also hastening the onset of dementia. Links between TBI and dementia are being increasingly made (Fakhran et al., 2013), with proteins implicated in dementias (e.g., amyloid-beta, amyloid precursor protein, tau), for example, found to accumulate in damaged axons and other neuronal compartments in the chronic stages of TBI (Bramlett et al., 1997b; Smith et al., 2003; Uryu et al., 2007; Johnson et al., 2012; Bennett et al., 2013).

Importantly, these candidate mechanisms of atrophy are empirically testable. Ultimately, an understanding is needed of whether a single mechanism or multiple mechanisms influence atrophy, whether different mechanisms affect different regions, and if multiple mechanisms do influence atrophy, whether they are additive or synergistic.

The findings in the current study favor some mechanisms over others, helping at least to constrain hypotheses for future research. The *ubiquity* of atrophy across patients would not support an exclusive genetic explanation of atrophy; for example, base rates of the e-4 allele that has been implicated in the relationship between TBI and dementia are considerably lower than the 96% incidence of patients who showed volume loss in this study.

With regard to neuroinflammation, Johnson et al. (2013) showed evidence of increasing neuroinflammation in the CC from the sub-acute to the more chronic stages of injury (i.e., 2 weeks to 1 year vs. > 1–18 years post-injury), and inflammation correlated with WM integrity losses and visible pathology. The prevalence of unequivocal markers of neuroinflammation appeared to be substantively lower than the 76.8% of patients in our study showing CC volume loss. However, neuroinflammation is likely one of multiple causes of volume loss in our study.

In humans, the identification of behavioral factors that may exacerbate or buffer against volume loss is of high importance given the potential for clinical intervention. It has been postulated that a downward spiral of negative neuroplastic change secondary to disuse may play a role in chronic decline (Evans, 2008; Miller et al., 2013). Supporting this putative mechanism, our group observed a significant negative correlation between self-reported hours of environmental enrichment in the first year post-injury and the degree of hippocampal atrophy observed from 5 to 20 months post-injury (Miller et al., 2013). Compounding disuse is physiological disconnection of healthy tissue from damaged tissue. Given that all of our patients had sustained brain damage and were therefore at risk of both disconnection and disuse, and moreover, that the CC and hippocampus are frequently affected acutely, and are associated with discrete cognitive functions, this explanation is consistent with the high prevalence of chronic atrophy observed. Within the substructures of the (right) hippocampus, the significant association observed is consistent with this interpretation, with the unique pattern of interconnectivity within the hippocampus meaning that damage to one area may deafferent another; if the disconnected tissue does not functionally re-organize, then it is vulnerable to transneuronal degeneration (McCarthy, 2003; Amaral et al., 2008).

However, other aspects of our findings do not support the interpretations above. For example, we found that hippocampal volume loss on the right was positively associated with volume loss on the left. Experience-dependent volume increases in the hippocampus (Draganski et al., 2006; Maguire et al., 2006) would have predicted that greater reliance on the less damaged hippocampus would result in volumetric increases to it, giving rise to a *negative* association between hippocampi. The positive association between hippocampi suggests a common mechanism deleteriously affecting both. One such mechanism is reduction in new neuronal growth, survival and integration. As is the case for many TBI patients, many of the patients in our cohort at 5 months post-injury and later, had residual physical impairments, reduced volition, had neither returned to work or school, were less socially engaged, and had limited access to resources (Frasca et al., 2013), Therefore, many underwent less physical activity, and many were engaged in less cognitively demanding activity. Since physical and cognitive enrichment have been associated, respectively, with enhanced neuronal proliferation and survivorship (Curlik and Shors, 2010, 2013), this reduced enrichment may have offset hippocampal growth. Moreover, widespread damage to networks might have further impeded integration of new neurons.

The array of possible interpretations for these findings indicates that much further research is needed to understand mechanisms of atrophy in sub-acute and chronic TBI. Such an understanding is critical for the development of treatment research to avert or abate this atrophy.

There were limitations of the current study. The size of the control group was relatively small and may have compromised the reliability of our findings. As well, because the timelines of the two assessments of controls and patients differed, we calculated monthly percent change to compare patients with controls. This calculation assumes a linear month-to-month change, which is not substantiated. There were significant education, but not age, differences between the patient and control groups. However, we speculate that this difference did not contribute to our findings. In a previous study by our group Miller et al. (2013) using overlapping participants, there was no relationship between years of education and degree of hippocampal atrophy. Moreover, the weight of evidence suggests that education confers protection against the clinical (cognitive) expression of disease, but not against the development of neuropathology or neurodegeneration itself (Members et al., 2010). As well, our findings do not permit us to distinguish between cell death versus volume loss without death. Other methodological approaches, including neuropathological ones, are needed to examine this distinction.

CONCLUSIONS

In the chronic stage of moderate-severe atrophy, loss of volume is substantive and ubiquitous across patients. Changes may be attributable to tissue shrinkage—the result of lost neuropil, protein and/or fluids—or to cell death, with disconnection and disuse, inflammation and delayed apoptosis contributing independently or interactively. Environmental enrichment could play a role in offsetting these changes, and in the chronic stages of injury is a "no-harm" intervention that warrants investigation. Further research is needed to identify precise mechanisms of atrophy that would help us to develop targeted clinical interventions.

ACKNOWLEDGMENTS

The authors acknowledge the support of the Canadian Institute of Health Research, Physicians Services Incorporated Foundation, Ontario Neurotrauma Foundation and the Canada Research Chairs Program.

REFERENCES

Adnan, A., Crawley, A., Mikulis, D., Moscovitch, M., Colella, B., and Green, R. E. (2013). Moderate-severe traumatic brain injury causes delayed loss of white matter integrity: evidence of fornix deterioration in the chronic stage of injury. *Brain Inj.* 27, 1415–1422. doi: 10.3109/02699052.2013.823659

Amaral, O. B., Vargas, R. S., Hansel, G., Izquierdo, I., and Souza, D. O. (2008). Duration of environmental enrichment influences the magnitude and per- sistence of its behavioral effects on mice. *Physiol. Behav.* 93, 388–394. doi: 10.1016/j.physbeh.2007.09.009

Analysisgroup. (2012). *FMRIB Software Library v4.0 [Online]. Oxford: Nuffield Department of Clinical Neurosciences, University of Oxford.* Accessed 2012. Available online at: http://www.fmrib.ox.ac.uk/fsl

Ariza, M., Serra-Grabulosa, J. M., Junqué, C., Ramírez, B., Mataró, M., Poca, A., et al. (2006). Hippocampal head atrophy after traumatic brain injury. *Neuropsychologia* 44, 1956–1961. doi: 10.1016/j.neuropsychologia.2005.11.007

Bendlin, B. B., Ries, M. L., Lazar, M., Alexander, A. L., Dempsey, R. J., Rowley, H. A., et al. (2008). Longitudinal changes in patients with traumatic brain injury assessed with diffusion-tensor and volumetric imaging. *Neuroimage* 42, 503–514. doi: 10.1016/j.neuroimage.2008.04.254

Bennett, R. E., Esparza, T. J., Lewis, H. A., Kim, E., Mac Donald, C. L., Sullivan, P. M., et al. (2013). Human apolipoprotein E4 worsens acute axonal pathology but not amyloid-beta immunoreactivity after traumatic brain injury in 3xTG-AD mice. *J. Neuropathol. Exp. Neurol.* 72, 396–403. doi: 10.1097/NEN.0b013e31828e24ab

Bigler, E. D. (2013a). Neuroinflammation and the dynamic lesion in traumatic brain injury. *Brain* 136, 9–11. doi: 10.1093/brain/aws342

Bigler, E. D. (2013b). Traumatic brain injury, neuroimaging, and neurodegeneration. *Front. Hum. Neurosci.* 7:395. doi: 10.3389/fnhum.2013.00395

Bramlett, H. M., Dietrich, W. D., Green, E. J., and Busto, R. (1997a). Chronic histopathological consequences of fluid-percussion brain injury in rats: effects of post-traumatic hypothermia. *Acta Neuropathol.* 93, 190–199. doi: 10.1007/s004010050602

Bramlett, H. M., Kraydieh, S., Green, E. J., and Dietrich, W. D. (1997b). Temporal and regional patterns of axonal damage following traumatic brain injury: a beta- amyloid precursor protein immunocytochemical study in rats. *J. Neuropathol. Exp. Neurol.* 56, 1132–1141. doi: 10.1097/00005072-199710000-00007

Colicos, M. A., Dixon, C. E., and Dash, P. K. (1996). Delayed, selective neuronal death following experimental cortical impact injury in rats: possible role in memory deficits. *Brain Res.* 739, 111–119. doi: 10.1016/S0006-8993(96)00819-0

Adnan,A., Collins, D. L., Neelin, P., Peters, T. M., and Evans, A. C. (1994). Automatic 3D intersubject registration of MR volumetric data in standardized Talairach space. *J. Comput. Assist. Tomogr.* 18, 192–205. doi: 10.1097/00004728-199403000- 00005

Coulson, E. J., May, L. M., Osborne, S. L., Reid, K., Underwood, C. K., Meunier, F. A., et al. (2008). p75 neurotrophin receptor mediates neuronal cell death by activating GIRK channels through phosphatidylinositol 4,5-bisphosphate. *J. Neurosci.* 28, 315–324. doi: 10.1523/JNEUROSCI.2699-07.2008

Curlik, D. M. 2nd., and Shors, T. J. (2010). Learning increases the survival of newborn neurons provided that learning is difficult to achieve and successful. *J. Cogn. Neurosci.* 23, 2159–2170. doi: 10.1162/jocn.2010.21597

Curlik, D. M. 2nd., and Shors, T. J. (2013). Training your brain: Do men- tal and physical (MAP) training enhance cognition through the process of neurogenesis in the hippocampus? *Neuropharmacology* 64, 506–514. doi: 10.1016/j.neuropharm.2012.07.027

Dixon, C. E., Kochanek, P. M., Yan, H. Q., Schiding, J. K., Griffith, R. G., Baum, E., et al. (1999). One-year study of spatial memory performance, brain morphol- ogy, and cholinergic markers after moderate controlled cortical impact in rats. *J. Neurotrauma* 16, 109–122. doi: 10.1089/neu.1999.16.109

Draganski, B., Gaser, C., Kempermann, G., Kuhn, H. G., Winkler, J., Buchel, C., et al. (2006). Temporal and spatial dynamics of brain structure changes during extensive learning. *J. Neurosci.* 26, 6314–6317. doi: 10.1523/JNEUROSCI.4628- 05.2006

Duering, M., Righart, R., Csanadi, E., Jouvent, E., Herve, D., Chabriat, H., et al. (2012). Incident subcortical infarcts induce focal thinning in connected cortical regions. *Neurology* 79, 2025–2028. doi: 10.1212/WNL.0b013e3182749f39

Evans, J. E. A. (2008). Research digest. *Neuropsychol. Rehabil.* 18, 372–384. doi: 10.1080/09602010801909153

Fakhran, S., Yaeger, K., and Alhilali, L. (2013). Symptomatic white matter changes in mild traumatic brain injury resemble pathologic features of early Alzheimer dementia. *Radiology* 269, 249–257. doi: 10.1148/radiol.13122343

Farbota, K. D., Bendlin, B. B., Alexander, A. L., Rowley, H. A., Dempsey, R. J., and Johnson, S. C. (2012). Longitudinal diffusion tensor imaging and neuropsychological correlates in traumatic brain injury patients. *Front. Hum. Neurosci.* 6:160. doi: 10.3389/fnhum.2012.00160

Frasca, D., Tomaszczyk, J., McFadyen, B. J., and Green, R. E. A. (2013). Traumatic brain injury and post-acute decline: what role does environmental enrichment play? A scoping review. *Front. Hum. Neurosci.* 7:31. doi: 10.3389/fnhum.2013.00031

Frisoni, G. B., Fox, N. C., Jack, C. R. Jr., Scheltens, P., and Thompson, P. M. (2010). The clinical use of structural MRI in Alzheimer disease. *Nat. Rev. Neurol.* 6, 67–77. doi: 10.1038/nrneurol.2009.215

Gennarelli, T. A., and Graham, D. I. (1998). Neuropathology of the head injuries. *Semin. Clin. Neuropsychiatry* 3, 160–175.

Gentleman, S. M., Leclercq, P. D., Moyes, L., Graham, D. I., Smith, C., Griffin, W. S. T., et al. (2004). Long-term intracerebral inflammatory response after trau- matic brain injury. *Forensic Sci. Int.* 146, 97–104. doi: 10.1016/j.forsciint.2004. 06.027

Green, R. E., Melo, B., Christensen, B., Ngo, L. A., Monette, G., and Bradbury, C. (2008). Measuring premorbid IQ in traumatic brain injury: an examina- tion of the validity of the Wechsler Test of Adult Reading (WTAR). *J. Clin. Exp. Neuropsychol.* 30, 163–172. doi: 10.1080/13803390701300524

Greenberg, G., Mikulis, D. J., Ng, K., Desouza, D., and Green, R. E. (2008). Use of diffusion tensor imaging to examine subacute white matter injury progres- sion in moderate to severe traumatic brain injury. *Arch. Phys. Med. Rehabil.* 89, S45–S50. doi: 10.1016/j.apmr.2008.08.211

Greer, J. E., Povlishock, J. T., and Jacobs, K. M. (2012). Electrophysiological abnormalities in both axotomized and nonaxotomized pyramidal neurons following mild traumatic brain injury. *J. Neurosci.* 32, 6682–6687. doi: 10.1523/JNEUROSCI.0881-12.2012

Griesbach, G. S., Gomez-Pinilla, F., and Hovda, D. A. (2007). Time window for voluntary exercise-induced increases in hippocampal neuroplasticity molecules after traumatic brain injury is severity dependent. *J. Neurotrauma* 24, 1161–1171. doi: 10.1089/neu.2006.0255

Hollingshead, A. B., and Redlich, F. C. (1958). *Social Class and Mental Illness.* New York, NY: John Wiley. doi: 10.1037/10645-000

Johnson, V. E., Stewart, J. E., Begbie, F. D., Trojanowski, J. Q., Smith, D. H., and Stewart, W. (2013). Inflammation and white matter degeneration per- sist for years after a single traumatic brain injury. *Brain* 136, 28–42. doi: 10.1093/brain/aws322

Johnson, V. E., Stewart, W., and Smith, D. H. (2012). Widespread tau and amyloid- Beta pathology many years after a single traumatic brain injury in humans. *Brain Pathol.* 22, 142–149. doi: 10.1111/j.1750-3639.2011.00513.x

Lezak, M. D. (2004). *Neuropsychological Assessment.* New York, NY: Oxford University Press.

Maguire, E. A., Woollett, K., and Spiers, H. J. (2006). London taxi drivers and bus drivers: a structural MRI and neuropsychological analysis. *Hippocampus* 16, 1091–1101. doi: 10.1002/hipo.20233

Maller, J. J., Daskalakis, Z. J., and Fitzgerald, P. B. (2007). Hippocampal volumetrics in depression: the importance of the posterior tail. *Hippocampus* 17, 1023–1027. doi: 10.1002/hipo.20339

Masel, B. E., and Dewitt, D. S. (2010). Traumatic brain injury: a disease process, not an event. *J. Neurotrauma* 27, 1529–1540. doi: 10.1089/neu.2010.1358

McCarthy, M. M. (2003). Stretching the truth. Why hippocampal neurons are so vulnerable following traumatic brain injury. *Exp. Neurol.* 184, 40–43. doi: 10.1016/j.expneurol.2003.08.020

Members, E. C. C., Brayne, C., Ince, P. G., Keage, H. A., McKeith, I. G., Matthews, F. E., et al. (2010). Education, the brain and dementia: neuro- protection or compensation? *Brain* 133, 2210–2216. doi: 10.1093/brain/ awq185

Miller, L. S., Colella, B., Mikulis, D., Maller, J., and Green, R. E. (2013). Environmental enrichment may protect against hippocampal atrophy in the chronic stages of traumatic brain injury. *Front. Hum. Neurosci.* 7:506. doi: 10.3389/fnhum.2013.00506

Millis, S. R., Rosenthal, M., Novack, T. A., Sherer, M., Nick, T. G., Kreutzer, J. S., et al. (2001). Long-term neuropsychological outcome after traumatic brain injury. *J. Head Trauma Rehabil.* 16, 343–355. doi: 10.1097/00001199-200108000-00005

Ng, K., Mikulis, D. J., Glazer, J., Kabani, N., Till, C., Greenberg, G., et al. (2008). Magnetic resonance imaging evidence of progression of subacute brain atro- phy in moderate to severe traumatic brain injury. *Arch. Phys. Med. Rehabil.* 89, S35–S44. doi: 10.1016/j.apmr.2008.07.006

Ponsford, J., McLaren, A., Schonberger, M., Burke, R., Rudzki, D., Olver, J., et al. (2011). The association between apolipoprotein E and traumatic brain injury severity and functional outcome in a rehabilitation sample. *J. Neurotrauma* 28, 1683–1692. doi: 10.1089/neu.2010.1623

Povlishock, J. T., and Katz, D. I. (2005). Update of neuropathology and neurological recovery after traumatic brain injury. *J. Head Trauma Rehabil.* 20, 76–94. doi: 10.1097/00001199-200501000-00008

Rodriguez-Paez, A. C., Brunschwig, J. P., and Bramlett, H. M. (2005). Light and electron microscopic assessment of progressive atrophy following mod- erate traumatic brain injury in the rat. *Acta Neuropathol.* 109, 603–616. doi: 10.1007/s00401-005-1010-z

Ross, D. E., Ochs, A. L., Seabaugh, J. M., Demark, M. F., Shrader, C. R., Marwitz, J. H., et al. (2012). Progressive brain atrophy in patients with chronic neuropsy- chiatric symptoms after mild traumatic brain injury: a preliminary study. *Brain Inj.* 26, 1500–1509. doi: 10.3109/02699052.2012.694570

Ruff, R. M., Young, D., Gautille, T., Marshall, L. F., Barth, J., Jane, J. A., et al. (1991). Verbal learning deficits following severe head injury: heterogeneity in recovery over 1 year. *J. Neurosurg.* 75, S50–S58.

Sidaros, A., Engberg, A. W., Sidaros, K., Liptrot, M. G., Herning, M., Petersen, P., et al. (2008). Diffusion tensor imaging during recovery from severe traumatic brain injury and relation to clinical outcome: a longitudinal study. *Brain* 131, 559–572. doi: 10.1093/brain/awm294

Sidaros, A., Skimminge, A., Liptrot, M. G., Sidaros, K., Engberg, A. W., Herning, M., et al. (2009). Long-term global and regional brain volume changes following severe traumatic brain injury: a longitudinal study with clinical correlates. *Neuroimage* 44, 1–8. doi: 10.1016/j.neuroimage.2008.08.030

Sled, J. G., Zijdenbos, A. P., and Evans, A. C. (1998). A nonparametric method for automatic correction of intensity nonuniformity in MRI data. *IEEE Trans. Med. Imaging* 17, 87–97. doi: 10.1109/42.668698

Smith, D. H., Johnson, V. E., and Stewart, W. (2013). Chronic neuropathologies of single and repetitive TBI: substrates of dementia? *Nat. Rev. Neurol.* 9, 211–221. doi: 10.1038/nrneurol.2013.29

Smith, D. H., Uryu, K., Saatman, K. E., Trojanowski, J. Q., and McIntosh, T. K. (2003). Protein accumulation in traumatic brain injury. *Neuromolecular Med.* 4, 59–72. doi: 10.1385/NMM:4:1-2:59

Talairach, J., and Tournoux, P. (1988). *Co-planar Stereotaxic Atlas of the Human Brain: 3-Dimensional Proportional System: an Approach to Cerebral Imaging.* New York, NY: Thieme Medical Publishers.

Tate, D. F., and Bigler, E. D. (2000). Fornix and hippocampal atrophy in traumatic brain injury. *Learn. Mem.* 7, 442–446. doi: 10.1101/lm.33000

Tate, D. F., Khedraki, R., Neeley, E. S., Ryser, D. K., and Bigler, E. D. (2011). Cerebral volume loss, cognitive deficit, and neuropsychological performance: comparative measures of brain atrophy: II. Traumatic brain injury.*J. Int. Neuropsychol. Soc.* 17, 308–316. doi: 10.1017/S1355617710001670

Till, C., Colella, B., Verwegen, J., and Green, R. E. (2008). Postrecovery cogni- tive decline in adults with traumatic brain injury. *Arch. Phys. Med. Rehabil.* 89, S25–S34. doi: 10.1016/j.apmr.2008.07.004

Underwood, C. K., and Coulson, E. J. (2008). The p75 neurotrophin receptor. *Int. J. Biochem. Cell Biol.* 40, 1664–1668. doi: 10.1016/j.biocel.2007.06.010

Uryu, K., Chen, X. H., Martinez, D., Browne, K. D., Johnson, V. E., Graham, D. I., et al. (2007). Multiple proteins implicated in neurodegenerative diseases accu- mulate in axons after brain trauma in humans. *Exp. Neurol.* 208, 185–192. doi: 10.1016/j.expneurol.2007.06.018

Watson, C., Andermann, F., Gloor, P., Jones-Gotman, M., Peters, T., Evans, A., et al. (1992). Anatomic basis of amygdaloid and hippocampal volume mea- surement by magnetic resonance imaging. *Neurology* 42, 1743–1750. doi: 10.1212/WNL.42.9.1743

Watson, C., Cendes, F., Fuerst, D., Dubeau, F., Williamson, B., Evans, A., et al. (1997). Specificity of volumetric magnetic resonance imaging in detecting hippocampal sclerosis. *Arch. Neurol.* 54, 67–73. doi: 10.1001/archneur.1997.00550130049015

Weschler, D. (2001). *Wechsler Test of Adult Reading (WTAR).* San Antonio, TX: Harcourt Assessment.

Wilde, E. A., Chu, Z., Bigler, E. D., Hunter, J. V., Fearing, M. A., Hanten, G., et al. (2006). Diffusion tensor imaging in the corpus callosum in children after moderate to severe traumatic brain injury. *J. Neurotrauma* 23, 1412–1426. doi: 10.1089/neu.2006.23.1412

Williams, S., Raghupathi, R., Mackinnon, M. A., McIntosh, T. K., Saatman, K. E., and Graham, D. I. (2001). *In situ* DNA fragmentation occurs in white matter up to 12 months after head injury in man. *Acta Neuropathol.* 102, 581–590. doi: 10.1007/s004010100410

Zijdenbos, A. P., Forghani, R., and Evans, A. C. (1998). "MRI brain data sets: validation of INSECT," in *Medical Image Computing and Computer-Assisted Intervention - Miccai '98*, eds W. M. Wells, A. Colchester, and S. Delps (Cambridge: Springer), 439–448.

3

Current understanding of the glial response to disorders of the aging CNS

Roger A Barker[1]* and Francesca Cicchetti[2,3]*

[1] *Department of Clinical Neuroscience, Cambridge Centre for Brain Repair, University of Cambridge, Cambridge, UK*
[2] *Centre de Recherche du CHUL (CHUQ), Axe Neurosciences, Québec, QC, Canada*
[3] *Département de Psychiatrie et Neurosciences, Université Laval, Québec, QC, Canada*

Edited by:
Ian M. Stanford, Aston University, UK

Reviewed by:
Jason B. Wu, Cedars-Sinai Medical Center, USA
Raja S. Settivari, The Dow Chemical Company, USA

****Correspondence:***
Roger A Barker, Cambridge Center for Brain Repair, University of Cambridge, Cambridge, CB2 0PY, UK.
e-mail: rab46@cam.ac.uk;
Francesca Cicchetti, Centre de recherche du CHUQ (pavillon CHUL), 2705 Boulevard Laurier, T2-50, Québec, QC, Canada.
e-mail: francesca.cicchetti@crchul.ulaval.ca

In this special issue of Frontiers in Pharmacology, we have asked leading experts to comment and review the evidence that inflammatory cells play a leading role in the pathological processes underlying neurodegenerative disorders. We now seek to draw these various observations together into a conclusion, with the hope that this will inform further work in this area and result in the identification of new therapeutic targets that will have a disease modifying effect.

Keywords: inflammation, microglia, Alzheimer's disease, Parkinson's disease, Huntington's disease, motorneuron disease

INTRODUCTION

For many years, chronic neurodegenerative disorders of the central nervous system (CNS) were thought of in terms of primary neuronal dysfunction and loss with secondary glial and inflammatory responses. These responses were defined by an astrogliosis and the presence of a few activated microglia, but of late this theory has required revision.

Microglia, which account for approximately 10% of the adult brain cell population, were first described by Pio Del Rio Hortega in 1919 (McGeer and McGeer, 2012) and their identity as a discrete cell population was met with great skepticism. Nevertheless, the recognition of microglia as a distinct cell type was taken on by Ralph van Furth who proposed that they may have some function akin to phagocytes found in other parts of the body. However, it was not until the late 1980s that this field came of age when, using the new technique of immunohistochemistry, the McGeers showed that within the Alzheimer's disease (AD) brain there were large numbers of activated HLA-DR II positive microglia (McGeer et al., 1987). This paper, which struggled to find its way into publication, has now been cited many hundreds of times and paved the way for a whole new area of work on the glial response in neurodegenerative disorders. This first demonstration of class II positive microglial cells in AD led to further discoveries of such cells in a whole range of different neurodegenerative disorders and with it the concept of neuroinflammation. The pioneering work of the McGeers was to radically change how these diseases were seen as they went on to show that microglia were not only intimately bound to central inflammatory responses and antigen presentation, but in fact the whole innate immune system itself had a role to play in these CNS disorders.

We now know that microglia continuously and actively survey the CNS microenvironment (Nimmerjahn et al., 2005), although their distribution is not uniform across the brain which may impact on their pathogenic capacity in different disease states (Lawson et al., 1990). They arise from the primitive myeloid progenitors and enter the developing CNS during embryogenesis and continue to be produced throughout life, sharing many similarities to peripheral macrophages. The original description of the phagocytic properties of microglia was taken to show that their primary function was to remove dying and dead cells and by so doing prevent the release of pro-inflammatory cytokines, chemoattractants, and infiltrating T-cells. However of late, Guy Brown and colleagues have shown that under certain conditions, activated microglia can actually phagocytose viable neurons and synapses and that this may be especially prominent in areas of CNS neuroinflammation as is seen in many, if not all, neurodegenerative disorders (Neher et al., 2012). This would fit well with their role in synaptic pruning in normal development as well as their emerging role in plasticity in the normal brain (Tremblay et al., 2011). In addition, microglia have an important role in adult neurogenesis through their ability to remove apoptotic cells and by so doing allow the integration of those cells that survive and mature into neurons [reviewed in Ekdahl (2012)]. Thus microglia have a repertoire of roles throughout life in the CNS.

MICROGLIA AND ALZHEIMER'S DISEASE

An appreciable number of brain diseases seem to share the common feature of a marked glial response and in this respect the role of microglia in AD has been particularly well studied following on from the original observations of the McGeers (McGeer et al.,

1987). This disorder, the most common of the chronic neurodegenerative diseases, typically presents with an evolving amnesic syndrome and is characterized pathologically by the deposition of extracellular beta-amyloid plaques and intracellularly by tau tangles. The way in which these two pathologies interact with each other to cause disease is unclear, as is how they relate to the inflammation seen within the brains of patients dying with AD. Nevertheless, it is known that inflammation starts early in the disease process, probably ahead of any obvious amyloid deposition [reviewed in Politis et al. (2012)] and at post-mortem there is a substantial inflammatory response especially around the Aβ plaques. Indeed, Aβ itself can activate microglia which in turn can phagocytose neurons, suggesting that microglia are a critical determinant of neuronal cell loss in this condition (Fuhrmann et al., 2010). Neuroinflammation has also been linked to tau-mediated neurodegeneration as well.

For many years, though, the role of inflammation in AD, whilst being recognized as being present, was always relegated to be a secondary or downstream event. However, the recent GWAS in AD have shown that a number of genetic loci linked to the disease possibly code for inflammatory factors (Harold et al., 2009), which implies that they may be much more intimately involved in the actual disease process. In this respect, it is of interest to note that systemic inflammation can also influence what happens within the CNS, which has led some investigators to propose that it may be a critical initiating factor in the genesis of disorders such as AD, and it is through this non-CNS route that the GWAS loci mediate their susceptibility effects (Ransohoff and Perry, 2009).

Whilst microglia responses can be thought to be detrimental to neuronal viability and survival, it is possible that some of the microglia responses may actually be neuroprotective by virtue of the fact that they could help clear Aβ, remove damaged cells and secrete a range of growth factors and anti-inflammatory agents [reviewed in Solito and Sastre (2012)]. Whilst all this may be the case in the young CNS, there is now an emerging concept that AD results primarily from microglial senescence and a progressive breakdown of innate CNS immunity. This is because the major function of microglia is a neuroprotective one given their ability to phagocytose pathogens, secrete neurotrophic factors as well as dampen down free radical production and sequester glutamate in conjunction with astrocytes. Indeed, the astrocytic response has an equally important role in AD pathogenesis with evidence that astrocytes and neurons can interact in a vicious cycle of chronic, sustained, progressive neuroinflammation and cell death. For example, in advanced stages of AD, it has been shown that TRAIL secreted from astrocytes binds to death receptors on neurons to trigger apoptosis (Li et al., 2011).

All of this complexity of action of inflammatory cells in an aging CNS presents a challenge in knowing how best to target them therapeutically in AD.

MICROGLIA AND PARKINSON'S DISEASE

Parkinson's disease (PD) has long been described clinically through its motor manifestations of a resting tremor, rigidity, and bradykinesia and, pathologically, by the formation of alpha synuclein positive Lewy bodies in the substantia nigra with the loss of the nigrostriatal dopaminergic projection. However, it is now clear that the pathology, and the clinical features of PD, are much more extensive and that the disease may even start outside the CNS (Ferrer et al., 2011). This change in our understanding of the extent and pattern of evolution of PD pathology has led to a re-examination of the pathogenic process and with this the potential role for inflammation and microglia, as first suggested by McGeer et al. (1988a) as early as 1988.

Several studies have now shown that microglial activation and elevated levels of inflammatory cytokines accompany neurodegeneration in PD patients (McGeer et al., 1988b; Mogi et al., 1994, 1995a,b; Banati et al., 1998). For example, Langston et al. (1999) in the post-mortem analysis of MPTP intoxicated patients and Brownell et al. (1999) in primates exposed to the same toxin, pointed to the possibility of an inflammatory and glial response in MPTP induced nigral cell death [also see review by McGeer et al. (2001)]. Subsequent studies have confirmed that activated microglia can be seen in the brains of patients with idiopathic PD both using PET imaging [reviewed in Politis et al. (2012)] and pathologically (reviewed in Huang and Halliday (2012)). These changes occur early in the disease course and thereafter remain stable, which suggests that they may be an important initiating event (Ouchi et al., 2005). In this respect, it has now been shown that in animal models of PD, dopaminergic cell loss can be induced solely by inflammatory insults (e.g., Lipopolysaccharide, LPS; Cicchetti et al., 2009a) and that in more traditional neurotoxin induced animal models of PD, inflammation may be necessary for the full expression of the lesion (e.g., Drouin-Ouellet et al., 2011). Furthermore, it has been shown that α- synuclein itself can directly activate microglia (Zhang et al., 2005), and that many of the gene products from the mendelian forms of PD, not only have a role in the intracellular handling of PD related proteins, but also in modulating innate immune signaling (Huang and Halliday, 2012). This sits well with the recent genetic studies linking PD to HLA (Hamza et al., 2010; Saiki et al., 2010). Finally it is worth noting that activated microglial cells in PD are predominantly found in proximity to a key sign of aging namely free neuromelanin (McGeer et al., 1988b) – again highlighting the complex interplay between microglia, disease processes, and an aging CNS.

Other inflammatory cells, such as astrocytes, may also be important in PD not only by virtue of their known ability to support normal neuronal function but also through a role in maintaining the integrity of the blood brain barrier (BBB; Halliday and Stevens, 2011). This may be especially important as abnormalities in this structure (namely the BBB) could allow other parts of the immune system to gain access to the CNS and by so doing contribute to the pathology seen in PD (Kortekaas et al., 2005).

MICROGLIA AND HUNTINGTON'S DISEASE

Huntington's disease (HD) is a rare autosomal dominant disorder characterized by motor, cognitive, and psychiatric problems with extensive pathology across the CNS. Driven by this dominant genetic mutation in the *huntingtin* gene, the neuropathological signs of HD are visible in many structures of the CNS, but predominantly within the striatum and cortex from an early stage of disease. This prominent neuronal loss is accompanied by protein aggregates composed of the mutated form of the huntingtin protein and with this there is significant activation of microglia (Sapp et al., 2001). This activation has been shown in both premanifest (Tai et al., 2007) and manifest HD patients (Sapp et al., 2001) and there appears to be a correlation between the level of microglial activation and disease severity (Pavese et al., 2006), all of which suggests that the microglia are intimately involved in the disease process in HD.

There is now emerging evidence that the ubiquitous expression of the mutant huntingtin protein affects the function of cells outside the CNS. In particular, the mutant huntingtin protein interacts with the immune system with accumulating evidence that changes in this system may critically contribute to the pathology of HD. However, the nature of this contribution remains unclear, to the extent that it is not even known whether the immune system plays a beneficial or detrimental role in HD patients (Soulet and Cicchetti, 2011). What is clear is that analysis of blood samples from HD patients shows abnormal release of pro-inflammatory cytokines in early stages of the disease (Bjorkqvist et al., 2008).

The astrocytic response in HD is substantial and in fact defined early descriptions of the pathology. Indeed the original grading system of striatal atrophy and disease severity by Vonsattel et al. (1985) used this response. This work also highlighted how the astrocytic response follows neuronal loss such that the striking striatal atrophy following a dorso-ventral pattern is mirrored by the intensity of the astrocytosis.

As in the other neurodegenerative conditions we have discussed, the glia are not passive bystanders to the disease process, but seem to be an integral part of the pathological process from the time of disease onset.

MICROGLIA AND MOTORNEURON DISEASE

Motorneuron disease covers a range of disorders all of which are characterized by the loss of motorneurons (MNs), and the extent to which this selectively targets the upper or lower MN defines the disease type, e.g., primary lateral sclerosis (PLS) for a pure upper motor neuron (UMN) disorder whilst spinal muscular atrophy (SMA) singles out the lower motorneurons (LMNs). However, the commonest type involves both UMN and LMNs and is termed amyotrophic lateral sclerosis (ALS), and whilst there are known genetic forms of this disorder, the vast majority are sporadic in nature (Talbot, 2011). Nevertheless, the rare genetic forms of ALS, especially those with mutations in SOD1, have been used to model the disease in the laboratory and of late this has led to studies where the mutant gene has been differentially expressed in various cellular compartments within the CNS. These studies have clearly shown that the effects of the mutant gene in non-neuronal cells is not insignificant, and coupled to the pathological findings in patients dying with ALS, has suggested that the disorder is one that is critically dependent on events in neurons, astrocytes, and microglia (Phani et al, submitted).

Within the MN itself, many pathogenic pathways, which compromise that cell – subsequently leading to dysfunction and death – have been postulated (Ince et al., 2011). These pathways involve the production of abnormal reactive oxidative species (ROS) which in turn compromises mitochondrial function, energy production, and cell integrity. This abnormal production of ROS is enhanced in SOD mutant cells and can further be exacerbated by excessive glutamate stimulation of the MNs and calcium influx. These latter processes may be in part mediated by abnormal glutamate handling by astrocytes, as further supported by studies demonstrating the beneficial effects of glial cell grafts in transgenic models of ALS (Lepore et al., 2008).

In addition, whilst the astrocyte-neuron interactions may be a critical component in the disease process, it is also known that in the brains of patients dying with ALS there is a marked microglial response. As is common to other neurodegenerative disorders, the question arises as to where this reaction lies in the causal cascade of pathogenic events and whether this changes over time. In this respect, there is evidence in animal models that minocycline can have deleterious effects on microglia and astrocytes once the disease has begun (Keller et al., 2011), which is in line with a clinical study of this drug in ALS showing that it was ineffective and even harmful (Gordon et al., 2007). As such, it is likely that the microglia, as with the astrocytes, do play a role in the loss of MNs in ALS, although the extent to which selectively targeting them therapeutically will truly change the disease course is less clear. What is clear however, is that in ALS, the disease is not localized to the motorneuronal compartment and as such, strategies designed around studying patient specific induced pluripotent stem cell derived MNs may only give partial answers. This is especially true if such assays are being used for patient selective drug screens (Ebert et al., 2009).

INFLAMMATORY CELL TARGETING FOR FUTURE THERAPEUTIC APPROACHES TO NEURODEGENERATIVE DISORDERS

Initial views on the role of microglia suggested that these cells were simply there to scavenge up debris and dead cells, while astrocytes fulfilled some supportive role in the CNS. However, microglia are now recognized to have a complex array of supportive and destructive roles in the CNS and that the balance between the two may be critical in driving some aspects of disease processes. Astrocytes are now seen as being fundamental in shaping and maintaining the developing and mature CNS, including a role in adult neurogenesis, axonal regeneration, and the BBB. The dynamic interplay between all of these different CNS compartments is becoming more evident, such that some neurodegenerative disorders of the CNS may have a pathology as much in the glial cells as in the neurons themselves. This all means that understanding what happens in disease states is far more complex than originally conceived and that targeting each element of the interaction may be the route by which true disease modification can be achieved.

In this special issue of Frontiers in Pharmacology we have repeatedly seen how the glia, immune response, and neurons interact to drive disease, and that our abilities to more accurately define and follow this *in vivo* has enabled us to better understand the temporal relationships that exist between these cellular players and when and how they can best be modulated for therapeutic benefit. Indeed, our capacity to better visualize the glial cells in patients with neurodegenerative disorders especially with respect to microglia is well covered by Politis et al. (2012). This is particularly important given the limitations of animal models of neurodegeneration which includes the fact that they often model disease using a transgenic approach, even though the commonest neurodegenerative disorders (AD and PD) are largely sporadic in nature. In addition, these animals typically develop disease over weeks and months when in patients they evolve over months or years, and thus short acute therapies in the laboratory may not be relevant to the clinic. Finally, our capacity to better define the heterogeneity of patient populations has meant that the therapeutic idea that "one size fits all" is no longer tenable, and that disease processes may follow very different trajectories in different patients and as such require completely different therapeutic approaches (see, e.g., Williams-Gray et al., 2009). A point reinforced by the heterogeneity of glial responses as a function of age and disease state.

As we move toward an era of ever more sophisticated therapeutic agents, our ability to better understand networks of disease pathogenesis will become increasingly important as our capacity to dissect the role of each component will be critical to the success of any such therapy. This is perhaps best shown in the world of cellular transplants for HD, where simply delivering a cell replacement therapy to a diseased brain may not be useful in itself, not because there is anything intrinsically wrong with replacing dysfunctional and lost neurons, but because the necessary support for those cells is no longer there and may even be replaced by a hostile environment (Cicchetti et al., 2009b, 2011). It has even been proposed and demonstrated that in some animal models of motorneuron disease, transplanting glial cells is better than trying to replace the MNs *per se*, as the former have a more critical role in disease pathogenesis through their handling of glutamate (Lepore et al., 2008).

In conclusion, there is now a growing body of evidence from many different sources demonstrating that glial and inflammatory responses are central to these diseases – this includes findings from epidemiological studies looking at anti-inflammatory drugs and the risk of PD and AD; the GWAS in AD and PD; pathological and imaging studies in patients as well as the study of peripheral markers of inflammation [e.g., in HD – reviewed in Wild et al. (2008)]. All of this makes for a very persuasive role for the glia and inflammation in chronic neurodegenerative disorders of the CNS, which will set the scene for a whole new approach to disease modifying therapeutics for a group of disorders that will become increasingly more common as the population ages. Exactly what form these agents will take is unresolved but may involve using drugs that are already in clinical use such as minocycline and non-steroidal anti-inflammatories (NSAIs). Indeed, the use of anti-inflammatory agents for treating AD has long been considered, outside of the amyloid immunization approach (Menendez-Gonzalez et al., 2011). Their efficacy has yet to be proven especially with respect to the commonly available NSAIs which appear to be much less effective in controlling the activation of aged, as compared to young microglia and are likely to be too wide-spectrum thereby suppressing both the detrimental (e.g., pro-inflammatory cytokines, oxidative stress, etc.) and beneficial roles (e.g., pro-repair processes, phagocytosis, and neuroprotection) of the immune cells (Soulet and Cicchetti, 2011). Thus selecting the right agent in the right aged patient group at the right stage of their disease will be critical, and as our understanding of the role of microglia, astrocytes and other related cells evolves, and how they relate to each other, so will our capacity to target them in disease settings.

REFERENCES

Banati, R. B., Daniel, S. E., and Blunt, S. B. (1998). Glial pathology but absence of apoptotic nigral neurons in long-standing Parkinson's disease. *Mov. Disord.* 13, 221–227.

Bjorkqvist, M., Wild, E. J., Thiele, J., Silvestroni, A., Andre, R., Lahiri, N., Raibon, E., Lee, R. V., Benn, C. L., Soulet, D., Magnusson, A., Woodman, B., Landles, C., Pouladi, M. A., Hayden, M. R., Khalili-Shirazi, A., Lowdell, M. W., Brundin, P., Bates, G. P., Leavitt, B. R., Moller, T., and Tabrizi, S. J. (2008). A novel pathogenic pathway of immune activation detectable before clinical onset in Huntington's disease. *J. Exp. Med.* 205, 1869–1877.

Brownell, A. L., Jenkins, B. G., and Isacson, O. (1999). Dopamine imaging markers and predictive mathematical models for progressive degeneration in Parkinson's disease. *Biomed. Pharmacother.* 53, 131–140.

Cicchetti, F., Drouin-Ouellet, J., and Gross, R. E. (2009a). Environmental toxins and Parkinson's disease: what have we learned from pesticide-induced animal models? *Trends Pharmacol. Sci.* 30, 475–483.

Cicchetti, F., Saporta, S., Hauser, R. A., Parent, M., Saint-Pierre, M., Sanberg, P. R., Li, X. J., Parker, J. R., Chu, Y., Mufson, E. J., Kordower, J. H., and Freeman, T. B. (2009b). Neural transplants in patients with Huntington's disease undergo disease-like neuronal degeneration. *Proc. Natl. Acad. Sci. U.S.A.* 106, 12483–12488.

Cicchetti, F., Soulet, D., and Freeman, T. B. (2011). Neuronal degeneration in striatal transplants and Huntington's disease: potential mechanisms and clinical implications. *Brain* 134, 641–652.

Drouin-Ouellet, J., Gibrat, C., Bousquet, M., Calon, F., Kriz, J., and Cicchetti, F. (2011). The role of the MYD88-dependent pathway in MPTP-induced brain dopaminergic degeneration. *J. Neuroinflammation* 8, 137.

Ebert, A. D., Yu, J., Rose, F. F. Jr., Mattis, V. B., Lorson, C. L., Thomson, J. A., and Svendsen, C. N. (2009). Induced pluripotent stem cells from a spinal muscular atrophy patient. *Nature* 457, 277–280.

Ekdahl, C. T. (2012). Microglia activation – tuning and pruning adult neurogenesis. *Front. Pharmacol.* 3:41. doi:10.3389/fphar.2012.00041

Ferrer, I., Martinez, A., Blanco, R., Dalfo, E., and Carmona, M. (2011). Neuropathology of sporadic Parkinson disease before the appearance of parkinsonism: preclinical Parkinson disease. *J. Neural Transm.* 118, 821–839.

Fuhrmann, M., Bittner, T., Jung, C. K., Burgold, S., Page, R. M., Mitteregger, G., Haass, C., LaFerla, F. M., Kretzschmar, H., and Herms, J. (2010). Microglial Cx3cr1 knockout prevents neuron loss in a mouse model of Alzheimer's disease. *Nat. Neurosci.* 13, 411–413.

Gordon, P. H., Moore, D. H., Miller, R. G., Florence, J. M., Verheijde, J. L., Doorish, C., Hilton, J. F., Spitalny, G. M., MacArthur, R. B., Mitsumoto, H., Neville, H. E., Boylan, K., Mozaffar, T., Belsh, J. M., Ravits, J., Bedlack, R. S., Graves, M. C., McCluskey, L. F., Barohn, R. J., and Tandan, R. (2007). Efficacy of minocycline in patients with amyotrophic lateral sclerosis: a phase III randomised trial. *Lancet Neurol.* 6, 1045–1053.

Halliday, G. M., and Stevens, C. H. (2011). Glia: initiators and progressors of pathology in Parkinson's disease. *Mov. Disord.* 26, 6–17.

Hamza, T. H., Zabetian, C. P., Tenesa, A., Laederach, A., Montimurro, J., Yearout, D., Kay, D. M., Doheny, K. F., Paschall, J., Pugh, E., Kusel, V. I., Collura, R., Roberts, J., Griffith, A., Samii, A., Scott, W. K., Nutt, J., Factor, S. A., and Payami, H. (2010). Common genetic variation in the HLA region is associated with late-onset sporadic Parkinson's disease. *Nat. Genet.* 42, 781–785.

Harold, D., Abraham, R., Hollingworth, P., Sims, R., Gerrish, A., Hamshere, M. L., Pahwa, J. S., Moskvina, V., Dowzell, K., Williams, A., Jones, N., Thomas, C., Stretton, A., Morgan, A. R., Lovestone, S., Powell, J., Proitsi, P., Lupton, M. K., Brayne, C., Rubinsztein, D. C., Gill, M., Lawlor, B., Lynch, A., Morgan, K., Brown, K. S., Passmore, P. A., Craig, D., McGuinness, B., Todd, S., Holmes, C., Mann, D., Smith, A. D., Love, S., Kehoe, P. G., Hardy, J., Mead, S., Fox, N., Rossor, M., Collinge, J., Maier, W., Jessen, F., Schurmann, B., van den Bussche, H., Heuser, I., Kornhuber, J., Wiltfang, J., Dichgans, M., Frolich, L., Hampel, H., Hull, M., Rujescu, D., Goate,

A. M., Kauwe, J. S., Cruchaga, C., Nowotny, P., Morris, J. C., Mayo, K., Sleegers, K., Bettens, K., Engelborghs, S., De Deyn, P. P., Van Broeckhoven, C., Livingston, G., Bass, N. J., Gurling, H., McQuillin, A., Gwilliam, R., Deloukas, P., Al-Chalabi, A., Shaw, C. E., Tsolaki, M., Singleton, A. B., Guerreiro, R., Muhleisen, T. W., Nothen, M. M., Moebus, S., Jockel, K. H., Klopp, N., Wichmann, H. E., Carrasquillo, M. M., Pankratz, V. S., Younkin, S. G., Holmans, P. A., O'Donovan, M., Owen, M. J., and Williams, J. (2009). Genome-wide association study identifies variants at CLU and PICALM associated with Alzheimer's disease. *Nat. Genet.* 41, 1088–1093.

Huang, Y., and Halliday, G. M. (2012). Aspects of innate immunity and Parkinson's disease. *Front. Pharmacol.* 3:33. doi:10.3389/fphar.2012.00033

Ince, P. G., Highley, J. R., Kirby, J., Wharton, S. B., Takahashi, H., Strong, M. J., and Shaw, P. J. (2011). Molecular pathology and genetic advances in amyotrophic lateral sclerosis: an emerging molecular pathway and the significance of glial pathology. *Acta Neuropathol.* 122, 657–671.

Keller, A. F., Gravel, M., and Kriz, J. (2011). Treatment with minocycline after disease onset alters astrocyte reactivity and increases microgliosis in SOD1 mutant mice. *Exp. Neurol.* 228, 69–79.

Kortekaas, R., Leenders, K. L., van Oostrom, J. C., Vaalburg, W., Bart, J., Willemsen, A. T., and Hendrikse, N. H. (2005). Blood-brain barrier dysfunction in parkinsonian midbrain in vivo. *Ann. Neurol.* 57, 176–179.

Langston, J. W., Forno, L. S., Tetrud, J., Reeves, A. G., Kaplan, J. A., and Karluk, D. (1999). Evidence of active nerve cell degeneration in the substantia nigra of humans years after 1-methyl-4-phenyl-1,2,3,6-tetrahydropyridine exposure. *Ann. Neurol.* 46, 598–605.

Lawson, L. J., Perry, V. H., Dri, P., and Gordon, S. (1990). Heterogeneity in the distribution and morphology of microglia in the normal adult mouse brain. *Neuroscience* 39, 151–170.

Lepore, A. C., Rauck, B., Dejea, C., Pardo, A. C., Rao, M. S., Rothstein, J. D., and Maragakis, N. J. (2008). Focal transplantation-based astrocyte replacement is neuroprotective in a model of motor neuron disease. *Nat. Neurosci.* 11, 1294–1301.

Li, C., Zhao, R., Gao, K., Wei, Z., Yin, M. Y., Lau, L. T., Chui, D., and Hoi Yu, A. C. (2011). Astrocytes: implications for neuroinflammatory pathogenesis of Alzheimer's disease. *Curr. Alzheimer Res.* 8, 67–80.

McGeer, P., and McGeer, E. (2012). History of innate immunity in neurodegenerative disorders. *Front. Pharmacol.* 2:77. doi:10.3389/fphar.2011.00077

McGeer, P. L., Itagaki, S., Akiyama, H., and McGeer, E. G. (1988a). Rate of cell death in parkinsonism indicates active neuropathological process. *Ann. Neurol.* 24, 574–576.

McGeer, P. L., Itagaki, S., Boyes, B. E., and McGeer, E. G. (1988b). Reactive microglia are positive for HLA-DR in the substantia nigra of Parkinson's and Alzheimer's disease brains. *Neurology* 38, 1285–1291.

McGeer, P. L., Itagaki, S., Tago, H., and McGeer, E. G. (1987). Reactive microglia in patients with senile dementia of the Alzheimer type are positive for the histocompatibility glycoprotein HLA-DR. *Neurosci. Lett.* 79, 195–200.

McGeer, P. L., Yasojima, K., and McGeer, E. G. (2001). Inflammation in Parkinson's disease. *Adv. Neurol.* 86, 83–89.

Menendez-Gonzalez, M., Perez-Pinera, P., Martinez-Rivera, M., Muniz, A. L., and Vega, J. A. (2011). Immunotherapy for Alzheimer's disease: rational basis in ongoing clinical trials. *Curr. Pharm. Des.* 17, 508–520.

Mogi, M., Harada, M., Kondo, T., Narabayashi, H., Riederer, P., and Nagatsu, T. (1995a). Transforming growth factor-beta 1 levels are elevated in the striatum and in ventricular cerebrospinal fluid in Parkinson's disease. *Neurosci. Lett.* 193, 129–132.

Mogi, M., Harada, M., Kondo, T., Riederer, P., and Nagatsu, T. (1995b). Brain beta 2-microglobulin levels are elevated in the striatum in Parkinson's disease. *J. Neural Transm. Park. Dis. Dement. Sect.* 9, 87–92.

Mogi, M., Harada, M., Kondo, T., Riederer, P., Inagaki, H., Minami, M., and Nagatsu, T. (1994). Interleukin-1 beta, interleukin-6, epidermal growth factor and transforming growth factor-alpha are elevated in the brain from parkinsonian patients. *Neurosci. Lett.* 180, 147–150.

Neher, J. J., Neniskyte, U., and Brown, G. C. (2012). Primary phagocytosis of neurons by inflamed microglia: potential roles in neurodegeneration. *Front. Pharmacol.* 3:27. doi:10.3389/fphar.2012.00027

Nimmerjahn, A., Kirchhoff, F., and Helmchen, F. (2005). Resting microglial cells are highly dynamic surveillants of brain parenchyma in vivo. *Science* 308, 1314–1318.

Ouchi, Y., Yoshikawa, E., Sekine, Y., Futatsubashi, M., Kanno, T., Ogusu, T., and Torizuka, T. (2005). Microglial activation and dopamine terminal loss in early Parkinson's disease. *Ann. Neurol.* 57, 168–175.

Pavese, N., Evans, A. H., Tai, Y. F., Hotton, G., Brooks, D. J., Lees, A. J., and Piccini, P. (2006). Clinical correlates of levodopa-induced dopamine release in Parkinson disease: a PET study. *Neurology* 67, 1612–1617.

Politis, M., Su, P., and Piccini, P. (2012). Imaging of microglia in patients with neurodegenerative disorders. *Front. Pharmacol.* 3:96. doi:10.3389/fphar.2012.00096

Ransohoff, R. M., and Perry, V. H. (2009). Microglial physiology: unique stimuli, specialized responses. *Annu. Rev. Immunol.* 27, 119–145.

Saiki, M., Baker, A., Williams-Gray, C. H., Foltynie, T., Goodman, R. S., Taylor, C. J., Compston, D. A., Barker, R. A., Sawcer, S. J., and Goris, A. (2010). Association of the human leucocyte antigen region with susceptibility to Parkinson's disease. *J. Neurol. Neurosurg. Psychiatr.* 81, 890–891.

Sapp, E., Kegel, K. B., Aronin, N., Hashikawa, T., Uchiyama, Y., Tohyama, K., Bhide, P. G., Vonsattel, J. P., and DiFiglia, M. (2001). Early and progressive accumulation of reactive microglia in the Huntington disease brain. *J. Neuropathol. Exp. Neurol.* 60, 161–172.

Solito, E., and Sastre, M. (2012). Microglia function in Alzheimer's disease. *Front. Pharmacol.* 3:14. doi:10.3389/fphar.2012.00014

Soulet, D., and Cicchetti, F. (2011). The role of immunity in Huntington's disease. *Mol. Psychiatry* 16, 889–902.

Tai, Y. F., Pavese, N., Gerhard, A., Tabrizi, S. J., Barker, R. A., Brooks, D. J., and Piccini, P. (2007). Microglial activation in presymptomatic Huntington's disease gene carriers. *Brain* 130, 1759–1766.

Talbot, K. (2011). Familial versus sporadic amyotrophic lateral sclerosis – a false dichotomy? *Brain* 134, 3429–3431.

Tremblay, M. E., Stevens, B., Sierra, A., Wake, H., Bessis, A., and Nimmerjahn, A. (2011). The role of microglia in the healthy brain. *J. Neurosci.* 31, 16064–16069.

Vonsattel, J. P., Myers, R. H., Stevens, T. J., Ferrante, R. J., Bird, E. D., and Richardson, E. P. Jr. (1985). Neuropathological classification of Huntington's disease. *J. Neuropathol. Exp. Neurol.* 44, 559–577.

Wild, E., Bjorkqvist, M., and Tabrizi, S. J. (2008). Immune markers for Huntington's disease? *Expert Rev. Neurother.* 8, 1779–1781.

Williams-Gray, C. H., Evans, J. R., Goris, A., Foltynie, T., Ban, M., Robbins, T. W., Brayne, C., Kolachana, B. S., Weinberger, D. R., Sawcer, S. J., and Barker, R. A. (2009). The distinct cognitive syndromes of Parkinson's disease: 5 year follow-up of the CamPaIGN cohort. *Brain* 132, 2958–2969.

Zhang, W., Wang, T., Pei, Z., Miller, D. S., Wu, X., Block, M. L., Wilson, B., Zhou, Y., Hong, J. S., and Zhang, J. (2005). Aggregated alpha-synuclein activates microglia: a process leading to disease progression in Parkinson's disease. *FASEB J.* 19, 533–542.

4

Is there evidence for neurodegenerative change following traumatic brain injury in children and youth?

Michelle L. Keightley[1,2,3,4,5]*, Katia J. Sinopoli[1,6], Karen D. Davis[7,8], David J. Mikulis[7], Richard Wennberg[9], Maria C. Tartaglia[9], Jen-Kai Chen[10] and Charles H. Tator[9]

[1] *Bloorview Research Institute, Holland Bloorview Kids Rehabilitation Hospital, Toronto, ON, Canada*
[2] *Department of Occupational Science and Occupational Therapy, University of Toronto, Toronto, ON, Canada*
[3] *Graduate Department of Rehabilitation Science, University of Toronto, ON, Canada*
[4] *Department of Psychology, University of Toronto, ON, Canada*
[5] *Cognitive Neurorehabilitation Sciences, Toronto Rehabilitation Institute, Toronto, ON, Canada*
[6] *Department of Psychology and Division of Neurology, Sickids Hospital for Sick Children, Toronto, ON, Canada*
[7] *Division of Brain, Imaging and Behaviour – Systems Neuroscience, Toronto Western Research Institute, University Health Network, Toronto, ON, Canada*
[8] *Department of Surgery and Institute of Medical Science, University of Toronto, Toronto, ON, Canada*
[9] *Krembil Neuroscience Centre, Toronto Western Hospital, University Health Network and University of Toronto, Toronto, ON, Canada*
[10] *Neuropsychology/Cognitive Neuroscience Unit, Montreal Neurological Institute, Montreal, QC, Canada*

Edited by:
James Blair, National Institute of Mental Health, USA

Reviewed by:
Jack Van Honk, Utrecht University, Netherlands
John Van Horn, University of California at Los Angeles, USA

****Correspondence:***
Michelle L. Keightley, Bloorview Research Institute, Holland Bloorview Kids Rehabilitation Hospital, 150 Kilgour Rd., Toronto, ON M4G 1R8, Canada
e-mail: mkeightley@hollandbloorview.ca

While generalized cerebral atrophy and neurodegenerative change following traumatic brain injury (TBI) is well recognized in adults, it remains comparatively understudied in the pediatric population, suggesting that research should address the potential for neurodegenerative change in children and youth following TBI. This focused review examines original research findings documenting evidence for neurodegenerative change following TBI of all severities in children and youth. Our relevant inclusion and exclusion criteria identified a total of 16 articles for review. Taken together, the studies reviewed suggest there is evidence for long-term neurodegenerative change following TBI in children and youth. In particular both cross-sectional and longitudinal studies revealed volume loss in selected brain regions including the hippocampus, amygdala, globus pallidus, thalamus, periventricular white matter, cerebellum, and brain stem as well as overall decreased whole brain volume and increased CSF and ventricular space. Diffusion Tensor Imaging (DTI) studies also report evidence for decreased cellular integrity, particularly in the corpus callosum. Sensitivity of the hippocampus and deep limbic structures in pediatric populations are similar to findings in the adult literature and we consider the data supporting these changes as well as the need to investigate the possibility of neurodegenerative onset in childhood associated with mild traumatic brain injury (mTBI).

Keywords: traumatic brain injury, neurodegeneration, magnetic resonance imaging

INTRODUCTION

One of the most commonly reported injuries in children who participate in sports is concussion or mild traumatic brain injury (mTBI) (Browne and Lam, 2006). Children and youth (<19 years) involved in organized contact sports are nearly six times more likely to suffer a severe concussion compared to other leisure physical activities (Browne and Lam, 2006). The recovery profile and breadth of consequences in children and youth remains largely unknown (McCrory et al., 2004). This dearth of literature is compounded by the recent scrutiny youth participation in competitive contact sports (such as boxing, hockey and football) has received, due primarily to case study and media reports linking repeat concussions to a distinct neurodegenerative disease known as chronic traumatic encephalopathy (CTE).

This condition was initially described in boxers in 1928 by Martland and known as dementia pugilistica (Martland, 1928). In some cases, a constellation of symptoms typical of neurodegenerative disease were observed in a syndrome, and Miller coined the term "CTE" (Miller, 1966). It is now recognized in many sports in which there are repetitive concussions. CTE is defined as a slowly progressive neurodegenerative disorder associated with repeated brain trauma that manifests years after implicated concussive events (McKee et al., 2009). CTE is a neurodegenerative disease with a distinct distribution of atrophy along the amygdalo-hippocampal-septo-hypothalamic-mesencephalic continuum (McKee et al., 2009). CTE shows some similarity to the chronic effects of moderate and severe traumatic brain injury (TBI). There is demonstrated evidence for neurodegeneration in the chronic phase of moderate to severe TBI, ensuing months to years after brain injury with sub-acute atrophy within the limbic system hippocampi (Ng et al., 2008) and elsewhere (Greenberg et al., 2008; Farbota et al., 2012; Green et al., 2014). The corpus callosum (unmyelinated axons in particular) is vulnerable to the deposition of protein post-TBI, suggesting commonality with CTE (Reeves et al., 2007). Thus, generalized cerebral atrophy is a well-established consequence of moderate-to-severe TBI in adults that can be quantified from MRI studies that assess total brain volume (e.g., Bigler et al., 2010).

To the best of our knowledge, there are currently no scientific studies published of CTE following repetitive concussions/mTBI in children. The popularity of competitive sports coupled with the dearth of literature investigating long-term outcomes following mTBI in the pediatric population, suggests that research addressing the potential for CTE in youth following multiple mTBIs should be a public priority. This mini-review examines the available evidence on atrophy and neurodegenerative change in children and adolescents (<19 years) in the chronic stages of mild, moderate and severe TBI compared to typically developing youths. Research findings describe widespread volume reductions (e.g., Levin et al., 2000; Verger et al., 2001; Serra-Grabulosa et al., 2005; Tasker et al., 2005; Wilde et al., 2005, 2006, 2007, 2010, 2012; Braga et al., 2007; Spanos et al., 2007; Yuan et al., 2007; Fearing et al., 2008; Bigler et al., 2010; Beauchamp et al., 2011a,b) and clearly indicate that childhood TBI disrupts normal age-related neuronal processes that may persist across the life-span (see Bigler, 2013).

METHODS

IDENTIFYING RELEVANT STUDIES

We chose a scoping review methodology (Mays et al., 2001) and entered the keywords mild, traumatic, brain, injury, MRI, child, chronic, long-term, and concussion combined with the Boolean operators AND and OR into PubMed, Ovid, PsychInfo, and Medline as the search engines. We also hand searched each reference list and included only published articles from January 1, 2000 to May 2, 2012 that contained human participants and were published in English. The start date of 2000 was chosen as studies published following this date contained imaging technology and methods sufficiently advanced in terms of sensitivity to detect more subtle structural changes. Foreign language material was excluded because of the cost and time in translating material. We adopted these methods for practical reasons and acknowledge that key articles may have been missed.

The various mechanisms for searching in our scoping study generated a total of 16 publications. No additional publications were identified as the study progressed. All publications were originally identified on the PubMed electronic databases and confirmed by subsequent databases searched.

STUDY SELECTION

Our initial examination of the studies indicated that our search strategy had identified a large number of irrelevant studies. Criteria to eliminate studies that did not address our central research question were developed *post-hoc* in three stages, based on increasing familiarity with the literature (Arksey and O'Malley, 2005). In Stage One we included original research articles and case studies that examined structural changes using MRI following mild, moderate and severe TBI. We included imaging studies examining adults only if the methods informed imaging techniques that could be applied to pediatric cases. We excluded meta-analyses and review articles as well as non-TBI forms of brain injury. These criteria identified 201 articles for review. During Stage Two, we narrowed our inclusion criteria to a TBI sustained during childhood and youth (defined as under the age of 19) and excluded metabolic studies which identified 71 articles. Finally during Stage Three we included only those studies that were cross-sectional or longitudinal in design and reported on neuroimaging findings of neurological degeneration obtained at least 1 year post-injury in order to identify those studies focused on the chronic effects following TBI for all subjects examined. We also excluded studies focusing solely on intentional brain trauma (i.e., inflicted abuse) to try and keep injury mechanism more similar to the biomechanical forces observed in concussion/mTBI. These criteria resulted in 16 articles for review.

Two reviewers (first and second authors) applied the inclusion and exclusion criteria to all the citations and copies of the full articles were obtained for those studies felt to "best fit" the research question. Having read the articles in full, all 16 articles were selected for inclusion in the review.

CHARTING THE DATA

We charted key items of information obtained from the primary research reports being reviewed (Arksey and O'Malley, 2005). We recorded information as follows:

- Author(s), year of publication and study location
- Study population (Brain Injury (TBI) Severity, Time Since Injury, and Mechanism)
- Study Population (Demographic Characteristics)
- Aims
- Study Design
- Structural Feature Assessed
- Behavioral Outcome Measure(s)
- Neurodegenerative Findings

RESULTS

NUMERICAL ANALYSIS OF THE EXTENT, NATURE, AND DISTRIBUTION OF STUDIES

Study design

Supplementary Table 1 summarizes the data obtained from each study. With respect to study design, 14 of the 16 studies reviewed utilized a cross-sectional design, of which 10 included a comparison group. Of the 10 studies containing a control group, seven studies individually matched participants across a number of demographic variables including age, sex, education (maternal or child), and socioeconomic status. One study matched on age and sex combined, with one study matching on age alone. Two studies described a control group consisting of children and youth of similar age who had sustained orthopedic injuries. All cross sectional studies included participants who were under the age of 19 years at the time of scanning. Two of the sixteen studies were prospective longitudinal investigations of the same cohort of children re-imaged at two time-points. One study re-imaged at 3 and 18 months post-injury while the second re-imaged at 3 and 36 months post-injury. Of these two longitudinal studies only one included a control group comprised of children of similar age who had sustained an orthopedic injury.

Of the 16 studies reviewed, eight examined volumetric properties of selected brain regions only, while three considered multiple brain regions and/or all gray and white matter (see **Figure 1**). Two studies report on diffusion tensor imaging (DTI) in selected brain regions (corpus callosum Wilde et al., 2006 and cingulum bundle Wilde et al., 2010, respectively), while one study used DTI to examine selected white matter regions including the corpus callosum, interior capsule, superior longitudinal fasciculus and inferior fronto-occipital fasciculus (Yuan et al., 2007). Two studies employed both volumetric and DTI methods to explore evidence for impaired brain growth across the whole brain following TBI.

Patient population

Of the sixteen studies reviewed, five present various findings from a single cohort of sixteen children and youth who previously sustained a moderate-severe TBI. Six studies in total considered the moderate to severe patient population. Three studies included mild, moderate and severe case while two included "complicated mTBI" [defined as children exhibiting focal pathology on acute computed tomography (CT), regardless of having GCS scores in the range of 13–15] in addition to children and youth survivors of moderate and severe TBI. One study considered the full spectrum of TBI including mild, moderate and severe TBI. One study defined their patient population as mild to moderate and severe, while a final three studies considered severe TBI only.

Behavioral outcome measures

Just over two thirds (11/16) of the studies correlated a measure of behavioral function with the MRI findings. A total of five studies did not include a behavioral outcome measure and three studies (Wilde et al., 2005, 2006; Yuan et al., 2007) correlated MRI findings with GCS or Glasgow Outcome Scale (GOS) alone (see Supplementary Table 1). Most studies that included a behavioral outcome measure reported positive correlations with the structural features assessed (see **Figure 2**). For example, Wilde et al. (2012) found a significant positive correlation between the emotional control subscale of the Behavior Rating Inventory of Executive Function (BRIEF) and right medial frontal and right anterior cingulate gyrus volume. Levin et al. (2000) reported that the uncorrected corpus callosum area was correlated with acute TBI severity and Vineland Adaptive Behavior Scale (VABS) score at 36 months postinjury. Wilde et al. (2010) reported a significant correlation between a low GCS score and high apparent diffusion coefficient (ADC). Furthermore, for the TBI group, significant correlations were found between DTI parameters and behavioral measures. Fearing et al. (2008) found a decreased baseline RT on the Sternberg task to be associated with total brainstem volume for both the control and TBI groups. Yuan et al. (2007) found GCS scores to be positively correlated with FA in several white matter areas including the inferior fronto-occipital fasciculus. Braga et al. (2007) observed lesion volume and presence of lesions left supramarginal gyrus in splenium to be significantly associated with dyscalculia. Wilde et al. (2006) found higher FA was related to increased cognitive processing speed and faster interference resolution. In the TBI patients, higher FA was also related to better functional outcome as measured by the GOS. Serra-Grabulosa et al. (2005) reported verbal long term memory to be significantly correlated with volume of cerebrospinal fluid (CSF) in the TBI group only. Hippocampal volume also correlated with visual and verbal long term recall for TBI subjects. Wilde et al. (2005) observed that greater tissue preservation predicted better recovery on the GOS. Finally, Verger et al. (2001) found that corpus callosum area strongly correlated with several measures involving processing speed and visuospatial function.

CHRONIC ATROPHY AND NEURODEGENERATIVE FINDINGS

Longitudinal studies

Cortical thickness and volumetric changes. Longitudinal investigation of cortical thickness revealed that at 18 months (relative to 3 months) post-injury, bilateral frontal, fusiform, and

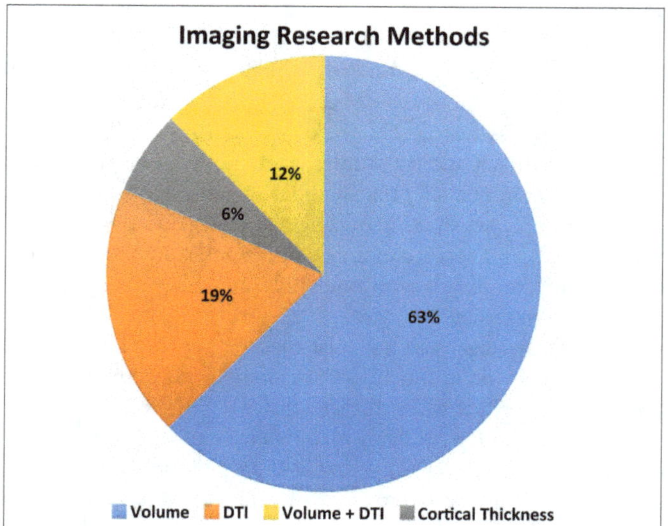

FIGURE 1 | Illustrative summary of imaging research methods.

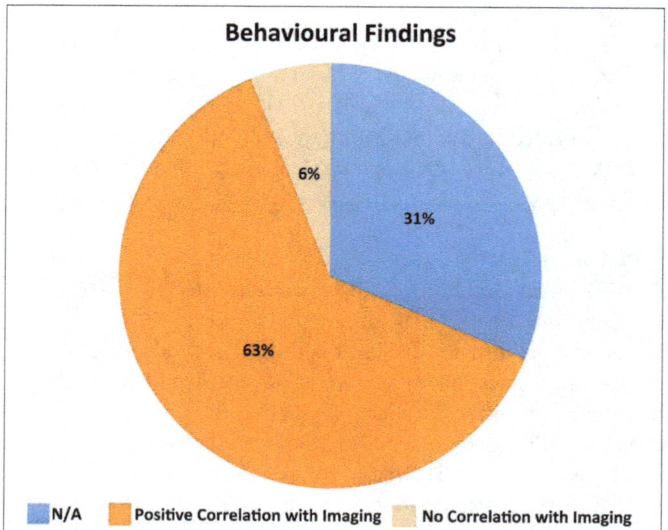

FIGURE 2 | Illustrative summary of behavioral findings.

lingual regions remained significantly decreased in TBI relative to orthopedic controls with additional areas of cortical thinning emerging in bilateral frontal regions, fusiform gyrus and left parietal regions. Wilde et al. (2012) found large bilateral regions of the medial aspects of the frontal lobes and anterior cingulate were attenuated. Most notably, there were also cortical thickness increases in aspects of the medial orbital frontal lobes and bilateral cingulate and right lateral orbital frontal lobe (Wilde et al., 2012) which could be interpreted as either compensatory hypertrophy or random effects. In addition, Levin et al. (2000) report that corpus callosum area decreased from 3 to 36 months in severely injured children and increased in the mild to moderate group. Uncorrected corpus callosum area was correlated with acute TBI severity and functional outcome at 36 months post-injury.

White matter integrity assessed by diffusion tensor imaging (DTI). None of the longitudinal studies examined this parameter.

Cross-sectional studies

Cortical thickness and volumetric changes. All eleven studies focusing on volumetric changes reported positive findings indicative of long-term degeneration in selected brain regions. More specifically, relative to a control group with similar demographic characteristics and in some cases, an orthopedic or extracranial injury, volume loss was evident in the hippocampus, amygdala, globus pallidus, thalamus (gray matter only), periventricular white matter, cerebellum, and the midbrain of the brainstem. Whole brain volume was found to be significantly decreased in TBI patients relative to controls while CSF and ventricular space was observed to be significantly greater. A number of studies attempted to control for the presence of focal lesions by analyzing volumes in brain regions with no focal lesions, as well as patients who did not have focal injuries. These, studies reported reduced volumes in selected brain regions suggesting that the degeneration was not secondary to acute injury and resulting atrophy. Finally in the one study that included mTBI and stratified results according to severity (Beauchamp et al., 2011a,b), significantly reduced gray matter and left hippocampal volume was reported for mild injuries as well as significantly increased CSF compared to an age and sex matched sample.

White matter integrity assessed by diffusion tensor imaging (DTI). All five studies employing DTI reported positive findings indicating compromised white matter integrity at least 1 year following TBI compared to demographically similar control subjects, some of whom sustained an orthopedic or extracranial injury. More specifically, fractional anisotropic (FA) values were significantly reduced in the genu, body and splenium of the corpus callosum, anterior limb of the posterior capsule, posterior limb of the anterior capsule, superior fronto-occipital fasciculus, superior longitudinal fasciculus, superior fronto-occipital fasciculus, and centrum semiovale. Moreover, FA values were significantly reduced bilaterally in the cingulum bundles, while ADC values were significantly increased. Similarly, TBI patients demonstrated significantly higher mean diffusivity in the right cerebral white matter, bilaterally in the forceps major and in the body and splenium of the corpus callosum.

DISCUSSION

Taken together, the studies reviewed suggest there is evidence for long-term neurodegenerative change following TBI in children and youth. In particular both cross-sectional and longitudinal studies revealed volume loss in selected brain regions including the hippocampus, amygdale, globus pallidus, thalamus, periventricular white matter, cerebellum, and brain stem as well as overall decreased whole brain volume and increased CSF and ventricular space. DTI studies also report evidence for decreased axonal integrity, particularly in the corpus callosum (Wilde et al., 2006; Yuan et al., 2007; Porto et al., 2011). Although fewer in number, longitudinal investigations are of critical importance and those reviewed here (i.e., Wilde et al., 2012) highlight the dynamic and disruptive interplay between childhood TBI and normal developmental neuronal processes such as axonal thinning and increased myelination (see Bigler, 2013).

Taken together, the findings appear to highlight a sensitivity of the hippocampus and deep limbic structures in pediatric populations, which like adults, show similarities to CTE where there is a distinct distribution of atrophy along the amygdalo-hippocampal-septo-hypothalamic-mesencephalic continuum (McKee et al., 2009). They also corroborate findings in the chronic phase of moderate to severe TBI in adults, where sub-acute atrophy within the limbic system hippocampi (Ng et al., 2008), corpus callosum (Reeves et al., 2007), and elsewhere (i.e., Greenberg et al., 2008; Bigler et al., 2010; Green et al., 2014) have been documented.

A major limitation of the studies reviewed is the lack of studies focused specifically on repetitive concussions or mTBIs. Only one study (Beauchamp et al., 2011a,b) reported results specific to mTBI where reduced gray matter and left hippocampal volume was reported for mild injuries as well as significantly increased CSF compared to an age and sex matched sample. The second important limitation is that the methods of only a subset of the studies speak directly to a progressive, and putatively neurodegenerative entity. Chronic findings in the rest of the studies reviewed may alternatively reflect the enduring effects of the initial injuries. These findings indicate that long-term investigation of neurodegenerative change following repetitive concussions and mTBIs in children is warranted (Tartaglia et al., 2014).

There is widespread belief that children are at an advantage to adults when inflicted with significant brain damage, such as repeat concussions or mTBIs, as the developing brain has a higher chance of reorganization or plasticity (McCrory et al., 2004). This view is becoming increasingly challenged. The developing brain is cognitively maturing throughout childhood and any impact may cause a disruption in this neuronal maturation (Anderson et al., 2001). Although the injury may occur in the same way, the outcome needs to be treated differently as the composition and mechanical properties of the head and brain differ in an adult and youth (Kirkwood et al., 2006). These differences include increased brain water content, decreased level of myelination, skull geometry, suture elasticity, and neck strength (Bauer and Fritz, 2004; Kirkwood et al., 2006).

In conclusion, the mini-review provides strong evidence for neurodegenerative change following TBI of all severities in children and youth while clearly highlighting repetitive and chronic mTBI in children and youth as an overlooked population. Future research should employ multi-centerd strategies to longitudinally investigate the possibility of neurodegenerative onset and CTE in childhood associated with repeat mTBIs by developing age specific normal databases for each of the imaging parameters under assessment.

REFERENCES

Anderson, V., Catroppa, C., Morse, S., Haritou, F., and Rosenfeld, J. (2001). Outcome from mild head injury in young children: a prospective study. *J. Clin. Exp. Neuropsychol.* 23, 705–717. doi: 10.1076/jcen.23.6.705.1015

Arksey, H., and O'Malley, L. (2005). Scoping studies: towards a meth- od- ological framework. *Int. J. Soc. Res. Methodol.* 8, 19–32. doi: 10.1080/1364557032000119616

Bauer, R., and Fritz, H. (2004). Pathophysiology of traumatic injury in the devel- oping brain: an introduction and short update. *Exp. Toxicol. Pathol.* 56, 65–73. doi: 10.1016/j.etp.2004.04.002

Beauchamp, M. H., Ditchfield, M., Catroppa, C., Kean, M., Godfrey, C., Rosenfeld, J. V., et al. (2011b). Focal thinning of the posterior corpus callosum: normal variant or post-traumatic? *Brain Inj.* 25, 950–957. doi: 10.3109/02699052.2011.589791

Beauchamp, M. H., Ditchfield, M., Maller, J. J., Catroppa, C., Godfrey, C., Rosenfeld, J. V., et al. (2011a). Hippocampus, amygdala and global brain changes 10 years after childhood traumatic brain injury. *Int. J. Dev. Neurosci.* 29, 137–143. doi: 10.1016/j.ijdevneu.2010.12.003

Bigler, E. D. (2013). Traumatic brain injury, neuroimaging, and neurodegeneration. *Front. Hum. Neurosci.* 7:395. doi: 10.3389/fnhum.2013.00395

Bigler, E. D., Abildskov, T. J., Wilde, E. A., McCauley, S. R., Li, X., Merkley, T. L., et al. (2010). Diffuse damage in pediatric traumatic brain injury: a comparison of automated versus operator-controlled quan- tification methods. *Neuroimage* 50, 1017–1026. doi: 10.1016/j.neuroimage.2010.01.003

Braga, L. W., Souza, L. N., Najjar, Y. J., and Dellatolas, G. (2007). Magnetic res- onance imaging (MRI) findings and neuropsychological sequelae in children after severe traumatic brain injury: the role of cerebellar lesion. *J. Child Neurol.* 22, 1084–1089. doi: 10.1177/0883073807306246

Browne, G. J., and Lam, L. T. (2006). Concussive head injury in children and ado- lescents related to sports and other leisure physical activities. *Br. J. Sports Med.* 40, 163–168. doi: 10.1136/bjsm.2005.021220

Farbota, K. D., Bendlin, B. B., Alexander, A. L., Rowley, H. A., Dempsey, R. J., and Johnson, S. C. (2012). Longitudinal diffusion tensor imaging and neuropsychological correlates in traumatic brain injury patients. *Front. Hum. Neurosci.* 6:160. doi: 10.3389/fnhum.2012.00160

Fearing, M. A., Bigler, E. D., Wilde, E. A., Johnson, J. L., Hunter, J. V., Li, X., et al. (2008). Morphometric MRI findings in the thalamus and brainstem in children after moderate to severe traumatic brain injury. *J. Child Neurol.* 23, 729–737. doi: 10.1177/0883073808314159

Green, R. E. A., Colella, B., Maller, J., Bayley, M., Glazer, J., and Mikulis, D. J. (2014). Scale and pattern of atrophy in the chronic stages of moderate-Severe traumatic brain injury. *Front. Hum. Neurosci.* 8:67. doi: 10.3389/fnhum.2014.00067

Greenberg, G., Mikulis, D. J., Ng, K., DeSouza, D., and Green, R. E. (2008). Use of diffusion tensor imaging to examine subacute white matter injury progres- sion in moderate to severe traumatic brain injury. *Arch. Phys. Med. Rehabil.* 89, S45–S50. doi: 10.1016/j.apmr.2008.08.211

Kirkwood, M., Yeates, K., and Wilson, P. (2006). Pediatric sport-related concussion: A review of the clinical management of an oft-neglected population. *Pediatrics* 117, 1359–1371. doi: 10.1542/peds.2005-0994

Levin, H. S., Benavidez, D., Verger-Maestre, K., Perachio, N., Song, J., Mendelsohn, D. B., et al. (2000). Reduction of corpus callosum growth after severe trau- matic brain injury in children. *Neurology* 54, 647–653 doi: 10.1212/WNL. 54.3.647

Martland, H. (1928). Punchdrunk. *JAMA* 91, 1103–1107. doi: 10.1001/jama.1928. 02700150029009

Mays, N., Roberts, E., and Popay, J. (2001). "Synthesising research evidence," in *Studying the Organisation and Delivery of Health Services: Research Methods*, eds N. Fulop, P. Allen, A. Clarke, and N. Black (London: Routledge), 188–220.

McCrory, P., Collie, A., Anderson, V., and Davis, G. (2004). Can we manage sport related concussion in children the same as in adults? *Br. J. Sports Med.* 38, 516–519. doi: 10.1136/bjsm.2004.014811

McKee, A. C., Cantu, R. C., Nowinski, C. J., Hedley-Whyte, E. T., Gavett, B. E., Budson, A. E., et al. (2009). Chronic traumatic encephalopathy in athletes: pro- gressive tauopathy after repetitive head injury. *J. Neuropathol. Exp. Neurol.* 68, 709–735. doi: 10.1097/NEN.0b013e3181a9d503

Miller, H. (1966). Mental after-effects of head injury. *Proc. R. Soc. Med.* 59, 257–261.

Ng, K., Mikulis, D. J., Glazer, J., Kabani, N., Till, C., Greenberg, G., et al. (2008). Magnetic resonance imaging evidence of progression of subacute brain atro- phy in moderate to severe traumatic brain injury. *Arch. Phys. Med. Rehabil.* 89, S35–S44. doi: 10.1016/j.apmr.2008.07.006

Porto, L., Jurcoane, A., Margerkurth, J., Althaus, J., Zanella, F., Hattingen, E., et al. (2011). Morphometry and diffusion MR imaging years after child- hood traumatic brain injury. *Eur. J. Paediatr. Neurol.* 15, 493–501. doi: 10.1016/j.ejpn.2011.06.004

Reeves, T. M., Phillips, L. L., Lee, N. N., and Povlishock, J. T. (2007). Preferential neuroprotective effect of tacrolimus (FK506) on unmyelinated axons following traumatic brain injury. *Brain Res.* 1154, 225–236. doi: 10.1016/j.brainres.2007.04.002

Serra-Grabulosa, J. M., Junqué, C., Verger, K., Salgado-Pineda, P., Mañeru, C., and Mercader, J. M. (2005). Cerebral correlates of declarative memory dysfunctions in early traumatic brain injury. *J. Neurol. Neurosurg. Psychiatry* 76, 129–131. doi: 10.1136/jnnp.2004.027631

Spanos, G. K., Wilde, E. A., Bigler, E. D., Cleavinger, H. B., Fearing, M. A., Levin, H. S., et al. (2007). Cerebellar atrophy after moderate-to-severe pediatric traumatic brain injury. *AJNR Am. J. Neuroradiol.* 28, 537–542.

Tartaglia, M. C., Hazrati, L., Davis, K. D., Green, R. E. A., Wennberg, R., Mikulis, D., et al. (2014). Chronic traumatic encephalopathy and other neurode- generative proteinopathies. *Front. Hum. Neurosci.* 8:30. doi: 10.3389/fnhum. 2014.00030

Tasker, R. C., Salmond, C. H., Westland, A. G., Pena, A., Gillard, J. H., Sahakian, B. J., et al. (2005). Head circumference and brain and hippocampal volume after severe traumatic brain injury in childhood. *Pediatr. Res.* 58, 302–308. doi: 10.1203/01.PDR.0000169965.08854.25

Verger, K., Junqué, C., Levin, H. S., Jurado, M. A., Pérez-Gómez, M., Bartrés-Faz, D., et al. (2001). Correlation of atrophy measures on MRI with neuropsycho- logical sequelae in children and adolescents with traumatic brain injury. *Brain Inj.* 15, 211–221. doi: 10.1080/02699050010004059

Wilde, E. A., Bigler, E. D., Hunter, J. V., Fearing, M. A., Scheibel, R. S., Newsome, M. R., et al. (2007). Hippocampus, amygdala, and basal gan- glia morphometrics in children after moderate-to-severe traumatic brain injury. *Dev. Med. Child Neurol.* 49, 294–299. doi: 10.1111/j.1469-8749. 2007.00294.x

Wilde, E. A., Chu, Z., Bigler, E. D., Hunter, J. V., Fearing, M. A., Hanten, G., et al. (2006). Diffusion tensor imaging in the corpus callosum in children after moderate to severe traumatic brain injury. *J. Neurotrauma* 23, 1412–1426. doi: 10.1089/neu.2006.23.1412

Wilde, E. A., Hunter, J. V., Newsome, M. R., Scheibel, R. S., Bigler, E. D., Johnson, L., et al. (2005). Frontal and temporal morphometric findings on MRI in children after moderate to severe traumatic brain injury. *J. Neurotrauma* 22, 333–344. doi: 10.1089/neu.2005.22.333

Wilde, E. A., Merkley, T. L., Bigler, E. D., Max, J. E., Schmidt, A. T., Ayoub, W., et al. (2012). Longitudinal changes in cortical thickness in children after traumatic brain injury and their relation to behavioral regulation and emotional control. *Int. J. Dev. Neurosci.* 30, 267–276. doi: 10.1016/j.ijdevneu.2012.01.003

Wilde, E. A., Ramos, M. A., Yallampalli, R., Bigler, E. D., McCauley, S. R., Chu, Z., et al. (2010). Diffusion tensor imaging of the cingulum bundle in children after traumatic brain injury. *Dev. Neuropsychol.* 35, 333–351. doi: 10.1080/87565641003696940

Yuan, W., Holland, S. K., Schmithorst, V. J., Walz, N. C., Cecil, K. M., Jones, B. V., et al. (2007). Diffusion tensor MR imaging reveals persistent white matter alteration after traumatic brain injury experienced during early childhood. *AJNR Am. J. Neuroradiol.* 28, 1919–1925. doi: 10.3174/ajnr.A0698

5

Cerebrospinal fluid biomarkers for differentiation of frontotemporal lobar degeneration from Alzheimer's disease

David J. Irwin[1,2], John Q. Trojanowski[1] and Murray Grossman[2]*

[1] Department of Pathology and Laboratory Medicine, Center for Neurodegenerative Disease Research, Alzheimer's Disease Core Center, Institute on Aging, University of Pennsylvania, Philadelphia, PA, USA

[2] Department of Neurology, Center for Frontotemporal Dementia, Perelman School of Medicine, University of Pennsylvania, Philadelphia, PA, USA

Edited by:
Manuel Menéndez-González, Hospital Álvarez-Buylla, Spain

Reviewed by:
Junming Wang, University of Mississippi Medical Center, USA
Angela de Iuliis, University of Padova, Italy

***Correspondence:**
Murray Grossman, Department of Neurology, University of Pennsylvania School of Medicine, Hospital of the University of Pennsylvania, 3400 Spruce Street, Philadelphia, PA 19104, USA.
e-mail: mgrossma@mail.med.upenn.edu

Accurate ante mortem diagnosis in frontotemporal lobar degeneration (FTLD) is crucial to the development and implementation of etiology-based therapies. Several neurodegenerative disease-associated proteins, including the major protein constituents of inclusions in Alzheimer's disease (AD) associated with amyloid-beta ($A\beta_{1-42}$) plaque and tau neurofibrillary tangle pathology, can be measured in cerebrospinal fluid (CSF) for diagnostic applications. Comparative studies using autopsy-confirmed samples suggest that CSF total-tau (t-tau) and $A\beta_{1-42}$ levels can accurately distinguish FTLD from AD, with a high t-tau to $A\beta_{1-42}$ ratio diagnostic of AD; however, there is also an urgent need for FTLD-specific biomarkers. These analytes will require validation in large autopsy-confirmed cohorts and face challenges of standardization of within- and between-laboratory sources of error. In addition, CSF biomarkers with prognostic utility and longitudinal study of CSF biomarker levels over the course of disease are also needed. Current goals in the field include identification of analytes that are easily and reliably measured and can be used alone or in a multi-modal approach to provide an accurate prediction of underlying neuropathology for use in clinical trials of disease modifying treatments in FTLD. To achieve these goals it will be of the utmost importance to view neurodegenerative disease, including FTLD, as a clinicopathological entity, rather than exclusively a clinical syndrome.

Keywords: cerebrospinal fluid, biomarker, tau, $A\beta_{1-42}$, frontotemporal dementia, primary progressive aphasia, Alzheimer's disease

INTRODUCTION

Most neurodegenerative diseases are characterized by specific abnormally-modified protein aggregates, with resulting neuronal cell loss and gliosis. The gold standard for diagnosis is microscopic examination at autopsy; however, there is considerable variability of clinical manifestations associated with underlying neuropathological diagnoses, as clinical symptoms most often reflect the regional burden of pathology within the central nervous system (CNS) rather than the specific underlying proteinopathy. This is especially true in the heterogeneous family of frontotemporal lobar degeneration (FTLD) clinical syndromes.

Two main pathologic FTLD subtypes exist (**Figures 1A, 2**): cases with inclusions formed from the microtubule-binding protein tau (FTLD-tau) and those with TAR DNA binding protein-43 (TDP-43) pathology (FTLD-TDP) (Mackenzie et al., 2010). FTLD-tau includes the following tauopathies (**Figures 2A–D**): Pick's disease (PiD), corticobasal degeneration (CBD), progressive supranuclear palsy (PSP), FTD and parkinsonism linked to chromosome 17 (pathogenic *MAPT* mutations; FTDP-17), and unclassifiable tauopathies (Mackenzie et al., 2010). FTLD-TDP (**Figures 2E–G**) can be subdivided into four subtypes (A–D) based on the morphology and distribution of lesions (Mackenzie et al., 2011) and can also be associated with TDP-43 inclusions in the anterior horn of the spinal cord and gliosis of the corticospinal tracts, suggesting a continuum of FTLD with amyotrophic lateral sclerosis (ALS; FTLD-ALS) (Geser et al., 2008, 2009). A smaller number of FTLD cases are associated with inclusions of another DNA-binding protein, fused-in-sarcoma protein (*FUS;* FTLD-FUS), or other rare, less-defined pathologies (FTLD-UPS, FTLD-ni) (Mackenzie et al., 2010). The major

Abbreviations: FTLD, frontotemporal lobar degeneration; AD, Alzheimer's disease; Aβ, amyloid-beta; CSF, cerebrospinal fluid; CNS, central nervous system; FTLD-tau, FTLD with tau pathology; TDP-43, TAR DNA binding protein-43; FTLD-TDP, FTLD with TDP pathology; PiD, Pick's disease; CBD, corticobasal degeneration; PSP, progressive supranuclear palsy; pathogenic *MAPT* mutations-FTDP-17, FTD and parkinsonism linked to chromosome 17; ALS, amyotrophic lateral sclerosis; FUS, fused-in-sarcoma protein; FTLD-FUS, FTLD with FUS pathology; FTLD-UPS, FTLD with tau- and TDP-43-negative ubiquitinated inclusions; FTLD-ni, FTLD in the absence of significant neuropathological inclusions; *GRN*, progranulin gene; *MAPT*, tau gene; *C9orf72*, C9orf72 gene; *VCP*, valosin-containing protein gene; *TARDBP*, TDP-43 gene; FTLD-ALS, clinical FTLD with ALS; *CHMP2B*, charged mutlivesciular body protein 2B gene; bvFTD, behavioral-variant frontotemporal dementia; PPA, primary progressive aphasia; lvPPA, logopenic-variant PPA; svPPA, semantic-variant PPA; naPPA, non-fluent aggramatic variant PPA; CBS, corticobasal syndrome; $A\beta_{1-42}$, β-amyloid; MCI, mild cognitive impairment; t-tau, total-tau; p-tau, phosphorylated-tau; $p\text{-tau}_{181}$, phosphorylated tau at serine 181; $p\text{-tau}_{231}$, phosphorylated tau at threonine 231; ELISA, enzyme-linked immunosorbent assay; xMAP, luminex flow immunoassay; MRI, magnetic resonance imaging; DIAN, dominantly-inherited AD network; MTBD, microtubule-binding domain; DTI, diffusion-tensor imaging; GM, gray matter; GWAS, genome-wide association studies.

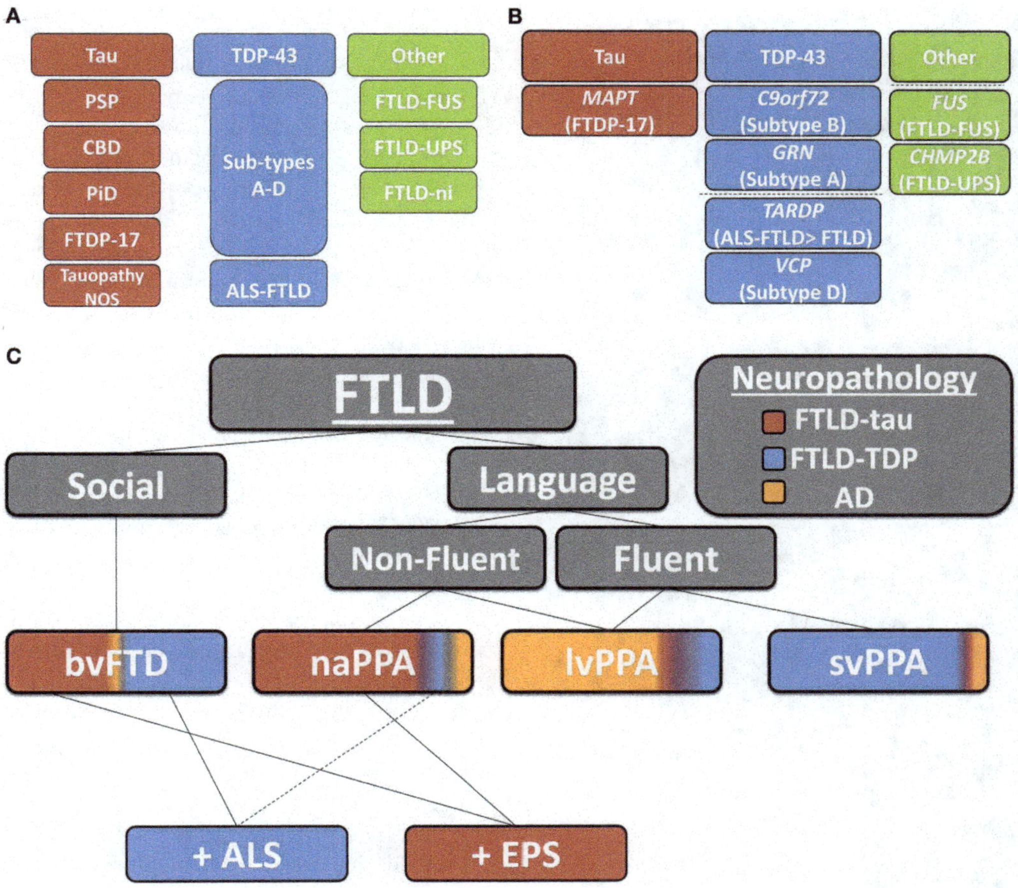

FIGURE 1 | Clinicopathological and genetic associations in FTLD. **(A)** Neuropathological classification of FTLD-tau and FTLD-TDP subtypes (PSP, progressive supranuclear palsy; CBD, corticobasal degeneration; PiD, Pick's disease; FTDP17, frontotemporal dementia with Parkinsonism linked to chromosome 17; Tauopathy NOS, unclassifiable tauopathy; Subtypes A–D, morphological subtypes of FTLD-TDP; ALS-FTLD, amyotrophic lateral sclerosis with FTLD-TDP; FTLD-FUS, FTLD with fused in sarcoma protein inclusions; FTLD-UPS, FTLD with tau- and TDP-43-negative ubiquitinated inclusions; FTLD-ni, FTLD in the absence of significant neuropathological inclusions), **(B)** pathogenic mutation associations with underlying neuropathology (dashed-line separates less common molecular etiologies of FTLD; *MAPT*, tau resulting in FTDP-17; *C90rf72*, pathogenic hexanucleotide expansion resulting in FTLD and/or ALS associated with FTLD-TDP B; *GRN*, progranulin resulting in FTLD-TDP type A; *TARDP*, TDP-43 resulting in ALS ± FTLD and less commonly FTLD; *VCP*, valosin-containing protein resulting in inclusion body myopathy with Paget's disease of bone and frontotemporal dementia with FTLD-TDP subtype D; *FUS*, fused-in sarcoma protein resulting in FTLD-FUS; and *CHMP2B*, charged mutlivesciular body protein 2B resulting in FTLD-UPS), **(C)** clinicopathological correlations of FTLD (colored regions of clinical syndromes represent relative percentages of neuropathological subtypes found in autopsy studies; AD, Alzheimer's disease; bvFTD, behavioral variant of FTLD; PPA, primary progressive aphasia; svPPA, semantic variant PPA; naPPA, nonfluent agrammatic variant PPA; lvPPA, logopenic variant PPA; +ALS, co-morbid amyotrophic lateral sclerosis; +EPS, co-morbid extra-pyramidal Parkinsonian symptoms: i.e., features of akinetic-rigid syndromes of PSP or corticobasal syndrome).

genetic etiologies resulting in FTLD are exclusively associated with specific underlying neuropathologies (**Figure 1B**), despite heterogeneous expression of FTLD clinical syndromes, and include pathogenic mutations in the gene for progranulin (*GRN*) (Baker et al., 2006; Cruts et al., 2006), tau (*MAPT*) (Hutton et al., 1998), and C9orf72 (*C9orf72*) (Dejesus-Hernandez et al., 2011; Renton et al., 2011). Less common genetic etiologies of FTLD include: valosin-containing protein (*VCP*) resulting in inclusion body myopathy with Paget's disease of bone and frontotemporal dementia with FTLD-TDP subtype D neuropathology, *TARDBP* coding for TDP-43 protein and causing ALS or ALS-FTLD (rarely FTLD-TDP alone), *CHMP2B* coding for charged mutlivesciular body protein 2B and resulting in FTLD-UPS, and mutations in *FUS* causing FTLD-FUS (**Figure 1B**) (Mackenzie et al., 2010).

Clinically, FTLD can be broadly divided into two main subtypes, those with predominant behavioral and social comportment disorder (behavioral-variant frontotemporal dementia, bvFTD) (Rascovsky et al., 2011) and those with primary language disturbances (primary progressive aphasia, PPA) (Mesulam, 1982, 2001). Among PPA patients, three subgroups have been recently divided (Gorno-Tempini et al., 2011) into the logopenic (lvPPA) (Gorno-Tempini et al., 2004, 2008), semantic (svPPA) (Hodges and Patterson, 2007), and non-fluent aggramatic variant (naPPA) (Turner et al., 1996). Clinicopathological correlations of these syndromes are complex (Josephs, 2008; Grossman, 2010). For example, large studies of autopsy-confirmed FTLD (behavioral and aphasic variants) find roughly equal numbers of FTLD-tau and FTLD-TDP (Hodges et al., 2004; Kertesz et al.,

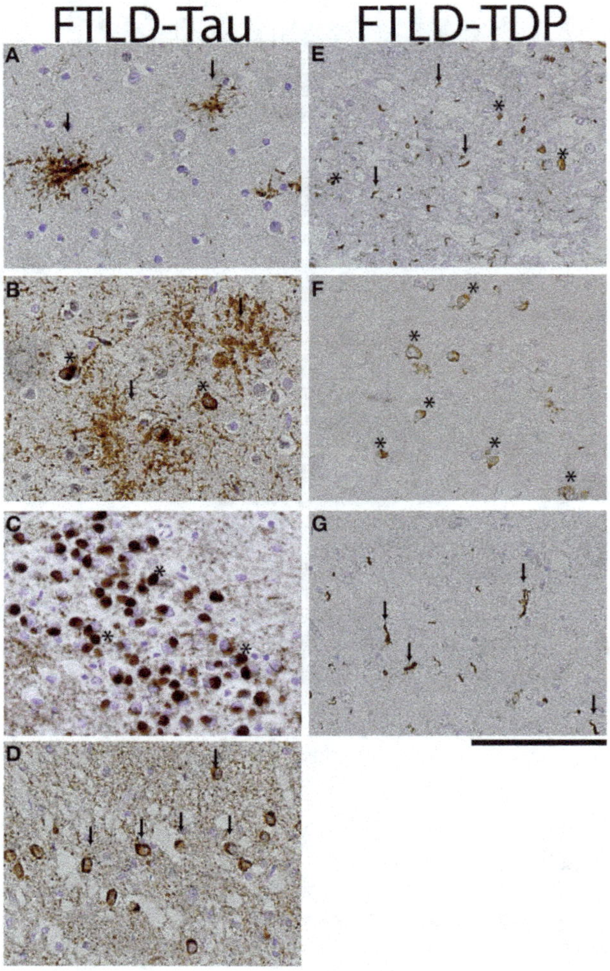

FIGURE 2 | FTLD-Tau and FTLD-TDP histology. Photomicrographs of FTLD-tau **(A–D)** and FTLD-TDP **(E–G)** visualized with immunohistochemistry (PHF-1 and pTDP 409/410 for tau and TDP, respectively). **(A)** PSP frontal cortex with tau-positive tufted astrocytes (arrows), **(B)** CBD temporal cortex with diffuse astrocytic plaques (arrows) and neuronal tangles (asterisks), **(C)** Pick's disease with round tau-positive Pick bodies (asterisks) in the dentate nucleus of the hippocampus, **(D)** FTDP-17 case with p.P301L pathogenic mutation with tau-positive neuronal tangles (arrows) and diffuse neuropil threads in temporal cortex, **(E)** FTLD-TDP subtype A with cytoplasmic neuronal inclusions (asterisks) and short dystrophic neurites (arrows) in superficial layers of frontal cortex, **(F)** FTLD-TDP subtype B with prominent cytoplasmic inclusions (asterisks) in deep temporal cortical layer, and **(G)** long dystrophic neurites (arrows) in superficial layers of mid-frontal cortex of a patient with FTLD-TDP subtype C. Scale bar = 100 μm.

2005; Knopman et al., 2005; Shi et al., 2005; Forman et al., 2006). Furthermore, a primary neuropathological diagnosis of Alzheimer's disease (AD) has been found in up to 30% of autopsy-confirmed clinically defined FTLD cohorts (Kertesz et al., 2005; Knopman et al., 2005; Forman et al., 2006; Knibb et al., 2006). Examination of focal presentations of AD found it to be the primary diagnosis in 7% of bvFTD, 44% of naPPA, 10% of svPPA, and 50% of the extrapyramidal and cognitive disorder, corticobasal syndrome (CBS) patients (Alladi et al., 2007). Others have also found a substantial proportion of AD in PPA cases (Forman et al., 2006; Knibb et al., 2006) especially in lvPPA (Grossman et al., 2008; Mesulam et al., 2008; Grossman, 2010) and also CBS (Lee et al., 2011). Thus, differentiation of AD and FTLD spectrum disorders poses a serious diagnostic challenge for clinicians.

Within the FTLD neuropathological spectrum, examination of the specific clinical subtypes finds varying degrees of association with FTLD-tau and FTLD-TDP (**Figure 1C**). FTLD-tau has been overrepresented in some naPPA cohorts (Hodges et al., 2004; Josephs et al., 2006a,b; Knibb et al., 2006; Snowden et al., 2007; Mesulam et al., 2008; Grossman et al., 2012), especially when associated with apraxia of speech (Josephs et al., 2006a; Snowden et al., 2007) and svPPA has been predominantly associated with TDP-43 pathology (Hodges et al., 2004; Josephs et al., 2006a; Snowden et al., 2007; Grossman et al., 2008); while bvFTD contains similar proportions of FTLD-tau and FTLD-TDP (Forman et al., 2006; Josephs et al., 2006b; Snowden et al., 2007). Extrapyramidal symptoms may predict a tauopathy (Forman et al., 2006; Josephs et al., 2006b) while co-morbid ALS is almost certainly due to TDP-43 aggregation (Shi et al., 2005; Forman et al., 2006; Josephs et al., 2006b). Clinicopathological associations from these large autopsy studies are summarized in **Figure 1C**.

A major challenge in the development and implementation of disease-modifying therapy in FTLD is the accurate identification of the neuropathological diagnosis during life, including differentiation from AD, so that patients may be triaged to the appropriate protein-targeted therapy (i.e., tau or TDP-43 targeted agents).

Biofluid biomarkers have the potential to optimize diagnostic accuracy and detect disease earlier in the course of an illness and possibly pre-symptomatically, such as prior to structural changes of neurodegeneration seen on neuroimaging (Hu et al., 2010a; Jack et al., 2010), making further exploration in this area promising for the development of disease modifying treatments. In addition, some clinical measures of disease progression in FTLD, including functional scales, may be limited by floor- and ceiling-effects (Knopman et al., 2008), so biofluid biomarkers are potentially attractive surrogate end points for use in clinical trials (Boxer et al., 2012b). The cerebrospinal fluid (CSF) is relatively easy to obtain and contains a direct connection to the pathological milieu in central nervous system, making it a desirable biofluid for study. In this review we will discuss the current state of CSF biomarker research in FTLD in terms of differentiation from AD and future directions and challenges for the field in development of FTLD-specific biomarkers.

ALZHEIMER'S DISEASE RELATED CSF BIOMARKERS: Aβ_{1-42} AND tau

STUDIES IN ALZHEIMER'S DISEASE

As a first step in biofluid-based biomarker assessment of neurodegenerative disease, it is valuable to distinguish broadly between AD and FTLD. CSF values of the major constituents of AD pathology, tau and β-amyloid, (Aβ_{1-42}) have been widely studied using immune-based analytical platforms in AD and amnestic mild cognitive impairment (MCI) patients, with lower Aβ_{1-42} values and higher levels of total- and phosphorylated-tau (t-tau, p-tau) compared with controls across multiple large studies (Shaw et al.,

2009, 2011; De Meyer et al., 2010; Trojanowski et al., 2010; Weiner et al., 2010). Furthermore, our group has shown prognostic utility of these markers by accurately predicting MCI conversion to AD (Shaw et al., 2009; De Meyer et al., 2010).

The majority of atypical clinical presentations of AD in early-onset patients consisting of predominantly visuo-spatial difficulties (i.e., consistent with poster cortical atrophy) or asymmetric apraxia/rigidity (i.e., consistent with CBS) may have a similar CSF biomarker profile to that of typical amnestic-AD (De Souza et al., 2011; Seguin et al., 2011), with a further elevated t-tau level in one study (Koric et al., 2010). Elevated CSF t-tau and low $A\beta_{1-42}$ levels have also been described in some PPA patients (i.e., lvPPA) (Bibl et al., 2011; De Souza et al., 2011) most likely due to underlying AD neuropathology in these individuals; however, to our knowledge no autopsy-confirmed studies of atypical clinical AD presentations have been performed.

The exact relationship between AD neuropathologic change (i.e., tau neurofibrillary pathology and $A\beta_{1-42}$ extracellular plaques) and observed measurement of these analytes in CSF is unclear; however, the total tau level is thought to reflect underlying neurodegeneration and neuron loss, as elevations are also seen in other CNS insults (Otto et al., 1997; Hesse et al., 2000; Jin et al., 2006; Ost et al., 2006; Krut et al., 2013). Lower $A\beta_{1-42}$ CSF levels may be the result of sequestration of soluble interstitial brain $A\beta_{1-42}$ into extracellular plaques as there is an inverse correlation of CSF $A\beta_{1-42}$ levels and the degree of cortical plaque pathology (Tapiola et al., 2009; Patel et al., 2012; Seppala et al., 2012) and *in vivo* neuroimaging evidence of amyloidosis (Fagan et al., 2006). Phosphorylated epitopes of tau (p-tau) can be measured in CSF as well; while most phospho-epitopes of tau are also found in healthy non-diseased brains and are not AD-specific, pathological tau species overall are highly phosphorylated in AD (Matsuo et al., 1994) and this altered state reflects the elevated levels of p-tau seen in AD. The most commonly studied p-tau epitopes are serine 181 (p-tau_{181}) (Vanmechelen et al., 2000), and threonine 231 (p-tau_{231}) (Buerger et al., 2002a,b).

STUDIES IN FRONTOTEMPORAL LOBAR DEGENERATION

FTLD is not characterized pathologically by cerebral $A\beta_{1-42}$ amyloidosis, and only FTLD-tau is characterized by significant tau inclusions. From this perspective, measures of CSF t-tau and $A\beta_{1-42}$ may have helpful diagnostic utility in excluding AD neuropathology. Indeed, in clinically-defined cohorts AD cases have higher levels of t-tau, p-tau_{181} and lower levels of $A\beta_{1-42}$ compared to FTLD and controls in group-wise comparisons (Blennow et al., 1995; Arai et al., 1997; Green et al., 1999; Sjogren et al., 2000a, 2001; Vanmechelen et al., 2000; Riemenschneider et al., 2002; Clark et al., 2003; Pijnenburg et al., 2004, 2007; Schoonenboom et al., 2004, 2012; Engelborghs et al., 2006; Bibl et al., 2007, 2011; Kapaki et al., 2008; Verwey et al., 2010; De Souza et al., 2011; Gabelle et al., 2011; Van Harten et al., 2011).

A major challenge in FTLD CSF biomarker studies is the heterogeneity of the condition (**Figure 1**), making autopsy-confirmation of diagnostic classification a crucial issue. As mentioned previously, up to 30% of clinically-defined FTLD cohorts may have underlying AD neuropathologic change as the etiology of their symptoms (Kertesz et al., 2005; Knopman et al., 2005; Forman et al., 2006; Knibb et al., 2006) and contamination with these atypical AD cases could influence results significantly. Indeed, examination of diagnostic accuracy of CSF t-tau and $A\beta_{1-42}$ in a large autopsy-confirmed dementia cohort found that use of the clinical diagnosis, rather than neuropathological diagnosis as the gold standard for biomarker performance resulted in a 10–20% underestimation of biomarker accuracy (Toledo et al., 2012). Furthermore, since 1995 there has been over a 10-fold increase in the number of FTLD manuscripts published (NLM/NIH, 2012) and due to this exponential increase in research in the field and our expanding knowledge of FTLD, clinical criteria (Gorno-Tempini et al., 2011; Rascovsky et al., 2011) have evolved resulting in refinement of our clinical definitions. Indeed, the emergence of the new clinical variant of PPA, lvPPA (Gorno-Tempini et al., 2008, 2011), which is most often associated with AD neuropathology (Mesulam et al., 2008; Rabinovici et al., 2008; Grossman, 2010) (**Figure 1C**), and therefore suggested to be excluded from FTLD clinical trials (Knopman et al., 2008), could influence group-wise CSF tau and $A\beta_{1-42}$ results. Thus, the makeup of clinical cohorts used in earlier studies may not be entirely translatable to newer studies, limiting the meaningful interpretation of the literature of clinically-derived cohorts.

As such, study of autopsy/genetic-confirmed cases has been a focus for our center. In an early study of autopsy-confirmed cases by our group, AD was differentiated from a mixed dementia cohort (including 13 FTLD cases) with reasonable sensitivity (72%) and specificity (69%) using CSF t-tau levels (Clark et al., 2003). Focused analysis of FTLD (with autopsy confirmation in 9 cases) in a later study found lower levels of t-tau and higher levels of $A\beta_{1-42}$ than AD, and roughly 30% of FTLD cases had significantly decreased t-tau from controls (Grossman et al., 2005). In a follow-up large autopsy/genetically confirmed FTLD series ($n = 30$) t-tau levels were significantly lower in FTLD than AD, while similar to controls on group-wise comparison; individual-case analysis revealed that a considerable subset of FTLD patients had markedly low t-tau values (Bian et al., 2008). Interestingly, FTLD cases with substantially lower t-tau levels included both FTLD-tau and FTLD-TDP (Bian et al., 2008), although a non-significant trend was found for lower t-tau in FTLD-tau (Hu et al., 2011). Furthermore, FTLD was differentiated from AD with high accuracy using the t-tau/$A\beta_{1-42}$ ratio; that is, FTLD cases had a lower ratio (lower t-tau and higher $A\beta_{1-42}$) (Bian et al., 2008).

Measurement of these analytes in the CSF in most studies utilizes one of two immune-based platforms: enzyme-linked immunosorbent assay (ELISA; Innotest, Innogenetics), and a multiplex assay based on flow-cytometry of antibody-coated fluorescent beads (INNO-BIA AlzBio3 xMAP; Luminex, Innogenetics). Absolute values obtained from these platforms differ because the coefficient of variance (%CV) with the xMAP Luminex platform is much narrower than with ELISA, but they are highly correlated (Olsson et al., 2005; Lewczuk et al., 2009; Fagan et al., 2011; Wang et al., 2012) and have similar levels of diagnostic accuracy for AD (Fagan et al., 2011; Wang et al., 2012) and differentiating AD from FTLD (Toledo et al., 2012). Thus, values from one platform can be effectively transformed into equivalent units of the other using a conversion factor (Fagan et al., 2011; Wang et al., 2012). Indeed, we were able to transform values obtained from ELISA to equivalent xMAP units using linear regression to create a larger autopsy/genetic-confirmed FTLD dataset and help confirm our pervious observations of the diagnostic utility of the t-tau/Aβ_{1-42} ratio to differentiate FTLD from AD (Irwin et al., 2012b). Maximizing available data is crucial for these extremely valuable and well-annotated research samples. In summary, in multiple large-scale autopsy-confirmed studies we have demonstrated the diagnostic utility of CSF t-tau, p-tau, and Aβ_{1-42} in differentiation of AD and FTLD (Bian et al., 2008; Irwin et al., 2012b; Toledo et al., 2012).

Few other CSF studies have used autopsy-confirmed cohorts of FTLD patients (**Table 1**). One study included 10 autopsy-confirmed FTLD patients and found similar results of lower t-tau and p-tau$_{181}$ levels in FTLD compared with AD, with high diagnostic accuracy of p-tau$_{181}$ (Koopman et al., 2009). Another study including 12 confirmed FTLD patients described "slightly elevated tau levels" in several patients compared to an age-dependent reference range and low compared to the majority of AD cases (Brunnstrom et al., 2010). Neuropathological subgroups of FTLD (FTLD-TDP, $n = 5$ and FTLD-tau, $n = 7$) had similar mean values, with 4/12 patients below the reference limit by >70 pg/ml (Brunnstrom et al., 2010). Thus, this study also found a subset of individual FTLD patients with lower than normal t-tau levels. The diagnostic utility of t-tau/Aβ_{1-42} in differentiating FTLD was not systematically explored in this small group of AD cases ($n = 8$). Finally, to our knowledge the only additional studies utilizing autopsy-confirmed FTLD cohorts included a small number of FTLD cases (<10) in a non-AD category, with no direct comparison of FTLD and AD (Engelborghs et al., 2008; Tapiola et al., 2009; Schoonenboom et al., 2012). Thus, further study is required in large prospective, autopsy-confirmed samples to confirm our observations.

The higher Aβ_{1-42} in FTLD compared to AD most likely reflects the absence of significant cerebral amyloidosis while the biological basis for observed low CSF t-tau in some FTLD patients is uncertain. One possibility is related to cortical tau depletion (Zhukareva et al., 2001, 2003; Grossman et al., 2005) through sequestration into the neuronal and glial inclusions in the absence of significant extracellular tau pathology (FTLD-tau) Dickson, 2004, such as extracellular "ghost tangles" as seen in AD (Schmidt et al., 1988), or altered post-translational stability of tau in FTLD-TDP (Zhukareva et al., 2001, 2003); furthermore, CSF t-tau does appear related to underlying FTLD pathophysiology as t-tau levels

Table 1 | Comparative studies of CSF biomarkers in autopsy/genetic-confirmed FTLD and AD cohorts.

Study	Patients	Aβ_{1-42}	t-tau	p-tau$_{181}$	Diagnostic accuracy (AD vs. FTLD)
Clark et al., 2003	(10) FTLD(74) AD*73 (4) CN	AD < FTLD, CN	CN < FTLD < AD	NA	No statistical analysis of FTLD diagnostic accuracy performed
Grossman et al., 2005	73 (11) FTLD(17) AD13 CN	AD < FTLD, CN	CN, FTLD < AD	CN, FTLD < AD	t-tau AUC = 0.86, sens = 74%, spec = 82.4%
Bian et al., 2008	(30) FTLD(19) AD13 CN	AD < FTLD, CN	CN, FTLD < AD	NA	t-tau/Aβ_{1-42} AUC = 0.93, sens = 78.9%, spec = 96.6%
Engelborghs et al., 2008	(2) FTLD(73) AD*100 CN	NA	NA	NA	No statistical analysis of FTLD diagnostic accuracy performed
Koopman et al., 2009	(10) FTLD(95) AD	AD < FTLD	FTLD < AD	FTLD < AD	p-tau$_{181}$ AUC = 0.85, sens = 91%, spec = 80%
Tapiola et al., 2009	(9) FTLD(83) AD	NA	NA	NA	No statistical analysis of FTLD diagnostic accuracy performed
Brunnstrom et al., 2010	(12) FTLD(8) AD*	NA	NA	NA	No statistical analysis of FTLD diagnostic accuracy performed
Irwin et al., 2012b	(20) FTLD(41) AD*	NA	NA	NA	t-tau/Aβ_{1-42} AUC = 0.99, sens = 90–100%, spec = 90–96%
Toledo et al., 2012	(71) AD(29) FTLD66 CN	AD < FTLD < CN	CN, FTLD < AD	CN, FTLD < AD	t-tau/Aβ_{1-42} (ELISA) AUC = 0.96, sens = 90, spec = 82% p-tau$_{181}$/Aβ_{1-42} (xMAP) AUC = 0.98, sens = 100%, spec = 88%

Other diagnostic groups that may be present in some studies are omitted and only direct comparisons of FTLD group to AD or CN are reported. "<" or ">" denotes significant difference between groups and "," denotes non-significant difference between groups, () denotes autopsy/genetic confirmed cohort.

*CN, non-demented controls; *, AD group contains cases with co-morbid Lewy Body or Vascular Disease; NA, Not assessed; AUC, Area under the curve for receiver operating curve analysis; ELISA, enzyme-linked immunosorbent assay; xMAP, luminex multiplex assay.*

in FTLD patients correlated to areas of frontal and temporal cortical atrophy on magnetic resonance imaging (MRI) (Grossman et al., 2005; McMillan et al., 2013). Further study of CSF protein dynamics in animal models of disease may help clarify these seemingly discordant associations of low tau levels with underlying neuropathology in FTLD-tau and FTLD-TDP.

Despite the clear distinction of t-tau and $A\beta_{1-42}$ levels between AD and FTLD, there is more variability in the literature for the relationship of these markers in FTLD compared with non-demented controls (**Table 1**). There are several reasons for these discrepancies; first, even in most autopsy-based studies, autopsy data on controls is lacking (**Table 1**) and a significant proportion of non-demented elderly can have underlying AD neuropathology (Davis et al., 1999), and thus influence CSF analyte measures. Next, even with pathologic confirmation, patient classification in FTLD is challenging, as another potential confounding issue is the presence of mixed pathologies in dementia patients. Indeed, our group has shown in a large autopsy-confirmed sample that mixed pathology is present in roughly 30% of cases, and that FTLD patients with significant AD neuropathologic change can influence the CSF t-tau and $A\beta_{1-42}$ levels, causing higher t-tau and lower $A\beta_{1-42}$ in cases with mixed FTLD and AD pathology compared to "pure" FTLD (Toledo et al., 2012). Additionally, a recent largely clinically-defined cohort study found an AD CSF biomarker profile in 30% of FTLD (Schoonenboom et al., 2012) which may be due, in part, to mixed pathology or inclusion of atypical AD cases mimicking the FTLD clinical syndrome (Toledo et al., 2012). Thus, the use of autopsy-confirmed samples is essential for in-depth study and validation of the diagnostic accuracy of potential biomarkers in FTLD.

Finally, variability in measurement between studies is another potential issue as significant variation between centers in absolute values measured in "spiked" pooled CSF control samples with known concentrations of analyte has been described (Shaw et al., 2011). These discrepancies are most likely due to sources of variation in CSF collection, handling and storage (pre-analytical), equipment, reagents and methods of analysis (analytical), and data management and interpretation (post-analytical) (Mattsson et al., 2011). For these reasons, large scale studies of measurement precision of these analytes and coordinated multi-center quality control programs with standard operating procedures to minimize these sources of variation have been conducted (Mattsson et al., 2011; Shaw et al., 2011).

Despite these issues, we have demonstrated (Bian et al., 2008; Irwin et al., 2012b; Toledo et al., 2012) that these AD-specific analytes (t-tau to $A\beta_{1-42}$ ratio) may perform within the range of sensitivity and specificity (>80%) for use in clinical trials (Trojanowski and Growdon, 1998) to differentiate FTLD from AD; however, these analytes are not as effective for differentiation of FTLD from normal controls (Bian and Grossman, 2007; Toledo et al., 2012). Although patients may present with decompensated psychiatric issues or other non-progressive non-degenerative etiologies resembling FTLD (phenocopy syndrome) (Kipps et al., 2010), these patients may be identified with serial clinical exams and neuroimaging (Kipps et al., 2010). The more urgent need is for FTLD-specific biomarkers and those that can differentiate between the two major neuropathologic subtypes (FTLD-tau and FTLD-TDP) (Hu et al., 2011).

FUTURE DIRECTIONS

FURTHER STUDY OF CSF tau AND $A\beta_{1-42}$

Previous work in large cross-sectional studies in AD suggests a temporal progression of dynamic biomarker change in AD (Jack et al., 2010, 2012), as $A\beta_{1-42}$ amyloidosis, and resultant lower CSF $A\beta_{1-42}$, is thought to occur decades before clinical symptoms emerge in AD, while increased CSF t-tau is thought to be a later event in disease progression and correlates more closely with cognitive decline. It is likely that t-tau, p-tau and potential novel CSF biomarkers could display similar changes throughout the course of disease in FTLD and could correlate with clinical symptoms. Few studies have examined the change in CSF biomarkers over time or their relation to clinical symptoms. One study included a follow up CSF analysis in one FTLD-tau patient, with similar t-tau and $A\beta_{1-42}$, roughly 18 months between CSF collections (Brunnstrom et al., 2010). Interestingly, a recent study of bvFTD patients found a significant correlation with $A\beta_{1-42}$ levels and cognitive performance, even after removal of patients with CSF profile suggestive of AD neuropathology (Koedam et al., 2012). These results could suggest an influence of co-morbid AD neuropathology; however autopsy information in these cases was lacking. Other studies in clinical series without autopsy confirmation found no association of these markers and clinical measures or disease severity (Riemenschneider et al., 2002; Engelborghs et al., 2006; De Souza et al., 2011). Further study of clinical correlates of CSF biomarkers and longitudinal profiles of CSF analyte change throughout the course of disease will be helpful.

Similar to the dominantly-inherited AD network (DIAN) initiative to study patients with known pathogenic mutations to cause AD (Bateman et al., 2012), study of prodromal FTLD patients with pathogenic mutations may provide additional insights into the temporal sequence of biomarkers in FTLD (Boxer et al., 2012a). Furthermore, CSF analyte levels in symptomatic patients with genetic forms of FTLD have not been explored in detail and could potentially differ from sporadic cases. Indeed, we found a more rapid rate of progression in cognitive measures corresponding to more severe neurodegeneration in *C9orf72*-associated FTLD (Irwin et al., 2013) and others have described unique neuroimaging patterns of atrophy across different genetic forms of FTLD (Whitwell et al., 2012). This evidence of biologic differences in genetic and sporadic FTLD suggest alterations in CSF biomarker profiles are also a possibility, although one study found similar levels of CSF tau and $A\beta_{1-42}$ in genetically-confirmed FTDP-17 ($n = 9$) compared to sporadic FTLD ($n = 17$) (Rosso et al., 2003).

DEVELOPMENT OF FTLD-SPECIFIC BIOMARKERS

In the context of disease-modifying therapies targeting a specific histopathologic abnormality, an important goal is to distinguish between FTLD due to TDP-43 and FTLD due to tau. Exploratory analyses for novel biomarkers that have diagnostic utility in FTLD are ongoing and include several basic approaches.

First, measurement of biologically relevant molecules is the most straightforward approach, as tau and $A\beta_{1-42}$ have been successful biomarker candidates in AD. Using this rationale, the two most obvious candidates for FTLD-specific biomarkers are TDP-43 progranulin. Indeed, TDP-43 has been detected in human CSF (Steinacker et al., 2008; Kasai et al., 2009) and serum (Foulds et al., 2008), suggesting elevated levels may occur in some patients with TDP-43 proteinopathies, but initial studies show limited diagnostic accuracy. Low serum progranulin may identify FTLD patients with a pathogenic *GRN* mutation resulting in progranulin haploinsufficiency (Ghidoni et al., 2008), which could be useful in monitoring potential progranulin-replacing therapies in development for FTLD (Boxer et al., 2012b).

Other biologically relevant potential biomarkers for FTLD include specific isoforms or neoepitopes of tau. Tau undergoes multiple post-translational modifications thought to contribute to tangle formation. Indeed, we found acetylation of tau at a specific residue in the microtubule-binding domain (MTBD) to be exclusively found in tauopathies, providing promise for this epitope as a useful marker of AD and FTLD-tau (Cohen et al., 2011; Irwin et al., 2012a). Translating these immunohistochemical observations to clinical assays may prove difficult, as levels of tau in CSF are near the lower limits of biologic detection (Hampel et al., 2010) limiting the further identification of a specific subset of tau in the form of a neoepitope; although one group has found promising evidence for diagnostic utility of specific C-truncated isoforms of tau in PSP through immunoprecipitation and western blotting techniques (Borroni et al., 2008, 2009) and others have developed assays to measure 3- and 4R tau in CSF (Luk et al., 2012). Alternatively-truncated forms of $A\beta_{1-42}$ may also have diagnostic importance in FTLD (Pijnenburg et al., 2007; Bibl et al., 2011, 2012; Gabelle et al., 2011) and cytoskeletal proteins, such as neurofilament have also been explored (Sjogren et al., 2000b; De Jong et al., 2007). These potential biomarkers warrant further study and validation.

Another, possible approach is to screen a large number of potential analytes without an a priori biologic rationale in a proteomic analysis of CSF in FTLD. Indeed, using an immune-based multiplex approach our group found promising CSF biomarker candidates to differentiate FTLD-TDP and FTLD-tau with high sensitivity and specificity, but these candidate analytes need further study to confirm their utility as FTLD biomarkers (Hu et al., 2010b). Finally, other non-immune based methods, such as mass-spectrometry are also being explored to identify novel biofluid biomarkers in FTLD (Mattsson et al., 2008).

Potential FTLD-specific biofluid biomarkers will be faced with the same challenges of testing reliability and sources of variation (i.e., analytical, pre-/post-analytical) currently experienced by CSF t-tau and $A\beta_{1-42}$ measurements. As such, coordinated and cooperative efforts between multiple centers will undoubtedly be necessary to help validate potential FTLD-specific CSF biomarkers prior to clinical use.

Most likely, a multimodal assessment incorporating potential novel biofluid biomarker values with clinical, neuroimaging and genetic markers may be the most effective approach to accurately identify FTLD subtypes. Neuropsychological testing can help differentiate AD from FTLD (Rascovsky et al., 2008; Libon et al., 2011) as routine cognitive measures may not be sensitive enough to detect the behavioral and language deficits in FTLD. Indeed, our group has explored quantitative approaches to language (Ash et al., 2006, 2009; Gunawardena et al., 2010) and social cognition (Massimo et al., 2009, 2013; Grossman et al., 2010; Eslinger et al., 2012; McMillan et al., 2012b) to examine brain-behavior relationships and improve diagnostic accuracy in FTLD. Neuroimaging is another potential method with diagnostic utility alone, or as an adjunct to clinical and biofluid biomarkers in FTLD; we have found combining neuropsychological testing and MRI can improve diagnostic accuracy in PPA (Hu et al., 2010c); and others find combination of CSF tau isoform levels and midbrain atrophy improve identification of PSP (Borroni et al., 2010). Multiple modalities of MRI methods, including diffusion-tensor imaging (DTI) of white matter may help identify FTLD patients in dementia cohorts. We have demonstrated increased diagnostic sensitivity to differentiate AD from FTLD cases using a combination of gray matter (GM) density and DTI measures (McMillan et al., 2012a). In addition, we have also discovered promising diagnostic utility for differentiating FTLD-tau and FTLD-TDP using DTI (unpublished data). Cortical atrophy and CSF biomarker levels appear to be highly correlated as we have recently demonstrated that GM density could predict CSF t-tau and $A\beta_{1-42}$ levels, and these predicted values could accurately distinguish AD and FTLD (McMillan et al., 2013). These results indicate that MRI could potentially serve as a surrogate for CSF, which would have significant utility for patients where lumbar puncture would be difficult or for clinical trial endpoints where repeated lumbar puncture may be needed. Finally, recent genome-wide association studies (GWAS) have found risk alleles associated with FTLD-TDP (Van Deerlin et al., 2010) and FTLD-tau (Hoglinger et al., 2011). Further knowledge of clinical, neuroimaging, and biofluid correlates of these risk alleles in FTLD could provide further useful diagnostic and prognostic information. Thus, comparative studies of clinical, genetic, biofluid, and neuroimaging biomarkers in longitudinally followed, well-annotated, autopsy-confirmed subjects will be a powerful method for improving our understanding of the pathophysiology of FTLD and further directing diagnostic and treatment efforts.

SUMMARY

CSF measurements of $A\beta_{1-42}$, t-tau, and p-tau in FTLD differ significantly from the abnormal levels seen in AD, and in a subset of both FTLD-tau and FTLD-TDP there are extremely low levels of t-tau of unclear etiology. These properties allow for accurate distinction of FTLD from AD in autopsy-confirmed cohorts, while FTLD-specific markers are still lacking.

As we move toward therapies that impact the progression of the disease and target the underlying pathophysiology in FTLD and other neurodegenerative disorders it will be essential for clinicians to view these disorders as clinicopathological entities with the underlying neuropathological substrate in mind. Indeed, new clinical criteria for AD incorporate this ideology with the designation of "pre-symptomatic AD" (Sperling et al., 2011). In the study of the complex clinicopathological spectrum of FTLD disorders, where heterogeneity is the rule, useful markers to develop homogenous clinical, genetic, and neuropathologic subgroups will be crucial to further our goals toward meaningful treatments that could potential slow disease progression and limit patient disability.

ACKNOWLEDGMENTS

We thank the patients studied here and their families who made the research reviewed here possible. Funding for this study was provided by the National Institutes of Health grants P30 AG10124, AG17586, and T32-AG000255 as well as the Wyncote Foundation.

REFERENCES

Alladi, S., Xuereb, J., Bak, T., Nestor, P., Knibb, J., Patterson, K., et al. (2007). Focal cortical presentations of Alzheimer's disease. *Brain* 130, 2636–2645.

Arai, H., Morikawa, Y., Higuchi, M., Matsui, T., Clark, C. M., Miura, M., et al. (1997). Cerebrospinal fluid tau levels in neurodegenerative diseases with distinct tau-related pathology. *Biochem. Biophys. Res. Commun.* 236, 262–264.

Ash, S., Moore, P., Antani, S., McCawley, G., Work, M., and Grossman, M. (2006). Trying to tell a tale: discourse impairments in progressive aphasia and frontotemporal dementia. *Neurology* 66, 1405–1413.

Ash, S., Moore, P., Vesely, L., Gunawardena, D., McMillan, C., Anderson, C., et al. (2009). Non-Fluent Speech in Frontotemporal Lobar Degeneration. *J. Neurolinguistics* 22, 370–383.

Baker, M., Mackenzie, I. R., Pickering-Brown, S. M., Gass, J., Rademakers, R., Lindholm, C., et al. (2006). Mutations in progranulin cause tau-negative frontotemporal dementia linked to chromosome 17. *Nature* 442, 916–919.

Bateman, R. J., Xiong, C., Benzinger, T. L., Fagan, A. M., Goate, A., Fox, N. C., et al. (2012). Clinical and biomarker changes in dominantly inherited Alzheimer's disease. *N. Engl. J. Med.* 367, 795–804.

Bian, H., and Grossman, M. (2007). Frontotemporal lobar degeneration: recent progress in antemortem diagnosis. *Acta Neuropathol.* 114, 23–29.

Bian, H., Van Swieten, J. C., Leight, S., Massimo, L., Wood, E., Forman, M., et al. (2008). CSF biomarkers in frontotemporal lobar degeneration with known pathology. *Neurology* 70, 1827–1835.

Bibl, M., Gallus, M., Welge, V., Esselmann, H., Wolf, S., Ruther, E., et al. (2012). Cerebrospinal fluid amyloid-beta 2-42 is decreased in Alzheimer's, but not in frontotemporal dementia. *J. Neural Transm.* 119, 805–813.

Bibl, M., Mollenhauer, B., Lewczuk, P., Esselmann, H., Wolf, S., Otto, M., et al. (2011). Cerebrospinal fluid tau, p-tau 181 and amyloid-beta38/40/42 in frontotemporal dementias and primary progressive aphasias. *Dement. Geriatr. Cogn. Disord.* 31, 37–44.

Bibl, M., Mollenhauer, B., Wolf, S., Esselmann, H., Lewczuk, P., Kornhuber, J., et al. (2007). Reduced CSF carboxyterminally truncated Abeta peptides in frontotemporal lobe degenerations. *J. Neural Transm.* 114, 621–628.

Blennow, K., Wallin, A., Agren, H., Spenger, C., Siegfried, J., and Vanmechelen, E. (1995). Tau protein in cerebrospinal fluid: a biochemical marker for axonal degeneration in Alzheimer disease? *Mol. Chem. Neuropathol.* 26, 231–245.

Borroni, B., Gardoni, F., Parnetti, L., Magno, L., Malinverno, M., Saggese, E., et al. (2009). Pattern of Tau forms in CSF is altered in progressive supranuclear palsy. *Neurobiol. Aging* 30, 34–40.

Borroni, B., Malinverno, M., Gardoni, F., Alberici, A., Parnetti, L., Premi, E., et al. (2008). Tau forms in CSF as a reliable biomarker for progressive supranuclear palsy. *Neurology* 71, 1796–1803.

Borroni, B., Malinverno, M., Gardoni, F., Grassi, M., Parnetti, L., Agosti, C., et al. (2010). A combination of CSF tau ratio and midsaggital midbrain-to-pons atrophy for the early diagnosis of progressive supranuclear palsy. *J. Alzheimers Dis.* 22, 195–203.

Boxer, A. L., Gold, M., Huey, E., Gao, F. B., Burton, E. A., Chow, T., et al. (2012a). Frontotemporal degeneration, the next therapeutic frontier: Molecules and animal models for frontotemporal degeneration drug development. *Alzheimers Dement.* doi: 10.1016/j.jalz.2012.03.002. [Epub ahead of print].

Boxer, A. L., Gold, M., Huey, E., Hu, W. T., Rosen, H., Kramer, J., et al. (2012b). The advantages of frontotemporal degeneration drug development (part 2 of frontotemporal degeneration: the next therapeutic frontier). *Alzheimers Dement.* doi: 10.1016/j.jalz.2012.03.003. [Epub ahead of print].

Brunnstrom, H., Rawshani, N., Zetterberg, H., Blennow, K., Minthon, L., Passant, U., et al. (2010). Cerebrospinal fluid biomarker results in relation to neuropathological dementia diagnoses. *Alzheimers Dement.* 6, 104–109.

Buerger, K., Teipel, S. J., Zinkowski, R., Blennow, K., Arai, H., Engel, R., et al. (2002a). CSF tau protein phosphorylated at threonine 231 correlates with cognitive decline in MCI subjects. *Neurology* 59, 627–629.

Buerger, K., Zinkowski, R., Teipel, S. J., Tapiola, T., Arai, H., Blennow, K., et al. (2002b). Differential diagnosis of Alzheimer disease with cerebrospinal fluid levels of tau protein phosphorylated at threonine 231. *Arch. Neurol.* 59, 1267–1272.

Clark, C. M., Xie, S., Chittams, J., Ewbank, D., Peskind, E., Galasko, D., et al. (2003). Cerebrospinal fluid tau and beta-amyloid: how well do these biomarkers reflect autopsy-confirmed dementia diagnoses? *Arch. Neurol.* 60, 1696–1702.

Cohen, T. J., Guo, J. L., Hurtado, D. E., Kwong, L. K., Mills, I. P., Trojanowski, J. Q., et al. (2011). The acetylation of tau inhibits its function and promotes pathological tau aggregation. *Nat. Commun.* 2:252. doi: 10.1038/ncomms1255

Cruts, M., Gijselinck, I., Van Der Zee, J., Engelborghs, S., Wils, H., Pirici, D., et al. (2006). Null mutations in progranulin cause ubiquitin-positive frontotemporal dementia linked to chromosome 17q21. *Nature* 442, 920–924.

Davis, D. G., Schmitt, F. A., Wekstein, D. R., and Markesbery, W. R. (1999). Alzheimer neuropathologic alterations in aged cognitively normal subjects. *J. Neuropathol. Exp. Neurol.* 58, 376–388.

De Jong, D., Jansen, R. W., Pijnenburg, Y. A., Van Geel, W. J., Borm, G. F., Kremer, H. P., et al. (2007). CSF neurofilament proteins in the differential diagnosis of dementia. *J. Neurol. Neurosurg. Psychiatry* 78, 936–938.

De Meyer, G., Shapiro, F., Vanderstichele, H., Vanmechelen, E., Engelborghs, S., De Deyn, P. P., et al. (2010). Diagnosis-independent Alzheimer disease biomarker signature in cognitively normal elderly people. *Arch. Neurol.* 67, 949–956.

De Souza, L. C., Lamari, F., Belliard, S., Jardel, C., Houillier, C., De Paz, R., et al. (2011). Cerebrospinal fluid biomarkers in the differential diagnosis of Alzheimer's disease from other cortical dementias. *J. Neurol. Neurosurg. Psychiatry* 82, 240–246.

Dejesus-Hernandez, M., Mackenzie, I. R., Boeve, B. F., Boxer, A. L., Baker, M., Rutherford, N. J., et al. (2011). Expanded GGGGCC hexanucleotide repeat in noncoding region of C9ORF72 causes chromosome 9p-linked FTD and ALS. *Neuron* 72, 245–256.

Dickson, D. (2004). "Sporadic tauopaties: Pick's disease, corticobasal degeneration, progressive supranuclear palsy and argyrophilic grain disease," in *The Neuropathology of Dementia 2nd Edn*, eds M. Esiri, V. M-Y. Lee, and J. Q. Trojanowski (New York, NY: Cambridge University Press), 227–256.

Engelborghs, S., De Vreese, K., Van De Casteele, T., Vanderstichele, H., Van Everbroeck, B., Cras, P., et al. (2008). Diagnostic performance of a CSF-biomarker panel in autopsy-confirmed dementia. *Neurobiol. Aging* 29, 1143–1159.

Engelborghs, S., Maertens, K., Vloeberghs, E., Aerts, T., Somers, N., Marien, P., et al. (2006). Neuropsychological and behavioural correlates of CSF biomarkers in dementia. *Neurochem. Int.* 48, 286–295.

Eslinger, P. J., Moore, P., Antani, S., Anderson, C., and Grossman, M. (2012). Apathy in frontotemporal dementia: behavioral and neuroimaging correlates. *Behav. Neurol.* 25, 127–136.

Fagan, A. M., Mintun, M. A., Mach, R. H., Lee, S. Y., Dence, C. S., Shah, A. R., et al. (2006). Inverse relation between *in vivo* amyloid imaging load and cerebrospinal fluid Abeta42 in humans. *Ann. Neurol.* 59, 512–519.

Fagan, A. M., Shaw, L. M., Xiong, C., Vanderstichele, H., Mintun, M. A., Trojanowski, J. Q., et al. (2011). Comparison of analytical platforms for cerebrospinal fluid measures of {beta}-amyloid 1-42, total tau, and P-tau181 for identifying alzheimer disease amyloid plaque pathology. *Arch. Neurol.* 68, 1137–1144.

Forman, M. S., Farmer, J., Johnson, J. K., Clark, C. M., Arnold, S. E., Coslett, H. B., et al. (2006). Frontotemporal dementia: clinicopathological correlations. *Ann. Neurol.* 59, 952–962.

Foulds, P., McAuley, E., Gibbons, L., Davidson, Y., Pickering-Brown, S. M., Neary, D., et al. (2008). TDP-43 protein in plasma may index TDP-43 brain pathology in Alzheimer's disease and frontotemporal lobar degeneration. *Acta Neuropathol.* 116, 141–146.

Gabelle, A., Roche, S., Geny, C., Bennys, K., Labauge, P., Tholance, Y., et al. (2011). Decreased sAbetaPPbeta, Abeta38, and Abeta40 cerebrospinal fluid levels in frontotemporal dementia. *J. Alzheimers Dis.* 26, 553–563.

Geser, F., Brandmeir, N. J., Kwong, L. K., Martinez-Lage, M., Elman, L., McCluskey, L., et al. (2008). Evidence of multisystem disorder in whole-brain map of pathological TDP-43 in amyotrophic lateral sclerosis. *Arch. Neurol.* 65, 636–641.

Geser, F., Martinez-Lage, M., Robinson, J., Uryu, K., Neumann, M., Brandmeir, N. J., et al. (2009). Clinical and pathological continuum of multisystem TDP-43 proteinopathies. *Arch. Neurol.* 66, 180–189.

Ghidoni, R., Benussi, L., Glionna, M., Franzoni, M., and Binetti, G. (2008). Low plasma progranulin levels predict progranulin mutations in frontotemporal lobar degeneration. *Neurology* 71, 1235–1239.

Gorno-Tempini, M. L., Brambati, S. M., Ginex, V., Ogar, J., Dronkers, N. F., Marcone, A., et al. (2008). The logopenic/phonological variant of primary progressive aphasia. *Neurology* 71, 1227–1234.

Gorno-Tempini, M. L., Dronkers, N. F., Rankin, K. P., Ogar, J. M., Phengrasamy, L., Rosen, H. J., et al. (2004). Cognition and anatomy in three variants of primary progressive aphasia. *Ann. Neurol.* 55, 335–346.

Gorno-Tempini, M. L., Hillis, A. E., Weintraub, S., Kertesz, A., Mendez, M., Cappa, S. F., et al. (2011). Classification of primary progressive aphasia and its variants. *Neurology* 76, 1006–1014.

Green, A. J., Harvey, R. J., Thompson, E. J., and Rossor, M. N. (1999). Increased tau in the cerebrospinal fluid of patients with frontotemporal dementia and Alzheimer's disease. *Neurosci. Lett.* 259, 133–135.

Grossman, M. (2010). Primary progressive aphasia: clinicopathological correlations. *Nat. Rev. Neurol.* 6, 88–97.

Grossman, M., Eslinger, P. J., Troiani, V., Anderson, C., Avants, B., Gee, J. C., et al. (2010). The role of ventral medial prefrontal cortex in social decisions: converging evidence from fMRI and frontotemporal lobar degeneration. *Neuropsychologia* 48, 3505–3512.

Grossman, M., Farmer, J., Leight, S., Work, M., Moore, P., Van Deerlin, V., et al. (2005). Cerebrospinal fluid profile in frontotemporal dementia and Alzheimer's disease. *Ann. Neurol.* 57, 721–729.

Grossman, M., Powers, J., Ash, S., McMillan, C., Burkholder, L., Irwin, D., et al. (2012). Disruption of large-scale neural networks in non-fluent/agrammatic variant primary progressive aphasia associated with frontotemporal degeneration pathology. *Brain Lang.* doi: 10.1016/j.bandl.2012.10.005. [Epub ahead of print].

Grossman, M., Xie, S. X., Libon, D. J., Wang, X., Massimo, L., Moore, P., et al. (2008). Longitudinal decline in autopsy-defined frontotemporal lobar degeneration. *Neurology* 70, 2036–2045.

Gunawardena, D., Ash, S., McMillan, C., Avants, B., Gee, J., and Grossman, M. (2010). Why are patients with progressive nonfluent aphasia nonfluent? *Neurology* 75, 588–594.

Hampel, H., Blennow, K., Shaw, L. M., Hoessler, Y. C., Zetterberg, H., and Trojanowski, J. Q. (2010). Total and phosphorylated tau protein as biological markers of Alzheimer's disease. *Exp. Gerontol.* 45, 30–40.

Hesse, C., Rosengren, L., Vanmechelen, E., Vanderstichele, H., Jensen, C., Davidsson, P., et al. (2000). Cerebrospinal fluid markers for Alzheimer's disease evaluated after acute ischemic stroke. *J. Alzheimers Dis.* 2, 199–206.

Hodges, J. R., Davies, R. R., Xuereb, J. H., Casey, B., Broe, M., Bak, T. H., et al. (2004). Clinicopathological correlates in frontotemporal dementia. *Ann. Neurol.* 56, 399–406.

Hodges, J. R., and Patterson, K. (2007). Semantic dementia: a unique clinicopathological syndrome. *Lancet Neurol.* 6, 1004–1014.

Hoglinger, G. U., Melhem, N. M., Dickson, D. W., Sleiman, P. M., Wang, L. S., Klei, L., et al. (2011). Identification of common variants influencing risk of the tauopathy progressive supranuclear palsy. *Nat. Genet.* 43, 699–705.

Hu, W. T., Chen-Plotkin, A., Arnold, S. E., Grossman, M., Clark, C. M., Shaw, L. M., et al. (2010a). Biomarker discovery for Alzheimer's disease, frontotemporal lobar degeneration, and Parkinson's disease. *Acta Neuropathol.* 120, 385–399.

Hu, W. T., Chen-Plotkin, A., Grossman, M., Arnold, S. E., Clark, C. M., Shaw, L. M., et al. (2010b). Novel CSF biomarkers for frontotemporal lobar degenerations. *Neurology* 75, 2079–2086.

Hu, W. T., McMillan, C., Libon, D., Leight, S., Forman, M., Lee, V. M., et al. (2010c). Multimodal predictors for Alzheimer disease in nonfluent primary progressive aphasia. *Neurology* 75, 595–602.

Hu, W. T., Trojanowski, J. Q., and Shaw, L. M. (2011). Biomarkers in frontotemporal lobar degenerations–progress and challenges. *Prog. Neurobiol.* 95, 636–648.

Hutton, M., Lendon, C. L., Rizzu, P., Baker, M., Froelich, S., Houlden, H., et al. (1998). Association of missense and 5'-splice-site mutations in tau with the inherited dementia FTDP-17. *Nature* 393, 702–705.

Irwin, D. J., Cohen, T. J., Grossman, M., Arnold, S. E., Xie, S. X., Lee, V. M., et al. (2012a). Acetylated tau, a novel pathological signature in Alzheimer's disease and other tauopathies. *Brain* 135, 807–818.

Irwin, D. J., McMillan, C. T., Toledo, J. B., Arnold, S. E., Shaw, L. M., Wang, L. S., et al. (2012b). Comparison of cerebrospinal fluid levels of tau and Abeta 1-42 in Alzheimer disease and frontotemporal degeneration using 2 analytical platforms. *Arch. Neurol.* 69, 1018–1025.

Irwin, D. J., McMillan, C. T., Brettschneider, J., Libon, D. J., Powers, J., Rascovsky, K., et al. (2013). Cognitive decline and reduced survival in C9orf72 expansion frontotemporal degeneration and amyotrophic lateral sclerosis. *J. Neurol. Neurosurg. Psychiatry.* 84, 163–169.

Jack, C. R. Jr., Knopman, D. S., Jagust, W. J., Shaw, L. M., Aisen, P. S., Weiner, M. W., et al. (2010). Hypothetical model of dynamic biomarkers of the Alzheimer's pathological cascade. *Lancet Neurol.* 9, 119–128.

Jack, C. R. Jr., Vemuri, P., Wiste, H. J., Weigand, S. D., Lesnick, T. G., Lowe, V., et al. (2012). Shapes of the trajectories of 5 major biomarkers of Alzheimer disease. *Arch. Neurol.* 69, 856–867.

Jin, K., Takeda, A., Shiga, Y., Sato, S., Ohnuma, A., Nomura, H., et al. (2006). CSF tau protein: a new prognostic marker for Guillain-Barre syndrome. *Neurology* 67, 1470–1472.

Josephs, K. A. (2008). Frontotemporal dementia and related disorders: deciphering the enigma. *Ann. Neurol.* 64, 4–14.

Josephs, K. A., Duffy, J. R., Strand, E. A., Whitwell, J. L., Layton, K. F., Parisi, J. E., et al. (2006a). Clinicopathological and imaging correlates of progressive aphasia and apraxia of speech. *Brain* 129, 1385–1398.

Josephs, K. A., Whitwell, J. L., Jack, C. R., Parisi, J. E., and Dickson, D. W. (2006b). Frontotemporal lobar degeneration without lobar atrophy. *Arch. Neurol.* 63, 1632–1638.

Kapaki, E., Paraskevas, G. P., Papageorgiou, S. G., Bonakis, A., Kalfakis, N., Zalonis, I., et al. (2008). Diagnostic value of CSF biomarker profile in frontotemporal lobar degeneration. *Alzheimer Dis. Assoc. Disord.* 22, 47–53.

Kasai, T., Tokuda, T., Ishigami, N., Sasayama, H., Foulds, P., Mitchell, D. J., et al. (2009). Increased TDP-43 protein in cerebrospinal fluid of patients with amyotrophic lateral sclerosis. *Acta Neuropathol.* 117, 55–62.

Kertesz, A., McMonagle, P., Blair, M., Davidson, W., and Munoz, D. G. (2005). The evolution and pathology of frontotemporal dementia. *Brain* 128, 1996–2005.

Kipps, C. M., Hodges, J. R., and Hornberger, M. (2010). Nonprogressive behavioural frontotemporal dementia: recent developments and clinical implications of the 'bvFTD phenocopy syndrome'. *Curr. Opin. Neurol.* 23, 628–632.

Knibb, J. A., Xuereb, J. H., Patterson, K., and Hodges, J. R. (2006). Clinical and pathological characterization of progressive aphasia. *Ann. Neurol.* 59, 156–165.

Knopman, D. S., Boeve, B. F., Parisi, J. E., Dickson, D. W., Smith, G. E., Ivnik, R. J., et al. (2005). Antemortem diagnosis of frontotemporal lobar degeneration. *Ann. Neurol.* 57, 480–488.

Knopman, D. S., Kramer, J. H., Boeve, B. F., Caselli, R. J., Graff-Radford, N. R., Mendez, M. F., et al. (2008). Development of methodology for conducting clinical trials in frontotemporal lobar degeneration. *Brain* 131, 2957–2968.

Koedam, E. L., Van Der Vlies, A. E., Van Der Flier, W. M., Verwey, N. A., Koene, T., Scheltens, P., et al. (2012). Cognitive correlates of cerebrospinal fluid biomarkers in frontotemporal dementia. *Alzheimers Dement.* doi: 10.1016/j.jalz.2011.12.007. [Epub ahead of print].

Koopman, K., Le Bastard, N., Martin, J. J., Nagels, G., De Deyn, P. P., and Engelborghs, S. (2009). Improved discrimination of autopsy-confirmed Alzheimer's disease (AD) from non-AD dementias using CSF P-tau(181P). *Neurochem. Int.* 55, 214–218.

Koric, L., Felician, O., Guedj, E., Hubert, A. M., Mancini, J., Boucraut, J., et al. (2010). Could clinical profile influence CSF biomarkers in early-onset Alzheimer disease? *Alzheimer Dis. Assoc. Disord.* 24, 278–283.

Krut, J. J., Zetterberg, H., Blennow, K., Cinque, P., Hagberg, L., Price, R. W., et al. (2013). Cerebrospinal fluid Alzheimer's biomarker profiles in CNS infections. *J. Neurol.* 260, 620–626.

Lee, S. E., Rabinovici, G. D., Mayo, M. C., Wilson, S. M., Seeley, W. W., Dearmond, S. J., et al. (2011). Clinicopathological correlations in corticobasal degeneration. *Ann. Neurol.* 70, 327–340.

Lewczuk, P., Zimmermann, R., Wiltfang, J., and Kornhuber, J. (2009). Neurochemical dementia diagnostics: a simple algorithm for interpretation of the CSF biomarkers. *J Neural Transm* 116, 1163–1167.

Libon, D. J., Rascovsky, K., Gross, R. G., White, M. T., Xie, S. X., Dreyfuss, M., et al. (2011). The Philadelphia Brief Assessment of Cognition (PBAC): a validated screening measure for dementia. *Clin. Neuropsychol.* 25, 1314–1330.

Luk, C., Compta, Y., Magdalinou, N., Marti, M. J., Hondhamuni, G., Zetterberg, H., et al. (2012). Development and assessment of sensitive immuno-PCR assays for the quantification of cerebrospinal fluid three- and four-repeat tau isoforms in tauopathies. *J. Neurochem.* 123, 396–405.

Mackenzie, I. R., Neumann, M., Baborie, A., Sampathu, D. M., Du Plessis, D., Jaros, E., et al. (2011). A harmonized classification system for FTLD-TDP pathology. *Acta Neuropathol.* 122, 111–113.

Mackenzie, I. R., Neumann, M., Bigio, E. H., Cairns, N. J., Alafuzoff, I., Kril, J., et al. (2010). Nomenclature and nosology for neuropathologic subtypes of frontotemporal lobar degeneration: an update. *Acta Neuropathol.* 119, 1–4.

Massimo, L., Libon, D. J., Chandrasekaran, K., Dreyfuss, M., McMillan, C. T., Rascovsky, K., et al. (2013). Self-appraisal in behavioural variant frontotemporal degeneration. *J. Neurol. Neurosurg. Psychiatry*, 84, 148–153.

Massimo, L., Powers, C., Moore, P., Vesely, L., Avants, B., Gee, J., et al. (2009). Neuroanatomy of apathy and disinhibition in frontotemporal lobar degeneration. *Dement. Geriatr. Cogn. Disord.* 27, 96–104.

Matsuo, E. S., Shin, R. W., Billingsley, M. L., Van Devoorde, A., O'Connor, M., Trojanowski, J. Q., et al. (1994). Biopsy-derived adult human brain tau is phosphorylated at many of the same sites as Alzheimer's disease paired helical filament tau. *Neuron* 13, 989–1002.

Mattsson, N., Andreasson, U., Persson, S., Arai, H., Batish, S. D., Bernardini, S., et al. (2011). The Alzheimer's association external quality control program for cerebrospinal fluid biomarkers. *Alzheimers Dement.* 7, 386–395. e386.

Mattsson, N., Ruetschi, U., Pijnenburg, Y. A., Blankenstein, M. A., Podust, V. N., Li, S., et al. (2008). Novel cerebrospinal fluid biomarkers of axonal degeneration in frontotemporal dementia. *Mol. Med. Report.* 1, 757–761.

McMillan, C. T., Avants, B., Irwin, D. J., Toledo, J. B., Wolk, D. A., Van Deerlin, V. M., et al. (2013). Can MRI screen for CSF biomarkers in neurodegenerative disease? *Neurology*, 80, 132–138.

McMillan, C. T., Brun, C., Siddiqui, S., Churgin, M., Libon, D., Yushkevich, P., et al. (2012a). White matter imaging contributes to the multimodal diagnosis of frontotemporal lobar degeneration. *Neurology* 78, 1761–1768.

McMillan, C. T., Rascovsky, K., Khella, M. C., Clark, R., and Grossman, M. (2012b). The neural basis for establishing a focal point in pure coordination games. *Soc. Cogn. Affect. Neurosci.* 7, 881–887.

Mesulam, M., Wicklund, A., Johnson, N., Rogalski, E., Leger, G. C., Rademaker, A., et al. (2008). Alzheimer and frontotemporal pathology in subsets of primary progressive aphasia. *Ann. Neurol.* 63, 709–719.

Mesulam, M. M. (1982). Slowly progressive aphasia without generalized dementia. *Ann. Neurol.* 11, 592–598.

Mesulam, M. M. (2001). Primary progressive aphasia. *Ann. Neurol.* 49, 425–432.

NLM/NIH. 2012. Available online at: http://www.ncbi.nlm.nih.gov/pubmed/ [Accessed 10/27/12 2012].

Olsson, A., Vanderstichele, H., Andreasen, N., De Meyer, G., Wallin, A., Holmberg, B., et al. (2005). Simultaneous measurement of beta-amyloid(1-42), total tau, and phosphorylated tau (Thr181) in cerebrospinal fluid by the xMAP technology. *Clin. Chem.* 51, 336–345.

Ost, M., Nylen, K., Csajbok, L., Ohrfelt, A. O., Tullberg, M., Wikkelso, C., et al. (2006). Initial CSF total tau correlates with 1-year outcome in patients with traumatic brain injury. *Neurology* 67, 1600–1604.

Otto, M., Wiltfang, J., Tumani, H., Zerr, I., Lantsch, M., Kornhuber, J., et al. (1997). Elevated levels of tau-protein in cerebrospinal fluid of patients with Creutzfeldt-Jakob disease. *Neurosci. Lett.* 225, 210–212.

Patel, S., Lee, E. B., Xie, S. X., Law, A., Jackson, E. M., Arnold, S. E., et al. (2012). Phosphorylated tau/amyloid beta 1-42 ratio in ventricular cerebrospinal fluid reflects outcome in idiopathic normal pressure hydrocephalus. *Fluids Barriers CNS* 9:7. doi: 10.1186/2045-8118-9-7

Pijnenburg, Y. A., Schoonenboom, N. S., Rosso, S. M., Mulder, C., Van Kamp, G. J., Van Swieten, J. C., et al. (2004). CSF tau and Abeta42 are not useful in the diagnosis of frontotemporal lobar degeneration. *Neurology* 62, 1649.

Pijnenburg, Y. A., Schoonenboom, S. N., Mehta, P. D., Mehta, S. P., Mulder, C., Veerhuis, R., et al. (2007). Decreased cerebrospinal fluid amyloid beta (1-40) levels in frontotemporal lobar degeneration. *J. Neurol. Neurosurg. Psychiatry* 78, 735–737.

Rabinovici, G. D., Jagust, W. J., Furst, A. J., Ogar, J. M., Racine, C. A., Mormino, E. C., et al. (2008). Abeta amyloid and glucose metabolism in three variants of primary progressive aphasia. *Ann. Neurol.* 64, 388–401.

Rascovsky, K., Hodges, J. R., Knopman, D., Mendez, M. F., Kramer, J. H., Neuhaus, J., et al. (2011). Sensitivity of revised diagnostic criteria for the behavioural variant of frontotemporal dementia. *Brain* 134, 2456–2477.

Rascovsky, K., Salmon, D. P., Hansen, L. A., and Galasko, D. (2008). Distinct cognitive profiles and rates of decline on the Mattis Dementia Rating Scale in autopsy-confirmed frontotemporal dementia and Alzheimer's disease. *J. Int. Neuropsychol. Soc.* 14, 373–383.

Renton, A. E., Majounie, E., Waite, A., Simon-Sanchez, J., Rollinson, S., Gibbs, J. R., et al. (2011). A hexanucleotide repeat expansion in C9ORF72 is the cause of chromosome 9p21-linked ALS-FTD. *Neuron* 72, 257–268.

Riemenschneider, M., Wagenpfeil, S., Diehl, J., Lautenschlager, N., Theml, T., Heldmann, B., et al. (2002). Tau and Abeta42 protein in CSF of patients with frontotemporal degeneration. *Neurology* 58, 1622–1628.

Rosso, S. M., Van Herpen, E., Pijnenburg, Y. A., Schoonenboom, N. S., Scheltens, P., Heutink, P., et al. (2003). Total tau and phosphorylated tau 181 levels in the cerebrospinal fluid of patients with frontotemporal dementia due to P301L and G272V tau mutations. *Arch. Neurol.* 60, 1209–1213.

Schmidt, M. L., Gur, R. E., Gur, R. C., and Trojanowski, J. Q. (1988). Intraneuronal and extracellular neurofibrillary tangles exhibit mutually exclusive cytoskeletal antigens. *Ann. Neurol.* 23, 184–189.

Schoonenboom, N. S., Pijnenburg, Y. A., Mulder, C., Rosso, S. M., Van Elk, E. J., Van Kamp, G. J., et al. (2004). Amyloid beta(1-42) and phosphorylated tau in CSF as markers for early-onset Alzheimer disease. *Neurology* 62, 1580–1584.

Schoonenboom, N. S., Reesink, F. E., Verwey, N. A., Kester, M. I., Teunissen, C. E., Van De Ven, P. M., et al. (2012). Cerebrospinal fluid markers for differential dementia diagnosis in a large memory clinic cohort. *Neurology* 78, 47–54.

Seguin, J., Formaglio, M., Perret-Liaudet, A., Quadrio, I., Tholance, Y., Rouaud, O., et al. (2011). CSF biomarkers in posterior cortical atrophy. *Neurology* 76, 1782–1788.

Seppala, T. T., Nerg, O., Koivisto, A. M., Rummukainen, J., Puli, L., Zetterberg, H., et al. (2012). CSF biomarkers for Alzheimer disease correlate with cortical brain biopsy findings. *Neurology* 78, 1568–1575.

Shaw, L. M., Vanderstichele, H., Knapik-Czajka, M., Clark, C. M., Aisen, P. S., Petersen, R. C., et al. (2009). Cerebrospinal fluid biomarker signature in Alzheimer's disease neuroimaging initiative subjects. *Ann. Neurol.* 65, 403–413.

Shaw, L. M., Vanderstichele, H., Knapik-Czajka, M., Figurski, M., Coart, E., Blennow, K., et al. (2011). Qualification of the analytical and clinical performance of CSF biomarker analyses in ADNI. *Acta Neuropathol.* 121, 597–609.

Shi, J., Shaw, C. L., Du Plessis, D., Richardson, A. M., Bailey, K. L., Julien, C., et al. (2005). Histopathological changes underlying frontotemporal lobar degeneration with clinicopathological correlation. *Acta Neuropathol.* 110, 501–512.

Sjogren, M., Davidsson, P., Tullberg, M., Minthon, L., Wallin, A., Wikkelso, C., et al. (2001). Both total and phosphorylated tau are increased in Alzheimer's disease. *J. Neurol. Neurosurg. Psychiatry* 70, 624–630.

Sjogren, M., Minthon, L., Davidsson, P., Granerus, A. K., Clarberg, A., Vanderstichele, H., et al. (2000a). CSF levels of tau, beta-amyloid(1-42) and GAP-43 in frontotemporal dementia, other types of dementia and normal aging. *J. Neural Transm.* 107, 563–579.

Sjogren, M., Rosengren, L., Minthon, L., Davidsson, P., Blennow, K., and Wallin, A. (2000b). Cytoskeleton proteins in CSF distinguish frontotemporal dementia from AD. *Neurology* 54, 1960–1964.

Snowden, J., Neary, D., and Mann, D. (2007). Frontotemporal lobar degeneration: clinical and pathological relationships. *Acta Neuropathol.* 114, 31–38.

Sperling, R. A., Aisen, P. S., Beckett, L. A., Bennett, D. A., Craft, S., Fagan, A. M., et al. (2011). Toward defining the preclinical stages of Alzheimer's disease: recommendations from the National Institute on Aging-Alzheimer's Association workgroups on diagnostic guidelines for Alzheimer's disease. *Alzheimers Dement.* 7, 280–292.

Steinacker, P., Hendrich, C., Sperfeld, A. D., Jesse, S., Von Arnim, C. A., Lehnert, S., et al. (2008). TDP-43 in cerebrospinal fluid of patients with frontotemporal lobar degeneration and amyotrophic lateral sclerosis. *Arch. Neurol.* 65, 1481–1487.

Tapiola, T., Alafuzoff, I., Herukka, S. K., Parkkinen, L., Hartikainen, P., Soininen, H., et al. (2009). Cerebrospinal fluid {beta}-amyloid 42 and tau proteins as biomarkers of Alzheimer-type pathologic changes in the brain. *Arch. Neurol.* 66, 382–389.

Toledo, J. B., Brettschneider, J., Grossman, M., Arnold, S. E., Hu, W. T., Xie, S. X., et al. (2012). CSF biomarkers cutoffs: the importance of coincident neuropathological diseases. *Acta Neuropathol.* 124, 23–35.

Trojanowski, J. Q., and Growdon, J. H. (1998). A new consensus report on biomarkers for the early antemortem diagnosis of Alzheimer disease: current status, relevance to drug discovery, and recommendations for future research. *J. Neuropathol. Exp. Neurol.* 57, 643–644.

Trojanowski, J. Q., Vandeerstichele, H., Korecka, M., Clark, C. M., Aisen, P. S., Petersen, R. C., et al. (2010). Update on the biomarker core of the Alzheimer's Disease Neuroimaging Initiative subjects. *Alzheimers Dement.* 6, 230–238.

Turner, R. S., Kenyon, L. C., Trojanowski, J. Q., Gonatas, N., and Grossman, M. (1996). Clinical, neuroimaging, and pathologic features of progressive nonfluent aphasia. *Ann. Neurol.* 39, 166–173.

Van Deerlin, V. M., Sleiman, P. M., Martinez-Lage, M., Chen-Plotkin, A., Wang, L. S., Graff-Radford, N. R., et al. (2010). Common variants at 7p21 are associated with frontotemporal lobar degeneration with TDP-43 inclusions. *Nat. Genet.* 42, 234–239.

Van Harten, A. C., Kester, M. I., Visser, P. J., Blankenstein, M. A., Pijnenburg, Y. A., Van Der Flier, W. M., et al. (2011). Tau and p-tau as CSF biomarkers in dementia: a meta-analysis. *Clin. Chem. Lab. Med.* 49, 353–366.

Vanmechelen, E., Vanderstichele, H., Davidsson, P., Van Kerschaver, E., Van Der Perre, B., Sjogren, M., et al. (2000). Quantification of tau phosphorylated at threonine 181 in human cerebrospinal fluid: a sandwich ELISA with a synthetic phosphopeptide for standardization. *Neurosci. Lett.* 285, 49–52.

Verwey, N. A., Kester, M. I., Van Der Flier, W. M., Veerhuis, R., Berkhof, H., Twaalfhoven, H., et al. (2010). Additional value of CSF amyloid-beta 40 levels in the differentiation between FTLD and control subjects. *J. Alzheimers Dis.* 20, 445–452.

Wang, L. S., Leung, Y. Y., Chang, S. K., Leight, S., Knapik-Czajka, M., Baek, Y., et al. (2012). Comparison of xMAP and ELISA assays for detecting cerebrospinal fluid biomarkers of Alzheimer's disease. *J. Alzheimers Dis.* 31, 439–445.

Weiner, M. W., Aisen, P. S., Jack, C. R. Jr., Jagust, W. J., Trojanowski, J. Q., Shaw, L., et al. (2010). The Alzheimer's disease neuroimaging initiative: progress report and future plans. *Alzheimers Dement.* 6, 202-211 e207.

Whitwell, J. L., Weigand, S. D., Boeve, B. F., Senjem, M. L., Gunter, J. L., Dejesus-Hernandez, M., et al. (2012). Neuroimaging signatures of frontotemporal dementia genetics: C9ORF72, tau, progranulin and sporadics. *Brain* 135, 794–806.

Zhukareva, V., Sundarraj, S., Mann, D., Sjogren, M., Blenow, K., Clark, C. M., et al. (2003). Selective reduction of soluble tau proteins in sporadic and familial frontotemporal dementias: an international follow-up study. *Acta Neuropathol.* 105, 469–476.

Zhukareva, V., Vogelsberg-Ragaglia, V., Van Deerlin, V. M., Bruce, J., Shuck, T., Grossman, M., et al. (2001). Loss of brain tau defines novel sporadic and familial tauopathies with frontotemporal dementia. *Ann. Neurol.* 49, 165–175.

6

Traumatic brain injury and post-acute decline: what role does environmental enrichment play?

Diana Frasca[1,2]*, Jennifer Tomaszczyk[2], Bradford J. McFadyen[3,4] and Robin E. Green[1,2]

[1] Graduate Department of Rehabilitation Science, University of Toronto, Toronto, ON, Canada
[2] Cognitive Neurorehabilitation Sciences Laboratory, Toronto Rehabilitation Institute, Toronto, ON, Canada
[3] Département de Réadaptation, Université Laval, Québec City, QC, Canada
[4] Centre Interdisciplinaire Recherche en Réadaptation et Intégration Sociale, Québec City, QC, Canada

Edited by:
Hauke R. Heekeren, Freie Universität Berlin, Germany

Reviewed by:
Barbara B. Bendlin, Wisconsin Alzheimer's Disease Research Center, USA
Lisa A. Brenner, University of Colorado Denver, USA

***Correspondence:**
Diana Frasca, Cognitive Neurorehabilitation Sciences Laboratory, Toronto Rehabilitation Institute, 550 University Ave, Room 11-207, Toronto, ON M5G 2A2, Canada.
e-mail: diane.frasca@uhn.ca

Objectives: While a growing number of studies provide evidence of neural and cognitive decline in traumatic brain injury (TBI) survivors during the post-acute stages of injury, there is limited research as of yet on environmental factors that may influence this decline. The purposes of this paper, therefore, are to (1) examine evidence that environmental enrichment (EE) can influence long-term outcome following TBI, and (2) examine the nature of post-acute environments, whether they vary in degree of EE, and what impact these variations have on outcomes.

Methods: We conducted a scoping review to identify studies on EE in animals and humans, and post-discharge experiences that relate to barriers to recovery.

Results: One hundred and twenty-three articles that met inclusion criteria demonstrated the benefits of EE on brain and behavior in healthy and brain-injured animals and humans. Nineteen papers on post-discharge experiences revealed that variables such as insurance coverage, financial, and social support, home therapy, and transition from hospital to home, can have an impact on clinical outcomes.

Conclusion: There is evidence to suggest that lack of EE, whether from lack of resources or limited ability to engage in such environments, may play a role in post-acute cognitive and neural decline. Maximizing EE in the post-acute stages of TBI may improve long-term outcomes for the individual, their family and society.

Keywords: traumatic brain injury, environmental enrichment, post-acute decline, adult, moderate to severe, post-discharge, transition home

INTRODUCTION

Moderate to severe traumatic brain injury (TBI) is a ubiquitous injury: studies suggest an annual incidence of upwards of 20–60 per 100,000 (Narayan et al., 2002; Bruns and Hauser, 2003; Cassidy et al., 2004; C.I.H.I., 2006). Many of these injuries are sustained in young adulthood (C.I.H.I., 2006; Faul et al., 2010) and result in significant impairment to cognitive, motor, and emotional functioning. Predominant and persisting deficits to executive functioning, attention, memory, and speed of processing compromise psychosocial functioning and quality of life (Sander et al., 2001; Hawthorne et al., 2009; Resch et al., 2009). Because these deficits prevent many TBI survivors from returning to pre-injury levels of activity and participation (Dikmen et al., 1983, 1995; Lezak, 2004; Christensen et al., 2008), successful community integration is now recognized as a primary goal of rehabilitation for persons with brain injury (Sander et al., 2010).

The consequences of brain injury are particularly concerning given the high incidence of TBI. Murray and Lopez (1997) predicted that by 2020, TBI will be the third leading cause of disability in the world. Considering that males aged 15–24 years have the highest incidence of TBI (Pickett et al., 2004; C.I.H.I., 2006; Faul et al., 2010), this can mean decades of disability and lost productivity. Not surprisingly, the annual burden of acute care and rehabilitation in North America is estimated to be in the billions of dollars (SMARTRISK, 2006; Faul et al., 2010).

A theoretically intriguing and clinically important question that is emerging from the literature is whether an impediment to recovery and a contributing factor to failed community integration after moderate to severe TBI is cognitive and brain deterioration in the post-acute stages after brain injury. TBI recovery studies typically show an asymptotic pattern of recovery, with rapid improvement within the first weeks and months of injury, followed by a slower rate of improvement and then a plateau with limited measureable recovery thereafter (Basso, 1989; Heinemann et al., 1995; Blatter et al., 1997; Holbrook et al., 1999; Christodoulou et al., 2001; Farne et al., 2004). However, not only do many fail to return to pre-injury levels of function when they reach that plateau (Christensen et al., 2008), but there is growing evidence that a subset of TBI survivors show cognitive deterioration.

A number of studies that have examined post-acute cognitive changes in TBI survivors have demonstrated that across domains of functioning, a combination of maintenance, further recovery and frank declines are observed (Ruff et al., 1991; Millis et al., 2001; Sander et al., 2001; Himanen et al., 2006; Salmond et al., 2006; Till et al., 2008). For example, Till et al. (2008) showed that nearly 30% of their sample of moderate-severe TBI patients showed clinically significant decline (as measured by the reliable change index) in two or more domains of cognitive functioning.

In examining changes of the brain during the post-acute stages of TBI, imaging studies have also shown evidence of deterioration, including decreased cerebral blood flow (Kim et al., 2010), declines in whole brain volume (Blatter et al., 1997; Mackenzie et al., 2002; Trivedi et al., 2007; Ng et al., 2008; Sidaros et al., 2009; Hudak et al., 2011), atrophy of discrete gray, and white matter structures including the hippocampus and corpus callosum (Wilson et al., 1988; Bigler et al., 1997; Levine et al., 2008; Ng et al., 2008; Sidaros et al., 2008), lesion expansion (Ng et al., 2008); and reduced white matter integrity as measured by diffusion tensor imaging (Bendlin et al., 2008; Greenberg et al., 2008; Sidaros et al., 2008; Warner et al., 2010; Farbota et al., 2012).

Correlations between brain and behavioral decline have also been observed. In one study, 24 TBI survivors underwent MRI scans at 8 weeks and 12 months post-injury. The authors not only demonstrated increased atrophy during this time period, but also negatively correlated outcomes on the Glasgow Outcome Scale (Sidaros et al., 2009). In other studies, Hudak et al. (2011) found that decreases in brain volume correlated with depressive symptoms in the post-acute phase, and Farbota et al. (2012) demonstrated that diffusion tensor imaging findings (fractional anisotropy values) and neuropsychological task performance were positively correlated.

Given mounting evidence revealing post-acute decline, we suggest that it is important at this stage of research to begin to consider what factors may hold the potential to influence, and in particular, offset this decline.

One factor that may play a role is "environmental enrichment" (EE). As we will discuss further in the next section, EE broadly refers to enhanced stimulation, associated with (1) environments that provide access to cognitive as well as physical and social stimulation, and (2) conditions that encourage maximal participation. An extensive body of literature shows positive correlations between EE and cognitive and neuronal status. (Scarmeas and Stern, 2003; Will et al., 2004; Simpson and Kelly, 2011). There have also been some findings to suggest that EE influences post-acute decline. In Till et al.'s (2008) study of post-injury cognitive decline, the authors found a relationship between hours of therapy at 5 months post-injury and degree of cognitive decline from 12 to 24 months. They concluded that lack of access to complex and enriched environments, due in part to limited access to resources, may play a critical a role in decline. In another study, Miller and Green (in press) found that greater hippocampal volume loss in the chronic stages of TBI (12–24 months post-injury) was negatively correlated with degree of cognitive stimulation reported at 5 months post-injury.

These few but important findings raise the question whether post-acute decline in these survivors was influenced by the extent of enrichment, or lack thereof, in the environments to which they were discharged following the early and intensive months of therapy. A reduction in the level of enrichment in the later stages of recovery from TBI might occur when the number and hours of therapies are reduced or when patients move from in-patient neurorehabilitation back to the home environment. Additionally, TBI survivors may return to environments that are indeed complex and enriched, but without the expertise of therapists actively providing supports and adaptations to the environments, patients may be unable to engage due to cognitive, emotional and/or physical impairments that render the environments overwhelming or inaccessible.

The purposes of this paper, therefore, are to (1) examine evidence that EE can influence long-term outcome following TBI, and (2) examine the nature of post-acute environments, whether they vary in degree of EE, and what impact these variations have on outcomes. To accomplish these aims, we will undertake a scoping review summarizing literature related to EE and post-acute environments.

SCOPING REVIEW METHODS

This paper addresses two of the reasons for undertaking a scoping review identified by Arksey and O'Malley (2005): to summarize and disseminate research findings and to identify research gaps in the existing literature. The scoping review typically unfolds in five steps: (1) identify the research question; (2) identify all pertinent studies; (3) select the studies for detailed analysis; (4) chart the data according to key concepts; and (5) collate and summarize the findings of the selected studies (Arksey and O'Malley, 2005; Rumrill et al., 2010):

IDENTIFY THE RESEARCH QUESTION

The research questions addressed in this paper are whether (1) EE can influence long-term recovery, and (2) post-discharge environments vary in degree of EE, and whether such variations influence outcomes.

IDENTIFY ALL PERTINENT STUDIES

The literature review aimed to identify a comprehensive set of articles detailing the effects of EE in animals and humans, and the post-discharge experiences related to recovery and regaining independence in the post-acute stages after TBI. Articles that addressed these topics were obtained through use of a traditional keyword-driven electronic search guided by the following terms: TBI; recovery; EE; environmental complexity; active lifestyle; stimulation; neuroplasticity; cognitive reserve; intervention; multi-disciplinary; multi-contextual; post-rehabilitation; transition home; barriers; community integration; re-engagement. Peer-reviewed journals were searched using the PubMed and Cochrane Collaboration research databases as well as the Google Scholar search engine, for articles published between 1987 and 2012. Additionally, hand searches were conducted of references from key articles to follow up on seminal work and promising literature that might not have been captured by the databases used.

SELECT STUDIES FOR DETAILED ANALYSIS

To be considered for inclusion in the review, articles had to meet the following criteria: (1) describe EE (or components of EE) in animals or adult humans or (2) describe the post-discharge experience, and more specifically, the transition from hospital to home in adult brain-injury survivors; and (3) be available in English. No methodological limitations were applied to screen for levels of evidence.

CHART DATA ACCORDING TO KEY CONCEPTS

Articles that met the inclusion criteria were reviewed in detail and categorized based on population examined, methodology, and study objectives to discover commonalities and provide connections between the sets of literatures reviewed.

COLLATE AND SUMMARIZE FINDINGS

The results are presented to correspond with the objectives of this paper. A numerical summary of the articles included is followed by a summary of the literature.

RESULTS

Database searches identified 2053 articles. Of these, 142 were included in the review based on the selection criteria listed above. **Table 1** provides a brief summary of the articles that were included. **Tables 2** and **3** provide a more detailed summary of the papers that specifically addressed EE in brain-injured animals and humans, as well as EE and post-discharge experiences, respectively. **Tables 2** and **3** detail the populations, methods, objectives, and main findings of the articles that were included.

ENVIRONMENTAL ENRICHMENT HAS BENEFICIAL EFFECTS ON BRAIN AND BEHAVIOR IN ANIMALS AND HUMANS

DEFINING ENVIRONMENTAL ENRICHMENT

A number of definitions have been proposed for EE, and it is often defined in relative terms. In animal studies, EEs (e.g., cages with running wheels, novel toys, several animals) are typically contrasted with standard or impoverished environments (e.g., cages with a single animal, and only the basic necessities for living). In these studies, researchers have stressed the importance of having cognitive, social and physical stimulation for environments to be considered enriched and a key property is the maintenance of novelty, for example through regularly changing toys and food (Diamond, 2001; Simpson and Kelly, 2011).

Kramer et al. (2004) have suggested that while numerous positive changes in cognitive functioning, neuroanatomy, and neurochemistry have been demonstrated as a result of exposure to EE in animals, we must examine the degree to which these findings translate to humans, and that an operational definition of EE applicable to humans needs to be established. Whereas novel toys and food, running wheels, and housing several animals together maps on well to cognitive, physical, and social stimulation in animals, identification of such concrete mappings in humans has proven more difficult. Subject factors, such as motivation and mental effort play a large role in reaping the benefits of EE. Thus, personality and earlier life experiences may influence engagement with the environment, such that what is a stimulating and engaging environment for one person may not be for another (Johansson, 2003). Thus, for humans, the definition of EE is more complex, addressing both the nature of the environment and factors that influence engagement with it.

Table 1 | Numerical summary of articles reviewed.

Literature topic	Number of studies	Methodologies	Populations
Beneficial effects of EE	123: animals—55; humans—68	*Animal literature*: quantitative, experimental; *Human literature*: quantitative, correlational, observational, intervention	Healthy and brain-injured animals, humans
Post-discharge experiences	19	Qualitative, observational, correlational, reviews, case study	Brain-injured humans

These ideas of Kramer et al. (2004) are consistent with earlier work by Schooler (1987), who defined the related concept of environmental complexity as being determined by stimulus and demand characteristics. He theorized that greater diversity of stimuli in one's environment could lead to more options/plans of action to consider and decisions to make. When cognitive efforts are reinforced and rewarded, people are motivated to continue engaging in complex environments, which in turn enhances cognitive functioning. Thus, enhancing cognitive functioning further promotes participation in complex environments, illustrating a dynamic facet of EE and its benefits. Enrichment, therefore, reflects environmental complexity (e.g., opportunity to participate in different sports, clubs or social networks, and to engage in intellectually demanding activities), one's inclination to participate in the environment, and the frequency of participation.

Given the limitations in defining, manipulating and controlling EE in human studies, animal studies have arguably provided the most compelling evidence for the causal effects of EE.

BENEFITS OF ENVIRONMENTAL ENRICHMENT

Environmental enrichment in healthy animals

In 1947, Hebb examined if rats exposed to EE would improve behaviorally on problem-solving tasks, compared to a control group (Hebb, 1947). EE rats were free to roam his home while control rats were housed in standard laboratory cages. Hebb found performance was superior in the EE group. Since then, more systematically controlled studies have had similar findings.

Exposure to EE has been associated with increases in cognitive functioning, specifically improvements in response selectivity, learning ability, spatial and problem solving skills, memory, and processing speed (Mohammed et al., 1990; Rosenzweig and Bennett, 1996; Nilsson et al., 1999; Van Praag et al., 2000; Kobayashi et al., 2002; Milgram, 2003; Valero et al., 2011; Leger et al., 2012; Speisman et al., 2012; Yang et al., 2013). Reductions in boredom (Meagher and Mason, 2012) and frustration (Latham and Mason, 2010) have been demonstrated as well. The benefits of EE are also observable at cellular and molecular levels. There is evidence of increased neurogenesis, synaptogenesis and dendritic spine density in parts of the brain associated with memory and learning (i.e., hippocampus, dentate gyrus and cerebellar Purkinje cells) in response to EE (Kolb and Whishaw, 1998; Johansson, 2000, 2002; Van Praag et al., 2000; Churchill et al., 2002; Kempermann et al., 2002; Valero et al., 2011; Eckert and Abraham, 2012; Jung and Herms, 2012; Leger et al., 2012; Speisman et al., 2012; Fares et al., 2013; Yang et al., 2013). Increases in brain weight and cortical thickness

Table 2 | Detailed summary of articles included in "Brain-injured animals and EE" and "Brain-injured humans and EE" scoping review.

Authors	Methods	(1) Main objectives and (2) Findings
BRAIN-INJURED ANIMALS AND EE		
Hamm et al., 1996	Brain-injured and sham-injured rats in EE and standard environment (SE)	(1) Determine whether exposure to EE would promote recovery of cognitive function; (2) Brain-injured rats in EE vs. SE: EE rats showed more improvement in Morris Water Maze task; Brain-injured rats in EE vs. sham-injured: performed at same level.
Johansson and Ohlsson, 1996	Brain-injured rats randomly assigned to EE, social-stimulation only or physical-stimulation only environment	(1) Determine relative importance of social and physical activity to EE; (2) No difference in infarct size between groups. EE group performed better than physical group in all tests, better than social group on rotating pole. With time EE group performed better than social group in limb placement, climbing, inclined plane. Social group performed better than physical group on inclined plane and in climbing at all times, by 13 weeks also in limb placement test and on beam.
Passineau et al., 2001	Brain-injured and sham-injured rats randomly assigned to EE and SE	(1) Examine effect of EE on behavior and on histological integrity of brain tissue selectively vulnerable to brain trauma; (2) Injured animals in EE showed shorter latencies to find platform in Morris Water Maze task vs. injured/SE animals on day 12 post-TBI. Both injured groups showed deficits vs. sham groups. At 14 days post-TBI, EE animals had approximately 2× smaller lesion areas in regions of cerebral cortex posterior to injury epicenter compared to injured/SE animals. Overall lesion volume for entire injured cortical hemisphere was smaller in animals recovering in EE.
Dobrossy and Dunnett, 2001	Brain-injured rodents; review	(1) Review degree to which housing conditions or behavioral training can modify survival, integration or function of transplanted tissue; (2) Behavioral training experience can promote behavioral, and functional compensation, and influence neuroplasticity at cellular, and systems levels of neuronal reorganization.
Johansson, 2003	Brain-injured rats; review	(1) Review influence of post-ischemic environmental factors, possible clinical implications; (2) EE improves functional outcome, increases dendrite branching, number of dendritic spines in contralateral cortex, influences expression of many genes, modifies lesion-induced stem cell differentiation in hippocampus.
Dobrossy and Dunnett, 2004	Brain-injured rats with and without neural grafts randomly assigned to EE and SE	(1) Examine effects of differential housing conditions on striatal graft morphology and functional recovery; (2) Functional recovery accompanied by reduction in infarct size and more afferent connections.
Will et al., 2004	Brain-injured rats; review	(1) Compare three main non-invasive therapeutic strategies for achieving rehabilitation after brain damage: EE, physical exercise, specific formal training; (2) EE increased neurogenesis in hippocampus and up-regulation of neurotropic factors (e.g., NGF) that result in decreased spontaneous apoptosis and increased neuronal survival.
Gobbo and O'Mara, 2004	Brain-injured rats housed under EE or SE, 6 weeks before, 4 weeks after surgery	(1) Investigate if EE can protect rats against the cognitive and neurological consequences of transient ischemia; (2) EE improved learning and memory; does not protect against actual loss of CA1 pyramidal cells. Brain-derived neurotrophic factor levels were increased.
Lippert-Gruener et al., 2007	Brain-injured and sham-injured rats assigned to EE, EE + multi-modal early onset stimulation (MEOS), or SE	(1) Investigate effects of EE, EE+ MEOS, and SE on cognitive and motor function, and cortical lesion volume; (2) Rats in EE and EE+MEOS demonstrated improvement over SE, but no change in lesion size.
Pereira et al., 2007	Brain-injured and sham-injured rats randomly assigned to EE and SE	(1) Examine effects of daily EE on memory deficits in water maze and cerebral damage; (2) Spatial reference, working memory impairments were completely reversed by EE; Reduction of both hippocampal volume and cortical area, ipsilateral to arterial occlusion, no EE effect on morphological measurements.
Hoffman et al., 2008	Brain-injured and sham-injured rats randomly assigned to early EE, delayed EE, continuous EE or no EE	(1) Examine whether EE-mediated benefits are dependent on exposure to EE during neurobehavioral training; (2) A3 cell loss significantly attenuated in TBI + continuous EE group vs. TBI + no EE group. Beam-walking was facilitated in TBI groups that received early or continuous EE vs. those receiving delayed or no EE. Cognitive training enhanced in TBI groups that received continuous or delayed EE vs. early or no EE groups.

(Continued)

Table 2 | Continued

Authors	Methods	(1) Main objectives and (2) Findings
Sozda et al., 2010	Brain-injured and sham-injured rats assigned to typical EE, EE –social, EE –stimuli, SE, SE +stimuli	(1) Investigate effects of typical EE, EE –social, EE –stimuli, SE, SE +stimuli on motor and cognitive function, lesion volume, brain volume loss; (2) Typical EE groups performed same as sham group, and showed most improvement compared to other TBI groups in terms of spatial learning and memory retention, lesion size reduction.
Sun et al., 2010	Brain-injured rats randomly assigned to EE or SE	(1) Investigate effects of EE on cognitive impairment, levels of BDNF and NMDA receptor subunit 1 (NR1) and subunit 2B (NR2B) in hippocampus; (2) EE exposure improved spatial cognitive performance and non-spatial memory performance. EE increased levels of BDNF and NR1 protein in hippocampus.
Matter et al., 2010	Brain-injured or sham-injured rats randomly assigned to 8 groups receiving continuous, early or delayed EE with either 1 or 2 weeks of exposure	(1) Further assess effects of time of initiation and duration of EE on neurobehavioral recovery by evaluating and directly comparing all the temporal permutations; (2) Motor ability was enhanced in TBI groups that received early EE (i.e., during testing) vs. standard housing. Acquisition of spatial learning facilitated in groups receiving delayed EE (i.e., during training).
De Witt et al., 2011	Brain-injured and sham-injured rats randomly assigned to EE, EE (2 h), EE (4 h), EE (6 h), or SE	(1) Determine whether abbreviated EE (i.e., rehab-relevant dose response) confers benefits similar to typical EE; (2) TBI + EE (2 h) and TBI + EE (4 h) groups not different from TBI + STD group in behavioral assessment. TBI + EE (6 h) group exhibited enhancement of motor and cognitive performance when compared with TBI + STD group, TBI + EE (2 h) and TBI + EE (4 h) groups, and did not differ from TBI + EE (typical) group.
Cheng et al., 2012	Brain-injured and sham-injured rats randomly assigned to 3 weeks of EE or SE. In phase 2: half of rats in EE transferred to SE conditions (TBI + EE + SE and sham + EE + SE; re-assessed 1/month for 6 months)	(1) Determine whether EE-mediated motor and cognitive benefits persist after its withdrawal; (2) TBI + EE and TBI + EE + STD groups performed better in the water maze than the TBI + STD group, did not differ from one another. Data replicate several studies showing that EE enhances recovery after brain injury, and extend by demonstrating that cognitive benefits are maintained for at least 6 months post-rehabilitation.
Shin et al., 2013	Brain-injured and sham-injured rats assigned to EE or SE	(1) Investigate effects of EE on substantia nigra gene expression; (2) EE-induced gene alterations after TBI included genes important for signal transduction, in particular calcium signaling pathways, membrane homeostasis, and metabolism.
Monaco et al., 2013	Brain-injured and sham-injured rats assigned to EE or SE	(1) Assess effect of EE on functional and histological outcome in female rats after TBI; (2) EE improved motor function and spatial learning; reduced lesion size and increased hippocampal cell survival.
BRAIN-INJURED HUMANS AND EE		
Blackerby, 1990	Acute moderate-severe TBI (*n* = 145); retrospective; quantitative	(1) Investigate effects of different levels of rehabilitation intensity on length of stay in two hospital-based coma and acute rehabilitation populations; (2) After increasing treatment intensity and changes in case management, patients were discharged an average of 1.5 months earlier than before changes.
Toglia, 1991	Brain injury; concept paper	(1) Review literature on learning and generalization and direct applications to treatment; (2) Five components identified in cognitive psychology literature as critical to process of generalization: (a) use of multiple environments, (b) identification of criteria for transfer, (c) meta-cognitive training, (d) emphasis on processing strategies, and (e) use of meaningful activities.
Spivack et al., 1992	Acute moderate-severe TBI (*n* = 95); prospective; quantitative: repeated measures	(1) Examine effects of intensity of treatment and length of stay during inpatient rehabilitation hospitalization; (2) Patients with longer length of stay (LOS) made more progress across all outcome variables than patients with shorter LOS; In long LOS group, two treatment-intensity groups initially equivalent, and at discharge high-intensity treatment group surpassed low-intensity treatment group.

(Continued)

Table 2 | Continued

Authors	Methods	(1) Main objectives and (2) Findings
Willer et al., 1999	Post-acute/chronic severe TBI ($n = 46$); prospective; quantitative: case control matched design, repeated measures	(1) Compare outcomes of a post-acute residential rehabilitation program with a matched sample receiving limited services in their homes or on an outpatient basis; (2) Individuals who received intensive rehabilitation services in community-based residential program exhibited considerable improvement in functional abilities (cognitive skills, motor skills). Treatment group showed greater improvement in community integration.
Sohlberg et al., 2000	Chronic moderate-severe TBI, ABI ($n = 14$); prospective; quantitative: repeated measures	(1) Compare attention processing training with an educational and support method; (2) 10 weeks of brain injury education seemed most effective in improving self-reports of psychosocial function. Attention process training influenced self-reports of cognitive function, had stronger influence on performance of executive attention tasks. Vigilance, orienting networks showed little specific improvement.
Cicerone et al., 2000	TBI/Stroke; review	(1) Establish evidence-based recommendations for clinical practice of cognitive rehabilitation from methodical review of scientific literature concerning effectiveness of cognitive rehabilitation; (2) Attention deficits: limited evidence exists for generalization of benefits attributable to attention remediation, tendency to observe gains on tasks most closely related to training tasks; Multi-modal interventions: can significantly improve neuropsychological performance in many skill areas. Maintenance, generalization of benefits from cognitive rehabilitation greatest when treatment is provided for appropriately long periods of time, when efforts are made by clinician and patient to identify and apply interventions to personally relevant areas of functioning, when patients are able to assume responsibility for using compensatory strategies in everyday functioning.
De Weerdt et al., 2000	Acute stroke ($n = 56$); prospective; quantitative: observational	(1) Observe how stroke patients spend their time in a rehabilitation unit; (2) Patients most frequently involved in therapeutic activities, Belgium: 28% of day, Switzerland: 45%. Belgian patients: 27% of day in own room, Swiss: 49% of day. Swiss patients spent nearly 1.5 h per day more in therapy. Differences between two settings could only partially be explained by more favorable patient-staff ratios in Swiss setting.
Fasotti et al., 2000	Post-acute/chronic severe TBI ($n = 22$); prospective; quantitative: repeated measures	(1) Compare the effectiveness of Time Pressure Management (TPM) training with concentration training in which verbal instruction was the key element; (2) TPM produces greater gains than concentration training and appears to generalize to other measures of speed and memory function.
Zhu et al., 2001	Post-acute moderate-severe TBI ($n = 36$); prospective; quantitative: repeated measures	(1) Evaluate effects of different levels of intensive rehabilitation treatment on functional outcome; (2) Increasing amount of rehabilitation from conventional 2–4 h/day improved functional outcome as measured by GOS. More patients in intensive group returned to gainful work, either original or modified job. Improvement most significant in early post-injury period at 2–3 months.
Shiel et al., 2001	Moderate-severe TBI ($n = 56$); prospective; quantitative: repeated measures	(1) Investigate effect of increased intensity of rehabilitation on rate at which independence was regained and duration of hospital admission; (2) Increasing hours per week of therapy can accelerate rate of recovery of personal independence and result in being discharged from hospital sooner. No evidence of ceiling effect of therapeutic intensity beyond which no further response observed.
Park and Ingles, 2001	ABI; meta-analysis	(1) Examine the efficacy of attention rehabilitation; (2) Direct-retraining methods produced only small non-significant improvements in performance. Few studies that attempted to rehabilitate specific skills requiring attention showed statistically significant improvements after training and had considerably larger effect sizes. Results suggest learning that occurs as a function of training is specific, does not tend to generalize or transfer to tasks that differ considerably from those used in training.

(Continued)

Table 2 | Continued

Authors	**Methods**	**(1) Main objectives and (2) Findings**
Powell et al., 2002	Post-acute/chronic severe TBI ($n = 94$); prospective; quantitative: RCT	(1) Evaluation of multidisciplinary community based outreach rehabilitation; (2) Outreach participants significantly more likely to show gains on Barthel Index, BICRO-39 total score, self-organization, psychological well-being subscales. Strong trends for BICRO personal care and mobility, on FIM+FAM for personal care and cognitive functions.
Slade et al., 2002	Acute stroke/TBI ($n = 161$); prospective; quantitative: RCT	(1) Examined if increased intensity of therapy would decrease length of stay; (2) Accounting for impairment/disability mix, and consequent response of therapy, enhanced levels of physiotherapy and occupational therapy led to benefits for experimental group, resulting in decrease length of stay.
Cifu et al., 2003	Moderate-severe TBI ($n = 491$); prospective; quantitative: RCT	(1) Identify factors relating to intensity of rehabilitation services received and to ascertain relation between injury outcomes, demographics, types of therapy, and intensity of rehabilitation services provided; (2) Findings support assertions that increased therapy intensity, particularly physical and psychological therapies, enhances functional outcomes.
Rath et al., 2003	Chronic mild-severe TBI ($n = 60$); prospective; quantitative: repeated measures	(1) Compare efficacy of a group-treatment protocol using a remedial programme that aims to reduce difficulties in emotional self-regulation, and to facilitate steps used in problem solving with a conventional neuropsychological rehabilitation programme; (2) Participants in innovative group improved in problem solving as assessed using a variety of measures, including (i) executive function, (ii) problem-solving self-appraisal, (iii) self-appraised emotional self-regulation and clear thinking, (iv) objective observer ratings of role-played scenarios. Improvements were maintained at follow-up.
Boman et al., 2004	Mild-moderate TBI ($n = 10$); prospective; experimental: repeated measures	(1) Examine efficacy of cognitive rehabilitation in the patient's home or vocational environment; (2) Positive effect on some measures on impairment level, no differences on activity or participation levels at follow-up; indicates home-based cognitive training improves some attentional and memory functions and facilitates learning of strategies.
Cicerone et al., 2004	Post-acute/chronic moderate-severe TBI ($n = 56$); prospective; quantitative: repeated measures	(1) Evaluate effectiveness of an intensive cognitive rehabilitation program (ICRP) compared with standard neurorehabilitation (SRP); (2) ICRP participants over twice as likely to show clinical benefit on Community Integration Questionnaire. ICRP participants showed improvement in overall neuropsychological functioning; participants with clinically significant improvement on Community Integration Questionnaire showed greater improvement of neuropsychological functioning. Satisfaction with cognitive functioning made significant contribution to post-treatment community integration.
De Wit et al., 2005	Stroke ($n = 60$); prospective; quantitative: observational	(1) Identify differences in use of time by stroke patients in 4 rehabilitation centers in 4 countries; (2) Patients in Belgium and UK spent more time in passive behavior, in rooms, without any interaction compared with patients in Germany and Switzerland. Latter centers had more structured rehabilitation program. May have resulted in more therapy time, more challenging environment for patients, physically and mentally.
Turner-Stokes et al., 2005	Mild-severe ABI; Cochrane review	(1) Assess effects of multi-disciplinary rehabilitation in adults aged 16–65 years; (2) For patients with moderate- severe ABI already in therapy, there was strong evidence that more intensive programmes are associated with earlier functional gains, and "moderate evidence" that continued outpatient therapy could help to sustain gains made in early post-acute rehabilitation.
Cicerone et al., 2005	TBI, stroke; review	(1) Update previous evidence-based recommendations of the Brain Injury Interdisciplinary Special Interest Group of the American Congress of Rehabilitation Medicine for cognitive rehabilitation; (2) Consensus that cognitive rehabilitation should focus on reducing disability, helping restore social role functioning, rather than exclusively on remediation of impairments. Most studies evaluated outcome of interventions at impairment level rather than effect on performance of activities or changes in social participation.

(Continued)

Table 2 | Continued

Authors	Methods	(1) Main objectives and (2) Findings
Zhu et al., 2007	Acute/post-acute moderate-severe TBI ($n = 68$); Prospective; RCT	(1) Evaluate the effects of an increase in the intensity of rehabilitation on functional outcome; (2) More patients in the high intensity group than in the control group who achieved a maximum FIM total score at the third month and a maximum Glasgow Outcome Scale score at the second and third months.
Kleim and Jones, 2008	Healthy adult/TBI; review	(1) Review 10 principles of experience-dependent neural plasticity and considerations in applying them to the damaged brain; (2) Optimism that the nature of brain plasticity can be capitalized upon to improve rehabilitation efforts and to optimize functional outcome.
Kennedy et al., 2008	TBI; Systematic review, meta-analysis	(1) Review studies that focused on executive functions of problem solving, planning, organizing and multitasking; (2) Compelling evidence from 10 intervention studies that using step-by-step meta-cognitive strategy instruction improves problem solving, etc. for personally relevant activities or problem situations; Changes more likely to be observed at level of activities and participation in daily living than on standardized tests (i.e., impairment outcomes).
Spikman et al., 2009	ABI ($n = 75$); prospective; quantitative: RCT, repeated measures	(1) Evaluate the effects of a treatment for dysexecutive problems on daily life functioning; (2) Experimental patients resumed previous roles significantly more than before treatment. From post-treatment to follow-up, only experimental group showed further improvement over time; DEX showed decrease of executive complaints similar for both groups. On DEX-therapist, significantly less executive problems after treatment for experimental group. Executive abilities observed by professionals improved more in experimental group.
Toglia et al., 2010	Chronic moderate TBI ($n = 4$); quantitative: single-subject design; repeated measures	(1) Refine, explore and provide preliminary testing of the multi-context approach in promoting strategy use across situations and increasing self-regulation, awareness and functional performance; (2) Participants demonstrated positive changes in self-regulatory skills and strategy use across tasks. Examination of individual participants revealed important, varying patterns of change in strategy use, learning transfer and self-awareness across intervention.
Cernich et al., 2010	Review; TBI	(1) Review of available evidence of cognition following TBI; (2) Recommendations: (i) Access to sub-acute rehabilitation that is holistic in nature and involves multi-disciplinary team to in work in an integrated fashion to support physical, cognitive and social skill retraining is vital to support positive outcome following TBI; (ii) Trials of medication to assist with attention, memory impairment appear well-supported by the available evidence; (iii) RCTs demonstrate utility of specific rehabilitation approached to attention retraining and retraining of executive function; (iv) Training in use of supportive devices to support individual's daily activities remains central to independent function.
Leon-Carrion et al., 2012	Acute severe TBI ($n = 19$); quantitative: observational	(1) Explore the course and timing of functional recovery in patients who have emerged from coma; (2) To achieve a good response and outcome nearing normalcy, a patient needs over 300 h of intensive rehabilitation.
Hayden et al., 2013	Acute-chronic mild-severe TBI ($n = 1274$); retrospective; quantitative	(1) Evaluate functional improvement after admission to post-acute rehabilitation; (2) Improved functioning after post-acute rehabilitation, regardless of severity of impairment or time since injury to admission to program. Rate of improvement greater for those admitted within 3 months of injury. Individuals with severe impairment demonstrated less improvement when admitted later in time after injury.

Acute, 0–3 months post-injury; post-acute, 3–12 months post-injury; chronic, greater than 12 months post-injury.

have also been demonstrated, as have increases in the amount of nerve growth factor, brain derived neurotropic factor, myelination, acetylcholinesterase activity, neurotransmitters, glial proliferation, blood vessels (number and size), and protein synthesis (Rosenzweig, 1966; West and Greenough, 1972; Bennett et al., 1974; Mohammed et al., 1990; Rosenzweig and Bennett, 1996; Kolb and Whishaw, 1998; Van Praag et al., 2000; Diamond, 2001; Churchill et al., 2002; Pietropaolo et al., 2004; Will et al., 2004; Bennett et al., 2006; Hoffman et al., 2008; Gabriel et al., 2009a,b; Lores-Arnaiz et al., 2010; Qiu et al., 2011, 2012; Williamson et al.,

Table 3 | Detailed summary of articles included in "Post-discharge experiences and EE" scoping review.

Authors	Methods	(1) Main objectives and (2) Findings
POST-DISCHARGE FACTORS THAT INFLUENCE STIMULATION		
Corrigan et al., 2004	Chronic mild-severe TBI ($n = 1802$); prospective; quantitative	(1) Provide population-based estimates of perceived needs following TBI and the prevalence of unmet needs; (2) Many reported still requiring help managing cognitive changes, emotional changes, and managing finances.
Staudenmayer et al., 2007	Post-acute severe TBI ($n = 211$); prospective; quantitative	(1) Determine whether there are specific types of functional deficits that disproportionately affect ethnic minorities after TBI; (2) Minorities demonstrated worse long-term functional outcome, less social and financial resources suggested as related/causal variables.
Shafi et al., 2007	Post-acute severe TBI ($n = 344$); prospective; quantitative	(1) Analyze whether racial or ethnic disparities exist in trauma care, specifically related to access to rehabilitation services and functional outcomes of patients with TBI; (2) Ethnic minorities less likely to be insured; more likely to have moderate-severe disability at follow-up. Data suggest insured patients less likely to be disabled, relationship strongest for private insurance.
Till et al., 2008	Post-acute moderate -severe TBI ($n = 33$); quantitative: observational cohort: 5, 12, 24 months post-injury	(1) Assess prospectively degree of post-acute long-term cognitive decline after TBI; (2) Amount of therapy received at 5 months post-injury significantly higher in group of non-decliners vs. decliners; individuals who were insured received more hours of therapy after discharge than those not insured.
Sander et al., 2009	Post-acute mild-severe TBI ($n = 151$); prospective; quantitative	(1) Determine contribution of race/ethnicity and income to community integration at approximately 6 months following TBI; (2) After controlling for age, education, injury severity, race/ethnicity, income made a significant contribution to variance in social integration, total score and scores on Belonging and Independent Participation scales of the Community Integral Measure. Lower income was associated with worse community integration.
Keightley et al., 2011	TBI, ABI + caregivers ($n = 17$); qualitative	(1) Explore barriers and enablers surrounding transition from health care to home community settings for Aboriginal clients recovering from ABI in northwestern Ontario; (2) Lack of awareness, education and resources acknowledged as key challenges to successful transitioning by clients and healthcare providers.
Sander et al., 2011	Post-acute mild-severe TBI ($n = 167$); prospective; mixed methods	(1) Investigate meaning of community integration in an ethnically diverse sample; (2) Financial issues, such as home ownership and insufficient funds, were perceived as contributing to decreased participation in the community.
Turner et al., 2009b	Post-acute mild-severe TBI, ABI + caregivers ($n = 38$); qualitative; pre-discharge, 1, 3 months post-discharge	(1) Explore people's lived experiences of reengagement in meaningful occupations during hospital-to-home transition phase after ABI; (2) Not being able to participate in desired occupations was source of stress and frustration. Many family caregivers reported participation in meaningful occupations was fundamental element of recovery gains. Other key elements: establishing routines or schedules and occupying one's time. Participation in meaningful occupations perceived to enhance functional recovery during transition.
POST-DISCHARGE FACTORS THAT INFLUENCE ENGAGEMENT		
Freeman, 1997	Severe TBI; Concept paper	(1) Explore methods used to establish a rehabilitation program in the home, the initial moves, the family dynamics, the advantages, and some of the programs required for the restoration of function of sensory, cognitive and motor abilities; (2) Family environment provides wide variety of activities, which are inclusive of person, guarantees provision of stimulation over a wide spectrum of inputs and activities.
Rotondi et al., 2007	Chronic moderate-severe TBI + caregivers ($n = 185$); qualitative	(1) Determine expressed needs of persons with TBI and their primary family caregivers; (2) Inadequate preparation of primary support persons and persons who experienced TBI for personality and behavioral sequelae prior to discharge from the hospital appeared to be a common complaint.
McCormack and Liddiard, 2009	Chronic severe TBI ($n = 1$); case study	(1) Examines a model of community rehabilitation; (2) Supportive and effective familial care system and specialist community interdisciplinary rehabilitation was effective in facilitating recovery.

(Continued)

Table 3 | Continued

Authors	Methods	(1) Main objectives and (2) Findings
Keightley et al., 2011	TBI, ABI + caregivers ($n = 17$); qualitative	(1) Explore barriers and enablers surrounding transition from health care to home community settings for Aboriginal clients recovering from ABI in north western Ontario; (2) Lack of awareness, education and resources acknowledged as key challenges to successful transitioning by clients and healthcare providers.
Sander et al., 2011	Post-acute mild-severe TBI ($n = 167$); prospective; mixed methods	(1) Investigate meaning of community integration in an ethnically diverse sample; (2) Feeling integrated into the community relates to aspects of the environment as much as to involvement in specific activities.
Turner et al., 2011b	Post-acute mild-severe TBI, ABI + caregivers ($n = 38$); qualitative; pre-discharge, 1, 3 months post-discharge	(1) Explore service and support needs of individuals with ABI and family caregivers during transition phase from hospital to home; (2) Individuals with ABI experience a range of service and support needs during the early transition phase, many of which are currently unmet. Findings also indicated that support for family caregivers and access to early community rehabilitation were the two areas in which participants most commonly reported experiencing unmet needs.
Rusconi and Turner-Stokes, 2003	Post-acute/chronic TBI, ABI, SCI ($n = 53$); quantitative: cross-sectional cohort survey	(1) Evaluate aftercare of patients discharged from specialist rehabilitation unit with respect to use of equipment and follow-up by therapy and care services and to assess change in dependency and care needs; (2) Many patients observed they were ill-prepared for sudden change from an intensive therapy programme on unit to a much less frequent and more self-reliant programme in community.
Rittman et al., 2004	Post-acute stroke + caregivers ($n = 51$); qualitative	(1) Evaluate the transition from hospital to home during the first month after discharge following acute stroke; (2) When routines are not re-established, survivors and caregivers experience more chaos, disruption during the transition. When talking about ways days are spent, most survivors describe problems with boredom and not having meaningful activities in their lives.
Turner et al., 2007	Chronic TBI, ABI + caregivers ($n = 24$); qualitative	(1) Explore transition experiences from hospital to home of a purposive sample of individuals with ABI; (2) Many participants found it difficult to locate and access suitable post-discharge therapy services. Friendship and social networks played important role during transition process. Post-discharge boredom, particularly during first 1–2 months at home, commonly expressed.
Turner et al., 2009b	Post-acute mild-severe TBI, ABI + caregivers ($n = 38$); qualitative; pre-discharge, 1, 3 months post-discharge	(1) Explore people's lived experiences of reengagement in meaningful occupations during hospital-to-home transition phase after ABI; (2) Not being able to participate in desired occupations was source of stress, frustration for many participants. Many family caregivers reported participation in meaningful occupations was fundamental element of recovery gains. Other key elements of transition success included establishing routines or schedules and occupying one's time. Results demonstrated participation in meaningful occupations was perceived to enhance functional recovery during transition; underscores importance of encouraging and facilitating participation in meaningful occupations.
Hoogerdijk et al., 2011	Chronic mild-severe TBI ($n = 4$); qualitative	(1) Better understand how individuals with TBI make sense of adaptation process and their performance of occupations within this process; (2) Results indicate adaptation process following TBI is a necessary struggle to gain new identity; facilitated by engagement in familiar occupations in familiar environments; a protracted learning process that continues long after rehabilitation ends; individual, situated.
Turner et al., 2011a	Post-acute mild-severe TBI, ABI + caregivers ($n = 38$); qualitative; pre-discharge, 1, 3 months post-discharge	(1) Explore perspectives of individuals with ABI and their family caregivers concerning recovery and adjustment during the early transition phase from hospital to home; (2) Findings highlight that while returning home was typically perceived to facilitate ongoing recovery, process of adjusting emotionally to life at home posed significant challenge for many participants during transition phase.

(Continued)

Table 3 | Continued

Authors	Methods	(1) Main objectives and (2) Findings
Nalder et al., 2012a	Post-acute moderate -severe TBI + caregivers ($n = 210$); prospective; quantitative: repeated measures: discharge, 1, 3, 6 months post-discharge	(1) Identify factors associated with perceived success of transition from hospital to home after TBI; (2) Greater perceived success of transition associated with higher levels of health-related quality of life, level of community integration, more severe injury. Sentinel events (e.g., returning to work, independent community access, changing living situation) associated with greater perceived success; financial strain, difficulty accessing therapy services associated with less success.
Nalder et al., 2012b	Post-acute moderate -severe TBI + caregivers ($n = 210$); prospective; quantitative: repeated measures: discharge, 1, 3, 6 months post-discharge	(1) Describe timing and factors associated with occurrence of sentinel events (financial strain, difficulty accessing therapy, return to work, accommodation change and independent transport use) during transition to community for individuals with TBI; (2) General positive sentinel events (e.g., regaining independence, returning to work) more likely experienced by individuals with higher levels of global functioning and psychosocial integration. Individuals with lower levels of functioning at greater risk of experiencing more negative sentinel events (e.g. financial strain). Individuals with more severe injury and poorer adjustment more likely to report difficulty accessing therapy.

Acute, 0–3 months post-injury; post-acute, 3–12 months post-injury; chronic, greater than 12 months post-injury.

2012; Fares et al., 2013; Vazquez-Sanroman et al., 2013; Yang et al., 2013).

In examining properties of EE that produce beneficial effects, factors such as *intensity* and *duration* emerge as critical for reaping the most benefits. Bennett et al. (2006) examined the effects of long-term continuous EE on memory performance in aged mice. Mice received a 10-week treatment of either 5 min of daily handling housed in impoverished environments (i.e., clear plastic shoe boxes), 3 h of daily exposure to a basic EE (i.e., small bin with fresh bedding, a running wheel, a plastic rodent dwelling, a plastic tube for climbing, a few toys), or continuous complex EE (i.e., larger bin to allow for more mice to be housed together, and for larger and more complex objects). Continuously enriched older mice performed significantly better than other groups of aged mice in spatial memory tasks, and were indistinguishable from younger control mice in their performance.

Amaral et al. (2008) examined durations of EE in mice and influences on behavioral changes (open field habituation and locomotion). They compared mice exposed to 1, 4, and 8 weeks of EE. While mice exposed to 4 and 8 weeks showed behavioral effects, the 1-week group did not. Furthermore, mice in the 4-week exposure group demonstrated effects lasting 2 months post-EE, but only mice in the 8-week EE group demonstrated effects lasting up to 6 months. The authors concluded that *(1) a minimum EE period is necessary to induce beneficial behavioral effects, (2) the effect of EE can persist at least partially for many months after its cessation, and (3) the degree of persistence is greater in animals exposed to longer durations of EE*. Relevant to the discharge environment of humans and the importance of ongoing therapy/stimulation, these findings showed that the benefits of EE are lost when animals are removed from enriched environments.

Environmental enrichment in healthy humans

Scarmeas and Stern (2003) undertook a review of the relationship between lifestyle and cognitive reserve, which they defined as the degree to which the brain can create and use networks or cognitive paradigms that are more efficient or flexible, and thus less susceptible to disruption. They asked whether exercising the brain had the same healthy effects as exercising the body. They found that greater participation in intellectual and social leisure activities was associated with less cognitive decline in healthy older adults and a lower incidence of dementia. These important "use it or lose it" findings support the need for EE in the sub-acute and chronic stages of TBI to avert decline. The authors proposed that leisure activities and an active lifestyle might buffer against cognitive decline by: (1) increasing synaptic density, which results in more efficient cognitive functioning of unaffected neurons; (2) more efficient use of the same brain networks; and (3) more efficient use of alternative brain networks. They also found that although it is a very active area of research, our understanding of the specific active ingredients that buffer against cognitive decline has not been fully elucidated.

In addition to studies examining how mentally active lifestyles are associated with cognitive benefits (Gribbin et al., 1980; Pushkar et al., 1997; Wang et al., 2002; Wilson et al., 2002, 2003; Crowe et al., 2003; Verghese et al., 2003; Newson and Kemps, 2005; Fujiwara et al., 2009), studies have also illustrated the benefits of maintaining physically active (Clarkson-Smith and Hartley, 1989; Schuit et al., 2001; Pignatti et al., 2002; Voss et al., 2011; Xu et al., 2011) and socially active lifestyles (Bassuk et al., 1999; Fratiglioni et al., 2000; Mahoney et al., 2000; Seeman et al., 2001). However, they are correlational in design and leave open the possibility that higher functioning people seek out the continuous exposure.

A number of further studies have shown the benefits of EE for healthy older adults (Huppert, 1991; Christensen and Mackinnon, 1993; Davidson and Bar-Yam, 2006; Sampson et al., 2009; Marioni et al., 2012a,b; Paillard-Borg et al., 2012). Winocur and Moscovitch (1990) compared cognitive functioning in community-dwelling and institutionalized older adults. After controlling for variables such as IQ, age, and health, they found that community-dwelling older adults had higher levels of cognitive functioning. They also identified a subgroup of high-functioning institutionalized older adults who performed similarly to the community-dwelling group. For this subgroup, they postulated that cognitive functioning may have been influenced by adjustment to institutional life, such that more social activity was correlated with better cognitive functioning, as was found in a prior study (Winocur et al., 1987). Winocur and Moscovitch suggested that lower cognitive functioning observed in the institutionalized group might be a result of an understimulating environment. This interpretation is also consistent with the position of Schooler and Mulatu (2001), who suggested that even if people have higher levels of education, it is the *continued practice* in complex activities that maintains their cognitive abilities—speaking directly to the thesis of this paper.

A number of studies have examined the benefits of continuous exposure (Blackerby, 1990; Spivack et al., 1992; Willer et al., 1999; De Weerdt et al., 2000; Shiel et al., 2001; Zhu et al., 2001; Cifu et al., 2003; De Wit et al., 2005), and interventions that incorporate many elements of EE, such as cognitive, social, and physical stimulation (Hayslip et al., 1995; Neely and Backman, 1995; Fasotti et al., 2000; Powell et al., 2002; Vance and Johns, 2002; Gunther et al., 2003; Rath et al., 2003; Noice and Noice, 2004; Van De Winckel et al., 2004; Green et al., 2006; Stine-Morrow et al., 2007; Spikman et al., 2009). These types of interventions can be contrasted with interventions involving manipulations over a discrete period of time that are designed to enhance a specific cognitive domain or skill. The former have broadly led to more generalizable gains, both cognitively and physically.

Brain-injured animals and environmental enrichment

Brain-injured animals show clear-cut benefits from exposure to EE. Studies comparing recovery in brain-injured animals reared in EEs to those reared in standard environments have demonstrated increased neurogenesis, upregulation of neurotrophic factors, increased neuronal survival, increased afferent innervation, as well as reductions in spontaneous apoptosis and infarct size (Van Praag et al., 2000; Dobrossy and Dunnett, 2001, 2004; Passineau et al., 2001; Gobbo and O'Mara, 2004; Will et al., 2004; Pereira et al., 2007; Hoffman et al., 2008; Sozda et al., 2010; Sun et al., 2010; Monaco et al., 2013; Shin et al., 2013). Superior performance on tasks of learning and memory, and spatial reference has also been found (Hamm et al., 1996; Johansson and Ohlsson, 1996; Passineau et al., 2001; Gobbo and O'Mara, 2004; Will et al., 2004; Lippert-Gruener et al., 2007; Pereira et al., 2007; Hoffman et al., 2008; Sozda et al., 2010; Monaco et al., 2013). Hamm et al. (1996) compared cognitive functioning in brain-injured and sham-brain-injured rats housed in EEs to those housed in standard environments. Rats housed in EEs were in social groups and had access to a variety of foods, novel toys, scented objects, and a running wheel. At 15 days post-injury, brain-injured rats exposed to EE performed significantly better than brain-injured rats in standard environments. Interestingly, they also found that brain-injured rats recovering in EE performed just as well as non-brain injured animals.

In an older but seminal study by Johansson and Ohlsson (1996), brain-injured rats recovering in comprehensive EE (i.e., cognitive, social, and physical enrichment) were compared to those recovering in either enriched social environments or enriched exercise environments. Rats in the EE group were placed in one cage with several other rats, and novel toys and objects that promoted exercise, whereas rats in the social-interaction group were caged with other rats without objects or toys, and rats in the exercise group were individually caged with access to a running wheel. The social-interaction group improved more than the exercise group; however, the EE group improved more than either group. More recently, Hoffman et al. (2008) demonstrated the importance of timing and duration of EE, comparing brain-injured rats exposed to continuous EE to those in early and temporary EE (immediately post-injury lasting 1 week), late EE (commencing 1 week post-injury) and no EE. The continuous EE group not only had significantly less hippocampal cell loss, but also performed better on motor and cognitive tests. Interestingly, they found an advantage of continuous and *early* EE for motor tasks, but an advantage of continuous and *delayed* EE for cognitive tasks. The benefits of increased EE-exposure in brain-injured rats have since been replicated (De Witt et al., 2011; Matter et al., 2010), and, moreover, shown to last for up to 6 months (Cheng et al., 2012).

These studies provide evidence that EE help animals to recover functions to levels that make them indistinguishable from healthy controls, and that *continual* EE is necessary to *maintain* both neural and cognitive improvements. The benefits of EE are substantial, but not permanent, thus highlighting the importance of ongoing stimulation. These findings are particularly relevant to the post-discharge environment, and the factors may contribute to decline.

Brain-injured humans and environmental enrichment

EE interventions for brain-injured humans can be grouped into two broad types: those that provide increased hours and duration of therapy (without prescription of specific content of therapies) and those that address discrete impairments and focus on improvement of a specific skill. Note that in clinical practice, the latter might be referred to as "training" rather than EE. However, we include them here as they entail increased cognitive stimulation.

While EE intervention designs have not been as comprehensive in human TBI studies, the effects of some of the classical properties of EE, such as novelty, intensity, and duration, have been examined. However, much like in healthy individuals, interventions for TBI survivors aimed at training specific skills have often resulted in poor generalization to everyday performance (Ruff et al., 1991; Cicerone et al., 2000, 2005; Sohlberg et al., 2000; Park and Ingles, 2001; Boman et al., 2004; Kennedy et al., 2008). In contrast to skills training, Cicerone et al. (2000) have suggested that cognitive rehabilitation should not focus exclusively on remediation of impairments, but should reduce disability and help restore social role functioning. In an earlier framework, Toglia (1991) proposed a "multi-context" treatment approach to enhance generalizability that contained hallmarks of what later became EE: namely, varied stimulation and environments that are meaningful to the person that thereby enhance engagement. Interventions that have incorporated such components have demonstrated better generalizability, as well as improvements in community integration (Fasotti et al., 2000; Powell et al., 2002; Vance and Johns, 2002; Rath et al., 2003; Van De Winckel et al., 2004; Toglia et al., 2010; Leon-Carrion et al., 2012).

The second broad category of interventions that are more intensive have also resulted in significant functional gains (Willer et al., 1999; Cicerone et al., 2004). Cicerone et al. (2004) compared the effectiveness of an intensive cognitive rehabilitation program to standard neurorehabilitation for persons with TBI. Participants in the intensive program demonstrated greater improvement in cognitive function (composite score based on attention, speed of processing, memory and executive function test scores) as well as greater improvement in community integration. Increasing hours of therapy has also led to greater functional and cognitive gains and faster recoveries (Blackerby, 1990; Spivack et al., 1992; De Weerdt et al., 2000; Shiel et al., 2001; Zhu et al., 2001; Slade et al., 2002; Cifu et al., 2003; De Wit et al., 2005; Zhu et al., 2007). Turner-Stokes et al.'s (2005) review of multi-disciplinary rehabilitation for brain injury recommended that "intensive intervention appears to lead to earlier gains." Therefore, they concluded that "Patients discharged from in-patient rehabilitation should have access to out-patient or community-based services appropriate to their needs." Cernich et al. (2010) provided a similar recommendation in their review of cognitive rehabilitation following TBI. Recently, Hayden et al. (2013) provided support for this recommendation, demonstrating functional gains for TBI survivors receiving rehabilitation services in the post-acute phase after brain injury.

ABSENCE OR REDUCTION OF ENVIRONMENTAL ENRICHMENT

If exposure to EE is beneficial at both behavioral and neural levels, it logically follows that the absence or reduction of EE would lead to poorer behavioral and neural health. Experience-dependent plasticity refers to changes in the brain that result from behavioral experiences. While stimulation can enhance or maintain neural pathways, the absence of stimulation can depress or weaken them with associated loss of a function that was previously acquired or mastered (Rubinov et al., 2009; Warraich and Kleim, 2010). Overall, there appears to be a growing consensus that maintaining and increasing neuroplasticity of the brain depends on continual and intensive cognitive, physical, and social stimulation (Kleim and Jones, 2008). TBI survivors transitioning from a rehabilitation setting to a home setting are therefore vulnerable to reversal of those gains made in the early and intensive therapeutic setting.

This assertion is supported by the flipside of EE experiments: animals that are exposed to less stimulating or impoverished environments do not fare as well. As described above, mice with less EE exposure have lower performances on spatial memory tasks, as compared to continuously enriched mice (Bennett et al., 2006), and rats that received less EE exposure maintain benefits for a shorter period of time (Amaral et al., 2008). Similarly, brain injured rats recovering in impoverished environments show poorer recovery of cognitive and motor functioning (Hamm et al., 1996; Hoffman et al., 2008; Matter et al., 2010; De Witt et al., 2011) and do not maintain benefits gained from short-term EE (Matter et al., 2010; De Witt et al., 2011; Cheng et al., 2012).

Furthermore, there is evidence that effects of environmental conditions are reversible (Bernstein, 1972; Winocur, 1998). Winocur (1998) demonstrated that when he transferred rats from impoverished to enriched environments, they improved significantly, whereas rats transferred from enriched and standard environments to impoverished ones declined. Similarly, more sedentary lifestyles have been linked to disease and disability, and overall poorer health (Huppert, 1991; Pushkar et al., 1997; Mackinnor et al., 2003; Salthouse, 2006; Shors et al., 2012).

ENVIRONMENTAL ENRICHMENT, POST-ACUTE DECLINE AND SUB-ACUTE ATROPHY

As therapies diminish in frequency over time (e.g., when patients move from in-patient neurorehabilitation to the home or a chronic-care facility), the amount of EE may also lessen. In the context of chronic TBI, Turner and Green (2008) examined the principles of negative neuroplasticity (maladaptive morphological changes to the brain in response to environmental factors), as described by Mahncke et al. (2006a,b), in the context of normal aging. These are: (1) reduced schedules of activity, (2) noisy processing in peripheral and central sensory systems, (3) alterations in neuromodulary control, and (4) negative learning. They suggest that a similar downward spiral of negative neuroplastic change may undermine long-term outcome in TBI due to similar environmental changes (as well as physiological changes) that result in withdrawal from communities and social networks, resulting in reduced stimulation. Such changes are withdrawal from the workforce (or school), physical losses that preclude travel, and perceptual and cognitive decrements that compromise communication.

As previously noted, in the case where neural pathways are under-stimulated, it is possible to lose the function that was acquired or mastered (Rubinov et al., 2009; Warraich and Kleim, 2010). Findings of increased neural representation after training (Cirillo et al., 2011; Cardinali et al., 2012) and different brain activation when comparing exposure vs. deprivation of stimulation (Klinge et al., 2012) provide evidence for experience-dependent neuroplasticity. This raises the question whether under-stimulation of neural pathways, due to disuse, may be responsible for post-acute neural degeneration seen in TBI survivors. If so, EE exposure may play a role in minimizing, or averting, this problem.

With respect to neural degeneration, mechanisms of apoptosis have been modeled in animals to understand the cascade of events that takes place after TBI (Raghupathi et al., 2000; Keane et al., 2001; Raghupathi, 2004). Coulson et al. (2004) provided support for their hypothesis that synaptic input may be the key to regulating neuronal survival and death pathways following neurotrauma. Synaptic activity regulates expression levels of neurotrophins and facilitates growth factor signaling. There is evidence that EE exposure enhances nerve growth factor and brain-derived neurotropic factor in animals (Clarkson-Smith and Hartley, 1989; Blackerby, 1990; Bassuk et al., 1999; De Weerdt et al., 2000; Mahoney et al., 2000; Wang et al., 2002; Wilson et al., 2002; Cifu et al., 2003; Johansson, 2003; Rath et al., 2003; Spikman et al., 2009). As well, animal studies have demonstrated that EE can enhance neurogenesis and attenuate apoptosis in the injured brain (Van Praag et al., 2000; Dobrossy and Dunnett, 2001, 2004; Passineau et al., 2001; Gobbo and O'Mara, 2004; Will et al., 2004; Pereira et al., 2007; Hoffman et al., 2008). Lastly, neurons deprived of synaptic input can be rescued from death by an increased supply of growth factors (Coulson et al., 2004). Taken together, these findings offer the possibility that EE can help to prevent neuronal death.

The relation between changes in brain structure and neuropsychological performance has also been recently explored (Farbota et al., 2012), providing further evidence that as we see declines at a neural levels, we also see parallel declines in cognitive functioning. Recent work from our laboratory has demonstrated that in TBI survivors, more engagement in EE, defined as participation in activities involving cognitive, physical, and social demands, is correlated with less hippocampal volume loss in the post-acute stages (Miller and Green, in press). While these findings are correlational, they provide preliminary evidence of the positive impact that an enriched environment can have in TBI survivors.

The research reviewed within this section of the scoping review supports that EE improves outcomes and that a dearth of EE results in poorer outcomes. Studies demonstrate continued and repeated EE exposure (Blackerby, 1990; Spivack et al., 1992; De Weerdt et al., 2000; Schooler and Mulatu, 2001; Shiel et al., 2001; Zhu et al., 2001, 2007; Cifu et al., 2003; De Wit et al., 2005; Amaral et al., 2008), which provides intensive cognitive, social, and physical stimulation is necessary to induce beneficial effects (Willer et al., 1999; Cicerone et al., 2004; Bennett et al., 2006). Furthermore, if this exposure is reduced or removed, the benefits will not be maintained and may diminish (Bernstein, 1972; Winocur, 1998; Cheng et al., 2012). Synaptic input may be necessary to maintain and strengthen neural pathways and connections, particularly those at risk after brain injury (Coulson et al., 2004; Turner and Green, 2008). Moreover, this research supports our contention that for the subset of people with moderate-severe TBI that show post-acute cognitive decline and neural deterioration in the post-acute phase, there may be some environmental variables that contribute to their negative outcomes.

POST-DISCHARGE EXPERIENCES AND ENVIRONMENTAL ENRICHMENT

In the first section, we discussed findings revealing that the brain atrophies and that cognitive abilities decline in the post-acute stages of brain injury. In the second section, we discussed findings that demonstrate that EE can alter the brain (both healthy and damaged), and perhaps most importantly that it has the potential to minimize atrophy after brain injury. Moreover, a mechanism of disuse-mediated atrophy has been proposed (i.e., synaptic input and neuronal survival) (Coulson et al., 2004).

A critical question, then, is to what extent do post-discharge factors reflect EE? This is important because it is possible that the post-discharge environment may be un-enriched, and this would in theory exacerbate/lead to post-acute cognitive and neural declines. Thus, it is of value to explore the factors that influence the environments in which people with brain injuries return with respect to level of enrichment, so that factors can be adjusted to provide *optimal levels of EE*. In the current section, we will discuss how post-discharge variables are conceptually related to EE and we will also discuss findings that show how these examples of EE (or lack thereof) correspond to human TBI outcomes.

WHAT IS ENVIRONMENTAL ENRICHMENT IN THE POST-DISCHARGE ENVIRONMENT?

Continued participation in environments that are challenging, yet at levels that allow people to participate and remain motivated to do so, is the crux of EE. In the section "Environmental Enrichment in Healthy Humans" we summarized findings demonstrating that people who (1) attend more social events, (2) are more physically active, and (3) engage in activities with continuous novelty (e.g., learning a new language, playing bridge) are mentally healthier. While demographic variables (i.e., age, premorbid intelligence, level of education) influence outcome after brain injury (Ruff et al., 1991; Green et al., 2008), environmental variables (e.g., access to insurance coverage) also play a vital role in recovery, as will be discussed. We contend that these variables map onto EE in that they provide cognitive, social, and physical stimulation through access to therapy, community resources, fostering return to meaningful occupations, and encouraging engagement in their environments.

POST-DISCHARGE ENVIRONMENTAL FACTORS THAT INFLUENCE MENTAL AND PHYSICAL STIMULATION

A number of factors influence the degree of cognitive, social, and physical stimulation TBI survivors experience either directly (e.g., presence of community resources such as a support groups or fitness centers) or indirectly (e.g., by influencing access to therapy). These include insurance, financial support, social support, and community resources.

Insurance

As recommended by Turner-Stokes et al. (2005), after discharge from in-patient rehabilitation, TBI survivors should have access to out-patient or community-based services appropriate to their needs to facilitate the recovery process. Till et al. (2008) demonstrated that post-acute cognitive decline was negatively correlated with hours of therapy, which was associated with insurance coverage. It has been widely demonstrated that individuals who have insurance coverage receive more access to therapy after discharge than those who do not (Pressman, 2007; Heffernan et al., 2011; Chen et al., 2012; Lundqvist and Samuelsson, 2012). Those that are insured have better access to post-acute medical care, which includes physical, occupational, and cognitive therapies, as well as home health and nursing needs, modification of living environment, vocational training, and job retraining (Shafi et al., 2007). In line with these findings, Shafi et al. (2007) found that ethnic minorities were less likely to be insured and more likely to have moderate to severe disability at follow-up.

Financial support

Diminished financial resources may reduce opportunities for accessing EEs. For example, Sander et al. (2009) reported that after controlling for age, education, injury severity, and race/ethnicity, income made a significant contribution to the variance in social integration, and in a more recent study, Sander et al. (2011) reported that TBI survivors perceived financial issues (e.g., home ownership, insufficient funds), as contributing to decreased participation in the community. Similar to Shafi et al. (2007) discussed previously, Staudenmayer et al. (2007) examined ethnic disparities in long-term functional outcomes after TBI. They concluded that less social and financial resources were likely implicated as an explanation. Additionally, in a study examining perceived needs after brain injury, many TBI survivors reported still requiring help managing money 1 year post-injury (Corrigan et al., 2004), which may compound the challenges of diminished finances after TBI. Increased financial burden can mean less access to expensive resources (e.g., therapy, participating in social activities, transportation).

Social support

Logically, a supportive social network influences participation in therapy (Sander et al., 2009; Turner et al., 2009b; Keightley et al., 2011), for example by providing transportation, accompaniment to therapies, supervision for recommended regimens for which safety is of concern (e.g., a gym program). Turner et al. (2007) found that those who had more supportive and closer networks at home had better transitions from the hospital setting to the home environment, as this was related to more access to social activities and transportation outside the home.

POST-DISCHARGE FACTORS THAT INFLUENCE ENGAGEMENT

Without private insurance, and with less social and financial resources, TBI survivors may be less able to engage in stimulating activities to facilitate recovery. However, as we will discuss, there are also factors that are purported to influence the level of engagement in the post-discharge environment, such as the amount of family support and patient education provided, as well as the structure and routine present in their home environment.

Family support

In Freeman's (1997) review of community-based rehabilitation for TBI survivors, he suggested that the level of care in the home setting, with a strong support network, can play a major role in successful rehabilitation. The family environment may provide a wide variety of activities that are inclusive, stimulating, and meaningful to the individual. Importantly, these are all properties found to be critical for experience-dependent plasticity (Kleim and Jones, 2008) and generalization of relearnt skills (Toglia, 1991). In a case study by McCormack and Liddiard (2009), a TBI survivor receiving community rehabilitation was followed for 3 years. The authors concluded that the supportive and effective care system in his family facilitated his recovery following severe TBI. His progress was attributed to active familial involvement that fostered goal setting and carry-over between sessions. Furthermore, learning took place in his home environment, increasing his ability to generalize skills. The authors concluded that these findings "add further weight . . . to the thesis that, with the right support, there is no place like home."

Post-discharge information and education

Several studies have indicated that the most often-reported barrier is adequate preparation prior to discharge (Rotondi et al., 2007; Sander et al., 2009; Keightley et al., 2011; Sander et al., 2011; Turner et al., 2011b). Many TBI survivors and their caregivers report that they were not given enough information regarding brain injuries (e.g., behavioral sequelae), how to access community resources (e.g., rehabilitation, emotional support, respite services), or how to access or implement home therapies (Rotondi et al., 2007; Sander et al., 2009, 2011; Keightley et al., 2011; Turner et al., 2011b). Corrigan et al. (2004) reported that TBI survivors who initially reported requiring help participating in recreation still did not have their perceived needs (viewed as a measure of quality of life) met 1 year post-injury. Likewise, Sander et al. (2011) reported that for TBI survivors, feeling more integrated into the community was related to greater participation in their environments. Without receiving appropriate assistance and information/educational resources to facilitate the post-discharge process, successful community integration will continue to be a challenge.

Routine and schedules

Many studies document that TBI survivors report feeling ill-prepared for the transition from hospital to home (Rusconi and Turner-Stokes, 2003). Several qualitative studies have explored the transition home, and the barriers or difficulties that TBI survivors experience (Rittman et al., 2004; Turner et al., 2007, 2009b, 2011a). Rittman et al. (2004) found that, post-discharge, commonly reported problems were increased idle time, boredom, and little-to-no engagement in meaningful activities. Survivors often reported, ". . . finding something new every day that they couldn't do . . ." What appears to influence the above is routine, or lack thereof. When routines were not re-established, survivors and caregivers experienced more chaos and disruption in the transition home. Turner et al. (2011a) examined perspectives concerning recovery and adjustment during the transition phase from hospital to home, and found that the process of adjusting emotionally to life at home posed significant challenges for many brain-injury survivors during this phase.

Turner et al.'s (2007) qualitative study of brain injury survivors' experiences with the transition from hospital to home made similar observations in terms of difficulty re-engaging in meaningful activities and occupations. However, those who were able to create a routine or structure once at home had better transitions. Essentially, this facilitated participation in their environments by providing organization in their daily schedules, which had been previously often provided for them in the rehabilitation setting.

Turner et al. (2009b) extended their work by examining re-engagement in meaningful occupations during the transition from hospital to home in brain-injury survivors. Many survivors reported that recovery sped up at home, and caregivers frequently attributed this to key elements such as creating routines and schedules, which enabled participation in meaningful activities. However, for those that did not have such experiences, not being able to participate in desired occupations led to stress and frustration. Turner et al. (2009b) found that "for some participants, the impact of this change in environment, coupled with the reality of not being able to engage in their desired occupations, led to a relatively unproductive lifestyle in which the main activity of their day involved little more than watching television or playing computer games." In Hoogerdijk et al.'s (2011) study of identity after TBI, the authors suggested that the adaptation process is a necessary struggle to gain new identity and it is facilitated by engagement in familiar occupations in familiar environments. In line with this finding, Nalder et al. (2012a,b) reported that TBI survivors that were able to reengage in meaningful occupations had greater perceived success of the transition from hospital to home. Reengagement in meaningful occupations was often experienced by individuals with higher levels of global functioning and psychosocial integration.

SUMMARY OF POST-DISCHARGE EXPERIENCES AND ENVIRONMENTAL ENRICHMMENT

The research presented in this section of the scoping review provides evidence that there are variables in the post-discharge environment that influence the amount stimulation and other variables that influence the level of engagement in EE. Largely, evidence suggests that those with better access and resources that map onto EE (i.e., insurance coverage, financial and social support) and those that are in environments that encourage participation (i.e., strong familial support, access to educational resources, more structure) have better functional outcomes.

DISCUSSION

The most direct (preliminary) evidence of the benefits of EE in the post-acute stages of recovery comes from work by Miller and Green (in press), where more engagement in enriched environments, defined as participation in activities involving cognitive, physical, and social demands, was correlated with less hippocampal volume loss. Further direct evidence of comes from Till et al.'s (2008) finding of a relationship between hours of therapy at 5 months post-injury and degree of cognitive decline, which the authors speculated was ay be due in part to lack of access to complex and enriched environments.

As we have discussed, a large corpus of studies have demonstrated the benefits of EE in healthy and brain-injured animals. There is evidence of neuroplastic change after EE exposure, with beneficial changes to neuroanatomy and neurochemistry (Kramer et al., 2004). These studies further support Coulson et al.'s (2004) hypothesis that synaptic input is critical to offset atrophy, in that increased input regulates neuronal survival, and prevents or attenuates apoptosis. This is of particular relevance to the neural decline observed in the post-acute stages after TBI. Turner and Green's (2008) re-formulation of the work of Mahncke et al. (2006a,b) in healthy older adults—that negative neuroplasticity (i.e., reduced activity schedules) may undermine long-term outcome in TBI—is also in accord with the hypothesis that EE may indeed play an important role in recovery.

In humans, engaging in cognitively, socially, and physically stimulating activities is related to better cognitive functioning in younger and older adults. Studies have also demonstrated that therapies for TBI survivors delivering continuous and intensified interventions result in better recovery at all levels of analysis, as well as better functional gains. These therapies have critical elements of EE, such as novelty, intensity, and prolonged periods of engagement in meaningful activities.

According to Schooler's (1987) model of environmental complexity, when cognitive efforts are reinforced and rewarded, people are motivated to continue engaging in complex environments, which in turn enhances cognitive functioning. However, TBI survivors may show reduced participation in complex environments, due to cognitive impairment, lack of psychological support/facilitation, or lack of resources, and thereby fail to obtain the emotional and neuromodulatory rewards for engaging. These conditions create a downward spiral of negative neuroplasticity (Turner and Green, 2008). Animal literature examining EE has provided critical evidence for the benefits of maintaining high levels of enrichment and stimulation post-discharge (Hamm et al., 1996; Bennett et al., 2006; Amaral et al., 2008; Hoffman et al., 2008). Findings that support the "Use it or Lose it" theory also suggest that continued engagement in mentally effortful activities is necessary to maintain cognitive functioning (Huppert, 1991; Pushkar et al., 1997; Mackinnor et al., 2003; Salthouse, 2006; Shors et al., 2012), and that an individual's environment (e.g., stressful or under-stimulating) can influence level of activity (Winocur and Moscovitch, 1990; Winocur, 1998). While TBI survivors may benefit from capacity-enhancing and intensified therapies provided in hospital, animal models have demonstrated that the effects of this enrichment will only continue to persist with longer exposure periods (Amaral et al., 2008). Furthermore, transitioning from a more stimulating/complex environment to a lesser one may result in a loss of benefits (Winocur, 1998).

The aim of this paper was to examine the question whether EE in the sub-acute and chronic stages of injury can influence progressive neural and cognitive decline. The aim of the first section was to establish the role of EE in long-term outcomes, and in particular, in offsetting decline; the aim of the second section was to illustrate that in the post-acute stages of injury, a number of factors influence the degree of EE. We have argued that post-discharge environments map onto conventional variables considered to create EE. Access to rehabilitative, social, and community resources, as well as strong support networks, provides essential cognitive, social, and physical stimulation. Moreover, these factors have shown to influence outcomes.

While there is strong evidence to suggest that TBI may be a progressive injury, more research needs to be conducted to further elucidate the role of EE in influencing this decline. It is important to note that the exact active ingredients of current interventions that incorporate multi-context environments and higher intensity therapies are still unclear, and how they compare to therapies that incorporate all elements of EE is still unknown. Furthermore, studies are needed that examine whether there is a correlation between post-acute brain changes and declines in function, as well as the type of environments that TBI survivors return to post-discharge. Turner et al. (2008) recommended that research is needed to explore the transition home after brain injury in order to "(1) Develop a comprehensive theoretical framework of the transition phase; and (2) facilitate both the validation of current intervention strategies and the development of innovative/tailored intervention approaches."

As reported by caregivers and TBI survivors, creating a routine and structure around daily activities facilitated engagement. Furthermore, activities that are meaningful and at an appropriate level (e.g., tailored to the individuals specific impairments) to facilitate participation are critical. Researchers that have examined the needs of TBI survivors and their caregivers in the post-acute phase have recommended increased education provided by health care institutions would be beneficial to ease the transition from hospital to home (Turner et al., 2007, 2009a, 2011b; Arango-Lasprilla et al., 2011). Based on the results of our scoping review, we suggest that more resources and guidelines on how to create structure and daily routines, as well as information regarding self-administered therapies and activities for the individual and their caregiver, would be beneficial. Further rehabilitation support during the post-acute stages of recovery, such as home assessments or on-going therapy maintenance, would also be optimal. Gan et al. (2010) examined the support needs after brain injury and made several recommendations for support services. They suggested that family systems-based services should be accessible, life-long, individualized and flexible, as well as efficient, and that support system-based services should include proper diagnoses, incorporate a multi-component approach, provide brain-injury-specific services that are responsive to needs with proactive follow-ups, and importantly, provide continuous education. The benefits of social peer-mentoring programs as an intervention to enhance improvements in social integration for TBI survivors has also shown promise in recent studies and is currently being further investigated (Struchen et al., 2011; Hanks et al., 2012).

TBI survivors often fail to return to pre-injury levels of cognitive function, as well as employment and income, and these factors have been shown to be related with life satisfaction, perceived quality of life, depression and social isolation (Christensen et al., 2008; Eriksson et al., 2009; Hawthorne et al., 2009; Resch et al., 2009; Shigaki et al., 2009; Strandberg, 2009; Tsaousides et al., 2009). Assuming that post-acute atrophy contributes to the failure to return to pre-injury levels of cognitive function and thus successful community integration, then the clinical consequences are notable.

While the elements that comprise EE may be different from one person to another, it is evident that engagement in such environments is beneficial at both the cognitive and neural level, and thus it is plausible that EE can offset post-acute deterioration. Providing information and support to ease the transition home, information about the benefits of an enriched environment and guidelines on how to successfully participate in enriched settings, may be key elements in improving recovery. Most importantly, it may be a critical factor to facilitate successful community integration.

REFERENCES

Amaral, O. B., Vargas, R. S., Hansel, G., Izquierdo, I., and Souza, D. O. (2008). Duration of environmental enrichment influences the magnitude and persistence of its behavioral effects on mice. *Physiol. Behav.* 93, 388–394.

Arango-Lasprilla, J. C., Nicholls, E., Villasenor Cabrera, T., Drew, A., Jimenez-Maldonado, M., and Martinez-Cortes, M. L. (2011). Health-related quality of life in caregivers of individuals with traumatic brain injury from Guadalajara, Mexico. *J. Rehabil. Med.* 43, 983–986.

Arksey, H., and O'Malley, L. (2005). Scoping studies: towards a methodological framework. *Int. J. Soc. Res. Methodol.* 8, 19–32.

Basso, A. (1989). "Spontaneous recovery and language rehabilitation," in *Cognitive Approaches in Neuropsychological Rehabilitation,* eds X. Seron and G. Deloche (Hillsdale, NJ: Lawrence Erlbaum), 17–37.

Bassuk, S., Glass, T., and Berkman, L. (1999). Social disengagement and incident cognitive decline in community-dwelling elderly persons. *Ann. Intern. Med.* 131, 165–173.

Bendlin, B. B., Ries, M. L., Lazar, M., Alexander, A. L., Dempsey, R. J., Rowley, H. A., et al. (2008). Longitudinal changes in patients with traumatic brain injury assessed with diffusion-tensor and volumetric imaging. *Neuroimage* 42, 503–514.

Bennett, E. L., Rosenzweig, M. R., Diamond, M. C., Morimoto, H., and Hebert, M. (1974). Effects of successive environments on brain measures. *Physiol. Behav.* 12, 621–631.

Bennett, J., McRae, P., Levy, L., and Frick, K. (2006). Long-term continuous, but not daily, environmental enrichment reduces spatial memory decline in aged male mice. *Neurobiol. Learn. Mem.* 85, 139–152.

Bernstein, L. (1972). The reversibility of learning deficits in early environmentally restricted rats as a function of amount of experience in later life. *J. Psychosom. Res.* 16, 71–73.

Bigler, E. D., Blatter, D. D., Anderson, C. V., Johnson, S. C., Gale, S. D., Hopkins, R. O., et al. (1997). Hippocampal volume in normal aging and traumatic brain injury. *AJNR Am. J. Neuroradiol.* 18, 11–23.

Blackerby, W. F. (1990). Intensity of rehabilitation and length of stay. *Brain Inj.* 4, 167–173.

Blatter, D. D., Bigler, E. D., Gale, S. D., Johnson, S. C., Anderson, C. V., Burnett, B. M., et al. (1997). MR-based brain and cerebrospinal fluid measurement after traumatic brain injury: correlation with neuropsychological outcome. *AJNR Am. J. Neuroradiol.* 18, 1–10.

Boman, I. L., Lindstedt, M., Hemmingsson, H., and Bartfai, A. (2004). Cognitive training in home environment. *Brain Inj.* 18, 985–995.

Bruns, J. Jr., and Hauser, W. A. (2003). The epidemiology of traumatic brain injury: a review. *Epilepsia* 44(Suppl. 10), 2–10.

Cardinali, L., Jacobs, S., Brozzoli, C., Frassinetti, F., Roy, A. C., and Farne, A. (2012). Grab an object with a tool and change your body: tool-use-dependent changes of body representation for action. *Exp. Brain Res.* 218, 259–271.

Cassidy, J. D., Carroll, L. J., Peloso, P. M., Borg, J., Von Holst, H., Holm, L., et al. (2004). Incidence, risk factors and prevention of mild traumatic brain injury: results of the WHO collaborating centre task force on mild traumatic brain injury. *J. Rehabil. Med.* 43(Suppl), 28–60.

Cernich, A. N., Kurtz, S. M., Mordecai, K. L., and Ryan, P. B. (2010). Cognitive rehabilitation in traumatic brain injury. *Curr. Treat. Options Neurol.* 12, 412–423.

Chen, A. Y., Zagorski, B., Parsons, D., Vander Laan, R., Chan, V., and Colantonio, A. (2012). Factors associated with discharge destination from acute care after acquired brain injury in Ontario, Canada. *BMC Neurol.* 12:16. doi: 10.1186/1471-2377-12-16

Cheng, J. P., Shaw, K. E., Monaco, C. M., Hoffman, A. N., Sozda, C. N., Olsen, A. S., et al. (2012). A relatively brief exposure to environmental enrichment after experimental traumatic brain injury confers long-term cognitive benefits. *J. Neurotrauma* 29, 2684–2688.

Christensen, B. K., Colella, B., Inness, E., Hebert, D., Monette, G., Bayley, M., et al. (2008). Recovery of cognitive function after traumatic brain injury: a multilevel modeling analysis of Canadian outcomes. *Arch. Phys. Med. Rehabil.* 89, S3–S15.

Christensen, H., and Mackinnon, A. (1993). The association between mental, social and physical activity and cognitive performance in young and old subjects. *Age Ageing* 22, 175–183.

Christodoulou, C., Deluca, J., Ricker, J. H., Madigan, N. K., Bly, B. M., Lange, G., et al. (2001). Functional magnetic resonance imaging of working memory impairment after traumatic brain injury. *J. Neurol. Neurosurg. Psychiatry* 71, 161–168.

Churchill, J. D., Galvez, R., Colcombe, S., Swain, R. A., Kramer, A. F., and Greenough, W. T. (2002). Exercise, experience and the aging brain. *Neurobiol. Aging* 23, 941–955.

Cicerone, K., Mott, T., Azulay, J., and Friel, J. (2004). Community integration and satisfaction with functioning after intensive cognitive rehabilitation for traumatic brain injury. *Arch. Phys. Med. Rehabil.* 85, 943–950.

Cicerone, K. D., Dahlberg, C., Kalmar, K., Langenbahn, D. M., Malec, J. F., Bergquist, T. F., et al. (2000).

Evidence-based cognitive rehabilitation: recommendations for clinical practice. *Arch. Phys. Med. Rehabil.* 81, 1596–1615.

Cicerone, K. D., Dahlberg, C., Malec, J. F., Langenbahn, D. M., Felicetti, T., Kneipp, S., et al. (2005). Evidence-based cognitive rehabilitation: updated review of the literature from 1998 through 2002. *Arch. Phys. Med. Rehabil.* 86, 1681–19692.

Cifu, D. X., Kreutzer, J. S., Kolakowsky-Hayner, S. A., Marwitz, J. H., and Englander, J. (2003). The relationship between therapy intensity and rehabilitative outcomes after traumatic brain injury: a multicenter analysis. *Arch. Phys. Med. Rehabil.* 84, 1441–1448.

C.I.H.I. (2006). Head injuries in Canada: a decade of change (1994-1995 to 2003-2004). *National Trauma Regist. Anal. Brief.* Available online at: http://secure.cihi.ca/cihiweb/dispPage.jsp?cw_page=bl_ntr_aug2006_e. [Accessed February 10, 2010].

Cirillo, J., Todd, G., and Semmler, J. G. (2011). Corticomotor excitability and plasticity following complex visuomotor training in young and old adults. *Eur. J. Neurosci.* 34, 1847–1856.

Clarkson-Smith, L., and Hartley, A. (1989). Relationships between physical exercise and cognitive abilities in older adults. *Psychol. Aging* 2, 183–189.

Corrigan, J. D., Whiteneck, G., and Mellick, D. (2004). Perceived needs following traumatic brain injury. *J. Head Trauma Rehabil.* 19, 205–216.

Coulson, E. J., Reid, K., Shipham, K. M., Morley, S., Kilpatrick, T. J., and Bartlett, P. F. (2004). The role of neurotransmission and the Chopper domain in p75 neurotrophin receptor death signaling. *Prog. Brain Res.* 146, 41–62.

Crowe, M., Andel, R., Pedersen, N., Johansson, B., and Gatz, M. (2003). Does participation in leisure activities lead to a reduced risk of Alzheimer's disease? A prospective study of Swedish twins. *J. Gerontol. Ser. B* 58B, 249–255.

Davidson, A., and Bar-Yam, Y. (2006). "Environmental complexity: information for human-environment well-being," in *Unifying Themes in Complex Systems*, eds A. Bar-Yam and Y. Minai (New England; Berlin; Heidelberg: Springer), 157–168.

De Weerdt, W., Selz, B., Nuyens, G., Staes, F., Swinnen, D., Van De Winckel, A., et al. (2000). Time use of stroke patients in an intensive rehabilitation unit: a comparison between a Belgian and a Swiss setting. *Disabil. Rehabil.* 22, 181–186.

De Wit, L., Putman, K., Dejaeger, E., Baert, I., Berman, P., Bogaerts, K., et al. (2005). Use of time by stroke patients: a comparison of four european rehabilitation centers. *Stroke* 36, 1977–1983.

De Witt, B. W., Ehrenberg, K. M., McAloon, R. L., Panos, A. H., Shaw, K. E., Raghavan, P. V., et al. (2011). Abbreviated environmental enrichment enhances neurobehavioral recovery comparably to continuous exposure after traumatic brain injury. *Neurorehabil. Neural Repair* 25, 343–350.

Diamond, M. (2001). Response of the brain to enrichment. *An. Acad. Bras. Cienc.* 73, 211–220.

Dikmen, S., Reitan, R. M., and Temkin, N. R. (1983). Neuropsychological recovery in head injury. *Arch. Neurol.* 40, 333–338.

Dikmen, S. S., Ross, B. L., Machamer, J. E., and Temkin, N. R. (1995). One year psychosocial outcome in head injury. *J. Int. Neuropsychol. Soc.* 1, 67–77.

Dobrossy, M. D., and Dunnett, S. B. (2001). The influence of environment and experience on neural grafts. *Nat. Rev. Neurosci.* 2, 871–879.

Dobrossy, M. D., and Dunnett, S. B. (2004). Environmental enrichment affects striatal graft morphology and functional recovery. *Eur. J. Neurosci.* 19, 159–168.

Eckert, M. J., and Abraham, W. C. (2012). "Effects of environmental enrichment exposure on synaptic transmission and plasticity in the hippocampus," in *Current Topics in Behavorial Neurosciences*, eds M. A. Geyer, B. A. Ellenbroek, and C. A. Marsden (Berlin; Heidelberg: Springer), 1–23.

Eriksson, G., Kottorp, A., Borg, J., and Tham, K. (2009). Relationship between occupational gaps in everyday life, depressive mood and life satisfaction after acquired brain injury. *J. Rehabil. Med.* 41, 187–194.

Farbota, K. D., Bendlin, B. B., Alexander, A. L., Rowley, H. A., Dempsey, R. J., and Johnson, S. C. (2012). Longitudinal diffusion tensor imaging and neuropsychological correlates in traumatic brain injury patients. *Front. Hum. Neurosci.* 6:160. doi: 10.3389/fnhum.2012.00160

Fares, R. P., Belmeguenai, A., Sanchez, P. E., Kouchi, H. Y., Bodennec, J., Morales, A., et al. (2013). Standardized environmental enrichment supports enhanced brain plasticity in healthy rats and prevents cognitive impairment in epileptic rats. *PLoS ONE* 8:e53888. doi: 10.1371/journal.pone.0053888

Farne, A., Buxbaum, L. J., Ferraro, M., Frassinetti, F., Whyte, J., Veramonti, T., et al. (2004). Patterns of spontaneous recovery of neglect and associated disorders in acute right brain-damaged patients. *J. Neurol. Neurosurg. Psychiatr.* 75, 1401–1410.

Fasotti, L., Kovacs, F., Eling, P., and Brouwer, W. (2000). Time pressure management as a compensatory strategy training after closed head injury. *Neuropsychol. Rehabil.* 10, 47–65.

Faul, M., Xu, L., Wald, M. M., and Coronado, V. G. (2010). Traumatic Brain Injury in the United States: Emergency Department Visits, Hospitalizations, and Deaths. Atlanta: Centers for Disease Control and Prevention, National Center for Injury Prevention and Control.

Fratiglioni, L., Wang, H., Ericsson, K., Maytan, M., and Winblad, B. (2000). Influence of social network on occurrence of dementia: a community-based longitudinal study. *Lancet* 355, 1315–1319.

Freeman, E. A. (1997). Community-based rehabilitation of the person with a severe brain injury. *Brain Inj.* 11, 143–153.

Fujiwara, Y., Chaves, P. H., Yoshida, H., Amano, H., Fukaya, T., Watanabe, N., et al. (2009). Intellectual activity and likelihood of subsequently improving or maintaining instrumental activities of daily living functioning in community-dwelling older Japanese: a longitudinal study. *Int. J. Geriatr. Psychiatry* 24, 547–555.

Gabriel, A., Paoletti, G., Della Seta, D., Panelli, R., Marcus, M., Farabollini, F., et al. (2009a). Enriched environment and the recovery from inflammatory pain: social versus physical aspects and their interaction. *Behav. Brain Res.* 208, 90–95.

Gabriel, A. F., Marcus, M. A., Honig, W. M., Helgers, N., and Joosten, E. A. (2009b). Environmental housing affects the duration of mechanical allodynia and the spinal astroglial activation in a rat model of chronic inflammatory pain. *Brain Res.* 1276, 83–90.

Gan, C., Gargaro, J., Brandys, C., Gerber, G., and Boschen, K. (2010). Family caregivers' support needs after brain injury: a synthesis of perspectives from caregivers, programs, and researchers. *NeuroRehabilitation* 27, 5–18.

Gobbo, O. L., and O'Mara, S. M. (2004). Impact of enriched-environment housing on brain-derived neurotrophic factor and on cognitive performance after a transient global ischemia. *Behav. Brain Res.* 152, 231–241.

Green, R. E., Colella, B., Christensen, B., Johns, K., Frasca, D., Bayley, M., et al. (2008). Examining moderators of cognitive recovery trajectories after moderate to severe traumatic brain injury. *Arch. Phys. Med. Rehabil.* 89, S16–S24.

Green, R. E., Melo, B., Christensen, B., Ngo, L., and Skene, C. (2006). Evidence of transient enhancement to cognitive functioning in healthy young adults through environmental enrichment: implications for rehabilitation after brain injury. *Brain Cogn.* 60, 201–203.

Greenberg, G., Mikulis, D. J., Ng, K., Desouza, D., and Green, R. E. (2008). Use of diffusion tensor imaging to examine subacute white matter injury progression in moderate to severe traumatic brain injury. *Arch. Phys. Med. Rehabil.* 89, S45–S50.

Gribbin, K., Schaie, K., and Parham, I. (1980). Complexity of life style and maintenance of intellectual abilities. *J. Soc. Issues* 36, 47–61.

Gunther, V. K., Schafer, P., Holzner, B. J., and Kemmler, G. W. (2003). Long-term improvements in cognitive performance through computer-assisted cognitive training: a pilot study in a residential home for older people. *Aging Ment. Health* 7, 200–206.

Hamm, R., Temple, M., O'Dell, D., Pike, B., and Lyeth, B. (1996). Exposure to environmental complexity promotes recovery of cognitive function after traumtic brain injury. *J. Neurotrauma* 13, 41–47.

Hanks, R. A., Rapport, L. J., Wertheimer, J., and Koviak, C. (2012). Randomized controlled trial of peer mentoring for individuals with traumatic brain injury and their significant others. *Arch. Phys. Med. Rehabil.* 93, 1297–1304.

Hawthorne, G., Gruen, R. L., and Kaye, A. H. (2009). Traumatic brain injury and long-term quality of life: findings from an Australian study. *J. Neurotrauma* 26, 1623–1633.

Hayden, M. E., Plenger, P., Bison, K., Kowalske, K., Masel, B., and Qualls, D. (2013). Treatment effect versus pretreatment recovery in persons with traumatic brain injury: a study regarding the effectiveness of postacute rehabilitation. *PM R.* doi: 10.1016/j.pmrj.2012.12.005. [Epub ahead of print].

Hayslip, B., Maloy, R. M., and Kohl, R. (1995). Long-term efficacy of fluid ability interventions with older adults. *J. Gerontol. Ser. B Psychol. Sci. Soc. Sci.* 50, P141–P149.

Hebb, D. O. (1947). The effects of early experience on problem solving in maturity. *Am. Psychol.* 2, 306–307.

Heffernan, D. S., Vera, R. M., Monaghan, S. F., Thakkar, R. K., Kozloff, M. S., Connolly, M. D., et al. (2011). Impact of socioethnic factors on outcomes following traumatic brain injury. *J. Trauma* 70, 527–534.

Heinemann, A. W., Hamilton, B., Linacre, J. M., Wright, B. D., and Granger, C. (1995). Functional status and therapeutic intensity during inpatient rehabilitation. *Am. J. Phys. Med. Rehabil.* 74, 315–326.

Himanen, L., Portin, R., Isoniemi, H., Helenius, H., Kurki, T., and Tenovuo, O. (2006). Longitudinal cognitive changes in traumatic brain injury: a 30-year follow-up study. *Neurology* 66, 187–192.

Hoffman, A., Malena, R., Westergoma, B., Luthra, P., Chenga, J., Aslama, H., et al. (2008). Environmental enrichment-mediated functional improvement after experimental traumatic brain injury is contingent on task-specific neurobehavioral experience. *Neurosci. Lett.* 431, 226–230.

Holbrook, T. L., Anderson, J. P., Sieber, W. J., Browner, D., and Hoyt, D. B. (1999). Outcome after major trauma: 12-month and 18-month follow-up results from the Trauma Recovery Project. *J. Trauma* 46, 765–771. discussion: 771–763.

Hoogerdijk, B., Runge, U., and Haugboelle, J. (2011). The adaptation process after traumatic brain injury an individual and ongoing occupational struggle to gain a new identity. *Scand. J. Occup. Ther.* 18, 122–132.

Hudak, A., Warner, M., Marquez De La Plata, C., Moore, C., Harper, C., and Diaz-Arrastia, R. (2011). Brain morphometry changes and depressive symptoms after traumatic brain injury. *Psychiatry Res.* 191, 160–165.

Huppert, F. (1991). *Age-Related Changes in Memory: Learning and Remembering New Information.* Amsterdam: Elsevier Science Publishers.

Johansson, B. B. (2000). Brain plasticity and stroke rehabilitation: the Willis lecture. *Stroke* 31, 223–230.

Johansson, B. B. (2002). "Environmental effects on recovery after stroke," in *Cerebrovascular Disease, 22nd Princeton Conference*, ed P. H. Chan (New York, NY: Cambridge University Press), 328–336.

Johansson, B. B. (2003). Environmental influence on recovery after brain lesions - experimental and clinical data. *J. Rehabil. Med.* 35, 11–16.

Johansson, B. B., and Ohlsson, A. L. (1996). Environment, social interaction, and physical activity as determinants of functional outcome after cerebral infarction in the rat. *Exp. Neurol.* 139, 322–327.

Jung, C. K., and Herms, J. (2012). Structural dynamics of dendritic spines are influenced by an environmental enrichment: an *in vivo* imaging study. *Cereb. Cortex.* doi: 10.1093/cercor/bhs317. [Epub ahead of print].

Keane, R. W., Kraydieh, S., Lotocki, G., Alonso, O. F., Aldana, P., and Dietrich, W. D. (2001). Apoptotic and antiapoptotic mechanisms after traumatic brain injury. *J. Cereb. Blood Flow Metab.* 21, 1189–1198.

Keightley, M., Kendall, V., Jang, S. H., Parker, C., Agnihotri, S., Colantonio, A., et al. (2011). From health care to home community: an Aboriginal community-based ABI transition strategy. *Brain Inj.* 25, 142–152.

Kempermann, M., Gast, G., and Gage, F. (2002). Neuroplasticity in old age: sustained fivefold induction of hippocampal neurogensis by long-term environmental enrichment. *Ann. Neurol.* 52, 135–143.

Kennedy, M., Coelho, C., Turkstra, L., Ylvisaker, M., Sohlberg, M., Yorkston, K., et al. (2008). Intervention for executive functions after traumatic brain injury: a systematic review, meta-analysis and clinical recommendations. *Neuropsychol. Rehabil.* 18, 257–299.

Kim, J., Whyte, J., Patel, S., Avants, B., Europa, E., Wang, J., et al. (2010). Resting cerebral blood flow alterations in chronic traumatic brain injury: an arterial spin labeling perfusion FMRI study. *J. Neurotrauma* 27, 1399–1411.

Kleim, J. A., and Jones, T. A. (2008). Principles of experience-dependent neural plasticity: implications for rehabilitation after brain damage. *J. Speech Lang. Hear. Res.* 51, S225–S239.

Klinge, C., Roder, B., and Buchel, C. (2012). Does training or deprivation modulate amygdala activation? *Neuroimage* 59, 1765–1771.

Kobayashi, S., Ohashi, Y., and Ando, S. (2002). Effects of enriched environments with different durations and starting times on learning capacity during aging in rats assessed by a refined procedure of the Hebb-Williams maze task. *J. Neurosci. Res.* 70, 340–346.

Kolb, B., and Whishaw, I. (1998). Brain plasticity and behaviour. *Annu. Rev. Psychol.* 49, 43–64.

Kramer, A. F., Bherer, L., Colcombe, S. J., Dong, W., and Greenough, W. T. (2004). Environmental influences on cognitive and brain plasticity during aging. *J. Gerontol. Ser. A Biol. Sci. Med. Sci.* 59, M940–M957.

Latham, N., and Mason, G. (2010). Frustration and perseveration in stereotypic captive animals: is a taste of enrichment worse than none at all? *Behav. Brain Res.* 211, 96–104.

Leger, M., Quiedeville, A., Paizanis, E., Natkunarajah, S., Freret, T., Boulouard, M., et al. (2012). Environmental enrichment enhances episodic-like memory in association with a modified neuronal activation profile in adult mice. *PLoS ONE* 7:e48043. doi: 10.1371/journal.pone.0048043

Leon-Carrion, J., Dominguez-Morales, M. R., Barroso Y Martin, J. M., and Leon-Dominguez, U. (2012). Recovery of cognitive function during comprehensive rehabilitation after severe traumatic brain injury. *J. Rehabil. Med.* 44, 505–511.

Levine, B., Kovacevic, N., Nica, E. I., Cheung, G., Gao, F., Schwartz, M. L., et al. (2008). The Toronto traumatic brain injury study: injury severity and quantified MRI. *Neurology* 70, 771–778.

Lezak, M. (2004). "The neuropsychological examination: procedures," in *Neuropsychological Assessment*, ed M. Lezak (New York, NY: Oxford University Press), 110–143.

Lippert-Gruener, M., Maegele, M., Garbe, J., and Angelov, D. N. (2007). Late effects of enriched environment (EE) plus multimodal early onset stimulation (MEOS) after traumatic brain injury in rats: ongoing improvement of neuromotor function despite sustained volume of the CNS lesion. *Exp. Neurol.* 203, 82–94.

Lores-Arnaiz, S., Lores Arnaiz, M. R., Czerniczyniec, A., Cuello, M., and Bustamante, J. (2010). Mitochondrial function and nitric oxide production in hippocampus and cerebral cortex of rats exposed to enriched environment. *Brain Res.* 1319, 44–53.

Lundqvist, A., and Samuelsson, K. (2012). Return to work after acquired brain injury: a patient perspective. *Brain Inj.* 26, 13–14.

Mackenzie, J. D., Siddiqi, F., Babb, J. S., Bagley, L. J., Mannon, L. J., Sinson, G. P., et al. (2002). Brain atrophy in mild or moderate traumatic brain injury: a longitudinal quantitative analysis. *AJNR Am. J. Neuroradiol.* 23, 1509–1515.

Mackinnor, A., Christensen, H., Hofer, S., Korten, A., and Jorm, A. (2003). Use it and still lose it? The association between activity and cognitive performance established using latent growth techniques in a community sample. *Aging Neuropsychol. Cogn.* 10, 215–229.

Mahncke, H., Connor, B., Appelman, J., Ahsanuddin, O., Hardy, J., Wood, R., et al. (2006a). Memory enhancement in healthy older adults using a brain plasticity-based training program: a randomized, controlled study. *Proc. Natl. Acad. Sci. U.S.A.* 103, 12523–12528.

Mahncke, H. W., Bronstone, A., and Merzenich, M. M. (2006b). Brain plasticity and functional losses in the aged: scientific bases for a novel intervention. *Prog. Brain Res.* 157, 81–109.

Mahoney, J., Eisner, J., Havighurst, T., Gray, S., and Palta, M. (2000). Problems of older adults living alone after hospitalization. *J. Gen. Int. Med.* 15, 611–619.

Marioni, R. E., Valenzuela, M. J., Van Den Hout, A., Brayne, C., and Matthews, F. E. (2012a). Active cognitive lifestyle is associated with positive cognitive health transitions and compression of morbidity from age sixty-five. *PLoS ONE* 7:e50940. doi: 10.1371/journal.pone.0050940

Marioni, R. E., Van Den Hout, A., Valenzuela, M. J., Brayne, C., and Matthews, F. E. (2012b). Active cognitive lifestyle associates with cognitive recovery and a reduced risk of cognitive decline. *J. Alzheimers Dis.* 28, 223–230.

Matter, A. M., Folweiler, K. A., Curatolo, L. M., and Kline, A. E. (2010). Temporal effects of environmental enrichment-mediated functional improvement after experimental traumatic brain injury in rats. *Neurorehabil. Neural Repair* 25, 558–564.

McCormack, E., and Liddiard, H. (2009). Home or away? Community rehabilitation following traumatic brain injury: a case report. *Physiother. Res. Int.* 14, 66–71.

Meagher, R. K., and Mason, G. J. (2012). Environmental enrichment reduces signs of boredom in caged mink. *PLoS ONE* 7:e49180. doi: 10.1371/journal.pone.0049180

Milgram, N. (2003). Cognitive experience and its effect on age-dependent cognitive decline in beagle dogs. *Neurochem. Res.* 2, 1677–1682.

Miller, L., and Green, R. E. (in press). Can environmental enrichment serve as a protective intervention for neurodegeneration in traumatic brain injury? *Front. Hum. Neurosci.*

Millis, S. R., Rosenthal, M., Novack, T. A., Sherer, M., Nick, T. G., Kreutzer, J. S., et al. (2001). Long-term neuropsychological outcome after traumatic brain injury. *J. Head Trauma Rehabil.* 16, 343–355.

Mohammed, A. K., Winblad, B., Ebendal, T., and Larkfors, L. (1990). Environmental influence on behaviour and nerve growth factor in the brain. *Brain Res.* 528, 62–72.

Monaco, C. M., Mattiola, V. V., Folweiler, K. A., Tay, J. K., Yelleswarapu, N. K., Curatolo, L. M., et al. (2013). Environmental enrichment promotes robust functional and histological benefits in female rats after controlled cortical impact injury. *Exp. Neurol.* doi: 10.1016/j.expneurol.2013.01.007. [Epub ahead of print].

Murray, C. J., and Lopez, A. D. (1997). Alternative projections of mortality and disability by cause 1990-2020: Global Burden of Disease Study. *Lancet* 349, 1498–1504.

Nalder, E., Fleming, J., Cornwell, P., Foster, M., and Haines, T. (2012a). Factors associated with the occurrence of sentinel events during transition from hospital to home for individuals with traumatic brain injury. *J. Rehabil. Med.* 44, 837–844.

Nalder, E., Fleming, J., Foster, M., Cornwell, P., Shields, C., and Khan, A. (2012b). Identifying factors associated with perceived success in the transition from hospital to home after brain injury. *J. Head Trauma Rehabil.* 27, 143–153.

Narayan, R. K., Michel, M. E., Ansell, B., Baethmann, A., Biegon, A., Bracken, M. B., et al. (2002). Clinical trials in head injury. *J. Neurotrauma* 19, 503–557.

Neely, A. S., and Backman, L. (1995). Effects of multifactorial memory training in old age: generalizability across tasks and individuals. *J. Gerontol. Ser. B Psychol. Sci. Soc. Sci.* 50, P134–P140.

Newson, R., and Kemps, E. (2005). General lifestyle activities as a predictor of current cognition and cognitive change in older adults: a cross-sectional and longitudinal examination. *J. Gerontol.* 60B, P113.

Ng, K., Mikulis, D. J., Glazer, J., Kabani, N., Till, C., Greenberg, G., et al. (2008). Magnetic resonance imaging evidence of progression of subacute brain atrophy in moderate to severe traumatic brain injury. *Arch. Phys. Med. Rehabil.* 89, S35–S44.

Nilsson, M., Perfilieva, E., Johansson, U., Orwar, O., and Eriksson, P. S. (1999). Enriched environment increases neurogenesis in the adult rat dentate gyrus and improves spatial memory. *J. Neurobiol.* 39, 569–578.

Noice, H., and Noice, T. (2004). A short term intervention to enhance cognitive and affective functioning in older adults. *J. Aging Health* 16, 562–585.

Paillard-Borg, S., Fratiglioni, L., Xu, W., Winblad, B., and Wang, H. X. (2012). An active lifestyle postpones dementia onset by more than one year in very old adults. *J. Alzheimers Dis.* 31, 835–842.

Park, N. W., and Ingles, J. L. (2001). Effectiveness of attention rehabilitation after an acquired brain injury: a meta-analysis. *Neuropsychology* 15, 199–210.

Passineau, M., Green, E., and Dalton, D. (2001). Therapeutic effects of environmental enrichment on cognitive function and tissue integrity following severe traumatic brain injury in rats. *Exp. Neurol.* 168, 373–384.

Pereira, L. O., Arteni, N. S., Petersen, R. C., Da Rocha, A. P., Achaval, M., and Netto, C. A. (2007). Effects of daily environmental enrichment on memory deficits and brain injury following neonatal hypoxia-ischemia in the rat. *Neurobiol. Learn. Mem.* 87, 101–108.

Pickett, W., Simpson, K., and Brison, R. J. (2004). Rates and external causes of blunt head trauma in Ontario: analysis and review of Ontario Trauma Registry datasets. *Chronic Dis. Can.* 25, 32–41.

Pietropaolo, S., Branchi, I., Cirulli, F., Chiarotti, F., Aloe, L., and Alleva, E. (2004). Long-term effects of the periadolescent environment on exploratory activity and aggressive behaviour in mice: social versus physical enrichment. *Physiol. Behav.* 81, 443–453.

Pignatti, F., Rozzini, R., and Trabucchi, M. (2002). Physical activity and cognitive decline in elderly persons. *Arch. Intern. Med.* 162, P361.

Powell, J., Heslin, J., and Greenwood, R. (2002). Community based rehabilitation after severe traumatic brain injury: a randomised controlled trial. *J. Neurol. Neurosurg. Psychiatr.* 72, 193–202.

Pressman, H. T. (2007). Traumatic brain injury rehabilitation: case management and insurance-related issues. *Phys. Med. Rehabil. Clin. N. Am.* 18, 165–174. viii.

Pushkar, D., Arbuckle, T., Conway, M., Chaikelson, J., and Maag, U. (1997). Everyday activity parameters and competence in older adults. *Psychol. Aging* 12, 600–609.

Qiu, X., Huang, C. X., Lu, W., Yang, S., Li, C., Shi, X. Y., et al. (2012). Effects of a 4 month enriched environment on the hippocampus and the myelinated fibers in the hippocampus of middle-aged rats. *Brain Res.* 1465, 26–33.

Qiu, X., Li, C., Jiang, R., Chen, L., Huang, C., Yang, S., et al. (2011). The effects of short-term enriched environment on capillaries of the middle-aged rat cortex. *Neurosci. Lett.* 505, 186–190.

Raghupathi, R. (2004). Cell death mechanisms following traumatic brain injury. *Brain Pathol.* 14, 215–222.

Raghupathi, R., Graham, D. I., and McIntosh, T. K. (2000). Apoptosis after traumatic brain injury. *J. Neurotrauma* 17, 927–938.

Rath, J., Simon, D., Langenbahn, D., Sherr, R., and Diller, L. (2003). Group treatment of problem-solving deficits in outpatients with traumatic brain injury: a randomised outcome study. *Neuropsychol. Rehabil.* 13, 461–488.

Resch, J. A., Villarreal, V., Johnson, C. L., Elliott, T. R., Kwok, O. M., Berry, J. W., et al. (2009). Trajectories of life satisfaction in the first 5 years following traumatic brain injury. *Rehabil. Psychol.* 54, 51–59.

Rittman, M., Faircloth, C., Boylstein, C., Gubrium, J. F., Williams, C., Van Puymbroeck, M., et al. (2004). The experience of time in the transition from hospital to home following stroke. *J. Rehabil. Res. Dev.* 41, 259–268.

Rosenzweig, M. (1966). Environmental complexity, cerebral change, and behavior. *Am. Psychol.* 21, 321–332.

Rosenzweig, M., and Bennett, E. (1996). Psychobiology of plasticity: effects of training and experience on brain and behaviour. *Behav. Brain Res.* 78, 57–65.

Rotondi, A. J., Sinkule, J., Balzer, K., Harris, J., and Moldovan, R. (2007). A qualitative needs assessment of persons who have experienced traumatic brain injury and their primary family caregivers. *J. Head Trauma Rehabil.* 22, 14–25.

Rubinov, M., McIntosh, A. R., Valenzuela, M. J., and Breakspear, M. (2009). Simulation of neuronal death and network recovery in a computational model of distributed cortical activity. *Am. J. Geriatr. Psychiatry* 17, 210–217.

Ruff, R., Barth, J., Kreutzer, J., Levin, H., and Foulkes, M. (1991). Verbal learning deficits following severe head injury: heterogeneity in recovery over 1 year. *J. Neurosurg.* 75, S50–S58.

Rumrill, P. D., Fitzgerald, S. M., and Merchant, W. R. (2010). Using scoping literature reviews as a means of understanding and interpreting existing literature. *Work* 35, 399–404.

Rusconi, S., and Turner-Stokes, L. (2003). An evaluation of aftercare following discharge from a specialist in-patient rehabilitation service. *Disabil. Rehabil.* 25, 1281–1288.

Salmond, C. H., Menon, D. K., Chatfield, D. A., Pickard, J. D., and Sahakian, B. J. (2006). Changes over time in cognitive and structural profiles of head injury survivors. *Neuropsychologia* 44, 1995–1998.

Salthouse, T. (2006). Mental exercise and mental aging: evaluating the validity of the "use it or lose it" hypothesis. *Perspect. Psychol. Sci.* 1, 68–87.

Sampson, E. L., Bulpitt, C. J., and Fletcher, A. E. (2009). Survival of community-dwelling older people: the effect of cognitive impairment and social engagement. *J. Am. Geriatr. Soc.* 57, 985–991.

Sander, A. M., Clark, A., and Pappadis, M. R. (2010). What is community integration anyway?: defining meaning following traumatic brain injury. *J. Head Trauma Rehabil.* 25, 121–127.

Sander, A. M., Pappadis, M. R., Clark, A. N., and Struchen, M. A. (2011). Perceptions of community integration in an ethnically diverse sample. *J. Head Trauma Rehabil.* 26, 158–169.

Sander, A. M., Pappadis, M. R., Davis, L. C., Clark, A. N., Evans, G., Struchen, M. A., et al. (2009). Relationship of race/ethnicity and income to community integration following traumatic brain injury: investigation in a non-rehabilitation trauma sample. *NeuroRehabilitation* 24, 15–27.

Sander, A. M., Roebuck, T. M., Struchen, M. A., Sherer, M., and High, W. M. (2001). Long-term maintenance of gains obtained in postacute rehabilitation by persons with traumatic brain injury. *J. Head Trauma Rehabil.* 16, 356–373.

Scarmeas, N., and Stern, Y. (2003). Cognitive reserve and lifestyle. *J. Clin. Exp. Neuropsychol.* 25, 625–633.

Schooler, C. (1987). "Psychological effects of complex environments during the life span: a review and theory," in *Cognitive Functioning and Social Structure Over the Life Course*, ed C. S. K. W. Schaie (Norwood, NJ: Ablex), 24–49.

Schooler, C., and Mulatu, M. (2001). The reciprocal effects of leisure time activities and intellectual functioning in older people: a longitudinal analysis. *Psychol. Aging* 16, 466–482.

Schuit, A., Feskens, E., Launer, L., and Kromhout, D. (2001). Physical activity and cognitive decline, the role of apolipoprotein e4 allele. *Med. Sci. Sports Exerc.* 33, 772–777.

Seeman, T., Lusignolo, T., Albert, M., and Berkman, L. (2001). Social relationships, social support, and patterns of cognitive aging in healthy, high-functioning older adults: MacArthur studies of successful aging. *Health Psychol.* 20, 243–255.

Shafi, S., Marquez De La Plata, C., Diaz-Arrastia, R., Shipman, K., Carlile, M., Frankel, H., et al. (2007). Racial disparities in long-term functional outcome after traumatic brain injury. *J. Trauma* 63, 1263–1268. discussion: 1268–1270.

Shiel, A., Burn, J. P., Henry, D., Clark, J., Wilson, B. A., Burnett, M. E., et al. (2001). The effects of increased rehabilitation therapy after brain injury: results of a prospective controlled trial. *Clin. Rehabil.* 15, 501–514.

Shigaki, C. L., Johnstone, B., and Schopp, L. H. (2009). Financial and vocational outcomes 2 years after traumatic brain injury. *Disabil. Rehabil.* 31, 484–489.

Shin, S. S., Bales, J. W., Yan, H. Q., Kline, A. E., Wagner, A. K., Lyons-Weiler, J., et al. (2013). The effect of environmental enrichment on substantia nigra gene expression after traumatic brain injury in rats. *J. Neurotrauma* 30, 259–270.

Shors, T. J., Anderson, M. L., Curlik, D. M. 2nd., and Nokia, M. S. (2012). Use it or lose it: how neurogenesis keeps the brain fit for learning. *Behav. Brain Res.* 227, 450–458.

Sidaros, A., Engberg, A. W., Sidaros, K., Liptrot, M. G., Herning, M., Petersen, P., et al. (2008). Diffusion tensor imaging during recovery from severe traumatic brain injury and relation to clinical outcome: a longitudinal study. *Brain* 131, 559–572.

Sidaros, A., Skimminge, A., Liptrot, M. G., Sidaros, K., Engberg, A. W., Herning, M., et al. (2009). Long-term global and regional brain volume changes following severe traumatic brain injury: a longitudinal study with clinical correlates. *Neuroimage* 44, 1–8.

Simpson, J., and Kelly, J. P. (2011). The impact of environmental enrichment in laboratory rats–behavioural and neurochemical aspects. *Behav. Brain Res.* 222, 246–264.

Slade, A., Tennant, A., and Chamberlain, M. A. (2002). A randomised controlled trial to determine the effect of intensity of therapy upon length of stay in a neurological rehabilitation setting. *J. Rehabil. Med.* 34, 260–266.

SMARTRISK. (2006). *The Economic Burden of Injury*. Toronto, ON: SMARTRISK.

Sohlberg, M. M., McLaughlin, K. A., Pavese, A., Heidrich, A., and Posner, M. I. (2000). Evaluation of attention process training and brain injury education in persons with acquired brain injury. *J. Clin. Exp. Neuropsychol.* 22, 656–676.

Sozda, C. N., Hoffman, A. N., Olsen, A. S., Cheng, J. P., Zafonte, R. D., and Kline, A. E. (2010). Empirical comparison of typical and atypical environmental enrichment paradigms on functional and histological outcome after experimental traumatic brain injury. *J. Neurotrauma* 27, 1047–1057.

Speisman, R. B., Kumar, A., Rani, A., Pastoriza, J. M., Severance, J. E., Foster, T. C., et al. (2012). Environmental enrichment restores neurogenesis and rapid acquisition in aged rats. *Neurobiol. Aging* 34, 263–274.

Spikman, J. M., Boelen, D. H., Lamberts, K. F., Brouwer, W. H., and Fasotti, L. (2009). Effects of a multifaceted treatment program for executive dysfunction after acquired brain injury on indications of executive functioning in daily life. *J. Int. Neuropsychol. Soc.* 16, 118–129.

Spivack, G., Spettell, C. M., Ellis, D. W., and Ross, S. E. (1992). Effects of intensity of treatment and length of stay on rehabilitation outcomes. *Brain Inj.* 6, 419–434.

Staudenmayer, K. L., Diaz-Arrastia, R., De Oliveira, A., Gentilello, L. M., and Shafi, S. (2007). Ethnic disparities in long-term functional outcomes after traumatic brain injury. *J. Trauma* 63, 1364–1369.

Stine-Morrow, E., Parisi, J., Morrow, D., Greene, J., and Park, D. (2007). An engagement model of cognitive optimization through adulthood. *J. Gerontol. Ser. B* 62B, 62–69.

Strandberg, T. (2009). Adults with acquired traumatic brain injury: experiences of a changeover process and consequences in everyday life. *Soc. Work Health Care* 48, 276–297.

Struchen, M. A., Davis, L. C., Bogaards, J. A., Hudler-Hull, T., Clark, A. N., Mazzei, D. M., et al. (2011). Making connections after brain injury: development and evaluation of a social peer-mentoring program for persons with traumatic brain injury. *J. Head Trauma Rehabil.* 26, 4–19.

Sun, H., Zhang, J., Zhang, L., Liu, H., Zhu, H., and Yang, Y. (2010). Environmental enrichment influences BDNF and NR1 levels in the hippocampus and restores cognitive impairment in chronic cerebral hypoperfused rats. *Curr. Neurovasc. Res.* 7, 268–280.

Till, C., Colella, B., Verwegen, J., and Green, R. E. (2008). Postrecovery cognitive decline in adults with traumatic brain injury. *Arch. Phys. Med. Rehabil.* 89, S25–S34.

Toglia, J., Johnston, M. V., Goverover, Y., and Dain, B. (2010). A multicontext approach to promoting transfer of strategy use and self regulation after brain injury: an exploratory study. *Brain Inj.* 24, 664–677.

Toglia, J. P. (1991). Generalization of treatment: a multicontext approach to cognitive perceptual impairment in adults with brain injury. *Am. J. Occup. Ther.* 45, 505–516.

Trivedi, M. A., Ward, M. A., Hess, T. M., Gale, S. D., Dempsey, R. J., Rowley, H. A., et al. (2007). Longitudinal changes in global brain volume between 79 and 409 days after traumatic brain injury: relationship with duration of coma. *J. Neurotrauma* 24, 766–771.

Tsaousides, T., Warshowsky, A., Ashman, T. A., Cantor, J. B., Spielman, L., and Gordon, W. A. (2009). The relationship between employment-related self-efficacy and quality of life following traumatic brain injury. *Rehabil. Psychol.* 54, 299–305.

Turner, B., Fleming, J., Cornwell, P., Worrall, L., Ownsworth, T., Haines, T., et al. (2007). A qualitative study of the transition from hospital to home for individuals with acquired brain injury and their family caregivers. *Brain Inj.* 21, 1119–1130.

Turner, B., Fleming, J., Cornwell, P., Haines, T., and Ownsworth, T. (2009a). Profiling early outcomes during the transition from hospital to home after brain injury. *Brain Inj.* 23, 51–60.

Turner, B., Ownsworth, T., Cornwell, P., and Fleming, J. (2009b). Reengagement in meaningful occupations during the transition from hospital to home for people with acquired brain injury and their family caregivers. *Am. J. Occup. Ther.* 63, 609–620.

Turner, B., Fleming, J., Ownsworth, T., and Cornwell, P. (2011a). Perceptions of recovery during the early transition phase from hospital to home following acquired brain injury: a journey of discovery. *Neuropsychol. Rehabil.* 21, 64–91.

Turner, B. J., Fleming, J., Ownsworth, T., and Cornwell, P. (2011b). Perceived service and support needs during transition from hospital to home following acquired brain injury. *Disabil. Rehabil.* 33, 818–829.

Turner, B. J., Fleming, J. M., Ownsworth, T. L., and Cornwell, P. L. (2008). The transition from hospital to home for individuals with acquired brain injury: a literature review and research recommendations. *Disabil. Rehabil.* 30, 1153–1176.

Turner, G. R., and Green, E. (2008). Cognitive remediation in aging and ABI: a question of negative plasticity? *Neuropsychol. Rehabil.* 18, 372–384.

Turner-Stokes, L., Disler, P. B., Nair, A., and Wade, D. T. (2005). Multidisciplinary rehabilitation for acquired brain injury in adults of working age. *Cochrane Database Syst. Rev.* 3:CD004170. doi: 10.1002/14651858.CD004170.pub2

Valero, J., Espana, J., Parra-Damas, A., Martin, E., Rodriguez-Alvarez, J., and Saura, C. A. (2011). Short-term environmental enrichment rescues adult neurogenesis and memory deficits in APP(Sw, Ind) transgenic mice. *PLoS ONE* 6:e16832. doi: 10.1371/journal.pone.0016832

Van De Winckel, A., Feys, H., De Weerdt, W., and Dom, R. (2004). Cognitive and behavioural effects of music-based exercises in patients with dementia. *Clin. Rehabil.* 18, 253–260.

Van Praag, H., Kempermann, G., and Gage, F. (2000). Neural consequences of environmental enrichment. *Neuroscience* 1, 191–198.

Vance, D., and Johns, R. (2002). Montessori improved cognitive domains in adults with Alzheimer's Disease. *Phys. Occup. Ther. Geriatr.* 20, 19–36.

Vazquez-Sanroman, D., Sanchis-Segura, C., Toledo, R., Hernandez, M. E., Manzo, J., and Miquel, M. (2013). The effects of enriched environment on BDNF expression in the mouse cerebellum depending on the length of exposure. *Behav. Brain Res.* 243C, 118–128.

Verghese, J., Lipton, R., Katz, M., Hall, C., Derby, C., Kuslansky, G., et al. (2003). Leisure activities and the risk of dementia in the elderly. *N. Engl. J. Med.* 348, 2508–2616.

Voss, M. W., Nagamatsu, L. S., Liu-Ambrose, T., and Kramer, A. F. (2011). Exercise, brain, and cognition across the life span. *J. Appl. Physiol.* 111, 1505–1513.

Wang, H., Karp, A., Wonblad, B., and Fratiglioni, L. (2002). Late-life engagement in social and leisure activities is associated with a decreased risk of dementia: a longitudinal study from the Kungsholmen project. *Am. J. Epidemiol.* 155, 1081–1087.

Warner, M. A., Marquez De La Plata, C., Spence, J., Wang, J. Y., Harper, C., Moore, C., et al. (2010). Assessing spatial relationships between axonal integrity, regional brain volumes, and neuropsychological outcomes after traumatic axonal injury. *J. Neurotrauma* 27, 2121–2130.

Warraich, Z., and Kleim, J. A. (2010). Neural plasticity: the biological substrate for neurorehabilitation. *PM R* 2, S208–S219.

West, R. W., and Greenough, W. T. (1972). Effect of environmental complexity on cortical synapses of rats: preliminary results. *Behav. Biol.* 7, 279–284.

Will, B., Galani, R., Kelche, C., and Rosenzweig, M. R. (2004). Recovery from brain injury in animals: relative efficacy of environmental enrichment, physical exercise or formal training (1990-2002). *Prog. Neurobiol.* 72, 167–182.

Willer, B., Button, J., and Rempel, R. (1999). Residential and home-based postacute rehabilitation of individuals with traumatic brain injury: a case control study. *Arch. Phys. Med. Rehabil.* 80, 399–406.

Williamson, L. L., Chao, A., and Bilbo, S. D. (2012). Environmental enrichment alters glial antigen expression and neuroimmune function in the adult rat hippocampus. *Brain Behav. Immun.* 26, 500–510.

Wilson, J. T., Wiedmann, K. D., Hadley, D. M., Condon, B., Teasdale, G., and Brooks, D. N. (1988). Early and late magnetic resonance imaging and neuropsychological outcome after head injury. *J. Neurol. Neurosurg. Psychiatr.* 51, 391–396.

Wilson, R., Barnes, L., and Bennett, D. (2003). Assessment of lifetime participation in cognitively stimulating activities. *J. Clin. Exp. Neuropsychol.* 25, 634–642.

Wilson, R. S., Mendes De Leon, C. F., Barnes, L. L., Schneider, J. A., Bienias, J. L., Evans, D. A., et al. (2002). Participation in cognitively stimulating activities and risk of incident Alzheimer disease. *J. Am. Med. Assoc.* 287, 742–748.

Winocur, G., and Moscovitch, M. (1990). A comparison of cognitive function in community-dwelling and institutionalized old people of normal intelligence. *Can. J. Psychol.* 44, 435–444.

Winocur, G., Moscovitch, M., and Freedman, J. (1987). An investigation of cognitive function in relation to psychosocial variables in institutionalized old people. *Can. J. Psychol.* 41, 257–269.

Winocur, G. (1998). Environmental influences on cognitive decline in aged rats. *Neurobiol. Aging* 19, 589–597.

Xu, L., Jiang, C. Q., Lam, T. H., Zhang, W. S., Thomas, G. N., and Cheng, K. K. (2011). Dose-response relation between physical activity and cognitive function: guangzhou biobank cohort study. *Ann. Epidemiol.* 21, 857–863.

Yang, S., Li, C., Qiu, X., Zhang, L., Lu, W., Chen, L., et al. (2013). Effects of an enriched environment on myelin sheaths in the white matter of rats during normal aging: a stereological study. *Neuroscience* 234C, 13–21.

Zhu, X. L., Poon, W. S., Chan, C. H., and Chan, S. H. (2001). Does intensive rehabilitation improve the functional outcome of patients with traumatic brain injury? Interim result of a randomized controlled trial. *Br. J. Neurosurg.* 15, 464–473.

Zhu, X. L., Poon, W. S., Chan, C. C., and Chan, S. S. (2007). Does intensive rehabilitation improve the functional outcome of patients with traumatic brain injury (TBI)? A randomized controlled trial. *Brain Inj.* 21, 681–690.

7

Aspects of innate immunity and Parkinson's disease

Yue Huang*[1,2] *and Glenda M. Halliday*[1,2]

[1] *Neuroscience Research Australia, Sydney, NSW, Australia*
[2] *University of New South Wales, Sydney, NSW, Australia*

Edited by:
Roger A. Barker, University of Cambridge and Addenbrooke's Hospital, UK

Reviewed by:
Jason B. Wu, Cedars-Sinai Medical Center, USA
Andreas Hartmann, Assistance Publique des Hopitaux de Paris, Hopital de la Pitie-Salpetriere, France
Tamas Revesz, Institute of Neurology, University College London, UK

****Correspondence:***
Glenda M. Halliday, Neuroscience Research Australia, Barker Street, Randwick, NSW 2031, Australia.
e-mail: g.halliday@neura.edu.au

Genetic studies on PARK genes have identified dysfunction in proteasomal, lysosomal, and mitochondrial enzymes as pathogenic for Parkinson's disease (PD). We review the role of these and similar enzymes in mediating innate immune signaling. In particular, we have identified that a number of PARK gene products as well as other enzymes have roles in innate immune signaling as well as DNA repair and regulation, ubiquitination, mitochondrial functioning, and synaptic trafficking. PD enzymatic dysfunction is likely to contribute to inadequate innate immune responses to a variety of extra- and intra-cellular stimuli, with a number of the innate immunity related enzymes found in the characteristic Lewy body pathology of PD. The decrease in innate immunity in PD is associated with an increase in markers of adaptive immunity, and recent GWAS studies have identified variants in human leukocyte antigen region as associated with late-onset sporadic PD (Hamza et al., 2010; Hill-Burns et al., 2011). Intriguing new data also suggest that peripheral immune responses may be involved, giving some potential to alleviate such peripheral dysfunction more directly in patients with PD. It is now important to identify the cell type specific immune responses contributing to the initial changes that occur in PD, as well as to the propagating immune responses important for the progression of PD pathology between cells and within the brain. Overall, a complex interplay between different types of immunity appear to be involved in the underlying pathology of PD.

Keywords: immunity, mitochondrial dysfunction, Parkinson's disease, synapse dysfunction, ubiquitination

INTRODUCTION

Although Parkinson's disease (PD) is the most common progressive movement disorder in the elderly, there is still considerable uncertainty about its etiology. Recent advances in genetics have identified a number of PARK genes in families with PD, which have pointed to common underlying intrinsically driven intracellular pathways (Corti et al., 2011). These include dysfunction of the proteosome (McNaught et al., 2001), lysosome (Shin et al., 2005), and mitochondria (Muqit et al., 2006). In particular, leucine repeat rich kinase 2 (LRRK2, PARK8) and PTEN-induced kinase 1 (PINK1, PARK6) are linked to familial dominant and recessive PD respectively. PINK1 deletion causes aberrant expression of genes that regulate innate immune responses (Akundi et al., 2011). LRRK2 expression is enriched in human immune cells and is a target gene of IFN-γ (Gardet et al., 2010). Increased LRRK2 expression occurs when an immune response is required (see below). As mutations in these proteins cause PD, this suggests that innate immunity may play a more fundamental role in PD. How these systems interact to cause the fundamental pathology of PD (intracellular Lewy body inclusions made from fibrilized α-synuclein protein) to occur within affected neurons needs to be addressed.

Despite considerable organelle dysfunction, neuronal death occurs slowly, initially, and selectively targeting certain brainstem regions with a predisposition for the substantia nigra (Fearnley and Lees, 1991). Neuronal death does not occur in isolation, but is accompanied by considerable neuroinflammation (Orr et al., 2002; Wilms et al., 2003) and intrinsically driven glial cell changes (Halliday and Stevens, 2011). These changes include the accumulation of α-synuclein in glia, with many of the PARK gene proteins also concentrating in glia in the human brain (LRRK2, PINK1, DJ-1, parkin; Gandhi et al., 2006; Huang et al., 2008; Halliday and Stevens, 2011; Song et al., 2011). As glia interact most closely with the immune system, we will review how innate immunity is involved in these processes.

The innate immune system is an immediate, non-specific, first line of defense against pathogen invasion, contrasting with the delayed and targeted adaptive immune response (Stone et al., 2009). The specific molecular structure of pathogens (pathogen-associated molecular patterns or PAMPs), like lipopolysaccharides (LPS) or the bacterial DNA motif polycytosine guanine (CpG), are directly recognized by phagocytes, granulocytes, and natural killer cells of the immune system (West et al., 2006). These PAMPs

Abbreviations: CARD, caspase recruitment domain; CpG, polycytosine guanine; ER, endoplasmic reticulum; HDAC, histone deacetylase; IKK, IκB kinase; IRAK, interleukin-1 receptor-associated kinase; JNK, c-Jun N-terminal kinase; LPS, lipopolysaccharides; LRRK2, leucine-rich repeat kinase 2; MAPK, mitogen-activated protein kinase; MAPKK, MAPK kinase; MAVS, mitochondrial antiviral signaling; Mda5, melanoma differentiation-associated gene 5; MPTP, 1-methyl-4-phenyl-1, 2,3,6-tetrahydropyridine; PAMPs, pathogen-associated molecular pattern; PARP, poly (ADP-ribose) polymerase; PD, Parkinson's disease; PINK1, PTEN-induced putative kinase 1; PKR, Protein kinase RNA-activated; RIG-I, RNA helicases protein retinoic acid-inducible gene I protein; TAK1, Transforming growth factor-beta-activated kinase 1; TBK-1, TANK-binding kinase 1; TLR, Toll-like receptor; TRAF6, tumor necrosis factor receptor-associated factor 6.

bind to Toll-like receptors (TLR) on cells, triggering a cascade of signaling that results in pro-inflammatory cytokine release and complement activation to clear the pathogen or the infected/dead cell through macroautophagy (West et al., 2006).

Pathogens activate cells by binding to specific TLRs through characteristic extracellular multiple leucine-rich repeats domains of TLR (Nguyen et al., 2002). The ultimate induction of interferons and inflammatory cytokines by different pathogens is led by several phosphorylation and subsequent ubiquitination events, with activation of TBK-1 and IKKε, JNK and p38 kinase, IKK, MAPK and MAPKK, IRAK, and TAK1 [detailed in previous reviews (Kawai and Akira, 2006; Seth et al., 2006)]. A major pathway is NF-κB activation by its release from IκB allowing its nuclear translocation and the subsequent activation of target genes to occur. IκB release occurs following IκB phosphorylation and consequent degradation through the lysine 48 linked ubiquitin–proteasome system (Silverman and Maniatis, 2001; Wu et al., 2006).

INNATE IMMUNITY AND PD

Classic PD is not considered an immune disease like multiple sclerosis, and can not be associated with common infectious agents. However, Parkinsonian symptoms can occur after Epstein–Barr virus (EBV) encephalitic infection in patients, with EBV DNA detected in the brain (Espay and Henderson, 2011). This shows that an immune activation in the brain can produce PD-like symptoms, and a number of genetic studies suggest the immune system is commonly involved. Genome-wide association studies (GWAS) show that common variants in human leukocyte antigen (HLA) region are associated with late-onset sporadic PD (Hamza et al., 2010; Hill-Burns et al., 2011). The brains of individuals with PD show upregulation of HLA-DR antigens and the presence of HLA-DR-immunopositive and highly reactive microglia (McGeer et al., 1988). Microglia are the only cells in the substantia nigra that express the initial recognition component of the complement cascade, C1q (Carlsson et al., 2011). Finally, nonsteroidal anti-inflammatory drugs reduce PD risk (Wahner et al., 2007; Steurer, 2011), further supporting some involvement of the immune system in PD.

From a PARK gene perspective, it is of interest that both parkin (PARK2) and LRRK2 (PARK8) are genes associated with leprosy (Cardoso et al., 2011), which is a chronic infectious disease of peripheral nerves. LRRK2 is also a risk gene for inflammatory bowel disease (Van Limbergen et al., 2009; Torkvist et al., 2010; Umeno et al., 2011), and there is much discussion about PD being initiated from peripheral neurons within the gut (enteric nervous system; Braak et al., 2003). In an animal model of ulcerative colitis, there is an alteration of the blood–brain-barrier (BBB) permeability that leads to more substantive cell loss to pathogen-induced cell loss of the substantia nigra (Villaran et al., 2010). Interestingly, treatment of the ulcerative colitis ameliorated cell loss in the brain in this model (Villaran et al., 2010). This could suggest a more direct link between immune defense mechanisms in peripheral neurons and the later onset of PD. Deletions within PINK1 (PARK6) or DJ-1 (PARK7) genes cause aberrant expression of genes involved in the p38 MAP kinase/NF-κB signaling pathway causing changes in the regulation of the innate immune response (Cornejo Castro et al., 2010; Akundi et al., 2011). This suggests that many PARK genes also have significant influence on the immune system which may be important for the onset and/or progression of PD.

A number of animal models of the neuronal loss in PD use direct initiation of the innate immune system to model this aspect of PD. Administration of LPS induces dramatic cell loss in primary neuronal cultures and direct injection of LPS into the substantia nigra produces progressive nigrostriatal degeneration and movement abnormalities in animal models of PD (Liu, 2006; Dutta et al., 2008). These LPS PD models trigger TLR4 mediated signaling pathways (Carvey et al., 2003; Visintin et al., 2003). Even intraperitoneal and *in utero* injections of LPS cause degeneration of the nigrostriatal system (Ling et al., 2002; Perry, 2004), consistent with peripheral effects causing PD-like neurodegeneration. These innate immunity models of PD cause neurodegeneration and microglial activation in a time and LPS dose dependent manner (Liu, 2006; Dutta et al., 2008). Similar direct injections of TLR3 into the substantia nigra produce nigrostriatal degeneration (Deleidi et al., 2010). These studies show that strong stimulators of the innate immune system and increased numbers of innate immune receptors can produce significant site-specific neurodegeneration, perhaps suggesting that the nigrostriatal system is particularly vulnerable to immune activation.

Innate immune signaling also plays a role in the abnormal deposition of α-synuclein. In α-synuclein overexpressing models, ablation of TLR4 augments the deposition of α-synculein due to disruption of the ability of microglia to adequately phagocytose α-synuclein (Stefanova et al., 2011). This suggests that certain aspects of innate immunity are required for initial protection from excessive extracellular α-synuclein. Whether these mechanisms play a role in patients is more difficult to determine. Overall, these studies suggest that the innate immune system can play both neuroprotective and neurotoxic roles depending on the circumstances.

ADAPTIVE IMMUNITY AND PD

In contrast to the "non-specific" innate immune system, the adaptive immune response is cell mediated and highly specialized to remove a specific antigen. It is mainly composed of two parts: humoral immunity, which is mediated by B-lymphocytes, and cell mediated immunity, which is mediated by T-lymphocytes. The CNS was traditionally considered as an "immune privileged" site due to its protection by the BBB, which prevents toxins and infections from reaching the CNS. However, in PD the BBB is disrupted due to activated microglia and monocytes in PD brain (Stone et al., 2009). IgG, but not IgM, has been shown bound to dopamine neurons in the substantia nigra of idiopathic and familial PD patients, but not in age-matched controls (Orr et al., 2005). In addition, LRRK2, a causative gene for PD (see above), regulates B2-lymphocyte function (Kubo et al., 2010). This suggests that adaptive immunity may also be involved in the progression of PD (**Figure 1**).

Apart from B-lymphocyte involvement in PD, both $CD4^+$ and $CD8^+$ T-lymphocytes have been found in the SN of PD patients, and $CD4^+$ T-lymphocytes are responsible for the T-cell-mediated immunopathology (Brochard et al., 2009). The expression of CD95 ligand (Fas) has been shown to be important for the capacity

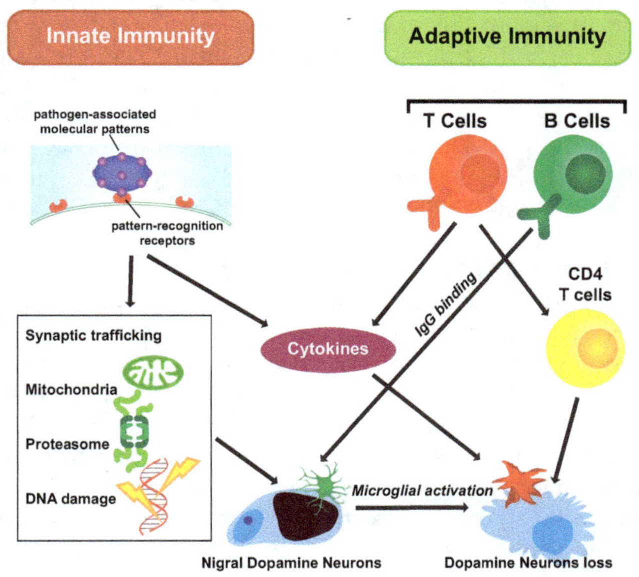

FIGURE 1 | Innate and adaptive immunity in PD. Innate and adaptive immunity are both thought to affect the cellular response to PD. Both produce cytokines facilitating microglial activation. Innate immune signaling is initiated by PAMP binding. Innate immunity influences cell functions through different organelles, such as the nucleus to affect DNA, the mitochondria and proteasome, and through impacting on synaptic trafficking. Adaptive immunity is a subsequent response. Antigen specific adaptive immune processes occur as immune cells survey the brain. In response to stimuli, B cells secrete IgG and CD4 T cells are activated impacting on selective neuronal degeneration.

of T-lymphocytes to induce neuronal death (Brochard et al., 2009). T-lymphocyte cells and T cell receptor (TCR) associated CD3, a polypeptide complex comprised of four distinct chains (CD3γ, CD3δ, CD3ε, and CD3ζ), are found in the PD characteristic Lewy body lesions (Castellani et al., 2011), providing another direct link between cell mediated immunity and PD pathology (**Figure 1**).

Through activation of both the adaptive and innate immune systems, cytokines are induced and secreted. Circulating IL-12 and IL-10 are significantly elevated in PD patients compared with controls (Rentzos et al., 2009) and our data show that the protein levels of IL-10 and GM-CSF are elevated in the cortex of patients with PD (unpublished data). Intercellular adhesion molecule-1 (ICAM-1)-positive glia are increased in the substantia nigra of PD brains (Miklossy et al., 2006). Further analysis of these immune responses in the brains of patients with PD may provide more specific cytokine targets for modifying detrimental immune responses in PD.

INNATE IMMUNITY AND DNA REPAIR AND REGULATION IN PD

The presence of genomic DNA single and double-strand breaks is very common in PD affected brain regions (Hegde et al., 2006). At early stages of DNA damage, DNA sensing molecules (such as PARP and ATM) activate and cause a signaling cascade for repair (Herceg and Wang, 2001). Histone deacetylases (HDAC) are important suppressors of gene transcription, but also deacetylates the p62 subunit of NF-κB increasing its binding to IκB and suppressing innate immunity and interferon-stimulated transcription (Babic et al., 2004; Into et al., 2010). HDACs have been localized to Lewy bodies in patients with PD (Takahashi-Fujigasaki and Fujigasaki, 2006), indicating that they are involved in PD pathogenesis. Inhibiting HDAC alleviates dopamine depletion in models of PD (Outeiro et al., 2007) and is protective by enhancing α-synuclein expression in neurons (Nusinzon and Horvath, 2003; Leng and Chuang, 2006), possibly in concert with an increased innate immune response.

Poly (ADP-ribose) polymerase catalyzes the attachment of ADP ribose units from NAD to nuclear proteins after DNA damage, resulting in three major outcomes, DNA repair, activation of transcription factors (notably NF-κB), and/or cell death due to NAD depletion and release of apoptosis releasing factor from mitochondria (Kauppinen and Swanson, 2007). PARP negatively regulates α-synuclein expression by binding to the α-synuclein promoter Rep1 region (Chiba-Falek et al., 2005) and α-synuclein protein suppresses PARP activity (Adamczyk and Kazmierczak, 2009). Inhibition of PARP activation protects mice from MPTP-induced parkinsonism (Mandir et al., 1999; Leng and Chuang, 2006). PARP may protect against PD through increasing innate immune signaling.

ATM is a kinase that is recruited to phosphorylate histones for DNA repair, signaling molecules for cell cycle arrest or apoptosis, and nuclear IKKγ (NF-κB essential modulator; Habraken and Piette, 2006; Hinz et al., 2010; Hadian and Krappmann, 2011). Phosphorylation of IKKγ leads to its ubiquitination and cytoplasmic translocation where it associates with the rest of the IKK complex, resulting in IKK activation followed by subsequent NF-κB activation and inflammatory cytokines production (Chen, 2005). ATM has also recently been shown to regulate proteasome-mediated protein turnover through suppression of the ISG15 pathway (Wood et al., 2011). ISG15 is an interferon-stimulated gene activated by viral infection and important in antiviral defense and innate immunity (Skaug and Chen, 2010). It is a ubiquitin-like protein that can be attached to both host and viral proteins (Skaug and Chen, 2010). ATM-deficient mice exhibit a selective loss of dopamine nigrostriatal neurons (Eilam et al., 1998), implicating dysfunction of ubiquitination as a factor in PD neurodegeneration, and specifically of ubiquitination in the innate immune system.

INNATE IMMUNITY AND UBIQUITINATION IN PD

The expression of ISG15 is increased in Crohn's disease (Labbe et al., 2011), an inflammatory bowel disorder sharing common genetic and environmental risk factors with PD (Bihari and Lees, 1987; Bialecka et al., 2007). Both ISG15 and LRRK2 (PARK8) are targets of interferon regulation (**Figure 2**). Interferon also regulates proteasome processing of ubiquitinated protein degradation into small peptides (Rivett et al., 2001; Piccinini et al., 2003; **Figure 2**). Ubiquitin is a small molecule and through lysine 48 and lysine 63 forms polyubiquitin chains for protein degradation and cellular localization (Ikeda and Dikic, 2008).

Among PARK genes, parkin has a variety of functions. It not only promotes lysine 48 linked ubiquitination for substrate degradation via the proteasome, but also functions in lysine 63 ubiquitin chain assembly to regulate diverse cellular processes, such as ribosome control, protein sorting and trafficking, and endocytosis of

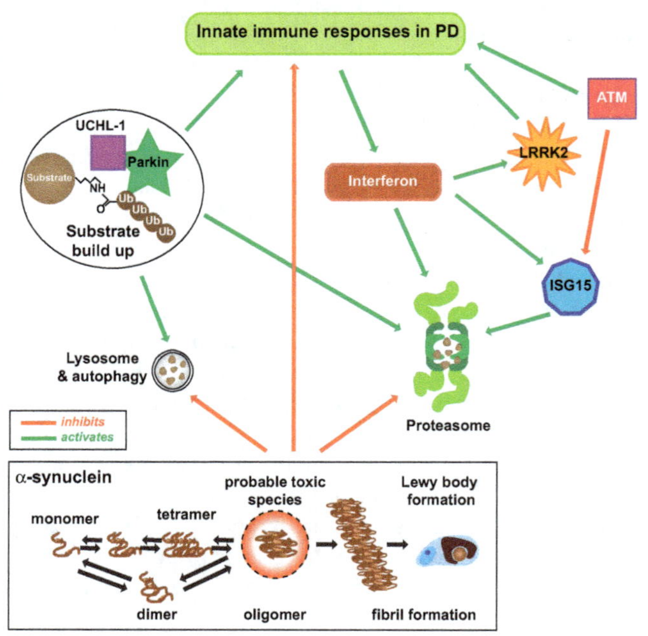

FIGURE 2 | Innate immunity and the ubiquitin–proteasome system in PD. Innate immunity is used by the cell to increase proteasome degradation of unwanted proteins by direct and indirect stimulation of the protesome through interferon-γ and ISG15, a ubiquitin-like protein that can be attached to both host and viral proteins. ATM (and appropriately functioning LRRK2) usually stimulates innate immune signaling when necessary. However, ATM also regulates proteasome-mediated protein turnover through suppression of the ISG15 pathway, and together with dysfunctional LRRK2 could decrease proteasome activity necessary for an adequate immune response and the degradation of normal cellular protein substrates, like dimer or tetramer forms of α-synuclein. As these forms are normally degraded through the ubiquitin/proteasome and lysosome/autophagy pathways, along with other cellular substrates, dysfunction in these pathways would increase α-synuclein to form toxic oligomeric species that also inhibit the proteasome and autophagy pathways, as well as innate immunity. This scenario would lead to the increase in toxic oligomers of α-synuclein that aggregate into fibrils to form Lewy bodies over time.

membrane proteins (Doss-Pepe et al., 2005). Lysine 63 linked ubiquitin chains promote the degradation of membrane proteins by the lysosome (Doss-Pepe et al., 2005). It is notable that α-synuclein is degraded via both the proteasome and lysosome pathways (Shin et al., 2005), suggestive that lysine 48 and lysine 63 linked ubiquitin chains are both important in the pathogenesis of PD (**Figure 2**). UCH-L1 has two opposing enzymatic activities, deubiquitination and ubiquityl ligase. The UCH-L1 ligase activity forms lysine 63 linked polyubiquitin chains (Liu et al., 2002). Lysine 63 multiubiquitin chains are also stimulated by α-synuclein (Doss-Pepe et al., 2005), and α-synuclein filaments and oligomers or its mutants inhibit proteasome function (Tanaka et al., 2001; Lindersson et al., 2004). These three genetically linked PD proteins all contribute to lysine 63 multiubiquitin chain formation. Dysfunction of this system is likely to decrease innate immune responses in PD.

Both lysine 48 and lysine 63 linked ubiquitin chains are known to be involved in anti-pathogen signaling cascades. In particular, lysine 63 linked ubiquitination is essential for NF-κB activation (detailed in review of Wu et al., 2006). Phosphorylation of IκB that releases NF-κB only occurs when the kinase IKKβ is released from its complex following IKKγ phosphorylation and lysine 63 linked degradation. Some other key immune response signaling molecules, such as TRAF6, also function as the lysine 63 linked ubiquitin E3 ligase to activate kinase activity (Kawai and Akira, 2006), and TRAF5 has been identified as a downstream target of VISA (see below) that mediates both IRF-3 and NF-κB activation (Tang and Wang, 2010).

INNATE IMMUNITY AND MITOCHONDRIAL FUNCTION IN PD

The proper functioning of mitochondria is crucial for adequate innate immune defense (Qi et al., 2007; Tang and Wang, 2010; West et al., 2011). Intracellular double-stranded RNA originating from viruses or virus replication is recognized by RIG-I and Mda5, which contain a caspase recruitment domain (CARD; **Figure 3**). Activated RIG-I/Mda5 passes the signal to mitochondrial antiviral signaling (MAVS/VISA) proteins via a CARD–CARD domain interaction (**Figure 3**). The C-terminal of MAVS/VISA bind to mitochondria to activate NF-κB and start interferon α and β production (Qi et al., 2007; **Figure 3**). Upon viral infection, MAVS/VISA immigrate from the outer membrane into the mitochondrial detergent-resistant membrane fraction, suggesting that mitochondria react and contribute to antiviral signaling (Qi et al., 2007; **Figure 3**). In addition to regulating antiviral signaling, there is mounting evidence that mitochondria facilitate antibacterial immunity by generating reactive oxygen species and contributing to innate immune activation following cellular damage and stress (Nakahira et al., 2011).

Most nuclear encoded PARK gene products are located within mitochondria (**Table 1**), such as PINK1, DJ-1, Omi/HtrA2, and LRRK2, suggesting mitochondrial dysfunction is common in PD. The mitochondrial complex I has been shown to be selectively reduced in PD vulnerable regions, such as the substantia nigra (Schapira et al., 1989). The mitochondrial complex I inhibitor rotenone and mitochondrial toxin MPTP (1-methyl 4-phenyl 1,2,3,6-tetrahydropyridine) induce selective dopamine neuron loss and a parkinsonian syndrome and have been used as a major model for studying the tissue aspects of PD (Langston and Ballard, 1984; Betarbet et al., 2000). These changes may decrease the cellular responses of the innate immune system in PD.

INNATE IMMUNITY AND SYNAPTIC TRAFFICKING IN PD

Most enveloped animal RNA and DNA viruses enter host cells via receptor-medicated endocytosis or viral membrane fusion with the plasma membrane in order to replicate. Endocytosis impinges on viral infection at a number of different cellular levels, from the plasma membrane to endosome to lysosome or alternatively to Golgi, and to ER (**Figure 4**; Hacker et al., 1998; Leadbetter et al., 2002; Diebold et al., 2004). Viral proteins accumulate in the ER during viral replication and elicit ER stress. Viral replication induced ER stress disturbs vesicle trafficking within the intracellular membranous web (Goodridge et al., 2011).

Many PARK genes are associated with endocytosis and synaptic vesicle trafficking. α-Synuclein, parkin and UCH-L1 concentrate in the presynapse and associate with synaptic vesicles, anchoring and regulating the undocked pool of presynaptic vesicles (Di Rosa et al., 2003; Ferrer, 2009). α-Synuclein acts as a molecular

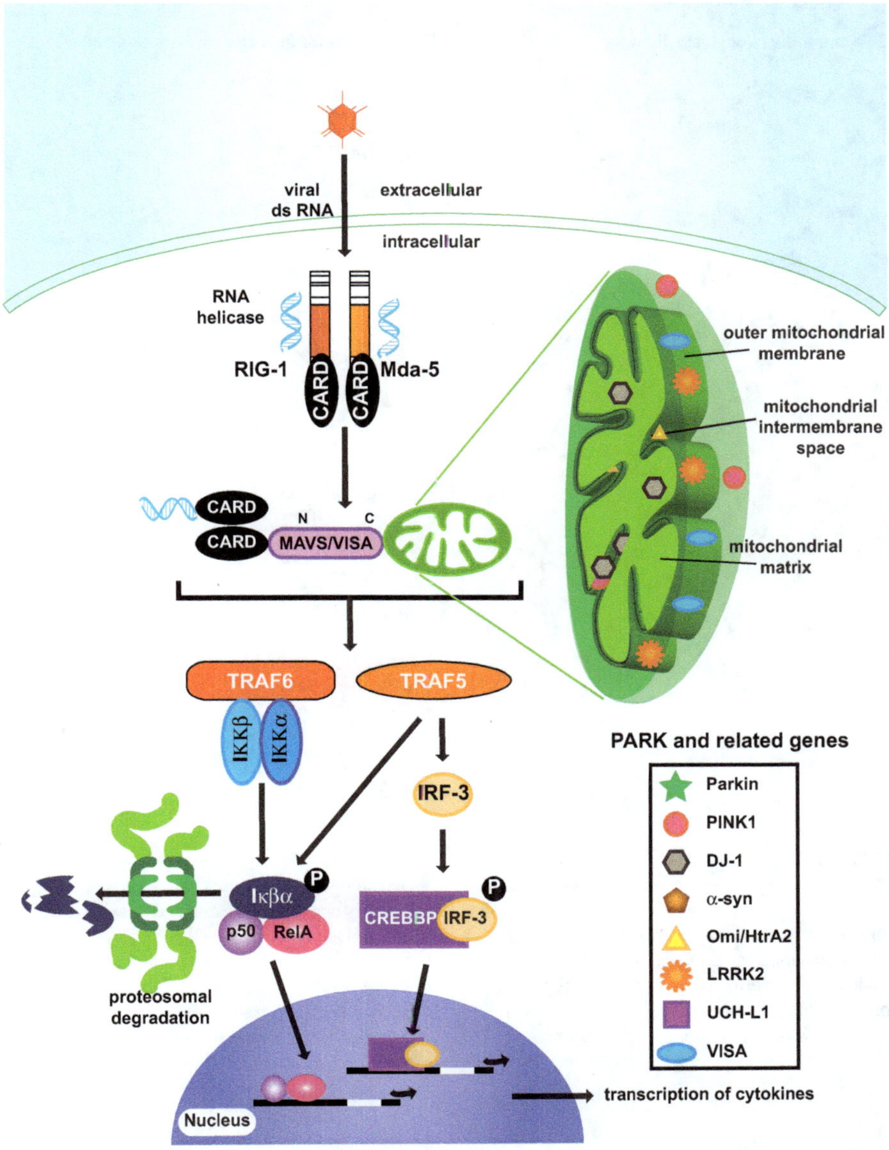

FIGURE 3 | Innate immunity and mitochondria in PD. Many PARK related gene products are located in mitochondria, implicating mitochondrial dysfunction in PD. Interestingly, MAVS/VISA that are attached to the outer membrane of mitochondria are involved in viral infection signaling by activating TRAF6 and TRAF5. Phosphorylation of Iκβα and IRF-3 leads to nuclear translocation of transcription factors and the production of cytokines.

Table 1 | Cellular localization and functions PARK and related genes

	Cellular location indicative functions in mitochondria and synaptic trafficking	Ubiquitination	Reference
Parkin	Outer mitochondrial membrane Synaptic vesicles and the synaptic membrane	Lysine 48-, 63-linked ubiquitin E3 ligase	Kubo et al. (2001); Darios et al. (2003)
DJ-1	Mitochondrial matrix and inter-membrane space	NA	Zhang et al., 2005)
PINK1	Mitochondria	Upstream of parkin	Valente et al. (2004)
Omi/HtrA2	Mitochondrial inter-membrane space	NA	Strauss et al. (2005)
LRRK2	Outer mitochondrial membrane	NA	West et al. (2005)
α-synuclein	Presynaptic terminal	Promote 63 linked ubiquitin assemble	Iwai et al. (1995)
UCH-L1	Synaptic vesicle	Lysine 63 linked ubiquitin E3 ligase	Liu et al. (2002)
VISA	Outer mitochondrial membrane	NA	Seth et al. (2005)

NA, not available.

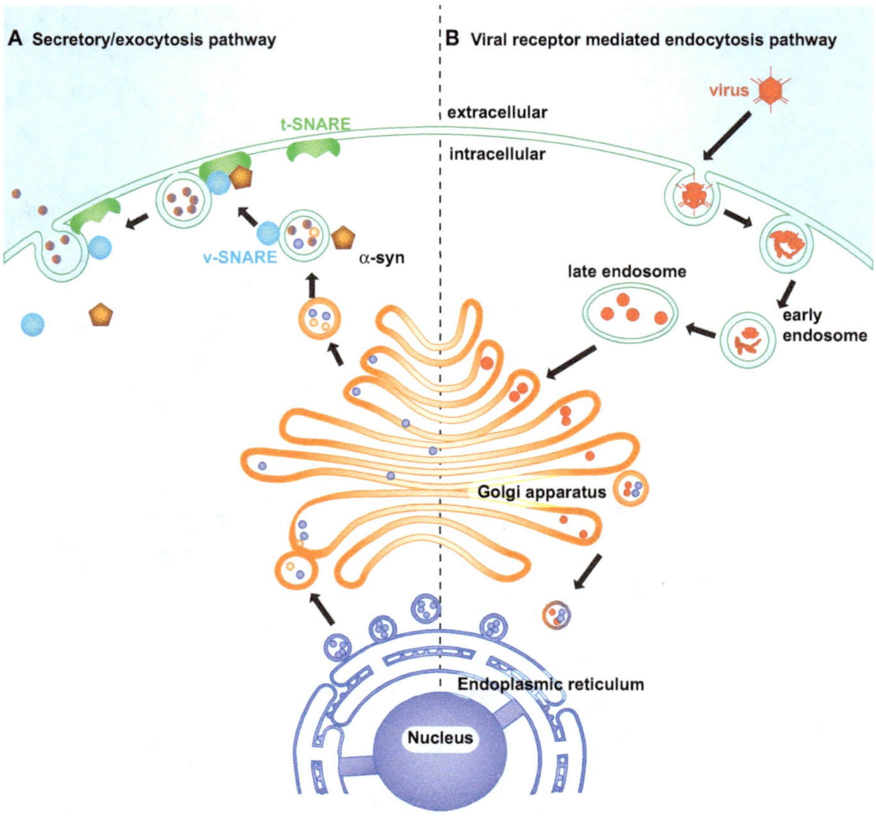

FIGURE 4 | Synaptic trafficking failure and viral intake leading to synaptic dysfunction in PD. Left: The endoplasmic reticulum is composed of a membranous network of tubes and cisternae enclosed in a membrane. It is continuous with the membrane surrounding the nuclear membrane and connects with the Golgi network via the vesicles carrying newly synthesized proteins. Certain vesicle-trafficking steps are required for the translocation of a vesicle from the Golgi apparatus to the plasma membrane. A transport vesicle is tethered and docked at the target membrane to form a tight SNARE complex, thus to merge the vesicle membrane with the target membrane and evacuate neurotransmitters into the extracellular space. The vesicle releasing process is under the assistance of α-synuclein, CDCrel-1, and synaptotagmin. Right: Viruses enter host cells through endosomes. Late endosomes fuse with or convert to lysosomes to degrade its contents, or alternatively it forms budding vesicles that pass to the trans-Golgi region and translocate to the Golgi and endoplasmic reticulum. The endoplasmic reticulum is coated with ribosomes, which assemble the viral amino acids into viral proteins.

chaperone, assisting in the folding and refolding of synaptic proteins called SNAREs, which are crucial for the release of neurotransmitters at the neuronal synapse, vesicle recycling, and synaptic integrity (Chandra et al., 2005). Upon the arrival of action potentials at the synaptic terminal, SNARE complexes, assembly of vesicle membrane (v-SNARE) and the presynaptic plasma membrane (t-SNARE), fuse the vesicle at the plasma membrane to release neurotransmitter into the synaptic cleft (Chandra et al., 2005; Fortin et al., 2005). Parkin ubiquitinates and regulates the turnover of the synaptic vesicle-associated protein, CDCrel-1, a synaptic vesicle-enriched septin GTPase implicated in the inhibition of exocytosis through its interactions with the SNARE complex component, syntaxin (Zhang et al., 2000). Another substrate of parkin is synaptotagmin XI, a member of the synaptotagmin family that is well characterized in vesicle formation and docking by interaction with SNAREs (Huynh et al., 2003). Loss of function of α-synuclein, parkin, or DJ-1 reduces neurotransmission and synaptic vesicle trafficking (Abeliovich et al., 2000; Goldberg et al., 2005). UCH-L1 deficient mice also show altered vesicle transport gene expression (Bonin et al., 2004). Reduced innate immunity allowing for pathogen replication would significantly exacerbate any loss of synaptic function caused by PARK gene products (**Figure 4**) precipitating frank degeneration.

CONCLUSION

A number of intrinsically driven cellular pathways shown to be dysfunctional in PD are important in mediating innate immune signaling. These important intracellular pathways have been identified through genetic studies in patients with PD. More recent genetic studies have also implicated immune pathways in the pathogenesis of PD. In particular, we have identified a number of PARK gene products as well as other enzymes that have dual roles in innate immune signaling as well as proteasome, lysosome, and mitochondrial functioning. The additional enzymes identified are important for DNA repair and regulation, ubiquitination, mitochondrial function, and synaptic trafficking. These pathways appear to lose their ability to mount an adequate innate immune response to PD and experimental manipulation of many of these intracellular molecules has been associated with characteristic PD pathologies in animal models. Intriguing new data also suggest that peripheral immune responses may be involved, with the potential to alleviate such peripheral dysfunction more directly in patients with PD.

Most important, the molecular pathways involved are likely to function in a cell type specific manner (Ledesma et al., 2002), a concept that has not yet been evaluated substantially in patients with PD. The cross-talk between neurons and glia is crucial for an adequate immune response, with astrocytes considered particularly important (Halliday and Stevens, 2011; Schmidt et al., 2011). Astrocytic endfeet form part of the BBB and may serve as ideal sentinel cells able to sense the appearance of toxins and viral pathogens (Scumpia et al., 2005), similar to their cousins found in the gut (Savidge et al., 2007; Daneman and Rescigno, 2009). Astroglia in both the brain and gut regulate barrier function and membrane permeability (Savidge et al., 2007; Daneman and Rescigno, 2009), functions which may be important for the cell to cell transfer of α-synuclein pathology as well as more traditional infectious agents. The increased expression of PARK gene proteins in astrocytes (see above) and their lack of activation to PD pathology in patients (Mirza et al., 2000; Halliday and Stevens, 2011) lends weight to a loss of innate immunity and BBB function in PD that potentially increases membrane and cellular permeability leading to increased toxin and pathogen infiltration in the brain. In addition to the direct cellular damage to vulnerable neurons this would initiate, pathogen exposure may also activate the alternate adaptive immune responses that are thought to participate in propagating the pathology of PD.

ACKNOWLEDGMENTS

We wish to thank Heidi Cartwight for the figurework. Yue Huang is funded by a University of New South Wales Goldstar award. Glenda M. Halliday is funded as a Senior Principal Research Fellow of the National Health and Medical Research Council of Australia.

REFERENCES

Abeliovich, A., Schmitz, Y., Farinas, I., Choi-Lundberg, D., Ho, W. H., Castillo, P. E., Shinsky, N., Verdugo, J. M., Armanini, M., Ryan, A., Hynes, M., Phillips, H., Sulzer, D., and Rosenthal, A. (2000). Mice lacking alpha-synuclein display functional deficits in the nigrostriatal dopamine system. *Neuron* 25, 239–252.

Adamczyk, A., and Kazmierczak, A. (2009). Alpha-synuclein inhibits poly (ADP-ribose) polymerase-1 (PARP-1) activity via NO-dependent pathway. *Folia Neuropathol.* 47, 247–251.

Akundi, R. S., Huang, Z., Eason, J., Pandya, J. D., Zhi, L., Cass, W. A., Sullivan, P. G., and Bueler, H. (2011). Increased mitochondrial calcium sensitivity and abnormal expression of innate immunity genes precede dopaminergic defects in Pink1-deficient mice. *PLoS ONE* 6, e16038. doi:10.1371/journal.pone.0016038

Babic, I., Jakymiw, A., and Fujita, D. J. (2004). The RNA binding protein Sam68 is acetylated in tumor cell lines, and its acetylation correlates with enhanced RNA binding activity. *Oncogene* 23, 3781–3789.

Betarbet, R., Sherer, T. B., Mackenzie, G., Garcia-Osuna, M., Panov, A. V., and Greenamyre, J. T. (2000). Chronic systemic pesticide exposure reproduces features of Parkinson's disease. *Nat. Neurosci.* 3, 1301–1306.

Bialecka, M., Kurzawski, M., Klodowska-Duda, G., Opala, G., Juzwiak, S., Kurzawski, G., Tan, E. K., and Drozdzik, M. (2007). CARD15 variants in patients with sporadic Parkinson's disease. *Neurosci. Res.* 57, 473–476.

Bihari, K., and Lees, A. J. (1987). Cigarette smoking, Parkinson's disease and ulcerative colitis. *J. Neurol. Neurosurg. Psychiatr.* 50, 635.

Bonin, M., Poths, S., Osaka, H., Wang, Y. L., Wada, K., and Riess, O. (2004). Microarray expression analysis of gad mice implicates involvement of Parkinson's disease associated UCH-L1 in multiple metabolic pathways. *Brain Res. Mol. Brain Res.* 126, 88–97.

Braak, H., Rub, U., Gai, W. P., and Del Tredici, K. (2003). Idiopathic Parkinson's disease: possible routes by which vulnerable neuronal types may be subject to neuroinvasion by an unknown pathogen. *J. Neural Transm.* 110, 517–536.

Brochard, V., Combadiere, B., Prigent, A., Laouar, Y., Perrin, A., Beray-Berthat, V., Bonduelle, O., Alvarez-Fischer, D., Callebert, J., Launay, J. M., Duyckaerts, C., Flavell, R. A., Hirsch, E. C., and Hunot, S. (2009). Infiltration of CD4+ lymphocytes into the brain contributes to neurodegeneration in a mouse model of Parkinson disease. *J. Clin. Invest.* 119, 182–192.

Cardoso, C. C., Pereira, A. C., De Sales Marques, C., and Moraes, M. O. (2011). Leprosy susceptibility: genetic variations regulate innate and adaptive immunity, and disease outcome. *Future Microbiol.* 6, 533–549.

Carlsson, T., Schindler, F. R., Hollerhage, M., Depboylu, C., Arias-Carrion, O., Schnurrbusch, S., Rosler, T. W., Wozny, W., Schwall, G. P., Groebe, K., Oertel, W. H., Brundin, P., Schrattenholz, A., and Hoglinger, G. U. (2011). Systemic administration of neuregulin-1beta1 protects dopaminergic neurons in a mouse model of Parkinson's disease. *J. Neurochem.* 117, 1066–1074.

Carvey, P. M., Chang, Q., Lipton, J. W., and Ling, Z. (2003). Prenatal exposure to the bacteriotoxin lipopolysaccharide leads to long-term losses of dopamine neurons in offspring: a potential, new model of Parkinson's disease. *Front. Biosci.* 8, s826–s837.

Castellani, R. J., Nugent, S. L., Morrison, A. L., Zhu, X., Lee, H. G., Harris, P. L., Bajic, V., Sharma, H. S., Chen, S. G., Oettgen, P., Perry, G., and Smith, M. A. (2011). CD3 in Lewy pathology: does the abnormal recall of neurodevelopmental processes underlie Parkinson's disease. *J. Neural Transm.* 118, 23–26.

Chandra, S., Gallardo, G., Fernandez-Chacon, R., Schluter, O. M., and Sudhof, T. C. (2005). Alpha-synuclein cooperates with CSPalpha in preventing neurodegeneration. *Cell* 123, 383–396.

Chen, Z. J. (2005). Ubiquitin signalling in the NF-kappaB pathway. *Nat. Cell Biol.* 7, 758–765.

Chiba-Falek, O., Kowalak, J. A., Smulson, M. E., and Nussbaum, R. L. (2005). Regulation of alpha-synuclein expression by poly (ADP ribose) polymerase-1 (PARP-1) binding to the NACP-Rep1 polymorphic site upstream of the SNCA gene. *Am. J. Hum. Genet.* 76, 478–492.

Cornejo Castro, E. M., Waak, J., Weber, S. S., Fiesel, F. C., Oberhettinger, P., Schutz, M., Autenrieth, I. B., Springer, W., and Kahle, P. J. (2010). Parkinson's disease-associated DJ-1 modulates innate immunity signaling in Caenorhabditis elegans. *J. Neural Transm.* 117, 599–604.

Corti, O., Lesage, S., and Brice, A. (2011). What genetics tells us about the causes and mechanisms of Parkinson's disease. *Physiol. Rev.* 91, 1161–1218.

Daneman, R., and Rescigno, M. (2009). The gut immune barrier and the blood-brain barrier: are they so different? *Immunity* 31, 722–735.

Darios, F., Corti, O., Lucking, C. B., Hampe, C., Muriel, M. P., Abbas, N., Gu, W. J., Hirsch, E. C., Rooney, T., Ruberg, M., and Brice, A. (2003). Parkin prevents mitochondrial swelling and cytochrome c release in mitochondria-dependent cell death. *Hum. Mol. Genet.* 12, 517–526.

Deleidi, M., Hallett, P. J., Koprich, J. B., Chung, C. Y., and Isacson, O. (2010). The Toll-like receptor-3 agonist polyinosinic:polycytidylic acid triggers nigrostriatal dopaminergic degeneration. *J. Neurosci.* 30, 16091–16101.

Di Rosa, G., Puzzo, D., Sant'Angelo, A., Trinchese, F., and Arancio, O. (2003). Alpha-synuclein: between synaptic function and dysfunction. *Histol. Histopathol.* 18, 1257–1266.

Diebold, S. S., Kaisho, T., Hemmi, H., Akira, S., and Reis E Sousa, C. (2004). Innate antiviral responses by means of TLR7-mediated recognition of single-stranded RNA. *Science* 303, 1529–1531.

Doss-Pepe, E. W., Chen, L., and Madura, K. (2005). Alpha-synuclein and parkin contribute to the assembly of ubiquitin lysine 63-linked multiubiquitin chains. *J. Biol. Chem.* 280, 16619–16624.

Dutta, G., Zhang, P., and Liu, B. (2008). The lipopolysaccharide Parkinson's disease animal model: mechanistic studies and drug discovery. *Fundam. Clin. Pharmacol.* 22, 453–464.

Eilam, R., Peter, Y., Elson, A., Rotman, G., Shiloh, Y., Groner, Y., and Segal, M. (1998). Selective loss of dopaminergic nigro-striatal neurons in brains of Atm-deficient mice. *Proc. Natl. Acad. Sci. U.S.A.* 95, 12653–12656.

Espay, A. J., and Henderson, K. K. (2011). Postencephalitic parkinsonism and basal ganglia necrosis due to Epstein-Barr virus infection. *Neurology* 76, 1529–1530.

Fearnley, J. M., and Lees, A. J. (1991). Ageing and Parkinson's disease: substantia nigra regional selectivity. *Brain* 114 (Pt 5), 2283–2301.

Ferrer, I. (2009). Early involvement of the cerebral cortex in Parkinson's disease: convergence of multiple metabolic defects. *Prog. Neurobiol.* 88, 89–103.

Fortin, D. L., Nemani, V. M., Voglmaier, S. M., Anthony, M. D., Ryan, T. A., and Edwards, R. H. (2005). Neural activity controls the synaptic accumulation of alpha-synuclein. *J. Neurosci.* 25, 10913–10921.

Gandhi, S., Muqit, M. M., Stanyer, L., Healy, D. G., Abou-Sleiman, P. M., Hargreaves, I., Heales, S., Ganguly, M., Parsons, L., Lees, A. J., Latchman, D. S., Holton, J. L., Wood, N. W., and Revesz, T. (2006). PINK1 protein in normal human brain and Parkinson's disease. *Brain* 129, 1720–1731.

Gardet, A., Benita, Y., Li, C., Sands, B. E., Ballester, I., Stevens, C., Korzenik, J. R., Rioux, J. D., Daly, M. J., Xavier, R. J., and Podolsky, D. K. (2010). LRRK2 is involved in the IFN-gamma response and host response to pathogens. *J. Immunol.* 185, 5577–5585.

Goldberg, M. S., Pisani, A., Haburcak, M., Vortherms, T. A., Kitada, T., Costa, C., Tong, Y., Martella, G., Tscherter, A., Martins, A., Bernardi, G., Roth, B. L., Pothos, E. N., Calabresi, P., and Shen, J. (2005). Nigrostriatal dopaminergic deficits and hypokinesia caused by inactivation of the familial Parkinsonism-linked gene DJ-1. *Neuron* 45, 489–496.

Goodridge, H. S., Reyes, C. N., Becker, C. A., Katsumoto, T. R., Ma, J., Wolf, A. J., Bose, N., Chan, A. S., Magee, A. S., Danielson, M. E., Weiss, A., Vasilakos, J. P., and Underhill, D. M. (2011). Activation of the innate immune receptor Dectin-1 upon formation of a 'phagocytic synapse'. *Nature* 472, 471–475.

Habraken, Y., and Piette, J. (2006). NF-kappaB activation by double-strand breaks. *Biochem. Pharmacol.* 72, 1132–1141.

Hacker, H., Mischak, H., Miethke, T., Liptay, S., Schmid, R., Sparwasser, T., Heeg, K., Lipford, G. B., and Wagner, H. (1998). CpG-DNA-specific activation of antigen-presenting cells requires stress kinase activity and is preceded by non-specific endocytosis and endosomal maturation. *EMBO J.* 17, 6230–6240.

Hadian, K., and Krappmann, D. (2011). Signals from the nucleus: activation of NF-kappaB by cytosolic ATM in the DNA damage response. *Sci. Signal.* 4, pe2.

Halliday, G. M., and Stevens, C. H. (2011). Glia: initiators and progressors of pathology in Parkinson's disease. *Mov. Disord.* 26, 6–17.

Hamza, T. H., Zabetian, C. P., Tenesa, A., Laederach, A., Montimurro, J., Yearout, D., Kay, D. M., Doheny, K. F., Paschall, J., Pugh, E., Kusel, V. I., Collura, R., Roberts, J., Griffith, A., Samii, A., Scott, W. K., Nutt, J., Factor, S. A., and Payami, H. (2010). Common genetic variation in the HLA region is associated with late-onset sporadic Parkinson's disease. *Nat. Genet.* 42, 781–785.

Hegde, M. L., Gupta, V. B., Anitha, M., Harikrishna, T., Shankar, S. K., Muthane, U., Subba Rao, K., and Jagannatha Rao, K. S. (2006). Studies on genomic DNA topology and stability in brain regions of Parkinson's disease. *Arch. Biochem. Biophys.* 449, 143–156.

Herceg, Z., and Wang, Z. Q. (2001). Functions of poly (ADP-ribose) polymerase (PARP) in DNA repair, genomic integrity and cell death. *Mutat. Res.* 477, 97–110.

Hill-Burns, E. M., Factor, S. A., Zabetian, C. P., Thomson, G., and Payami, H. (2011). Evidence for more than one Parkinson's disease-associated variant within the HLA region. *PLoS ONE* 6, e27109. doi:10.1371/journal.pone.0027109

Hinz, M., Stilmann, M., Arslan, S. C., Khanna, K. K., Dittmar, G., and Scheidereit, C. (2010). A cytoplasmic ATM-TRAF6-cIAP1 module links nuclear DNA damage signaling to ubiquitin-mediated NF-kappaB activation. *Mol. Cell* 40, 63–74.

Huang, Y., Song, Y. J., Murphy, K., Holton, J. L., Lashley, T., Revesz, T., Gai, W. P., and Halliday, G. M. (2008). LRRK2 and parkin immunoreactivity in multiple system atrophy inclusions. *Acta Neuropathol.* 116, 639–646.

Huynh, D. P., Scoles, D. R., Nguyen, D., and Pulst, S. M. (2003). The autosomal recessive juvenile Parkinson disease gene product, parkin, interacts with and ubiquitinates synaptotagmin XI. *Hum. Mol. Genet.* 12, 2587–2597.

Ikeda, F., and Dikic, I. (2008). Atypical ubiquitin chains: new molecular signals. "Protein Modifications: Beyond the Usual Suspects" review series. *EMBO Rep.* 9, 536–542.

Into, T., Inomata, M., Niida, S., Murakami, Y., and Shibata, K. (2010). Regulation of MyD88 aggregation and the MyD88-dependent signaling pathway by sequestosome 1 and histone deacetylase 6. *J. Biol. Chem.* 285, 35759–35769.

Iwai, A., Masliah, E., Yoshimoto, M., Ge, N., Flanagan, L., De Silva, H. A., Kittel, A., and Saitoh, T. (1995). The precursor protein of non-A beta component of Alzheimer's disease amyloid is a presynaptic protein of the central nervous system. *Neuron* 14, 467–475.

Kauppinen, T. M., and Swanson, R. A. (2007). The role of poly (ADP-ribose) polymerase-1 in CNS disease. *Neuroscience* 145, 1267–1272.

Kawai, T., and Akira, S. (2006). Innate immune recognition of viral infection. *Nat. Immunol.* 7, 131–137.

Kubo, M., Kamiya, Y., Nagashima, R., Maekawa, T., Eshima, K., Azuma, S., Ohta, E., and Obata, F. (2010). LRRK2 is expressed in B-2 but not in B-1 B cells, and downregulated by cellular activation. *J. Neuroimmunol.* 229, 123–128.

Kubo, S. I., Kitami, T., Noda, S., Shimura, H., Uchiyama, Y., Asakawa, S., Minoshima, S., Shimizu, N., Mizuno, Y., and Hattori, N. (2001). Parkin is associated with cellular vesicles. *J. Neurochem.* 78, 42–54.

Labbe, C., Boucher, G., Foisy, S., Alikashani, A., Nkwimi, H., David, G., Beaudoin, M., Goyette, P., Charron, G., Xavier, R. J., and Rioux, J. D. (2011). Genome-wide expression profiling implicates a MAST3-regulated gene set in colonic mucosal inflammation of ulcerative colitis patients. *Inflamm. Bowel Dis.* doi: 10.1002/ibd.21887. [Epub ahead of print].

Langston, J. W., and Ballard, P. (1984). Parkinsonism induced by 1-methyl-4-phenyl-1,2,3,6-tetrahydropyridine (MPTP): implications for treatment and the pathogenesis of Parkinson's disease. *Can. J. Neurol. Sci.* 11, 160–165.

Leadbetter, E. A., Rifkin, I. R., Hohlbaum, A. M., Beaudette, B. C., Shlomchik, M. J., and Marshak-Rothstein, A. (2002). Chromatin-IgG complexes activate B cells by dual engagement of IgM and Toll-like receptors. *Nature* 416, 603–607.

Ledesma, M. D., Galvan, C., Hellias, B., Dotti, C., and Jensen, P. H. (2002). Astrocytic but not neuronal increased expression and redistribution of parkin during unfolded protein stress. *J. Neurochem.* 83, 1431–1440.

Leng, Y., and Chuang, D. M. (2006). Endogenous alpha-synuclein is induced by valproic acid through histone deacetylase inhibition and participates in neuroprotection against glutamate-induced excitotoxicity. *J. Neurosci.* 26, 7502–7512.

Lindersson, E., Beedholm, R., Hojrup, P., Moos, T., Gai, W., Hendil, K. B., and Jensen, P. H. (2004). Proteasomal inhibition by alpha-synuclein filaments and oligomers. *J. Biol. Chem.* 279, 12924–12934.

Ling, Z., Gayle, D. A., Ma, S. Y., Lipton, J. W., Tong, C. W., Hong, J. S., and Carvey, P. M. (2002). In utero bacterial endotoxin exposure causes loss of tyrosine hydroxylase neurons in the postnatal rat midbrain. *Mov. Disord.* 17, 116–124.

Liu, B. (2006). Modulation of microglial pro-inflammatory and neurotoxic activity for the treatment of Parkinson's disease. *AAPS J.* 8, E606–E621.

Liu, Y., Fallon, L., Lashuel, H. A., Liu, Z., and Lansbury, P. T. Jr. (2002). The UCH-L1 gene encodes two opposing enzymatic activities that affect alpha-synuclein degradation and Parkinson's disease susceptibility. *Cell* 111, 209–218.

Mandir, A. S., Przedborski, S., Jackson-Lewis, V., Wang, Z. Q., Simbulan-Rosenthal, C. M., Smulson, M. E., Hoffman, B. E., Guastella, D. B., Dawson, V. L., and Dawson, T. M. (1999). Poly (ADP-ribose) polymerase activation mediates 1-methyl-4-phenyl-1,2,3,6-tetrahydropyridine (MPTP)-induced parkinsonism. *Proc. Natl. Acad. Sci. U.S.A.* 96, 5774–5779.

McGeer, P. L., Itagaki, S., Boyes, B. E., and McGeer, E. G. (1988). Reactive microglia are positive for HLA-DR in the substantia nigra of Parkinson's and Alzheimer's disease brains. *Neurology* 38, 1285–1291.

McNaught, K. S., Olanow, C. W., Halliwell, B., Isacson, O., and Jenner, P. (2001). Failure of the ubiquitin-proteasome system in Parkinson's disease. *Nat. Rev. Neurosci.* 2, 589–594.

Miklossy, J., Doudet, D. D., Schwab, C., Yu, S., Mcgeer, E. G., and Mcgeer, P. L. (2006). Role of ICAM-1 in persisting inflammation in Parkinson disease and MPTP monkeys. *Exp. Neurol.* 197, 275–283.

Mirza, B., Hadberg, H., Thomsen, P., and Moos, T. (2000). The absence of reactive astrocytosis is indicative of a unique inflammatory process in Parkinson's disease. *Neuroscience* 95, 425–432.

Muqit, M. M., Gandhi, S., and Wood, N. W. (2006). Mitochondria in Parkinson disease: back in fashion with a little help from genetics. *Arch. Neurol.* 63, 649–654.

Nakahira, K., Haspel, J. A., Rathinam, V. A., Lee, S. J., Dolinay, T., Lam, H. C., Englert, J. A., Rabinovitch, M., Cernadas, M., Kim, H. P., Fitzgerald, K. A., Ryter, S. W., and Choi, A. M. (2011). Autophagy proteins regulate innate immune responses by inhibiting the release of mitochondrial DNA mediated by the NALP3 inflammasome. *Nat. Immunol.* 12, 222–230.

Nguyen, M. D., Julien, J. P., and Rivest, S. (2002). Innate immunity: the missing link in neuroprotection and neurodegeneration? *Nat. Rev. Neurosci.* 3, 216–227.

Nusinzon, I., and Horvath, C. M. (2003). Interferon-stimulated transcription and innate antiviral immunity require deacetylase activity and histone deacetylase 1. *Proc. Natl. Acad. Sci. U.S.A.* 100, 14742–14747.

Orr, C. F., Rowe, D. B., and Halliday, G. M. (2002). An inflammatory review of Parkinson's disease. *Prog. Neurobiol.* 68, 325–340.

Orr, C. F., Rowe, D. B., Mizuno, Y., Mori, H., and Halliday, G. M. (2005). A possible role for humoral immunity in the pathogenesis of Parkinson's disease. *Brain* 128, 2665–2674.

Outeiro, T. F., Kontopoulos, E., Altmann, S. M., Kufareva, I., Strathearn, K. E., Amore, A. M., Volk, C. B., Maxwell, M. M., Rochet, J. C., Mclean, P. J., Young, A. B., Abagyan, R., Feany, M. B., Hyman, B. T., and Kazantsev, A. G. (2007). Sirtuin 2 inhibitors rescue alpha-synuclein-mediated toxicity in models of Parkinson's disease. *Science* 317, 516–519.

Perry, V. H. (2004). The influence of systemic inflammation on inflammation in the brain: implications for chronic neurodegenerative disease. *Brain Behav. Immun.* 18, 407–413.

Piccinini, M., Mostert, M., Croce, S., Baldovino, S., Papotti, M., and Rinaudo, M. T. (2003). Interferon-gamma-inducible subunits are incorporated in human brain 20S proteasome. *J. Neuroimmunol.* 135, 135–140.

Qi, B., Huang, Y., Rowe, D., and Halliday, G. (2007). VISA – a pass to innate immunity. *Int. J. Biochem. Cell Biol.* 39, 287–291.

Rentzos, M., Nikolaou, C., Andreadou, E., Paraskevas, G. P., Rombos, A., Zoga, M., Tsoutsou, A., Boufidou, F., Kapaki, E., and Vassilopoulos, D. (2009). Circulating interleukin-10 and interleukin-12 in Parkinson's disease. *Acta Neurol. Scand.* 119, 332–337.

Rivett, A. J., Bose, S., Brooks, P., and Broadfoot, K. I. (2001). Regulation of proteasome complexes by gamma-interferon and phosphorylation. *Biochimie* 83, 363–366.

Savidge, T. C., Sofroniew, M. V., and Neunlist, M. (2007). Starring roles for astroglia in barrier pathologies of gut and brain. *Lab. Invest.* 87, 731–736.

Schapira, A. H., Cooper, J. M., Dexter, D., Jenner, P., Clark, J. B., and Marsden, C. D. (1989). Mitochondrial complex I deficiency in Parkinson's disease. *Lancet* 1, 1269.

Schmidt, S., Linnartz, B., Mendritzki, S., Sczepan, T., Lubbert, M., Stichel, C. C., and Lubbert, H. (2011). Genetic mouse models for Parkinson's disease display severe pathology in glial cell mitochondria. *Hum. Mol. Genet.* 20, 1197–1211.

Scumpia, P. O., Kelly, K. M., Reeves, W. H., and Stevens, B. R. (2005). Double-stranded RNA signals antiviral and inflammatory programs and dysfunctional glutamate transport in TLR3-expressing astrocytes. *Glia* 52, 153–162.

Seth, R. B., Sun, L., and Chen, Z. J. (2006). Antiviral innate immunity pathways. *Cell Res.* 16, 141–147.

Seth, R. B., Sun, L., Ea, C. K., and Chen, Z. J. (2005). Identification and characterization of MAVS, a mitochondrial antiviral signaling protein that activates NF-kappaB and IRF 3. *Cell* 122, 669–682.

Shin, Y., Klucken, J., Patterson, C., Hyman, B. T., and Mclean, P. J. (2005). The co-chaperone carboxyl terminus of Hsp70-interacting protein (CHIP) mediates alpha-synuclein degradation decisions between proteasomal and lysosomal pathways. *J. Biol. Chem.* 280, 23727–23734.

Silverman, N., and Maniatis, T. (2001). NF-kappaB signaling pathways in mammalian and insect innate immunity. *Genes Dev.* 15, 2321–2342.

Skaug, B., and Chen, Z. J. (2010). Emerging role of ISG15 in antiviral immunity. *Cell* 143, 187–190.

Song, Y. J., Huang, Y., and Halliday, G. M. (2011). Clinical correlates of similar pathologies in parkinsonian syndromes. *Mov. Disord.* 26, 499–506.

Stefanova, N., Fellner, L., Reindl, M., Masliah, E., Poewe, W., and Wenning, G. K. (2011). Toll-like receptor 4 promotes alpha-synuclein clearance and survival of nigral dopaminergic neurons. *Am. J. Pathol.* 179, 954–963.

Steurer, J. (2011). [Nonsteroidal analgesics have a protective effect against Parkinson disease]. *Praxis (Bern 1994)* 100, 617–618.

Stone, D. K., Reynolds, A. D., Mosley, R. L., and Gendelman, H. E. (2009). Innate and adaptive immunity for the pathobiology of Parkinson's disease. *Antioxid. Redox Signal.* 11, 2151–2166.

Strauss, K. M., Martins, L. M., Plun-Favreau, H., Marx, F. P., Kautzmann, S., Berg, D., Gasser, T., Wszolek, Z., Muller, T., Bornemann, A., Wolburg, H., Downward, J., Riess, O., Schulz, J. B., and Kruger, R. (2005). Loss of function mutations in the gene encoding Omi/HtrA2 in Parkinson's disease. *Hum. Mol. Genet.* 14, 2099–2111.

Takahashi-Fujigasaki, J., and Fujigasaki, H. (2006). Histone deacetylase (HDAC) 4 involvement in both Lewy and Marinesco bodies. *Neuropathol. Appl. Neurobiol.* 32, 562–566.

Tanaka, Y., Engelender, S., Igarashi, S., Rao, R. K., Wanner, T., Tanzi, R. E., Sawa, A., V, L. D., Dawson, T. M., and Ross, C. A. (2001). Inducible expression of mutant alpha-synuclein decreases proteasome activity and increases sensitivity to mitochondria-dependent apoptosis. *Hum. Mol. Genet.* 10, 919–926.

Tang, E. D., and Wang, C. Y. (2010). TRAF5 is a downstream target of MAVS in antiviral innate immune signaling. *PLoS ONE* 5, e9172. doi:10.1371/journal.pone.0009172

Torkvist, L., Halfvarson, J., Ong, R. T., Lordal, M., Sjoqvist, U., Bresso, F., Bjork, J., Befrits, R., Lofberg, R., Blom, J., Carlson, M., Padyukov, L., D'Amato, M., Seielstad, M., and Pettersson, S. (2010). Analysis of 39 Crohn's disease risk loci in Swedish inflammatory bowel disease patients. *Inflamm. Bowel Dis.* 16, 907–909.

Umeno, J., Asano, K., Matsushita, T., Matsumoto, T., Kiyohara, Y., Iida, M., Nakamura, Y., Kamatani, N., and Kubo, M. (2011). Meta-analysis of published studies identified eight additional common susceptibility loci for Crohn's disease and ulcerative colitis. *Inflamm. Bowel. Dis.* 17, 2407–2415.

Valente, E. M., Abou-Sleiman, P. M., Caputo, V., Muqit, M. M., Harvey, K., Gispert, S., Ali, Z., Del Turco, D., Bentivoglio, A. R., Healy, D. G., Albanese, A., Nussbaum, R., Gonzalez-Maldonado, R., Deller, T., Salvi, S., Cortelli, P., Gilks, W. P., Latchman, D. S., Harvey, R. J., Dallapiccola, B., Auburger, G., and Wood, N. W. (2004). Hereditary early-onset Parkinson's disease caused by mutations in PINK1. *Science* 304, 1158–1160.

Van Limbergen, J., Wilson, D. C., and Satsangi, J. (2009). The genetics of Crohn's disease. *Annu. Rev. Genomics Hum. Genet.* 10, 89–116.

Villaran, R. F., Espinosa-Oliva, A. M., Sarmiento, M., De Pablos, R. M., Arguelles, S., Delgado-Cortes, M. J., Sobrino, V., Van Rooijen, N., Venero, J. L., Herrera, A. J., Cano, J., and Machado, A. (2010). Ulcerative colitis exacerbates lipopolysaccharide-induced damage to the nigral dopaminergic system: potential risk factor in Parkinson's disease. *J. Neurochem.* 114, 1687–1700.

Visintin, A., Latz, E., Monks, B. G., Espevik, T., and Golenbock, D. T. (2003). Lysines 128 and 132 enable lipopolysaccharide binding to MD-2, leading to Toll-like receptor-4 aggregation and signal transduction. *J. Biol. Chem.* 278, 48313–48320.

Wahner, A. D., Bronstein, J. M., Bordelon, Y. M., and Ritz, B. (2007). Nonsteroidal anti-inflammatory drugs may protect against Parkinson disease. *Neurology* 69, 1836–1842.

West, A. B., Moore, D. J., Biskup, S., Bugayenko, A., Smith, W. W., Ross, C. A., Dawson, V. L., and Dawson, T. M. (2005). Parkinson's disease-associated mutations in leucine-rich repeat kinase 2 augment kinase activity. *Proc. Natl. Acad. Sci. USA* 102, 16842–16847.

West, A. P., Koblansky, A. A., and Ghosh, S. (2006). Recognition and signaling by Toll-like receptors. *Annu. Rev. Cell Dev. Biol.* 22, 409–437.

West, A. P., Shadel, G. S., and Ghosh, S. (2011). Mitochondria in innate immune responses. *Nat. Rev. Immunol.* 11, 389–402.

Wilms, H., Rosenstiel, P., Sievers, J., Deuschl, G., Zecca, L., and Lucius, R. (2003). Activation of microglia by human neuromelanin is NF-kappaB dependent and involves p38 mitogen-activated protein kinase: implications for Parkinson's disease. *FASEB J.* 17, 500–502.

Wood, L. M., Sankar, S., Reed, R. E., Haas, A. L., Liu, L. F., Mckinnon, P., and Desai, S. D. (2011). A novel role for ATM in regulating proteasome-mediated protein degradation through suppression of the ISG15 conjugation pathway. *PLoS ONE* 6, e16422. doi:10.1371/journal.pone.0016422

Wu, C. J., Conze, D. B., Li, T., Srinivasula, S. M., and Ashwell, J. D. (2006). NEMO is a sensor of Lys 63-linked polyubiquitination and functions in NF-kappaB activation. *Nat. Cell Biol.* 8, 398–406.

Zhang, Y., Gao, J., Chung, K. K., Huang, H., Dawson, V. L., and Dawson, T. M. (2000). Parkin functions as an E2-dependent ubiquitin- protein ligase and promotes the degradation of the synaptic vesicle-associated protein, CDCrel-1. *Proc. Natl. Acad. Sci. U.S.A.* 97, 13354–13359.

Zhang, L., Shimoji, M., Thomas, B., Moore, D. J., Yu, S. W., Marupudi, N. I., Torp, R., Torgner, I. A., Ottersen, O. P., Dawson, T. M., and Dawson, V. L. (2005). Mitochondrial localization of the Parkinson's disease related protein DJ-1: implications for pathogenesis. *Hum. Mol. Genet.* 14, 2063–2073.

8

Chronic traumatic encephalopathy and other neurodegenerative proteinopathies

Maria Carmela Tartaglia[1,2,3]*, Lili-Naz Hazrati[2,3,4], Karen D. Davis[3,5,6,7,8], Robin E. A. Green[3,9], Richard Wennberg[1,3], David Mikulis[3,10], Leo J. Ezerins[3,11], Michelle Keightley[3,9,12,13,14,15] and Charles Tator[3,16]

[1] Division of Neurology, Krembil Neuroscience Centre, University Health Network, University of Toronto, Toronto, ON, Canada
[2] Tanz Centre for Research in Neurodegenerative Disease, University of Toronto, Toronto, ON, Canada
[3] Canadian Sports Concussion Project, Toronto, ON, Canada
[4] Department of Laboratory Medicine and Pathobiology, University of Toronto, Toronto, ON, Canada
[5] Division of Neurosurgery, University Health Network, University of Toronto, Toronto, ON, Canada
[6] Division of Brain, Imaging and Behaviour – Systems Neuroscience, Toronto Western Research Institute, University Health Network, Toronto, ON, Canada
[7] Department of Surgery, University of Toronto, Toronto, ON, Canada
[8] Institute of Medical Science, University of Toronto, Toronto, ON, Canada
[9] Toronto Rehabilitation Institute, Toronto, ON, Canada
[10] Division of Neuroradiology, Joint Department of Medical Imaging, Toronto Western Hospital, The University of Toronto, Toronto, ON, Canada
[11] Executive Director, Canadian Football League Alumni Association, Toronto, ON, Canada
[12] Bloorview Research Institute, Holland Bloorview Kids Rehabilitation Hospital, Toronto, ON, Canada
[13] Department of Occupational Science and Occupational Therapy, University of Toronto, Toronto, ON, Canada
[14] Graduate Department of Rehabilitation Science, University of Toronto, Toronto, ON, Canada
[15] Department of Psychology, University of Toronto, Toronto, ON, Canada
[16] Division of Neurosurgery, Krembil Neuroscience Centre, Toronto Western Hospital, University of Toronto, Toronto, ON, Canada

Edited by:
Hauke R. Heekeren, Freie Universität Berlin, Germany

Reviewed by:
Jerome J. Maller, Monash Alfred Psychiatry Research Centre, Australia
Hal S. Wortzel, Veterans Health Administration, USA
Barbara B. Bendlin, University of Wisconsin, USA

***Correspondence:**
Maria Carmela Tartaglia, Memory Clinic - Toronto Western Hospital, Tanz Centre for Research in Neurodegenerative Disease, University of Toronto, West Wing 5-449, 399 Bathurst St., Toronto, ON M5T 2S8, Canada
e-mail: carmela.tartaglia@uhn.on.ca

"Chronic traumatic encephalopathy" (CTE) is described as a slowly progressive neurodegenerative disease believed to result from multiple concussions. Traditionally, concussions were considered benign events and although most people recover fully, about 10% develop a post-concussive syndrome with persisting neurological, cognitive and neuropsychiatric symptoms. CTE was once thought to be unique to boxers, but it has now been observed in many different athletes having suffered multiple concussions as well as in military personal after repeated blast injuries. Much remains unknown about the development of CTE but its pathological substrate is usually tau, similar to that seen in Alzheimer's disease (AD) and frontotemporal lobar degeneration (FTLD). The aim of this "perspective" is to compare and contrast clinical and pathological CTE with the other neurodegenerative proteinopathies and highlight that there is an urgent need for understanding the relationship between concussion and the development of CTE as it may provide a window into the development of a proteinopathy and thus new avenues for treatment.

Keywords: concussions, chronic traumatic encephalopathy, neurodegenerative disease, Alzheimer's disease, frontotemporal lobar degeneration, tau

CONCUSSIONS: AN EVOLUTION IN OUR UNDERSTANDING

"Chronic traumatic encephalopathy" (CTE) is described as a slowly progressive neurodegenerative disease with pathological tau accumulation at the depths of the sulci in superficial layers of the cortex. Clinically CTE is believed to include neuropsychiatric, cognitive and motor deficits that manifest years after implicated concussive or subconcussive events (McKee et al., 2009). It is believed to be a consequence of repeated mild brain traumas also known as concussions. Although the majority of concussions are fully resolved within 3 months (Iverson, 2007), and conventional neuroimaging and neuropsychological testing are typically normal (Broglio and Puetz, 2008), the notion of concussion as a completely benign event (e.g., "bell-ringer") is outdated. Most people return to baseline after a single concussion but an estimated 10% of cases result in serious and persisting somatic, affective, cognitive, and/or movement sequelae (Wood, 2004). There is growing clinical and societal concern about the effects of multiple concussions (Jordan, 2013) although one meta-analyses revealed no significant effects after multiple concussions (Belanger et al., 2010). CTE was first described in Miller (1966) as a constellation of symptoms typical of neurodegenerative disease. Clinically and pathologically it bears resemblance to other neurodegenerative diseases, now thought of as proteinopathies, which includes Alzheimer's disease (AD) and frontotemporal lobar degeneration (FTLD). Although widespread media attention has spawned a dogma on the *delayed* effects of multiple concussions (Corsellis and Brierley, 1959; Corsellis et al., 1973; Omalu et al., 2005, 2010a; Gavett et al., 2010; Costanza et al., 2011; Stern et al., 2011; Goldstein et al., 2012; McKee et al., 2013), there remains much to be known on the clinical and pathophysiology of CTE. A better understanding of the differences and similarities of CTE and the other proteinopathies may help guide future studies.

MULTIPLE CONCUSSIONS AND CHRONIC TRAUMATIC ENCEPHALOPATHY

PUNCH DRUNK SYNDROME, DEMENTIA PUGILISTICA, CHRONIC TRAUMATIC ENCEPHALOPATHY

In 1928, Martland introduced the term "punch-drunk" state (Martland, 1928) in reference to the chronic motor and psychiatric consequences of blows to the head in boxing. Millspaugh (1937) coined "dementia pugilistica" to describe similar cases. A few decades later, Critchley (1957) reported on 69 cases of progressive neurological disease in boxers and proposed "chronic progressive traumatic encephalopathy of boxers." He described an insidious and gradual development of mental and physical anomalies marked by a "euphoric dementia" with emotional lability, little insight, progressive bradyphrenia, and memory deficits, along with changes in behavior. Critchley added that many patients displayed mood-swings, intense irritability, and occasionally, uninhibited violent behavior. He noted "fatuous cheerfulness" as the commonest mood finding but also reported paranoid depression. Motor findings included pyramidal, extra-pyramidal, and cerebellar signs, with tremor and dysarthria the most frequently reported. Sensory perceptual findings included deafness and poor vision. His patients also complained of persistent dull headaches, postural dizziness, and unsteady gait, reminiscent of acute concussion and post-concussive syndrome. In 1969, Roberts reported on 224 former boxers and found that 17% suffered from significant memory loss, aggression, confusion, or depression and that there was direct correlation of incidence to number of fights and overall length of boxing career (Roberts, 1969). Many observational studies, some prospective, have also been undertaken, including a systematic review of 36 of an initial 943 studies on the chronic effects of amateur boxing (Loosemore et al., 2007).

The early literature on the chronic effects of multiple concussions focused on boxing, but multiple concussions sustained under different circumstances can also produce chronic effects. The term CTE has been coined to encompass progressive neurodegenerative effects observed after multiple concussions sustained in any context (Miller, 1966).

Clinical CTE cases overlap with punch-drunk syndrome. CTE is usually described as an evolving constellation of cognitive, psychiatric and motor symptoms (McKee et al., 2009). Cognitive findings may precede, co-occur or follow psychiatric findings, and can include impaired concentration, attention, and memory along with disorientation, confusion, and speech abnormalities later on McKee et al. (2009). Emotional lability, inappropriate behavior, paranoia, outbursts of aggressive behavior and explosivity, mood disturbance, disinhibition, psychosis, and dysexecutive symptoms are observed. Dizziness and headaches are frequent (McKee et al., 2009). Psychiatric symptoms are observable at all stages of CTE, with no clear dose response between extent of neuropathology and clinical symptoms (McKee et al., 2013). Parkinsonian symptoms of tremor, masked facies, wide based gait, poor speech, ocular abnormalities, bradykinesia, and dementia appear as the disease progresses (Omalu et al., 2011a; McKee et al., 2013).

WHO IS AT RISK?

The majority of cases of suspected CTE have been reported in athletes in contact sports, including boxing, hockey, wrestling, soccer, and North American football (Corsellis et al., 1973; Omalu et al., 2006, 2010b; McKee et al., 2009; Dekosky et al., 2010; Gavett et al., 2011; Neselius et al., 2012). CTE has also been associated with physical abuse and epilepsy (McKee et al., 2009). More recently, CTE was reported in a war veteran having suffered blast-injury without signs of overt concussion (Omalu et al., 2011b).

CTE requires post-mortem assessment and all post-mortem studies to date contain samples that are not representative of either the general population or even of multiply concussed populations. McKee et al. (2009) reported that 46/51 (90%) of neuropathologically confirmed CTE cases occurred in athletes who had played contact sports. However, in general, brains referred for autopsy are those of individuals who displayed overt neurological signs at the time of death and therefore were at elevated risk of underlying pathology compared to the large number of athletes who play contact sports but do not show neurological signs throughout their life.

McKee et al. (2013) recently published an expansion of her previous study with 85 brains from former athletes, veterans and civilians with a history of multiple concussions. Importantly, there was no evidence of CTE despite repetitive concussion in 17/85 (20%) of cases, and in 15/85 cases (37%) there was significant comorbid pathology of AD, Lewy body disease (LBD), motor neuron disease (MND), or FTLD. In advanced cases, a comorbid condition such as AD, LBD, or FTLD was present in almost half the cases (10/25) These findings converge with a recent study undertaken by our group, which showed that even with a history of multiple concussions from contact sport *and* a positive clinical presentation before death, a diagnosis of CTE is not inevitable on neuropathological examination. Our case series included the brains of six retired professional players of the Canadian Football League with a history of multiple concussions (Hazrati et al., 2013) and all clinically symptomatic before death. While each case displayed significant neuropathological changes on post-mortem examination, only three showed pathology consistent with CTE. In the other three cases, the neuropathological diagnoses were Parkinson's Disease (PD), Amyotrophic Lateral Sclerosis (ALS), and AD. Even the cases with CTE had co-pathology, including AD, PD, or vasculopathy. This study demonstrates that there is not always a direct relationship between multiple concussions, clinical symptomology, and CTE.

In a recent retrospective analysis a higher incidence of mortality from neurodegenerative disease including AD- and ALS was reported among former National Football League players, compared to the general population (Lehman et al., 2012). Notably, however, players (vs. the rest of the general US population studied), and in particular players in speed positions, showed the *lowest* death rate for other causes of death including cardiovascular disease and cancer, the largest killers of the general US population. These data may thus inflate the apparent risk of neurodegenerative disease and argue for prospective research into the biological effects of multiple concussions.

AGE OF ONSET

Critchley (1957) reports age of onset on 11 cases of punch-drunk syndrome: two were still boxing, six were in their 20 s, two were in their 30 s, and one was 61 years old. McKee et al. (2009) reported CTE symptom onset at ages ranging from 25 to 76 years; one-third were symptomatic at retirement and half were symptomatic within 4 years of their retirement. Although Omalu et al. (2011a) proposed an asymptomatic period between playing of the sport and symptom onset, in his series of 10 cases, four were in their 30 s, three were in their 40 s, and three were in their 50 s. Thus, very few of the players had a prolonged asymptomatic or latent period. There has been no differentiation between the delayed onset of CTE-associated symptoms and the more immediate onset observed in boxers. Importantly, in the absence of serial, longitudinal evaluations in the above studies, we cannot rule out symptom onset prior to formal diagnosis.

Whether CTE and the punch-drunk syndrome are dissociable entities is still unclear. While both syndromes can be associated with the cumulative effects of concussion, it is conceivable that CTE reflects a delayed onset entity, while the punch-drunk syndrome represents a continuation and progression of symptoms from an acute concussive state (Gardner et al., 2014). Also uncertain is whether some players are in a prolonged or more severe postconcussive syndrome that may have a different pathophysiology than the players who develop symptoms decades after their last concussion.

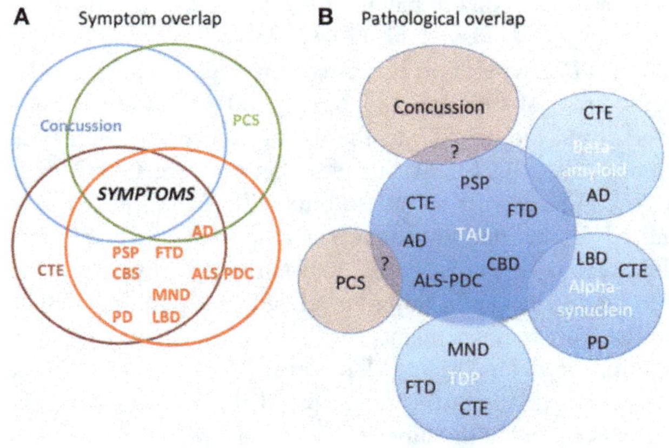

FIGURE 1 | The interrelationships between concussion, post-concussion syndrome (PCS), chronic traumatic encephalopathy (CTE), and all the neurodegenerative diseases. (A) There is considerable symptom overlap between concussion, PCS, CTE, and the neurodegenerative diseases. **(B)** Pathologically the relationship between concussion, PCS, CTE, and all the neurodegenerative diseases is unclear. In CTE there is substantial evidence for overlapping pathology of tau, TDP-43, amyloid, and alpha-synuclein with neurodegenerative diseases. In neurodegenerative diseases such as AD, PD, and LBD, there is also overlapping pathology. The pathology of concussion and PCS and their relationship to CTE remains to be explored. AD, Alzheimer's Disease; ALS-PDC, amyotrophic lateral sclerosis-parkinson's dementia complex (Guam); CBD, corticobasal degeneration; CBS, corticobasal syndrome; CTE, chronic traumatic encephalopathy; LBD, Lewy Body Disease; FTD, frontotemporal dementia; MND, motor neuron disease; PCS, Post-concussive syndrome; PSP, progressive supranuclear palsy; PD, Parkinson's disease. "?" indicates uncertainty about overlap.

CHRONIC TRAUMATIC ENCEPHALOPATHY vs. OTHER PROTEINOPATHIES

CLINICAL COMPARISONS

The clinical diagnosis of CTE is currently not feasible due to the overlap with other neurodegenerative conditions. AD is the most common neurodegenerative disease in those over age 65 (Prince et al., 2013) and most often presents with impaired learning and recall of recently learned information (McKhann et al., 2011). Neuropsychiatric symptoms including depression, apathy, agitation, and irritability, as in CTE, are not uncommon (Cummings, 1997).

FTLD is the most common neurodegenerative disease in those less than 65, and includes several clinical syndromes involving changes in behavior, language, and motor function. The main clinical phenotypes are: behavioral variant frontotemporal dementia (bvFTD), primary progressive aphasia, FTD-motor neuron disease (FTD-MND), progressive supranuclear palsy (PSP), and corticobasal syndrome (CBS). Although these syndromes strongly overlap in clinical, genetic, and pathological features their syndrome specific clinical expression differs markedly due to focal pathology (Brun, 1993) (**Figure 1A**). bvFTD, as its name implies, is primarily a behavioral syndrome characterized by dramatic personality and behavioral changes. The apathy, loss of social norms, and decreased empathy seen in bvFTD are frequent symptoms in traumatic brain injury (TBI) including moderate-severe TBI, concussion, and CTE and are attributed to frontal lobe degeneration (Damasio et al., 1991; Stuss et al., 2001; Jordan, 2013) in particular orbitofrontal and ventromedial prefrontal cortex, as well as insula (Rosen et al., 2005). The language variants, as well as CBS (a progressive, asymmetric, akinetic-rigid syndrome) and PSP (cognitive and behavioral deficits and prominent oculomotor and movement impairments) (Litvan et al., 1996) have less in common with CTE. bvFTD-like symptoms can co-occur in patients with MND (Lomen-Hoerth et al., 2003), and some patients with CTE have presented with MND phenotype and a TAR-DNA binding protein 43 (TDP-43) pathology (McKee et al., 2010). Parkinsonism and cognitive deficits as seen in LBD and PD are also seen in CTE and there are cases of LBD and PD subsequent to multiple concussions (Hazrati et al., 2013; McKee et al., 2013).

The overlap in signs and symptoms of CTE and other neurodegenerative diseases, especially bvFTD, is likely a result of focal involvement of frontal networks that subserve numerous higher functions including personality/emotional life, executive function, and motivation (Stuss and Levine, 2002). A better understanding of the pathophysiology of any of the neurodegenerative diseases may shed light on the risk factors for developing CTE.

PATHOLOGICAL SIGNS OF CTE vs. OTHER NEURODEGENERATIVE DISEASE

Only a limited number of cases of suspected CTE have undergone pathological examination but post-mortem assessments show a distinct pattern from other proteinopathies including dilated ventricles, a fenestrated, and cavum septum pellucidum, significant atrophy of the medial temporal lobes, thalamus, and mammillary bodies and occasionally pallor of the locus coeruleus and substantia nigra (McKee et al., 2009; Gavett et al., 2011; Stern et al., 2011). Hyperphosphorylated tau deposits in neurons of specific areas of the brains of boxers and professional football players, thus adding CTE to the list of known tauopathies that includes PSP, CBD, FTLD, Guam-Parkinson Dementia Complex, and AD. Tau is a protein that binds to and stabilizes microtubules required for maintaining neuronal shape and for transport of cellular cargo (Brunden et al., 2009). The distribution of these pathological changes is along the amygdalo-hippocampal-septo-hypothalamic-mesencephalic continuum, which is part of the emotional or visceral brain (McKee et al., 2009). The pathological changes are greatest in the depths of sulci, perivascularly around small vessels, and in the superficial cortical layers (II/III). This tau distribution pattern is distinct from other tauopathies. In AD, the neurofibrillary tangles (NFTs) are more regular, are primarily in layers III and V of the cortex, and are neither perivascular nor primarily at the depths of the sulci. In PSP, the NFTs are mainly in the basal ganglia and hindbrain structures. Other distinguishing patterns of tau deposition seen in CTE include irregular and patchy distributions and also prominence in the periventricular and subpial areas. Unlike AD, CTE usually lacks significant amounts of beta-amyloid plaque deposition (Braak and Braak, 1997; McKee et al., 2009; Gavett et al., 2011; Stern et al., 2011).

In select cases of CTE, widespread TDP-43 immunopositive inclusions have been observed (McKee et al., 2010). Lesions involving the corticospinal tracts and the anterior horns of the spinal cord are associated with clinical motor findings of spasticity, weakness, and fasciculations similar to those seen in ALS (McKee et al., 2010). The pathological accumulation of TDP-43 is also seen in FTLD and like tau can cause various FTLD syndromes (Whitwell and Josephs, 2011). Alpha-synuclein positive Lewy bodies as seen in PD and LBD and Alzheimer's beta-amyloid pathology has also occasionally been reported in CTE (McKee et al., 2013).

Similarities exist between CTE and the chronic effects of moderate and severe TBI, in which there can be neurodegeneration in the chronic phase months to years after TBI with sub-acute atrophy within the hippocampi (Ng et al., 2008) and elsewhere (Green et al., 2010). Interestingly, the corpus callosum (unmyelinated axons in particular) is vulnerable to protein deposition post-TBI, suggesting commonality with CTE (Reeves et al., 2005, 2012).

Recently Omalu et al. (2011a) proposed four histomorphologic phenotypes in CTE based on the distribution of NFTs and neuritic threads in the cortex, brainstem, subcortical nuclei, basal ganglia, and cerebellum, and they include amyloid plaques in one phenotype. In contrast, McKee et al. (2013) proposed a staging scheme for CTE severity based on tau distribution which would range from focal epicentres of phosphorylated tau (p-tau) usually in the frontal cortex and typically around small vessels at the depths of sulci to widespread p-tau pathology in a patchy irregular distribution in cortical areas and medial temporal lobe as well as in thalamus, hypothalamus, mammillary bodies, basal ganglia, brainstem and in white matter tracts. Currently, the clinical-pathological relationship is unknown and questions as to whether differences relate to different types of CTE, different types of injury and/or different clinical syndromes remain. There is some evidence for pathological and clinical differences between the classic CTE cases and the "modern" form described in the last few years (Gardner et al., 2014). These authors argue that the classic form of CTE does not appear to advance in a predictable and sequential series of stages, and progression of physical symptoms is only present in approximately one-third of cases. Clearly long-term, prospective clinical studies followed by detailed neuropathological examination are needed to help unravel this issue.

It has become increasingly apparent that CTE frequently coexists with other pathologies. In our series of six cases, the three patients with CTE also exhibited other neurodegenerative pathology as noted above (Hazrati et al., 2013). McKee's recent case series (McKee et al., 2013) found co-pathology of CTE with AD, LBD or both in 17 cases and CTE and MND in eight cases. The relative contribution of the different pathological substrates to the clinical symptoms is currently unknown and requires further study. A recent review of the contemporary cases in the literature found that over 50% had copathology with CTE and only 20% had pure CTE (Gardner et al., 2014).

In vivo diagnosis of the specific proteinopathy responsible for a neurodegenerative disease is now the goal. Currently, amyloid imaging and cerebrospinal fluid (CSF) biomarkers of amyloid and tau for the *in vivo* diagnosis of AD are available although not in clinical use (Sperling and Johnson, 2013). Regarding the other neurodegenerative diseases, neither imaging nor fluid biomarkers are available for their diagnosis although there are some experimental data coming out in PD (Parnetti et al., 2013; Schapira, 2013) and FTLD (Hu et al., 2010, 2013). In CTE, concussion, and post-concussion syndrome there are a few studies suggesting abnormalities including elevated levels of CSF tau (Neselius et al., 2012; Shenton et al., 2012; Zetterberg et al., 2013) but these lack pathological confirmation and haven't been reproduced. CTE is still in its infancy with regard to defining the clinical syndrome and determining *in vivo* biomarkers of the underlying pathology.

SUMMARY AND CONCLUSIONS: MUCH REMAINS TO BE KNOWN

Tau deposition and pathological changes in a particular distribution have been observed in cases of multiple concussions. The evidence to date concerning CTE, its association with multiple concussions, and its clinical signs and symptoms comes from case reports, cases series, and retrospective analyses (Graves et al., 1990; Schofield et al., 1997; Mehta et al., 1999; McKee et al., 2013). The symptoms described in CTE overlap with those described in concussion, PCS and the neurodegenerative diseases. **Figure 1A**. There is a selection bias for many of the reported cases, some died from violent deaths such as suicide or drug overdose and/or were otherwise clinically symptomatic with cognitive symptoms. There are now an increasing number of reports of cases with multiple concussions but no evidence of CTE at autopsy (Hazrati et al., 2013; McKee et al., 2013). The exact relationship between multiple concussions and CTE is ambiguous. Moreover, one must distinguish clinically and pathologically between static, non-progressive cumulative effects of multiple concussions vs. progressive findings of symptomatic neurodegenerative disease. Complicating the situation are cases of a single, but more serious TBI associated with increased risk of dementia (Blennow et al., 2012; Sayed et al., 2013) as well as atrophy and loss of white matter integrity in the sub-acute and chronic stages of injury (Greenberg et al., 2008; Ng et al., 2008; Whitwell and Josephs, 2011; Adnan et al., 2013)

Prospective, longitudinal studies with neuropathological analysis that sample a broader cross section of individuals, including those with a history of multiple concussions but without positive clinical neurological findings prior to death are critically needed. Understanding the relationship of multiple concussions to CTE as well as possible modifiers is paramount for preventing or ameliorating this illness and for finding a cure. Furthermore, and most importantly, by evoking a diagnosis of CTE as a cause of the symptoms and signs and symptoms in multiple concussions, and failing to address treatable and potentially reversible causes of the suffering is a disservice to the patient and a lost opportunity to understand their sequelae (Wortzel et al., 2013).

CTE now joins the family of tauopathies that includes PSP, bvFTD, and AD but there a number of cases of associated TDP and amyloid pathology, which requires further study and clinical correlate (**Figure 1B**). As well, the pathological relationship of CTE with concussion and post-concussion syndrome remains to be explored. As we move toward protein specific treatments, *in vivo* diagnosis of CTE at an early stage will be imperative for implementing appropriate treatments and to delay, halt, or reverse its progression. In order to do this, good clinical-pathological studies will be required and appropriate biomarkers will have to be developed.

REFERENCES

Adnan, A., Crawley, A., Mikulis, D., Moscovitch, M., Colella, B., and Green, R. (2013). Moderate-severe traumatic brain injury causes delayed loss of white matter integrity: evidence of fornix deterioration in the chronic stage of injury. *Brain Inj.* 27, 1415–1422. doi: 10.3109/02699052.2013.823659

Belanger, H. G., Spiegel, E., and Vanderploeg, R. D. (2010). Neuropsychological performance following a history of multiple self-reported concus- sions: a meta-analysis. *J. Int. Neuropsychol. Soc.* 16, 262–267. doi: 10.1017/S1355617709991287

Blennow, K., Hardy, J., and Zetterberg, H. (2012). The neuropathology and neurobiology of traumatic brain injury. *Neuron* 76, 886–899. doi: 10.1016/j.neuron.2012.11.021

Braak, H., and Braak, E. (1997). Staging of Alzheimer-related cortical destruc- tion. *Int. Psychogeriatr.* 9(Suppl. 1), 257–261. discussion: 269–272. doi: 10.1017/S1041610297004973

Broglio, S. P., and Puetz, T. W. (2008). The effect of sport concussion on neurocog- nitive function, self-report symptoms and postural control: a meta-analysis. *Sports Med.* 38, 53–67. doi: 10.2165/00007256-200838010-00005

Brun, A. (1993). Frontal lobe degeneration of non-Alzheimer type revisited. *Dementia* 4, 126–131. doi: 10.1159/000107311

Brunden, K. R., Ballatore, C., Crowe, A., Smith, A. B., 3rd, Lee, V. M., and Trojanowski, J. Q. (2009). Tau-directed drug discovery for Alzheimer's disease and related tauopathies: a focus on tau assembly inhibitors. *Exp. Neurol.* 223, 304–310. doi: 10.1016/j.expneurol.2009.08.031

Corsellis, J. A., and Brierley, J. B. (1959). Observations on the pathology of insidious dementia following head injury. *J. Ment. Sci.* 105, 714–720.

Corsellis, J. A., Bruton, C. J., and Freeman-Browne, D. (1973). The aftermath of boxing. *Psychol. Med.* 3, 270–303. doi: 10.1017/S0033291700049588

Costanza, A., Weber, K., Gandy, S., Bouras, C., Hof, P. R., Giannakopoulos, P., et al. (2011). Review: Contact sport-related chronic traumatic encephalopathy in the elderly: clinical expression and structural substrates. *Neuropathol. Appl. Neurobiol.* 37, 570–584. doi: 10.1111/j.1365-2990.2011.01186.x

Critchley, M. (1957). Medical Aspects of Boxing, Particularly from a neurological standpoint. *BMJ* 1, 357–362. doi: 10.1136/bmj.1.5015.357

Cummings, J. L. (1997). The Neuropsychiatric Inventory: assessing psy- chopathology in dementia patients. *Neurology* 48, S10–S16. doi: 10.1212/WNL.48.5_Suppl_6.10S

Damasio, A. R., Tranel, D., and Damasio, H. C. (1991). "Somatic markers and guid- ance of behavior: theory and preliminary testing," in *Frontal Lobe Function and Dysfunction,* eds H.M.E. H. S. Levin and A. L. Benton. (New York, NY: Oxford University Press), 217–229.

Dekosky, S. T., Ikonomovic, M. D., and Gandy, S. (2010). Traumatic brain injury- football, warfare, and long-term effects. *N. Engl. J. Med.* 363, 1293–1296. doi: 10.1056/NEJMp1007051

Gardner, A., Iverson, G. L., and McCrory, P. (2014). Chronic traumatic encephalopathy in sport: a systematic review. *Br. J. Sports Med.* 48, 84–90. doi: 10.1136/bjsports-2013-092646

Gavett, B. E., Stern, R. A., Cantu, R. C., Nowinski, C. J., and McKee, A. C. (2010). Mild traumatic brain injury: a risk factor for neurodegeneration. *Alzheimers Res. Ther.* 2, 18. doi: 10.1186/alzrt42

Gavett, B. E., Stern, R. A., and McKee, A. C. (2011). Chronic trau- matic encephalopathy: a potential late effect of sport-related concussive and subconcussive head trauma. *Clin. Sports Med.* 30, 179–188, xi. doi: 10.1016/j.csm.2010.09.007

Goldstein, L. E., Fisher, A. M., Tagge, C. A., Zhang, X. L., Velisek, L., Sullivan, J. A., et al. (2012). Chronic traumatic encephalopathy in blast-exposed military veterans and a blast neurotrauma mouse model. *Sci. Transl. Med.* 4, 134ra160. doi: 10.1126/scitranslmed.3003716

Graves, A. B., White, E., Koepsell, T. D., Reifler, B. V., Van Belle, G., Larson, E. B., et al. (1990). The association between head trauma and Alzheimer's disease. *Am. J. Epidemiol.* 131, 491–501.

Green, R., Koshimori, Y., and Turner, G. (2010). Research digest. Understanding the organic basis of persistent complaints in mTBI: findings from func- tional and structural neuroimaging. *Neuropsychol. Rehabil.* 20, 471–478. doi: 10.1080/09602011003693298

Greenberg, G., Mikulis, D. J., Ng, K., Desouza, D., and Green, R. E. (2008). Use of diffusion tensor imaging to examine subacute white matter injury progres- sion in moderate to severe traumatic brain injury. *Arch. Phys. Med. Rehabil.* 89, S45–S50. doi: 10.1016/j.apmr.2008.08.211

Hazrati, L. N., Tartaglia, M. C., Diamandis, P., Davis, K. D., Green, R. E., Wennberg, R., et al. (2013). Absence of chronic traumatic encephalopathy in retired foot- ball players with multiple concussions and neurological symptomatology. *Front. Hum. Neurosci.* 7:222. doi: 10.3389/fnhum.2013.00222

Hu, W. T., Chen-Plotkin, A., Grossman, M., Arnold, S. E., Clark, C. M., Shaw, L. M., et al. (2010). Novel CSF biomarkers for frontotemporal lobar degenerations. *Neurology* 75, 2079–2086. doi: 10.1212/WNL.0b013e318200d78d

Hu, W. T., Watts, K., Grossman, M., Glass, J., Lah, J. J., Hales, C., et al. (2013). Reduced CSF p-Tau181 to Tau ratio is a biomarker for FTLD-TDP. *Neurology* 81, 1945–1952. doi: 10.1212/01.wnl.0000436625.63650.27

Iverson, G. (2007). Predicting slow recovery from sport-related concussion: the new simple-complex distinction. *Clin. J. Sport Med.* 17, 31–37. doi: 10.1097/JSM.0b013e3180305e4d

Jordan, B. D. (2013). The clinical spectrum of sport-related traumatic brain injury. *Nat. Rev. Neurol.* 9, 222–230. doi: 10.1038/nrneurol.2013.33

Lehman, E. J., Hein, M. J., Baron, S. L., and Gersic, C. M. (2012). Neurodegenerative causes of death among retired National Football League players. *Neurology* 79, 1970–1974. doi: 10.1212/WNL.0b013e31826daf50

Litvan, I., Agid, Y., Calne, D., Campbell, G., Dubois, B., Duvoisin, R. C., et al. (1996). Clinical research criteria for the diagnosis of progressive supranuclear palsy (Steele-Richardson-Olszewski syndrome): report of the NINDS-SPSP international workshop. *Neurology* 47, 1–9. doi: 10.1212/WNL.47.1.1

Lomen-Hoerth, C., Murphy, J., Langmore, S., Kramer, J. H., Olney, R. K., and Miller, B. (2003). Are amyotrophic lateral sclerosis patients cognitively normal? *Neurology* 60, 1094–1097. doi: 10.1212/01.WNL.0000055861.95202.8D

Loosemore, M., Knowles, C. H., and Whyte, G. P. (2007). Amateur boxing and risk of chronic traumatic brain injury: systematic review of observational studies. *BMJ* 335, 809. doi: 10.1136/bmj.39342.690220.55

Martland, H. (1928). Punch drunk. *JAMA* 91, 1103–1107. doi: 10.1001/jama.1928.02700150029009

McKee, A. C., Cantu, R. C., Nowinski, C. J., Hedley-Whyte, E. T., Gavett, B. E., Budson, A. E., et al. (2009). Chronic traumatic encephalopathy in athletes: pro- gressive tauopathy after repetitive head injury. *J. Neuropathol. Exp. Neurol.* 68, 709–735. doi: 10.1097/NEN.0b013e3181a9d503

McKee, A. C., Gavett, B. E., Stern, R. A., Nowinski, C. J., Cantu, R. C., Kowall, N. W., et al. (2010). TDP-43 proteinopathy and motor neuron disease in chronic traumatic encephalopathy. *J. Neuropathol. Exp. Neurol.* 69, 918–929. doi: 10.1097/NEN.0b013e3181ee7d85

McKee, A. C., Stern, R. A., Nowinski, C. J., Stern, R. A., Daneshvar, D. H., Alvarez, V. E., et al. (2013). The spectrum of disease in chronic traumatic encephalopathy. *Brain* 136, 43–64. doi: 10.1093/brain/aws307

McKhann, G. M., Knopman, D. S., Chertkow, H., Hyman, B. T., Jack, C. R., Jr., Kawas, C. H., et al. (2011). The diagnosis of dementia due to Alzheimer's disease: recommendations from the National Institute on Aging-Alzheimer's Association workgroups on diagnostic guidelines for Alzheimer's disease. *Alzheimers Dement.* 7, 263–269. doi: 10.1016/j.jalz.2011.03.005

Mehta, K. M., Ott, A., Kalmijn, S., Slooter, A. J., Van Duijn, C. M., Hofman, A., et al. (1999). Head trauma and risk of dementia and Alzheimer's disease: the Rotterdam Study. *Neurology* 53, 1959–1962. doi: 10.1212/WNL.53.9.1959

Miller, H. (1966). Mental after-effects of head injury. *Proc. R. Soc. Med.* 59, 257–261.

Millspaugh, J. (1937). Dementia pugilistica. *U.S. Naval Med. Bull.* 35, 297–303. Neselius, S., Brisby, H., Theodorsson, A., Blennow, K., Zetterberg, H., and

Marcusson, J. (2012). CSF-biomarkers in Olympic boxing: diagnosis and effects of repetitive head trauma. *PLoS ONE* 7:e33606. doi: 10.1371/jour- nal.pone.0033606

Ng, K., Mikulis, D. J., Glazer, J., Kabani, N., Till, C., Greenberg, G., et al. (2008). Magnetic resonance imaging evidence of progression of subacute brain atro- phy in moderate to severe traumatic brain injury. *Arch. Phys. Med. Rehabil.* 89, S35–S44. doi: 10.1016/j.apmr.2008.07.006

Omalu, B., Bailes, J., Hamilton, R. L., Kamboh, M. I., Hammers, J., Case, M., et al. (2011a). Emerging histomorphologic phenotypes of chronic traumatic encephalopathy in American athletes. *Neurosurgery* 69, 173–183. discussion: 183. doi: 10.1227/NEU.0b013e318212bc7b

Omalu, B., Hammers, J. L., Bailes, J., Hamilton, R. L., Kamboh, M. I., Webster, G., et al. (2011b). Chronic traumatic encephalopathy in an Iraqi war veteran with posttraumatic stress disorder who committed suicide. *Neurosurg. Focus* 31, E3. doi: 10.3171/2011.9.FOCUS11178

Omalu, B. I., Bailes, J., Hammers, J. L., and Fitzsimmons, R. P. (2010a). Chronic traumatic encephalopathy, suicides and parasuicides in professional American athletes: the role of the forensic pathologist. *Am. J. Forensic Med. Pathol.* 31, 130–132. doi: 10.1097/PAF.0b013e3181ca7f35

Omalu, B. I., Hamilton, R. L., Kamboh, M. I., Dekosky, S. T., and Bailes, J. (2010b). Chronic traumatic encephalopathy (CTE) in a National Football League Player: Case report and emerging medicolegal practice questions. *J. Forensic Nurs.* 6, 40–46. doi: 10.1111/j.1939-3938.2009.01064.x

Omalu, B. I., Dekosky, S. T., Hamilton, R. L., Minster, R. L., Kamboh, M. I., Shakir, A. M., et al. (2006). Chronic traumatic encephalopathy in a national football league player: part II. *Neurosurgery* 59, 1086–1092. discussion: 1092–1083. doi: 10.1227/01.NEU.0000245601.69451.27

Omalu, B. I., Dekosky, S. T., Minster, R. L., Kamboh, M. I., Hamilton, R. L., and Wecht, C. H. (2005). Chronic traumatic encephalopathy in a National Football League player. *Neurosurgery* 57, 128–134. discussion: 128–134. doi: 10.1227/01.NEU.0000163407.92769.ED

Parnetti, L., Castrioto, A., Chiasserini, D., Persichetti, E., Tambasco, N., El-Agnaf, O., et al. (2013). Cerebrospinal fluid biomarkers in Parkinson disease. *Nat. Rev. Neurol.* 9, 131–140. doi: 10.1038/nrneurol.2013.10

Prince, M., Bryce, R., Albanese, E., Wimo, A., Ribeiro, W., and Ferri, C. P. (2013). The global prevalence of dementia: a systematic review and metaanalysis. *Alzheimers Dement.* 9, 63–75 e62. doi: 10.1016/j.jalz.2012.11.007

Reeves, T. M., Phillips, L. L., and Povlishock, J. T. (2005). Myelinated and unmyeli- nated axons of the corpus callosum differ in vulnerability and functional recovery following traumatic brain injury. *Exp. Neurol.* 196, 126–137. doi: 10.1016/j.expneurol.2005.07.014

Reeves, T. M., Smith, T. L., Williamson, J. C., and Phillips, L. L. (2012). Unmyelinated axons show selective rostrocaudal pathology in the corpus callosum after traumatic brain injury. *J. Neuropathol. Exp. Neurol.* 71, 198–210. doi: 10.1097/NEN.0b013e3182482590

Roberts, A. (1969). *Brain Damage in Boxers: a Study of the Prevalence of Traumatic Encephalopathy among Ex-Professional Boxers.* London: Pitman Medical and Scientific Publishing Co., Ltd.

Rosen, H. J., Allison, S. C., Schauer, G. F., Gorno-Tempini, M. L., Weiner, M. W., and Miller, B. L. (2005). Neuroanatomical correlates of behavioural disorders in dementia. *Brain* 128, 2612–2625. doi: 10.1093/brain/awh628

Sayed, N., Culver, C., Dams-O'Connor, K., Hammond, F., and Diaz-Arrastia, R. (2013). Clinical phenotype of dementia after traumatic brain injury. *J. Neurotrauma* 30, 1117–1122. doi: 10.1089/neu.2012.2638

Schapira, A. H. (2013). Recent developments in biomarkers in Parkinson disease. *Curr. Opin. Neurol.* 26, 395–400. doi: 10.1097/WCO.0b013e3283633741

Schofield, P. W., Tang, M., Marder, K., Bell, K., Dooneief, G., Chun, M., et al. (1997). Alzheimer's disease after remote head injury: an incidence study. *J. Neurol. Neurosurg. Psychiatr.* 62, 119–124. doi: 10.1136/jnnp.62.2.119

Shenton, M. E., Hamoda, H. M., Schneiderman, J. S., Bouix, S., Pasternak, O., Rathi, Y., et al. (2012). A review of magnetic resonance imaging and diffusion tensor imaging findings in mild traumatic brain injury. *Brain Imaging Behav.* 6, 137–192. doi: 10.1007/s11682-012-9156-5

Sperling, R., and Johnson, K. (2013). Biomarkers of Alzheimer disease: current and future applications to diagnostic criteria. *Continuum (Minneap. Minn.).* 19, 325–338. doi: 10.1212/01.CON.0000429181.60095.99

Stern, R. A., Riley, D. O., Daneshvar, D. H., Nowinski, C. J., Cantu, R. C., and Mckee, A. C. (2011). Long-term consequences of repetitive brain trauma: chronic traumatic encephalopathy. *PMR* 3, S460–S467. doi: 10.1016/j.pmrj.2011.08.008

Stuss, D. T., Gallup, G. G., Jr., and Alexander, M. P. (2001). The frontal lobes are necessary for 'theory of mind.' *Brain* 124, 279–286. doi: 10.1093/brain/124.2.279 Stuss, D. T., and Levine, B. (2002). Adult clinical neuropsychology: lessons from studies of the frontal lobes. *Annu. Rev. Psychol.* 53, 401–433. doi: 10.1146/annurev.psych.53.100901.135220

Whitwell, J. L., and Josephs, K. A. (2011). Neuroimaging in frontotemporal lobar degeneration–predicting molecular pathology. *Nat. Rev. Neurol.* 8, 131–142. doi: 10.1038/nrneurol.2012.7

Wood, R. L. (2004). Understanding the 'miserable minority': a diasthesis-stress paradigm for post-concussional syndrome. *Brain Inj.* 18, 1135–1153. doi: 10.1080/02699050410001675906

Wortzel, H. S., Brenner, L. A., and Arciniegas, D. B. (2013). Traumatic brain injury and chronic traumatic encephalopathy: a forensic neuropsychiatric perspective. *Behav. Sci. Law.* doi: 10.1002/bsl.2079. [Epub ahead of print].

Zetterberg, H., Smith, D. H., and Blennow, K. (2013). Biomarkers of mild

traumatic brain injury in cerebrospinal fluid and blood. *Nat. Rev. Neurol.* 9, 201–210. doi: 10.1038/nrneurol.2013.9

9

Microglia function in Alzheimer's disease

Egle Solito*[1] *and Magdalena Sastre*[2]

[1] *Centre for Translational Medicine and Therapeutics, William Harvey Research Institute, Barts and The London, Queen Mary's School of Medicine and Dentistry, London, UK*

[2] *Centre for Neuroscience, Division of Experimental Medicine, Imperial College London, London, UK*

Edited by:
Roger A. Barker, University of Cambridge and Addenbrooke' Hospital, UK

Reviewed by:
Emmanuel Planel, Centre Hospitalier de l'Université Laval, Canada
Mariela Fermanda Perez, Universidad Nacional de Cordoba, Argentina

****Correspondence:***
Magdalena Sastre, Centre for Neuroscience, Division of Experimental Medicine, Imperial College London, Hammersmith Hospital, Du Cane Road, London W12 0NN, UK.
e-mail: m.sastre@imperial.ac.uk

Contrary to early views, we now know that systemic inflammatory/immune responses transmit to the brain. The microglia, the resident "macrophages" of the brain's innate immune system, are most responsive, and increasing evidence suggests that they enter a hyper-reactive state in neurodegenerative conditions and aging. As sustained over-production of microglial pro-inflammatory mediators is neurotoxic, this raises great concern that systemic inflammation (that also escalates with aging) exacerbates or possibly triggers, neurological diseases (Alzheimer's, prion, motoneuron disease). It is known that inflammation has an essential role in the progression of Alzheimer's disease (AD), since amyloid-β (Aβ) is able to activate microglia, initiating an inflammatory response, which could have different consequences for neuronal survival. On one hand, microglia may delay the progression of AD by contributing to the clearance of Aβ, since they phagocyte Aβ and release enzymes responsible for Aβ degradation. Microglia also secrete growth factors and anti-inflammatory cytokines, which are neuroprotective. In addition, microglia removal of damaged cells is a very important step in the restoration of the normal brain environment, as if left such cells can become potent inflammatory stimuli, resulting in yet further tissue damage. On the other hand, as we age microglia become steadily less efficient at these processes, tending to become over-activated in response to stimulation and instigating too potent a reaction, which may cause neuronal damage in its own right. Therefore, it is critical to understand the state of activation of microglia in different AD stages to be able to determine the effect of potential anti-inflammatory therapies. We discuss here recent evidence supporting both the beneficial or detrimental performance of microglia in AD, and the attempt to find molecules/biomarkers for early diagnosis or therapeutic interventions.

Keywords: microglia, amyloid-β, Alzheimer's disease, inflammation, NSAIDs, annexin A1, immunity

INTRODUCTION

For many years, the central nervous system (CNS) was considered to be immune privileged, neither susceptible nor contributing to infection/inflammation. It is now evident that CNS infection and neurological diseases trigger local inflammation and consequently activation of the immune response. In particular, the response to aggression is driven by the resident immune cells, the microglia distributed throughout the normal adult brain (Perry and Andersson, 1992; Nimmerjahn et al., 2005). Specifically, Alzheimer's disease (AD) is characterized by an inflammatory response to Amyloid-β (Aβ), inducing the activation of microglia and the recruitment of astrocytes to the sites where Aβ deposits occur (Sastre et al., 2006a).

It is nowadays accepted that there is a dynamic microglia turnover in the brain and that microglia phenotype may change depending on aging, stage of the disease, and/or the presence of peripheral inflammation. In the brain there are also infiltrated macrophages, which play an essential role in the immune response.

The purpose of this review is first, to describe microglia as a cell of the immune system and the effects of peripheral inflammation on their activation. Secondly, our aim is to describe how this system is altered in a neurodegenerative disease, such as AD. Therefore, targeting microglia could serve as a potential therapy to treat AD patients.

MICROGLIA THE INNATE IMMUNITY CELL COMPONENT

ROLE OF MICROGLIA AND MACROPHAGES IN THE BRAIN

- Microglia represent around 10% of the cells in the nervous system. Although there are many theories concerning the origin of microglia, the general consensus today is its hematopoietic origin, derived from myeloid precursor cells, which enter the developing CNS during embryogenesis. Many questions remain about the recruitment and the life of the resident microglial in adult and aging brain (Chan et al., 2007).

Microglia constitute the first line of defense against invading pathogens or other types of brain tissue injury. The general agreement is that microglia are the "sentinels" of the CNS. Their fundamental role is sensing both pathogen- and host-derived ligands within the CNS. By detecting the type of insult and consequently directing the innate to the adaptive immune response (e.g., removal of pathogen) they are fundamental to the resolution of inflammation. Under pathological situations, such as neurodegenerative disease, stroke, and tumor invasion, microglia become activated, surround damaged and dead cells, and clear cellular debris from the area, in analogy to phagocytic macrophages of the immune system (Fetler and Amigorena, 2005). This process plays a fundamental part in the reorganization of neural circuitry and repair mechanisms that arise following injury (Neumann et al., 2009; Neher et al., 2011). As part of a beneficial role microglial phagocytosis is a highly regulated process, with activated microglia expressing a wide, and redundant, variety of distinct receptors for the removal of pathogenic organisms, e.g., Toll-like receptors (TLRs; Neumann et al., 2009), or of apoptotic cell debris, e.g., CD36 and integrins (Napoli and Neumann, 2009; Lue et al., 2010). The microglial phagocytic response is thus a central part of the brain's defense mechanisms, and is a powerful contributor to the systems in place that ensure healthy neural function.

Activated microglia also up-regulate other cell-surface receptors, including the major histocompatibility complex and complement receptors (Liu and Hong, 2003). Microglia experience dramatic morphological changes from ramified cells to activated amoeboid microglia (Kreutzberg, 1996). In addition, when microglia become activated they generate inflammatory mediators like cytokines, chemokines, prostaglandins, inducible nitric oxide synthase (iNOS), cyclooxygenase-2 (COX-2), free radicals, and stimulating an adaptive immune response (Nimmerjahn et al., 2005; Ransohoff and Perry, 2009). The principal goals of such reactions include the repair and the restoration of the homeostasis, but complications often arise, resulting in detrimental effects and actual exacerbation of the occurring damage (Lehnardt, 2010).

- Apart from resident microglia, in the brain there are monocyte-derived macrophages (Schwartz and Shechter, 2010). Perivascular macrophages have a phagocytic role and are also implicated in the presentation of antigens to T cells that have been activated in the periphery, thereby facilitating the recognition of CNS antigens (Perry et al., 2010). The macrophage and microglia phenotype has been defined as M1 (classically activated via TLRs or interferon γ) and M2 (alternatively activated by interleukin 4 or interleukin 13), although it is assumed that a mixed population of both phenotypes exists (Cameron and Landreth, 2010; Perry et al., 2010). Because most techniques are unable to differentiate between both populations of microglia and macrophages in the brain, they are collectively referred as microglia. However, both microglia and infiltrated monocytes are not functionally redundant and have different properties, so they are both necessary to display functions such as brain repair.

IMPACT OF PERIPHERAL INFLAMMATION IN THE BRAIN

Inflammation is a response mounted by the innate immune system in response to injury and infections in order to promote recovery. It was long thought that the brain was protected from systemic inflammation. However, growing evidence shows that systemic inflammatory stimuli, such as infection, also trigger a central response through microglia with consequent release of pro-inflammatory mediators (cytokines, lipid metabolites, free radicals). As part of the host-defense process, this stimulates autonomic, neuroendocrine, and behavioral responses that promote recovery. Under normal conditions the neuroinflammatory response resolves and microglia resume their "resting" state and role of monitoring the microenvironment. However, increasing experimental and clinical evidence indicates that systemic inflammation can worsen, or possibly trigger, neurological diseases (Weller et al., 2005; Ransohoff and Perry, 2009). These include stroke (McColl et al., 2007), Alzheimer's, prion, and motoneuron diseases (Nguyen et al., 2004; Perry, 2004; Rogers et al., 2007). Although the underlying mechanisms are not clear, mounting evidence suggests that microglia enter a primed/hyper-sensitive state in neurodegenerative conditions. This pre-disposes to an exaggerated production of toxic pro-inflammatory mediators in response to systemic inflammogens, thereby exacerbating neuronal loss (Streit et al., 2004; Godbout et al., 2005; Perry et al., 2007).

Understanding the routes of communication between peripheral immune responses and the brain has not been an easy challenge (Perry et al., 2007). The general belief is that immune messages are passed to the brain mainly through three different pathways: first, peripherally derived signals (mainly pro-inflammatory cytokines like IL-1β, TNF-α, and IL-6) and even pathogen-associated molecular patterns (PAMPs; for example the lipopolysaccharide (LPS), the main cell-wall component of Gram-negative bacteria) can access the nervous system through brain sites that lack a proper blood brain barrier (BBB), or through fenestrated capillaries (Rivest, 2003); secondly, on-going peripheral reactions can be sensed and transmitted to the brain via neural afferent pathways, mainly through the vagus nerve (Gao et al., 2008); lastly, the BBB itself, through the role of its numerous cellular components like endothelial cells and perivascular macrophages can sense circulating signals and respond to them, affecting behavior of neurons, astrocytes, and especially resident microglia population (Rivest, 2009; **Figure 1**).

MICROGLIA IN AGING

Despite the similarities with the innate immune response in the peripheral system, there are important differences with brain environment, where the microglia activity could be sometimes deleterious for the brain. This in-balance phenotype is determined by the fact that neuroinflammation may be chronic or acute (Colton, 2009). Both chronic low-grade peripheral inflammation (Ouchi et al., 2005) and microglial priming/hypersensitivity are associated with aging.

It is well known that microglia exhibit significant phenotypic changes during normal aging. Microglia cells from both aged humans and rodents show profoundly altered morphology, characterized by dystrophic processes, and abnormal clustering (Perry et al., 1996; Streit et al., 2008). These changes in morphology are accompanied by increased expression of activation markers such as MHCII and RAGE (Perry et al., 1993), raised basal production of the pro-inflammatory cytokines TNFα, IL-6, and IL-1β (Ye and Johnson, 1999; Xie et al., 2003; Sierra et al., 2007), and hyper-responsiveness to inflammatory stimulation (Njie et al., 2012), together suggesting that microglia become progressively dysfunctional with age. A likely explanation for this fact lies in the loss of endogenous factors which would normally control/drive prevent excessive microglial activation, and promote the beneficial, anti-inflammatory, phenotype. We could further hypothesize that microglia turnover with aging is reduced and that newly attracted

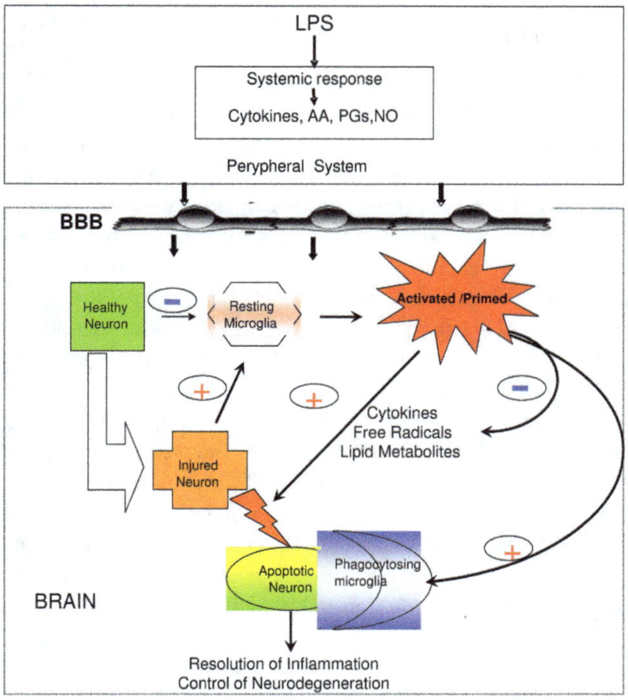

FIGURE 1 | Peripheral infection/inflammation causes the release of pro-inflammatory mediators, including cytokines (TNF-α, IL-1β, IL-6), arachidonic acid (AA), prostaglandins (PGs), and nitric oxide (NO) synthesis. The brain also mounts an inflammatory response to systemic inflammation, as well as to local injury (neurodegeneration, trauma, stroke), with the microglial cells responding soonest and with production of the greatest amounts of pro-inflammatory mediators. However, the central response appears to be under tighter control than the peripheral response in that it is delayed and more modest, probably in order to avoid the dire consequences of a full-blown inflammatory response within the confines of the skull. Modified after Solito et al. (2008).

monistic cells may acquire a wrong phenotype once enriched the brain environment (Kofler and Wiley, 2011).

In summary, microglial activation presents a double-edged sword: from one side we can define it as neuroprotective, forming the first line of defense in the CNS; from the other, it can become a neurodegenerative force, when its power is excessive and to represent risk factors for developing age-associated neurodegenerative disease (AD), contributing to the worsening of symptoms that occur after systemic infection (Perry et al., 2007). Understanding the shift between these two opposite and the changes that occurring with aging will allow us to minimize the harmful and capitalize the beneficial effects and consequently the treatment of neurodegenerative diseases (Yong and Rivest, 2009).

MICROGLIA IN ALZHEIMER'S DISEASE

IMPLICATIONS OF AD PATHOGENESIS IN MICROGLIA ACTIVATION

Inflammation has been implicated in neuronal damage, increased Aβ generation, increased phosphorylation of tau, and cognitive impairment in AD. Cause or consequence of disease progression is still not clear. Clinical work and studies in animal models suggest that microglial activation precede amyloid plaques and tangles formation (Griffin et al., 1989; Heneka et al., 2005a) while PET studies have reported inflammatory changes in one-third of amnestic mild cognitive impairment (MCI; Cagnin et al., 2001; Okello et al., 2009).

Many of the cytokines and chemokines secreted by microglia such as IL-1β, IL-6, TNF-α, IL-8, TGF-β, and macrophage inflammatory protein-1α (MIP-1α) have been found to have altered expression in AD patients compared to control individuals (Sastre et al., 2006a). Animal models of AD, including the APP transgenic line Tg2567 carrying the Swedish mutation, also show elevated levels for TNF-α, IL-1β, IL-1α, chemoattractant protein-1, COX-2, and complement component 1q (Benzing et al., 2000; Matsuoka et al., 2001). In addition, an increased risk of AD has been associated with several polymorphisms of pro-inflammatory genes, including IL-1 (Nicoll et al., 2000), IL-6 (Capurso et al., 2004), TNF-α (McCusker et al., 2001; Perry et al., 2001), and α1-antichymotrypsin (Kamboh et al., 1995).

Amyloid peptides and their precursor protein (APP) are strong glial activators (Barger and Harmon, 1997) and knockdown of APP gene and its proteolytic products delay and decrease microglial activation (DeGiorgio et al., 2002). The extent of astrocytosis and microglial activation is directly dependent on the amyloid load, and treatment with β-sheet breaker peptides leads to reduced brain inflammation (Permanne et al., 2002). Aβ is able to activate a NFκB-dependent pathway that is required for cytokine production (Combs et al., 2001). In addition, the C-terminal (CT) 100 amino acids of βAPP, which is also present in senile plaques, can induce gliosis and neuronal death. CT100 exposure results in activation of mitogen-activated protein kinase (MAPK) pathways as well as NFκB (Bach et al., 2001). At the same time, inflammation may increase Aβ generation by affecting the transcription of the β-secretase (BACE1), the main enzyme responsible for Aβ generation (Sastre et al., 2006b, 2008), therefore creating a feed-forward cycle.

In addition, neuroinflammation participates in tau-mediated neurodegeneration (Jaworski et al., 2011). Animal models of tauopathy such as the P301S tau transgenic mice exhibit accumulation of activated microglial cells around tau-positive nerve cells (Yoshiyama et al., 2007). Eventually, pro-inflammatory cytokines are also able to modify the activity of kinases involved in Tau phosphorylation (Arnaud et al., 2006). Products of inflammation might change the substrate specificity of kinases/phosphatases leading to tau phosphorylation at pathological sites. It was shown recently that inflammation induced by infection increased GSK3 activity in the triple-transgenic mouse model of AD, associated with a shift of tau from the detergent-soluble to the detergent-insoluble fraction (Sy et al., 2011).

On the other hand, other proteins involved in AD, such as presenilin, have been implicated in inflammation. Presenilin conditional knockout mice present differential up-regulation of inflammatory markers in the cerebral cortex, such as strong microglial activation, and elevated levels of glial fibrillary acidic protein (GFAP), complement component C1q, and cathepsin S (Beglopoulos et al., 2004). In fact, γ-secretase inhibitors have been reported to impair microglial activity as measured in gene expression, protein levels, and migration ability, which resulted in a reduction of soluble β-amyloid phagocytosis. Moreover, microglia deficient in presenilin 1 and 2 showed impairment in phagocytosis of soluble β-amyloid (Farfara et al., 2011).

MECHANISMS OF Aβ-INDUCED MICROGLIAL ACTIVATION

As indicated above, Aβ is able to bind and activate microglia. The mechanism of action for this is through interaction with pattern recognition receptors (PRRS). Microglia express many PRRs (Farina et al., 2007; Falsig et al., 2008), which recognize and bind to both PAMPs, or danger-associated molecular patterns (DAMPs), such as Aβ (Salminen et al., 2009). Interaction of microglia with Aβ, via PRRs provokes their inflammatory actions.

Toll-like receptors

Toll-like receptors are a type-1 integral glycoproteins (Pancer and Cooper, 2006; Miyake, 2007). Among the cell-surface TLRs, TLR2 and 4 can recognize Aβ (Carty and Bowie, 2011). Several studies have confirmed that TLR4 mediates microglial-induced neurotoxicity both *in vivo* and *in vitro* (Lehnardt et al., 2003; Walter et al., 2007).

Toll-like receptor activation is regulated by co-receptors, including MD-2, CD14, and CD36 (Akashi-Takamura and Miyake, 2006). Research using knockout mice for TLR4 or TLR2 demonstrated an increase in Aβ deposition and acceleration in cognitive decline (Tahara et al., 2006; Richard et al., 2008). These results suggest that TLR2 and TLR4 may be involved in Aβ clearance *in vivo* and hence provide neuroprotection in AD. In fact, it was shown that response of microglial cells to fibrillar forms of Aβ requires the participation of TLRs and the co-receptor CD14 (Reed-Geaghan et al., 2009). However, microglia internalize soluble Aβ through a non-saturable, fluid phase macropinocytic mechanism that is distinct from phagocytosis and receptor-mediated endocytosis (Mandrekar et al., 2009).

Receptor for advanced end glycation products (RAGE)

RAGE is a member of the immunoglobulin superfamily of cell-surface proteins (Schmidt et al., 2001; Chavakis et al., 2003; Bierhaus et al., 2005). It is a multiligand receptor, which recognizes Aβ peptides and fibrils (Knapp and Prince, 2007). Interestingly, RAGE-expressing microglia are upregulated in AD, and microglial RAGE is reported to mediate the pro-inflammatory effects of Aβ (Yan et al., 1996; Lue et al., 2001; Arancio et al., 2004). This is supported by recent work whereby it was demonstrated in transgenic AD models that the interaction of microglial RAGE with Aβ activates signal transduction cascades (MAP kinase, p38, and ERK1/2), enhances cytokines production (IL-β and TNF-α), and accelerates or amplifies the inflammatory response, leading to recruitment or activation of microglia and astrocytes (Fang et al., 2010).

Scavenger receptors

Scavenger receptor (SR) type-A (SR-A), type B1 (SR-B1), CD36, and CD40 are established receptors for insoluble fibrillar Aβ aggregates, and are expressed by activated microglia, mediating the endocytosis of oligomeric and fibrillar Aβ (El Khoury et al., 1996; Paresce et al., 1996; Coraci et al., 2002; Husemann et al., 2002). Microglial adherence via SR-A binding to fibrillar Aβ leads to microglial immobilization, production of ROS, secretion of cytokines such as TNF-α and complement proteins (El Khoury et al., 1996).

Formyl peptide receptors

Aβ can also bind to members of the seven-transmembrane G protein coupled receptors known as formyl peptide receptors (FPRs; Le et al., 2002). FPR, FPR-like 1 (FPRL-1), and FPR-like 2 (FPRL2) have been characterized as series of receptors, for which the main endogenous ligand is Annexin A1 (ANXA1; Solito et al., 2008). These receptors bind with high affinity to N-formylated bacterial peptides. FPRs are expressed on several immune cells including leukocytes, monocytes, and microglia. Among them the FPRL-1 mediates the chemotactic activity of Aβ42 for mononuclear phagocytes and therefore appear to be pathophysiologically relevant in the AD (Iribarren et al., 2005). In addition, Aβ bound to FPRL-1 is rapidly internalized into the cytoplasmic region as ligand/receptor complexes in mononuclear phagocytes. This process may represent responses of host-defense aiming at the clearance of abnormally elevated, pathogenic Aβ. However, the Aβ interaction with FPRL-1 is clearly associated with cell activation (Cui et al., 2002) and the release of pro-inflammatory and neurotoxic mediators (Pan et al., 2011). Interestingly FPRL-1 is highly express in mononuclear phagocytes surrounding and infiltrating Congo red-positive plaques in AD patients' brain tissue (Le et al., 2001).

Complement receptors

Complement receptors are one of the categories of cell-surface molecules on microglia that are upregulated in response to the activation of these cells (Liu and Hong, 2003). Aβ-induced complement activation leads to generation of C1q, C4, and C3 activation fragments around the plaques. Here microglia express complement proteins C1q, C3, and receptors C1qR, CR3, CR4, and C5aR, which support phagocytic uptake (Keene et al., 2011). Inhibition of the complement system results in an increase of Aβ plaque formation and neurodegeneration in AD transgenic mice (Shen and Meri, 2003).

In contrast, lack of C1q in mice models of AD results in decrease pathology (Hafer-Macko et al., 2000). This indicates that one mechanism by which microglia could recruit further reactive cells to the site of a plaque and cause neurotoxic damage is by activating the classic complement pathway and the inflammatory machinery associated with it (pro-inflammatory cytokines, oxidative products) through production of C1q (McGeer and McGeer, 1998; Bonifati and Kishore, 2007).

The demonstration that the peripheral benzodiazepine receptor is upregulated in activated microglia led to the development of a ligand, $[^{11}C](R)$-PK11195, which binds to this receptor also known as the 18-kDa translocator protein (TSPO). Extensive amyloid deposition and microglial activation can be demonstrated in the same group of AD patients *in vivo* by PET using $[^{11}C]$PK11195 and a negative correlation between microglial activation and levels of cognition has been reported. Both amyloid deposition and microglial activation can be detected *in vivo* with PET in around 50% of patients with MCI. However, amyloid deposition and microglial activation are not necessarily correlated in MCI suggesting both can occur in the absence of the other (Okello et al., 2009; Sastre et al., 2011). On the other hand, a significant age-dependent increase in specific $[^{3}H](R)$-PK11195 binding was also demonstrated in a transgenic mouse model of AD (TASTPM:

APPswxPS1M146V; Roberts et al., 2009). This was consistent with immunohistochemical data showing age-dependent increases in CD68 immunoreactivity co-localized with Aβ deposits. CD68 is a 110-kDa transmembrane glycoprotein, expressed by monocyte/macrophage lineages and serves as a marker for microglia. Interestingly, an antibody to human TSPO revealed induction of TSPO-positive microgliosis by tau fibrils in tauopathy brains. In addition, in transgenic PS19 mice, carrying the P301S Tau mutation, radiolabeling of TSPO with $[^{11}C]$AC-5216 was linearly proportional to the amount of phospho-tau immunolabeling (Maeda et al., 2011). The results of that study indicated that TSPO immunoreactivities are associated with NFTs, neuropil threads, and plaque neuritis rather than Aβ deposits. All together, the analysis of microglia by PET in AD and MCI patients plus the studies of microglial activation over time in animal models suggest that microglia activation occurs before Aβ deposition and correlates better with cognitive deficits and tau phosphorylation.

MICROGLIAL ACTIVATION IN DIFFERENT STAGES OF AD

It has been hypothesized that early microglial activation in AD delays disease progression by promoting clearance of Aβ before formation of senile plaques. It is conceivable that glial activation is protective early in the disease (Wyss-Coray et al., 2003; Maragakis and Rothstein, 2006; Wyss-Coray, 2006). In fact, studies have shown that blood derived macrophages (BMDM) are able to efficiently eliminate amyloid and confer neuroprotection by secretion of growth factors such as the glia-derived neurotrophic factor (GDNF), which are potentially beneficial to the survival of neurons (Liu and Hong, 2003). Activated microglia in early stages of AD can reduce Aβ accumulation by increasing its phagocytosis, clearance, and degradation (Frautschy et al., 1998; Qiu et al., 1998). The mechanism by which Aβ is phagocytosed depends on the physical properties of Aβ and whether it is soluble or fibrillar. Secreted Aβ1-40 and Aβ1-42 peptides are constitutively degraded by neprilysin and the insulin degrading enzyme (IDE), a metalloprotease released by microglia and other neural cells, whose enzymatic activity is enhanced by inflammatory events, such as LPS stimulation (Qiu et al., 1997).

In later stages, with persistent production of pro-inflammatory cytokines, microglia lose their protective effect (Hickman et al., 2008; Jimenez et al., 2008) and may become detrimental through the release of cytokines and chemokines (Hickman et al., 2008). These inflammatory mediators modulate immune and inflammatory function and may also alter neuronal function. In addition, microglia from old transgenic mice have a decrease in the expression of the Aβ-binding SR-A, CD36 and RAGE, and the Aβ degrading enzymes IDE, neprilysin, and matrix metalloprotease 9 (MMP9), compared with wild-type controls (Hickman et al., 2008). Therefore, all the evidences support the idea that over-activated microglia could cause uncontrolled inflammation that may drive the chronic progression of AD by exacerbating Aβ deposition and stimulating neuronal death (Mrak and Griffin, 2005; Gao and Hong, 2008). This concept constitutes the "Neuroinflammatory hypothesis."

By comparison, the "Microglial dysfunction hypothesis" stipulates that rather than an increase of inflammatory function there is a loss of the microglial neuroprotective function in AD (Polazzi and Monti, 2010). Research has shown that the phagocytic abilities of microglia are altered in aging and impaired in neurodegenerative diseases. Therefore this "senescent" or dystrophic microglia can also contribute to the onset of sporadic AD (Streit et al., 2004, 2009).

In addition, other studies have shown that inadequate recruitment of blood monocytes with aging might be a critical event that leads to disease onset. Because the dynamics of the local and systemic inflammatory response may vary with aging and stage of the disease, this would important for the outcome of immunosuppressive treatments (Schwartz and Shechter, 2010).

Studies with animal models have provided controversial data regarding the role of microglia in AD. Experiments crossing APP animal models with Iba1-TK mice, leading to nearly complete ablation of microglia, did not display differences in plaque formation (Grathwohl et al., 2009). These results suggest that microglia may not have a direct role on Aβ deposition, but affect neuronal function. These results also reinforce the role of blood monocytes, which may support the phagocytic function of microglia. However, another study, using two-photon microscopy, performed in triple-transgenic mice crossed with the microglial chemokine receptor CX3CR1 knockout mouse, revealed that microglia is involved in neuron elimination, indicated by locally increased number and migration velocity of microglia around lost neurons (Fuhrmann et al., 2010). Microglia were recruited to the neuron before and not after the elimination of the neuron. Furthermore, CX3CR1 knockout prevented neuronal loss, indicating that neuronal loss depends on the communication between neurons and microglia (Fuhrmann et al., 2010).

MICROGLIA AS TARGET FOR AD THERAPY

Anti-inflammatory drugs

Microglia associated with the senile plaques is thought to be a potential target of non-steroidal anti-inflammatory drugs (NSAIDs). A study by Mackenzie and Muñoz (1998) carried out in non-demented patients showed that those treated with NSAIDs had three times less activated microglia as non-treated controls. These data have been confirmed by *in vivo* treatment with NSAIDs such as ibuprofen in mouse models of AD, which have shown decreases in microglial activation and in inflammatory mediators such as iNOS, cyclooxygenase (COX), and cytokines (Lim et al., 2000; Heneka et al., 2005b). Experiments performed using cultured microglia have revealed that incubation with NSAIDs decreased the secretion of pro-inflammatory cytokines and may increase Aβ phagocytosis (Lleo et al., 2007). However, the reduction of activated microglia and astroglia by NSAIDs was not significant in AD patients, indicating an age or stage dependent difference in the glial response, i.e., in their activation rate (Alafuzoff et al., 2000). Microglia in aged or diseased brains are primed and usually behave differently to those in younger individuals (Gao and Hong, 2008). Thus, it is likely that microglia do not respond equally to anti-inflammatory therapy in old age and therefore, treatment of patients with NSAIDs in advanced stages of the disease may not produce any benefit. In this regard, NSAIDs have been shown to have beneficial effects in young individuals with robust immune systems. In aged patients, these drugs may affect the weak systemic immune response of the patients, exacerbating the local damage by eliminating the capacity of the immune system to introduce disease-modifying factors to the inflamed area (Sastre and Gentleman, 2010) (**Figure 2**).

A potential downstream target of some NSAIDs such as ibuprofen, indomethacin, and naproxen is the peroxisome proliferator-activated receptor-γ (PPAR-γ; Lehmann et al., 1997; Willson et al., 2000). Several PPAR-γ activators including NSAIDs, drugs of the thiazolidinedione class, and the natural ligand prostaglandin J2 (15d-PGJ2) have been shown to be able to inhibit the β-amyloid-stimulated secretion of pro-inflammatory products by microglia and monocytes responsible for neurotoxicity and astrocyte activation (Combs et al., 2000). Furthermore 15d-PGJ(2) caused microglial death, which terminates brain inflammation (Yang et al., 2006).

Interestingly, anti-TNFα treatment reduced Aβ and Tau phosphorylation in transgenic mice. Treatment with the antibody against TNF-α Infliximab increased the number of CD11c-positive dendritic-like cells and the expression of CD11c. These data suggested that the CD11c-positive dendritic-like cells might contribute to the Infliximab-induced reduction of AD-like pathology (Shi et al., 2011).

Therapeutic vaccination with Aβ antibodies in mice evidenced the Fc-mediated uptake and clearance of Aβ antibody complexes by local activated microglia (Bard et al., 2000; Weiner and Selkoe, 2002). Therefore, it was proposed that microglial activation by active immunization might be a valid mechanism for clearance of senile plaques (Gelinas et al., 2004).

Endogenous molecule for the control of microglia detrimental action

The major breakthrough in the therapy of neurodegenerative disease would be controlling the switch between the beneficial versus the detrimental microglia phenotype in order to control inflammation.

Because Aβ stimulates microglia phagocytosis with consequent release of toxic factors, many studies have reported possible mechanism of action implicating receptors on microglia surface. In this regard, therapeutic agents that are able to disrupt the interaction between Aβ42 and FPR may prove beneficial in the treatment of AD.

We have recently published data providing strong indication for a protective role of a protein called annexin A1 (ANXA1), a glucocorticoid anti-inflammatory mediator in the peripheral system (Perretti and D'Acquisto, 2009). ANXA1 plays a key role in ensuring the effective and selective removal of apoptotic neuron-like cells under inflammatory and non-inflammatory conditions which is a ligand for FPRL-1 receptor (McArthur et al., 2010).

Our studies have shown that ANXA1 is upregulated in human microglia in AD, supporting a possible role for the protein in regulating the microglial response to amyloid plaques and inflammatory response in neurodegeneration. This view is strongly supported by further findings in which recombinant ANXA1 administration *in vitro* suppress microglial activation following an inflammatory challenge (McArthur et al., 2010).

The identification of microglial FPRL-1 as a receptor for ANXA1, together with our identification of strong expression of ANXA1 in neuritic plaque-associated microglia in AD, suggests a fascinating connection with published data indicating a link between Aβ and FPRL-1 (Heurtaux et al., 2010). Microglia have clearly been shown to phagocytose Aβ through this receptor, but they appear unable to digest this protein, leading to persistent internalization of Aβ/FPRL-1 complexes and culminating in intracellular fibril formation and apoptosis (Pan et al., 2011). The binding of ANXA1 to FPRL-1 in microglia may thus be able to disrupt the interaction of the receptor with Aβ, potentially being of significant benefit in the treatment of AD (**Figure 3**).

CONCLUSION

Microglia effects on AD seem to have double component. On one hand their activation seems to be neuroprotective at early stages of the disease but at older ages and in severely ill patients the effects could be counterproductive. There is therefore the need

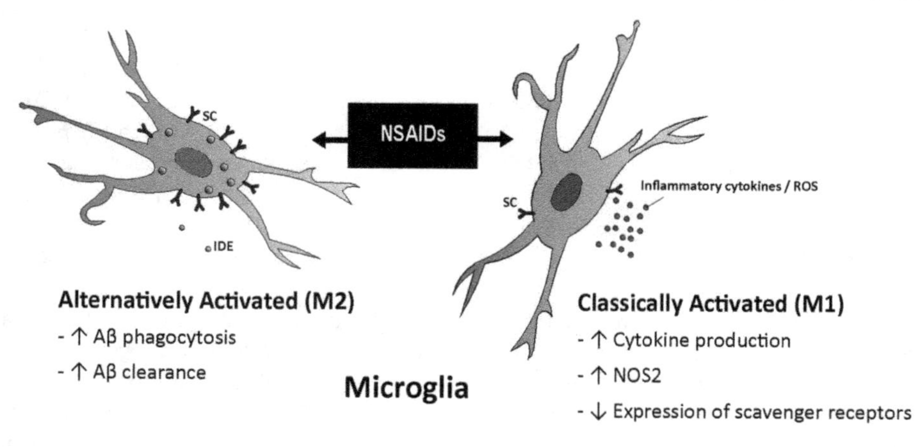

FIGURE 2 | Different effects of NSAIDs on microglia. The response to NSAIDs may differ depending on whether they are used in early stages of disease, in which microglia present an alternatively activated phenotype compared with late stages which is associated with a classical microglia phenotype. (Adapted from Sastre and Gentleman, 2010). Abbreviations: ROS, reactive oxygen species; NOS2, same as iNOS; IDE, insulin degrading enzyme; SC, scavenger receptors.

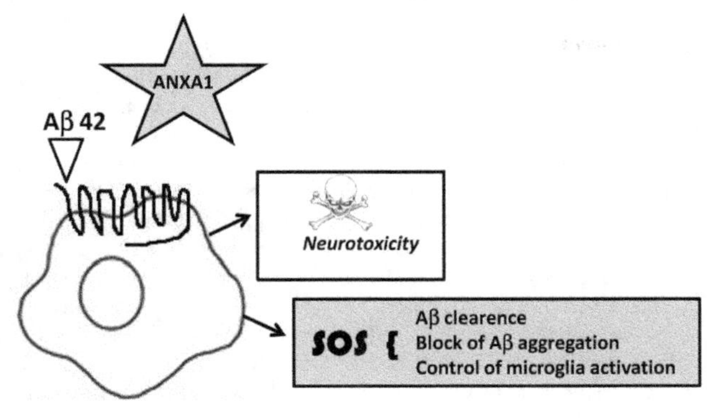

FIGURE 3 | Hypothetical annexin A1- FPRLI mechanism of action in microglia. Annexin A1 binds to FPRL-1 triggering an SOS signaling limiting microglia response to Aβ and preventing a constant uptake and apoptosis, altering microglia pro-inflammatory phenotype.

to investigate the changes in phenotype of resident microglia and how they react to anti-inflammatory therapy over age. In addition, it would be relevant to determine the role of monocyte-derived macrophages along different stages of the disease. One could speculate that the use of BMDM, which are more effective at degrading Aβ could compensate the defective functions of senescent resident microglia (Davoust et al., 2008).

In the future, the combined use of amyloid and microglial imaging should allow one to determine how different anti-amyloid strategies exert their therapeutic effects. Follow-up and further imaging of patients at risk of developing AD with radiotracers that bind to the TSPO/peripheral benzodiazepine receptor will enable a better understanding of both the pattern and the time course of microglial activation and will also provide the opportunity to monitor the pathophysiological effects of anti-inflammatory agents in these patients *in vivo.*

ACKNOWLEDGMENTS

We would like to thank Prof. Glenda Gillies (Imperial College London) for critical reading of the manuscript and the Alzheimer's Research UK for their support. We also thank The Wellcome Trust.

REFERENCES

Akashi-Takamura, S., and Miyake, K. (2006). Toll-like receptors (TLRs) and immune disorders. *J. Infect. Chemother.* 12, 233–240.

Alafuzoff, I., Overmyer, M., Helisalmi, S., and Soininen, H. (2000). Lower counts of astroglia and activated microglia in patients with Alzheimer's disease with regular use of nonsteroidal anti-inflammatory drugs. *J. Alzheimers Dis.* 2, 37–46.

Arancio, O., Zhang, H. P., Chen, X., Lin, C., Trinchese, F., Puzzo, D., Liu, S., Hegde, A., Yan, S. F., Stern, A., Luddy, J. S., Lue, L. F., Walker, D. G., Roher, A., Buttini, M., Mucke, L., Li, W., Schmidt, A. M., Kindy, M., Hyslop, P. A., Stern, D. M., and Du Yan, S. S. (2004). RAGE potentiates Abeta-induced perturbation of neuronal function in transgenic mice. *EMBO J.* 23, 4096–4105.

Arnaud, L., Robakis, N. K., and Figueiredo-Pereira, M. E. (2006). It may take inflammation, phosphorylation and ubiquitination to 'tangle' in Alzheimer's disease. *Neurodegener. Dis.* 3, 313–319.

Bach, J. H., Chae, H. S., Rah, J. C., Lee, M. W., Park, C. H., Choi, S. H., Choi, J. K., Lee, S. H., Kim, Y. S., Kim, K. Y., Lee, W. B., Suh, Y. H., and Kim, S. S. (2001). C-terminal fragment of amyloid precursor protein induces astrocytosis. *J. Neurochem.* 78, 109–120.

Bard, F., Cannon, C., Barbour, R., Burke, R. L., Games, D., Grajeda, H., Guido, T., Hu, K., Huang, J., Johnson-Wood, K., Khan, K., Kholodenko, D., Lee, M., Lieberburg, I., Motter, R., Nguyen, M., Soriano, F., Vasquez, N., Weiss, K., Welch, B., Seubert, P., Schenk, D., and Yednock, T. (2000). Peripherally administered antibodies against amyloid beta-peptide enter the central nervous system and reduce pathology in a mouse model of Alzheimer disease. *Nat. Med.* 6, 916–919.

Barger, S. W., and Harmon, A. D. (1997). Microglial activation by Alzheimer amyloid precursor protein and modulation by apolipoprotein E. *Nature* 388, 878–881.

Beglopoulos, V., Sun, X., Saura, C. A., Lemere, C. A., Kim, R. D., and Shen, J. (2004). Reduced b-amyloid production and increased inflammatory responses in presenilin conditional knock-out mice. *J. Biol. Chem.* 279, 46907–46914.

Benzing, W. C., Wujek, J. R., Ward, E. K., Shaffer, D., Ashe, K. H., Younkin, S. G., and Brunden, K. R. (2000). Evidence for glial-mediated inflammation in aged APPSw transgenic mice. *Neurobiol. Aging* 16, 523–530.

Bierhaus, A., Humpert, P. M., Morcos, M., Wendt, T., Chavakis, T., Arnold, B., Stern, D. M., and Nawroth, P. P. (2005). Understanding RAGE, the receptor for advanced glycation end products. *J. Mol. Med. (Berl.)* 83, 876–886.

Bonifati, D. M., and Kishore, U. (2007). Role of complement in neurodegeneration and neuroinflammation. *Mol. Immunol.* 44, 999–1010.

Cagnin, A., Brooks, D. J., Kennedy, A. M., Gunn, R. N., Myers, R., Turkheimer, F. E., Jones, T., and Banati, R. B. (2001). In-vivo measurement of activated microglia in dementia. *Lancet* 358, 461–467.

Cameron, B., and Landreth, G. E. (2010). Inflammation, microglia, and Alzheimer's disease. *Neurobiol. Dis.* 37, 503–509.

Capurso, C., Solfrizzi, V., D'Introno, A., Colacicco, A. M., Capurso, S. A;.,Capurso, A., and Panza, F. (2004). Interleukin 6-174 G/C promoter gene polymorphism and sporadic Alzheimer's disease: geographic allele and genotype variations in Europe. *Exp. Gerontol.* 39, 1567–1573.

Carty, M., and Bowie, A. G. (2011). Evaluating the role of Toll-like receptors in diseases of the central nervous system. *Biochem. Pharmacol.* 81, 825–837.

Chan, W. Y., Kohsaka, S., and Rezaie, P. (2007). The origin, and cell lineage of microglia: new concepts. *Brain Res. Rev.* 53, 344–354.

Chavakis, T., Bierhaus, A., Al-Fakhri, N., Schneider, D., Witte, S., Linn, T., Nagashima, M., Morser, J., Arnold, B., Preissner, K. T., and Nawroth, P. P. (2003). The pattern recognition receptor (RAGE) is a counterreceptor for leukocyte integrins: a novel pathway for inflammatory cell recruitment. *J. Exp. Med.* 198, 1507–1515.

Colton, C. A. (2009). Heterogeneity of microglial activation in the innate immune response in the brain. *J. Neuroimmune Pharmacol.* 4, 399–418.

Combs, C. K., Johnson, D. E., Karlo, J. C., Cannady, S. B., and Landreth, G. E. (2000). Inflammatory mechanisms in Alzheimer's disease: inhibition of b-amyloid stimulated proinflammatory responses and neurotoxicity by PPARg agonists. *J. Neurosci.* 20, 558–567.

Combs, C. K., Karlo, J. C., Kao, S. C., and Landreth, G. E. (2001). b-Amyloid stimulation of microglia and monocytes results in TNFa-dependent expression of inducible nitric oxide synthase and neuronal apoptosis. *J. Neurosci.* 21, 1179–1188.

Coraci, I. S., Husemann, J., Berman, J. W., Hulette, C., Dufour, J. H., Campanella, G. K., Luster, A. D., Silverstein, S. C., and El-Khoury, J. B. (2002). CD36, a class B scavenger receptor, is expressed on microglia in Alzheimer's disease brains and can mediate production of reactive oxygen species in response to beta-amyloid fibrils. *Am. J. Pathol.* 160, 101–112.

Cui, Y., Le, Y., Yazawa, H., Gong, W., and Wang, J. M. (2002). Potential role of the formyl peptide receptor-like 1 (FPRL1) in inflammatory aspects of Alzheimer's disease. *J. Leukoc. Biol.* 72, 628–635.

Davoust, N., Vuaillat, C., Androdias, G., and Nataf, S. (2008). From bone marrow to microglia: barriers and avenues. *Trends Immunol.* 29, 227–234.

DeGiorgio, L. A., Shimizu, Y., Chun, H. S., Kim, Y. S., Sugama, S., Son, J. H., Joh, T. H., and Volpe, B. T. (2002). Amyloid precursor protein gene disruption attenuates degeneration of substantia nigra compacta neurons following axotomy. *Brain Res.* 938, 38–44.

El Khoury, J., Hickman, S. E., Thomas, C. A., Cao, L., Silverstein, S. C., and Loike, J. D. (1996). Scavenger receptor-mediated adhesion of microglia to beta-amyloid fibrils. *Nature* 382, 716–719.

Falsig, J., van Beek, J., Hermann, C., and Leist, M. (2008). Molecular basis for detection of invading pathogens in the brain. *J. Neurosci. Res.* 86, 1434–1447.

Fang, F., Lue, L. F., Yan, S., Xu, H., Luddy, J. S., Chen, D., Walker, D. G., Stern, D. M., Yan, S., Schmidt, A. M., Chen, J. X., and Yan, S. S. (2010). RAGE-dependent signaling in microglia contributes to neuroinflammation, Abeta accumulation, and impaired learning/memory in a mouse model of Alzheimer's disease. *FASEB J.* 24, 1043–1055.

Farfara, D., Trudler, D., Segev-Amzaleg, N., Galron, R., Stein, R., and Frenkel, D. (2011). γ-Secretase component presenilin is important for microglia β-amyloid clearance. *Ann. Neurol.* 69, 170–180.

Farina, C., Aloisi, F., and Meinl, E. (2007). Astrocytes are active players in cerebral innate immunity. *Trends Immunol.* 28, 138–145.

Fetler, L., and Amigorena, S. (2005). Neuroscience. Brain under surveillance: the microglia patrol. *Science* 309, 392–393.

Frautschy, S. A., Yang, F., Irrizarry, M., Hyman, B., Saido, T. C., Hsiao, K., and Cole, G. M. (1998). Microglial response to amyloid plaques in APPsw transgenic mice. *Am. J. Pathol.* 152, 307–317.

Fuhrmann, M., Bittner, T., Jung, C. K., Burgold, S., Page, R. M., Mitteregger, G., Haass, C., Laferla, F. M., Kretzschmar, H., and Herms, J. (2010). Microglial Cx3cr1 knockout prevents neuron loss in a mouse model of Alzheimer's disease. *Nat. Neurosci.* 13, 411–413.

Gao, H. M., and Hong, J. S. (2008). Why neurodegenerative diseases are progressive: uncontrolled inflammation drives disease progression. *Trends Immunol.* 29, 357–365.

Gao, H. M., Kotzbauer, P. T., Uryu, K., Leight, S., Trojanowski, J. Q., and Lee, V. M. (2008). Neuroinflammation and oxidation/nitration of alpha-synuclein linked to dopaminergic neurodegeneration. *J. Neurosci.* 28, 7687–7698.

Gelinas, D. S., DaSilva, K., Fenili, D., St George-Hyslop, P., and McLaurin, J. (2004). Immunotherapy for Alzheimer's disease. *Proc. Natl. Acad. Sci. U.S.A.* 101(Suppl. 2), 14657–14662.

Godbout, J. P., Chen, J., Abraham, J., Richwine, A. F., Berg, B. M., Kelley, K. W., and Johnson, R. W. (2005). Exaggerated neuroinflammation and sickness behavior in aged mice following activation of the peripheral innate immune system. *FASEB J.* 19, 1329–1331.

Grathwohl, S. A., Kälin, R. E., Bolmont, T., Prokop, S., Winkelmann, G., Kaeser, S. A., Odenthal, J., Radde, R., Eldh, T., Gandy, S., Aguzzi, A., Staufenbiel, M., Mathews, P. M., Wolburg, H., Heppner, F. L., and Jucker, M. (2009). Formation and maintenance of Alzheimer's disease beta-amyloid plaques in the absence of microglia. *Nat. Neurosci.* 12, 1361–1363.

Griffin, W. S., Stanley, L. C., Ling, C., White, L., MacLeod, V., Perrot, L. J., White, C. L. III, and Araoz, C. (1989). Brain interleukin 1 and S-100 immunoreactivity are elevated in down syndrome and Alzheimer disease. *Proc. Natl. Acad. Sci. U.S.A.* 86, 7611–7615.

Hafer-Macko, C. E., Dyck, P. J., and Koski, C. L. (2000). Complement activation in acquired and hereditary amyloid neuropathy. *J. Peripher. Nerv. Syst.* 5, 131–139.

Heneka, M. T., Sastre, M., Dumitrescu-Ozimek, L., Dewachter, I., Walter, J., Klockgether, T., and Van Leuven, F. (2005a). Focal glial activation coincides with increased BACE1 activation and precedes amyloid plaque deposition in APP(V717I) transgenic mice. *J. Neuroinflammation* 2, 22.

Heneka, M. T., Sastre, M., Dumitrescu-Ozimek, L., Kreutz, A., Dewachter, I., Kuiperi, C., Klockgether, T., Van Leuven, F., and Landreth, G. (2005b). The PPARγ agonist pioglitazone reduces inflammation and Aβ1-42 levels in APP V717I transgenic mice. *Brain* 128, 1442–1453.

Heurtaux, T., Michelucci, A., Losciuto, S., Gallotti, C., Felten, P., Dorban, G., Grandbarbe, L., Morga, E., and Heuschling, P. (2010). Microglial activation depends on beta-amyloid conformation: role of the formylpeptide receptor 2. *J. Neurochem.* 114, 576–586.

Hickman, S. E., Allison, E. K., and El Khoury, J. (2008). Microglial dysfunction and defective beta-amyloid clearance pathways in aging Alzheimer's disease mice. *J. Neurosci.* 28, 8354–8360.

Husemann, J., Loike, J. D., Anankov, R., Febbraio, M., and Silverstein, S. C. (2002). Scavenger receptors in neurobiology and neuropathology: their role on microglia and other cells of the nervous system. *Glia* 40, 195–205.

Iribarren, P., Zhou, Y., Hu, J., Le, Y., and Wang, J. M. (2005). Role of formyl peptide receptor-like 1 (FPRL1/FPR2) in mononuclear phagocyte responses in Alzheimer disease. *Immunol. Res.* 31, 165–176.

Jaworski, T., Lechat, B., Demedts, D., Gielis, L., Devijver, H., Borghgraef, P., Duimel, H., Verheyen, F., Kügler, S., and Van Leuven, F. (2011). Dendritic degeneration, neurovascular defects, and inflammation precede neuronal loss in a mouse model for tau-mediated neurodegeneration. *Am. J. Pathol.* 179, 2001–2015.

Jimenez, S., Baglietto-Vargas, D., Caballero, C., Moreno-Gonzalez, I., Torres, M., Sanchez-Varo, R., Ruano, D., Vizuete, M., Gutierrez, A., and Vitorica, J. (2008). Inflammatory response in the hippocampus of $PS1_{M146L}/APP_{751SL}$ mouse model of Alzheimer's disease: age-dependent switch in the microglial phenotype from alternative to classic. *J. Neurosci.* 28, 11650–11661.

Kamboh, M. I., Sanghera, D. K., Ferrell, R. E., and DeKosky, S. T. (1995). APOE*4-associated Alzheimer's disease risk is modified by alpha 1-antichymotrypsin polymorphism. *Nat. Genet.* 10, 486–488.

Keene, C. D., Cudaback, E., Li, X., Montine, K. S., and Montine, T. J. (2011). Apolipoprotein E isoforms and regulation of the innate immune response in brain of patients with Alzheimer's disease. *Curr. Opin. Neurobiol.* 21, 920–928.

Knapp, M., and Prince, M. (2007). *Dementia UK the Full Report.* London: Alzheimer's Society.

Kofler, J., and Wiley, C. A. (2011). Microglia: key innate immune cells of the brain. *Toxicol. Pathol.* 39, 103–114.

Kreutzberg, G. W. (1996). Microglia: a sensor for pathological events in the CNS. *Trends Neurosci.* 19, 312–318.

Le, Y., Gong, W., Tiffany, H. L., Tumanov, A., Nedospasov, S., Shen, W., Dunlop, N. M., Gao, J. L., Murphy, P. M., Oppenheim, J. J., and Wang, J. M. (2001). Amyloid (beta)42 activates a G-protein-coupled chemoattractant receptor, FPR-like-1. *J. Neurosci.* 21, RC123.

Le, Y., Murphy, P. M., and Wang, J. M. (2002). Formyl-peptide receptors revisited. *Trends Immunol.* 23, 541–548.

Lehmann, J. M., Lenhard, J. M., Oliver, B. B., Ringold, G. M., and Kliewer, S. A. (1997). Peroxisome proliferator-activated receptors α and γ are activated by indomethacin and other non-steroidal anti-inflammatory drugs. *J. Biol. Chem.* 272, 3406–3410.

Lehnardt, S. (2010). Innate immunity and neuroinflammation in the CNS: the role of microglia in Toll-like receptor-mediated neuronal injury. *Glia* 58, 253–263.

Lehnardt, S., Massillon, L., Follett, P., Jensen, F. E., Ratan, R., Rosenberg, P. A., Volpe, J. J., and Vartanian, T. (2003). Activation of innate immunity in the CNS triggers neurodegeneration through a Toll-like receptor 4-dependent pathway. *Proc. Natl. Acad. Sci. U.S.A.* 100, 8514–8519.

Lim, G. P., Yang, F., Chu, T., Chen, P., Beech, W., Teter, B., Tran, T., Ubeda, O., Ashe, K. H., Frautschy, S. A., and Cole, G. M. (2000). Ibuprofen suppresses plaque pathology and inflammation in a mouse model for Alzheimer's disease. *J. Neurosci.* 20, 5709–5714.

Liu, B., and Hong, J.-S. (2003). Role of microglia in inflammation-mediated neurodegenerative diseases: mechanisms and strategies for therapeutic intervention. *J. Pharmacol. Exp. Ther.* 304, 1–7.

Lleo, A., Galea, E., and Sastre, M. (2007). Molecular targets of non-steroidal anti-inflammatory drugs in neurodegenerative diseases. *Cell. Mol. Life Sci.* 64, 1403–1418.

Lue, L. F., Kuo, Y. M., Beach, T., and Walker, D. G. (2010). Microglia activation and anti-inflammatory regulation in Alzheimer's disease. *Mol. Neurobiol.* 41, 115–128.

Lue, L. F., Walker, D. G., Brachova, L., Beach, T. G., Rogers, J., Schmidt, A. M., Stern, D. M., and Yan, S. D. (2001). Involvement of microglial receptor for advanced glycation endproducts (RAGE) in Alzheimer's disease: identification of a cellular activation mechanism. *Exp. Neurol.* 171, 29–45.

Mackenzie, I. R., and Muñoz, D. G. (1998). Nonsteroidal anti-inflammatory drug use and Alzheimer-type pathology in aging. *Neurology* 50, 986–990.

Maeda, J., Zhang, M. R., Okauchi, T., Ji, B., Ono, M., Hattori, S., Kumata, K., Iwata, N., Saido, T. C., Trojanowski, J. Q., Lee, V. M., Staufenbiel, M., Tomiyama, T., Mori, H., Fukumura, T., Suhara, T and Higuchi, M. (2011). In vivo positron emission tomographic imaging of glial responses to amyloid-beta and tau pathologies in mouse models of Alzheimer's disease and related disorders. *J. Neurosci.* 31, 4720–4730.

Mandrekar, S., Jiang, Q., Lee, C. Y., Koenigsknecht-Talboo, J.,

Holtzman, D. M., and Landreth, G. E. (2009). Microglia mediate the clearance of soluble Abeta through fluid phase macropinocytosis. *J. Neurosci.* 29, 4252–4262.

Maragakis, N. J., and Rothstein, J. D. (2006). Mechanisms of disease: astrocytes in neurodegenerative disease. *Nat. Clin. Pract. Neurol.* 2, 679–689.

Matsuoka, Y., Picciano, M., Malester, B., LaFrancois, J., Zehr, C., Daeschner, J. M., Olschowka, J. A., Fonseca, M. I., O'Banion, M. K., Tenner, A. J., Lemer, C. A., and Duff, K. (2001). Inflammatory responses to amyloidosis in a transgenic mouse model of Alzheimer's disease. *Am. J. Pathol.* 158, 1345–1354.

McArthur, S., Cristante, E., Paterno, M., Christian, H., Roncaroli, F., Gillies, G. E., and Solito, E. (2010). Annexin A1: a central player in the anti-inflammatory and neuroprotective role of microglia. *J. Immunol.* 185, 6317–6328.

McColl, B. W., Rothwell, N. J., and Allan, S. M. (2007). Systemic inflammatory stimulus potentiates the acute phase and CXC chemokine responses to experimental stroke and exacerbates brain damage via interleukin-1- and neutrophil-dependent mechanisms. *J. Neurosci.* 27, 4403–4412.

McCusker, S. M., Curran, M. D., Dynan, K. B., McCullagh, C. D., Urquhart, D. D., Middleton, D., Patterson, C. C., McIlroy, S. P., and Passmore, A. P. (2001). Association between polymorphism in regulatory region of gene encoding tumour necrosis factor alpha and risk of Alzheimer's disease and vascular dementia: a case-control study. *Lancet* 357, 436–439.

McGeer, P. L., and McGeer, E. G. (1998). Mechanisms of cell death in Alzheimer disease – immunopathology. *J. Neural Transm. Suppl.* 54, 159–166.

Miyake, K. (2007). Innate immune sensing of pathogens and danger signals by cell surface toll-like receptors. *Semin. Immunol.* 19, 3–10.

Mrak, R. E., and Griffin, W. S. T. (2005). Glia and their cytokines in progression of neurodegeneration. *Neurobiol. Aging* 26, 349–354.

Napoli, I., and Neumann, H. (2009). Microglial clearance function in health and disease. *Neuroscience* 158, 1030–1038.

Neher, J. J., Neniskyte, U., Zhao, J. W., Bal-Price, A., Tolkovsky, A. M., and Brown, G. C. (2011). Inhibition of microglial phagocytosis is sufficient to prevent inflammatory neuronal death. *J. Immunol.* 186, 4973–4983.

Neumann, H., Kotter, M. R., and Franklin, R. J. (2009). Debris clearance by microglia: an essential link between degeneration and regeneration. *Brain* 132, 288–295.

Nguyen, M. D., D'Aigle, T., Gowing, G., Julien, J. P., and Rivest, S. (2004). Exacerbation of motor neuron disease by chronic stimulation of innate immunity in a mouse model of amyotrophic lateral sclerosis. *J. Neurosci.* 24, 1340–1349.

Nicoll, J. A., Mrak, R. E., Graham, D. I., Stewart, J., Wilcock, G., MacGowan, S., Esiri, M. M., Murray, L. S., Dewar, D., Love, S., Moss, T., and Griffin, W. S. (2000). Association of interleukin-1 gene polymorphisms with Alzheimer's disease. *Ann. Neurol.* 47, 365–368.

Nimmerjahn, A., Kirchhoff, F., and Helmchen, F. (2005). Resting microglial cells are highly dynamic surveillants of brain parenchyma in vivo. *Science* 308, 1314–1318.

Njie, E. G., Boelen, E., Stassen, F. R., Steinbusch, H. W., Borchelt, D. R., and Streit, W. J. (2012). Ex vivo cultures of microglia from young and aged rodent brain reveal age-related changes in microglial function. *Neurobiol. Aging* 33, 195.e1–195.e12.

Okello, A., Edison, P., Archer, H. A., Turkheimer, F. E., Kennedy, J., Bullock, R., Walker, Z., Kennedy, A., Fox, N., Rossor, M., and Brooks, D. J. (2009). Microglial activation and amyloid deposition in mild cognitive impairment: a PET study. *Neurology* 72, 56–62.

Ouchi, Y., Yoshikawa, E., Sekine, Y., Futatsubashi, M., Kanno, T., Ogusu, T., and Torizuka, T. (2005). Microglial activation and dopamine terminal loss in early Parkinson's disease. *Ann. Neurol.* 57, 168–175.

Pan, X. D., Zhu, Y. G., Lin, N., Zhang, J., Ye, Q. Y., Huang, H. P., and Chen, X. C. (2011). Microglial phagocytosis induced by fibrillar beta-amyloid is attenuated by oligomeric beta-amyloid: implications for Alzheimer's disease. *Mol. Neurodegener.* 6, 45.

Pancer, Z., and Cooper, M. D. (2006). The evolution of adaptive immunity *Annu. Rev. Immunol.* 24, 497–518.

Paresce, D. M., Ghosh, R. N., and Maxfield, F. R. (1996). Microglial cells internalize aggregates of the Alzheimer's disease amyloid beta-protein via a scavenger receptor. *Neuron* 17, 553–565.

Permanne, B., Adessi, C., Saborio, G. P., Fraga, S., Frossard, M. J., Van Dorpe, J., Dewachter, I., Banks, W. A., Van Leuven, F., and Soto, C. (2002). Reduction of amyloid load and cerebral damage in a transgenic mouse model of Alzheimer's disease by treatment with a b-sheet breaker peptide. *FASEB J.* 16, 860–862.

Perretti, M., and D'Acquisto, F. (2009). Annexin A1 and glucocorticoids as effectors of the resolution of inflammation. *Nat. Rev. Immunol.* 9, 62–70.

Perry, R. T., Collins, J. S., Wiener, H., Acton, R., and Go, R. C. P. (2001). The role of TNF and its receptors in Alzheimer's disease. *Neurobiol. Aging* 22, 873–883.

Perry, V. H. (2004). The influence of systemic inflammation on inflammation in the brain: implications for chronic neurodegenerative disease. *Brain Behav. Immun.* 18, 407–413.

Perry, V. H., and Andersson, P. B. (1992). The inflammatory response in the CNS. *Neuropathol. Appl. Neurobiol.* 18, 454–459.

Perry, V. H., Anthony, D. C., Bell, M. D., Lawson, L. J., Reid, D. M., and Gordon, S. (1996). Microglia activation and inflammation in the CNS. *J. Neurochem.* 66, S70.

Perry, V. H., Cunningham, C., and Holmes, C. (2007). Systemic infections and inflammation affect chronic neurodegeneration. *Nat. Rev. Immunol.* 7, 161–167.

Perry, V. H., Matyszak, M. K., and Fearn, S. (1993). Altered antigen expression of microglia in the aged rodent CNS. *Glia* 7, 60–67.

Perry, V. H., Nicoll, J. A., and Holmes, C. (2010). Microglia in neurodegenerative disease. *Nat. Rev. Neurol.* 6, 193–201.

Polazzi, E., and Monti, B. (2010). Microglia and neuroprotection: from in vitro studies to therapeutic applications. *Prog. Neurobiol.* 92, 293–315.

Qiu, W. Q., Walsh, D. M., Ye, Z., Vekrellis, K., Zhang, J., Podlisny, M. B., Rosner, M. R., Safavi, A., Hersh, L. B., and Selkoe, D. J. (1998). Insulin-degrading enzyme regulates extracellular levels of amyloid b-protein by degradation. *J. Biol. Chem.* 273, 32730–32738.

Qiu, W. Q., Ye, Z., Kholodenko, D., Seubert, P., and Selkoe, D. J. (1997). Degradation of amyloid b-protein by a metalloprotease secreted by microglia and other neural and non-neural cells. *J. Biol. Chem.* 272, 6641–6646.

Ransohoff, R. M., and Perry, V. H. (2009). Microglial physiology: unique stimuli, specialized responses. *Annu. Rev. Immunol.* 27, 119–145.

Reed-Geaghan, E. G., Savage, J. C., Hise, A. G., and Landreth, G. E. (2009). CD14 and toll-like receptors 2 and 4 are required for fibrillar A{beta}-stimulated microglial activation. *J. Neurosci.* 29, 11982–11992.

Richard, K. L., Filali, M., Préfontaine, P., and Rivest, S. (2008). Toll-like receptor 2 acts as a natural innate immune receptor to clear amyloid beta 1-42 and delay the cognitive decline in a mouse model of Alzheimer's disease. *J. Neurosci.* 28, 5784–5793.

Rivest, S. (2003). Molecular insights on the cerebral innate immune system. *Brain Behav. Immun.* 17, 13–19.

Rivest, S. (2009). Regulation of innate immune responses in the brain. *Nat. Rev. Immunol.* 9, 429–439.

Roberts, J. C., Friel, S. L., Roman, S., Perren, M., Harper, A., Davis, J. B., Richardson, J. C., Virley, D., and Medhurst, A. D. (2009). Autoradiographical imaging of PPARgamma agonist effects on PBR/TSPO binding in TASTPM mice. *Exp. Neurol.* 216, 459–470.

Rogers, J., Mastroeni, D., Leonard, B., Joyce, J., and Grover, A. (2007). Neuroinflammation in Alzheimer's disease and Parkinson's disease: are microglia pathogenic in either disorder? *Int. Rev. Neurobiol.* 82, 235–246.

Salminen, A., Ojala, J., Kauppinen, A., Kaarniranta, K., and Suuronen, T. (2009). Inflammation in Alzheimer's disease: amyloid-beta oligomers trigger innate immunity defence via pattern recognition receptors. *Prog. Neurobiol.* 87, 181–194.

Sastre, M., and Gentleman, S. M. (2010). NSAIDs: how they work and their prospects as therapeutics in Alzheimer's disease. *Front. Aging Neurosci.* 2:20. doi:10.3389/fnagi.2010.00020

Sastre, M., Klockgether, T., and Heneka, M. T. (2006a). Contribution of inflammatory processes to Alzheimer's disease: molecular mechanisms. *Int. J. Dev. Neurosci.* 24, 167–176.

Sastre, M., Roßner, S., Bogdanovic, N., Rosen, E., Dewachter, I., Thal, D., Evert, B., Klockgether, T., van Leuven, F., and Heneka, M. T. (2006b). Non-steroidal anti-inflammatory drugs repress beta-secretase gene promoter activity by the activation of PPARgamma. *Proc. Natl. Acad. Sci. U.S.A.* 103, 443–448.

Sastre, M., Richardson, J., Gentleman, S. M., and Brooks, D. (2011). Inflammatory risk factors and pathologies associated with Alzheimer's disease. *Curr. Alzheimer Res.* 8, 132–141.

Sastre, M., Walter, J., and Gentleman, S. M. (2008). Interactions between APP secretases and inflammatory mediators. *J. Neuroinflammation* 5, 25.

Schmidt, A. M., Yan, S. D., Yan, S. F., and Stern, D. M. (2001). The multiligand receptor RAGE as a progression factor amplifying immune and inflammatory responses. *J. Clin. Invest.* 108, 949–955.

Schwartz, M., and Shechter, R. (2010). Systemic inflammatory cells fight off neurodegenerative disease. *Nat. Rev. Neurol.* 6, 405–410.

Shen, Y., and Meri, S. (2003). Yin and Yang: complement activation and regulation in Alzheimer's disease. *Prog. Neurobiol.* 70, 463–472.

Shi, J. Q., Shen, W., Chen, J., Wang, B. R., Zhong, L. L., Zhu, Y. W., Zhu, H. Q., Zhang, Q. Q., Zhang, Y. D., and Xu, J. (2011). Anti-TNF-α reduces amyloid plaques and tau phosphorylation and induces CD11c-positive dendritic-like cell in the APP/PS1 transgenic mouse brains. *Brain Res.* 1368, 239–247.

Sierra, A., Gottfried-Blackmore, A. C., McEwen, B. S., and Bulloch, K. (2007). Microglia derived from aging mice exhibit an altered inflammatory profile. *Glia* 55, 412–424.

Solito, E., McArthur, S., Christian, H., Gavins, F., Buckingham, J. C., and Gillies, G. E. (2008). Annexin A1 in the brain – undiscovered roles? *Trends Pharmacol. Sci.* 29, 135–142.

Streit, W., Braak, H., Xue, Q. S., and Bechmann, I. (2009). Dystrophic (senescent) rather than activated microglial cells are associated with tau pathology and likely precede neurodegeneration in Alzheimer's disease. *Acta Neuropathol.* 118, 475–485.

Streit, W. J., Miller, K. R., Lopes, K. O., and Njie, E. (2008). Microglial degeneration in the aging brain – bad news for neurons? *Front. Biosci.* 13, 3423–3438.

Streit, W. J., Sammons, N. W., Kuhns, A. J., and Sparks, D. L. (2004). Dystrophic microglia in the aging human brain. *Glia* 45, 208–212.

Sy, M., Kitazawa, M., Medeiros, R., Whitman, L., Cheng, D., Lane, T. E., and Laferla, F. M. (2011). Inflammation induced by infection potentiates tau pathological features in transgenic mice. *Am. J. Pathol.* 178, 2811–2822.

Tahara, K., Kim, H. D., Jin, J. J., Maxwell, J. A., Li, L., and Fukuchi, K. (2006). Role of toll-like receptor signalling in Abeta uptake and clearance. *Brain* 129, 3006–3019.

Walter, S., Letiembre, M., Liu, Y., Heine, H., Penke, B., Hao, W., Bode, B., Manietta, N., Walter, J., Schulz-Schuffer, W., and Fassbender, K. (2007). Role of the toll-like receptor 4 in neuroinflammation in Alzheimer's disease. *Cell. Physiol. Biochem.* 20, 947–956.

Weiner, H. L., and Selkoe, D. J. (2002). Inflammation and therapeutic vaccination in CNS diseases. *Nature* 420, 879–884.

Weller, C., Oxlade, N., Dobbs, S. M., Dobbs, R. J., Charlett, A., and Bjarnason, I. T. (2005). Role of inflammation in gastrointestinal tract in aetiology and pathogenesis of idiopathic parkinsonism. *FEMS Immunol. Med. Microbiol.* 44, 129–135.

Willson, T. M., Brown, P. J., Sternbach, D. D., and Henke, B. R. (2000). The PPARs: from orphan receptors to drug discovery. *J. Med. Chem.* 43, 527–550.

Wyss-Coray, T. (2006). Inflammation in Alzheimer disease: driving force, bystander or beneficial response? *Nat. Med.* 12, 1005–1015.

Wyss-Coray, T., Loike, J. D., Brionne, T. C., Lu, E., Anankov, R., Yan, F., Silverstein, S. C., Husemann, J. (2003). Adult mouse astrocytes degrade amyloid-beta in vitro and in situ. *Nat. Med.* 9, 453–457.

Xie, Z., Morgan, T. E., Rozovsky, I., and Finch, C. E. (2003). Aging and glial responses to lipopolysaccharide in vitro: greater induction of IL-1 and IL-6, but smaller induction of neurotoxicity. *Exp. Neurol.* 182, 135–141.

Yan, S. D., Chen, X., Fu, J., Chen, M., Zhu, H., Roher, A., Slattery, T., Zhao, L., Nagashima, M., Morser, J., Migheli, A., Nawroth, P., Stern, D., and Schmidt, A. M. (1996). RAGE and amyloid-beta peptide neurotoxicity in Alzheimer's disease. *Nature* 382, 685–691.

Yang, M. S., Ji, K. A., Jeon, S. B., Jin, B. K., Kim, S. U., Jou, I., and Joe, E. (2006). Interleukin-13 enhances cyclooxygenase-2 expression in activated rat brain microglia: implications for death of activated microglia. *J. Immunol.* 177, 1323–1329.

Ye, S. M., and Johnson, R. W. (1999). Increased interleukin-6 expression by microglia from brain of aged mice. *J. Neuroimmunol.* 93, 139–148.

Yong, V. W., and Rivest, S. (2009). Taking advantage of the systemic immune system to cure brain diseases. *Neuron* 64, 55–60.

Yoshiyama, Y., Higuchi, M., Zhang, B., Huang, S. M., Iwata, N., Saido, T. C., Maeda, J., Suhara, T., Trojanowski, J. Q., and Lee, V. M. (2007). Synapse loss and microglial activation precede tangles in a P301S tauopathy mouse model. *Neuron* 53, 337–351.

Absence of chronic traumatic encephalopathy in retired football players with multiple concussions and neurological symptomatology

Lili-Naz Hazrati[1,2*], Maria C. Tartaglia[2,3], Phedias Diamandis[1], Karen D. Davis[4,5,6,7], Robin E. Green[8], Richard Wennberg[3], Janice C. Wong[1,2], Leo Ezerins[9] and Charles H. Tator[4,7]

[1] Department of Laboratory Medicine and Pathobiology, University of Toronto, Toronto, ON, Canada
[2] Tanz Centre for Research in Neurodegenerative Diseases, University of Toronto, Toronto, ON, Canada
[3] Division of Neurology, Krembil Neuroscience Centre, University Health Network, University of Toronto, Toronto, ON, Canada
[4] Division of Neurosurgery, Krembil Neuroscience Centre, University Health Network, University of Toronto, Toronto, ON, Canada
[5] Division of Brain, Imaging, and Behaviour – Systems Neuroscience, Toronto Western Research Institute, University Health Network, Toronto, ON, Canada
[6] Department of Surgery, University of Toronto, Toronto, ON, Canada
[7] Institute of Medical Science, University of Toronto, Toronto, ON, Canada
[8] Research, Cognitive Neurorehabilitation Sciences Lab, Toronto Rehabilitation Institute, University of Toronto, Toronto, ON, Canada
[9] Executive Director, Canadian Football League Alumni Association, Members of the Canadian Sports Concussion Project at the Krembil Neuroscience Centre, Toronto Western Hospital and University of Toronto, Toronto, ON, Canada

Edited by:
Alvaro Pascual-Leone, Beth Israel Deaconess Medical Center, USA

Reviewed by:
Donna R. Roberts, Medical University of South Carolina, USA
Giuliana Lucci, IRCCS Santa Lucia of Rome, Italy

****Correspondence:***
Lili-Naz Hazrati, Tanz Center for Research in Neurodegenerative Diseases, Tanz Neuroscience Building, University of Toronto, 6 Queen's Park Crescent West, Toronto, ON M5S 3H2, Canada.
e-mail: lilinaz.hazrati@utoronto.ca

Background: Chronic traumatic encephalopathy (CTE) is the term coined for the neurodegenerative disease often suspected in athletes with histories of repeated concussion and progressive dementia. Histologically, CTE is defined as a tauopathy with a distribution of tau-positive neurofibrillary tangles (NFTs) that is distinct from other tauopathies, and usually shows an absence of beta-amyloid deposits, in contrast to Alzheimer's disease (AD). Although the connection between repeated concussions and CTE-type neurodegeneration has been recently proposed, this causal relationship has not yet been firmly established. Also, the prevalence of CTE among athletes with multiple concussions is unknown.

Methods: We performed a consecutive case series brain autopsy study on six retired professional football players from the Canadian Football League (CFL) with histories of multiple concussions and significant neurological decline.

Results: All participants had progressive neurocognitive decline prior to death; however, only 3 cases had post-mortem neuropathological findings consistent with CTE. The other 3 participants had pathological diagnoses of AD, amyotrophic lateral sclerosis (ALS), and Parkinson's disease (PD). Moreover, the CTE cases showed co-morbid pathology of cancer, vascular disease, and AD.

Discussion: Our case studies highlight that not all athletes with history of repeated concussions and neurological symptomology present neuropathological changes of CTE. These preliminary findings support the need for further research into the link between concussion and CTE as well as the need to expand the research to other possible causes of taupathy in athletes. They point to a critical need for prospective studies with good sampling methods to allow us to understand the relationship between multiple concussions and the development of CTE.

Keywords: chronic traumatic encephalopathy, repetitive brain injury, professional athletes, dementia, neurodegenerative disease

INTRODUCTION

Sport-related concussions affect millions of people in North America annually (Pickett et al., 2004). Among Canadian university hockey players, concussion accounts for 13% of all injures, ranking as the second most common injury after sprains or strains (Rishiraj et al., 2009). Although concussions were previously considered reversible injuries with transient symptoms, a number of recent studies have emerged linking repeated concussions and possibly asymptomatic subconcussive impacts with long-term neurodegenerative changes (McKee et al., 2009, 2010; Omalu et al., 2011; Stern et al., 2011).

The clinical neurocognitive impact of repetitive head injury was described by Martland in 1928 in "poorly skilled boxers" who withstood multiple blows to the head in efforts to position themselves in close proximity to their opponents to land a punch; subsequent symptoms included ataxia, amnesia, dementia, dysarthria, parkinsonism, and other motor and coordination deficits (Martland, 1928; Parker, 1934). In addition, behavioral and personality changes, aggression, jealousy, paranoia, and an increased incidence of physical domestic disputes and suicide were noted (Parker, 1934; Mendez, 1995; McKee et al., 2009; Omalu et al., 2010a).

Recently, the term chronic traumatic encephalopathy (CTE) was coined to refer to the clinical constellation of neurocognitive decline in conjunction with neuropathological findings of abnormal hyperphosphorylated-tau neuronal deposits in a pattern distinguishable from other tauopathies. CTE has been associated with many contact sports, including football, wrestling, hockey, and rugby (Corsellis et al., 1973; Omalu et al., 2005, 2006, 2010a,b,c, 2011; McKee et al., 2009, 2010; Gavett et al., 2011; Stern et al., 2011).

Because of the clinical and social ramifications of CTE and its putative relationship to concussion history, further research is critically needed to better understand the prevalence and risk factors for CTE. As well, the relationship between multiple concussions, positive clinical symptoms and the presence of CTE is also unclear. The current case series examines this relationship.

CTE can only be definitively diagnosed post-mortem. Given the relative rarity of cases of CTE, and the even rarer opportunity for post-mortem examination of individuals with a history of concussions at risk for CTE, it is important to provide a description of these clinical cases as they emerge.

On gross neuropathological examination, typical advanced CTE findings include dilated ventricles, fenestrated cavum septi pellucidi, and significant atrophy of the medial temporal lobes, thalamus, and mammillary bodies (McKee et al., 2009; Gavett et al., 2011; Stern et al., 2011). There can also be pallor of the locus coeruleus and substantia nigra (McKee et al., 2009; Gavett et al., 2011; Stern et al., 2011). Microscopically, CTE typically features tau-positive NFTs and astrocytic tangles, and neuropil neurites in a distribution distinctly different from other tauopathies such as Progressive Supranuclear Palsy, Corticobasal degeneration, and Alzheimers' Disease (AD) (McKee et al., 2009; Omalu et al., 2011). In CTE, these changes are patchy, localized to the depths of sulci, perivascularly around small vessels, in subpial areas and in the superficial cortical layers (II/III) (McKee et al., 2009; Omalu et al., 2011). In contrast to AD, CTE, as defined in recent literature (McKee et al., 2009; Omalu et al., 2011) lacks significant amounts of Alzheimer's-like beta-amyloid plaques (McKee et al., 2009; Gavett et al., 2011; Omalu et al., 2011; Stern et al., 2011). The neuropathology of CTE has been recently expanded to encompass in some cases the possible presence of widespread TDP-43-positive inclusions in the brainstem, basal ganglia, and cortex (McKee et al., 2010). In such cases, the presence of these lesions in the corticospinal tract and anterior horn of the spinal cord may be associated with clinical findings of spasticity, weakness, and fasciculations, similar to the clinical presentation ALS (McKee et al., 2010).

Here, we report on the clinical and pathological case histories for 6 retired Canadian Football League (CFL) athletes who underwent autopsies limited to the central nervous system. We address the question whether retired professional athletes with a history of multiple concussions and the presence of neurological findings will invariably manifest as CTE (alone or with co-morbid pathology) or whether this history can be associated with other diagnoses.

METHODS

This study was approved by the Ethics Review Board of the University Health Network. Informed consent to participate in this study was provided by each participant or the participant's designated next of kin.

PARTICIPANTS

The brains of six adults consecutively referred for autopsy were examined. Participants comprised a convenience sample of adults who played professional football (CFL) with a history of multiple concussions and medically- or family-member documented histories of progressive cognitive, psychiatric, and/or motor symptoms (see **Table 1**).

DESIGN

This was a retrospective, case series design of consecutively referred brains for autopsy. Analyses are descriptive, using the following possible primary outcomes: neuropathological diagnosis of (i) CTE alone, (ii) CTE plus other neurological disorder, (iii) other neurodegenerative disorder and (iv) no neurodegenerative disorder.

PROCEDURES

Clinical details were collected from next of kin, treating physicians, and medical records. The clinical data was obtained through structured interviews of the family members as well through clinical consult notes sent by treating physicians. The brain autopsy was authorized by next of kin.

Neuropathological analysis protocol

The post-mortem time varied from 4 to 72 h. At autopsy, the brains were immediately placed in neutral formalin and sectioned after two weeks. At the time of autopsy, a piece of frontal lobe was snap frozen for future proteomic/genetic studies. The brains were photographed and extensively sampled from several cortical, subcortical, cerebellar and brainstem areas. Tissue blocks were processed and embedded in paraffin. Six micron coronal sections were stained with Luxol fast blue and hematoxylin and eosin (H&E/LFB), Bielschowsky silver impregnation or Gallyas silver stain, and by immunohistochemistry with the following antibodies: hyperphosphorylated-tau (mouse monoclonal AT8; Pierce Endogen, Rockford IL; 1:2000), [alpha]-synuclein (rabbit polyclonal; Chemicon, Temecula, CA; 1:15,000), and A[beta] (mouse monoclonal, Dako North America Inc., Carpinteria, CA; 1:2000) (after formic acid pretreatment). Other antibodies used for immunostaining were: glial fibrillary acidic protein (GFAP-Chemicon; 1:2000), TDP-43 (rabbit polyclonal to TAR DNA-binding protein, 1:1000; Abcam, Cambridge, MA), and ubiquitin (rabbit polyclonal, 1:2000; Dako North America Inc., Carpinteria, CA). The neuropathological diagnoses were based on most recent neuropathological criteria provided by consensus studies for AD (Hyman et al., 2012), Parkinson's disease (PD) (Dickson, 2012) and fronto-temporal dementia (Cairns et al., 2007). CTE diagnosis was based on recent publications (McKee et al., 2009; Omalu et al., 2011).

Table 1 | Summary of clinical histories of professional football athletes in study cohort.

Case	Age at onset (yrs)	Initial symptoms	Progressive dementia	Behavioral changes	Language	Memory decline	Executive function	VSP	Motor impairment	Disease duration (yrs)	Concussions	Family history	Pathological diagnosis
1	70	Apathy, Memory deficits, decreased concentration, getting lost, language deficits	Yes	Apathy; rummaging through garbage, irritable, aggressive late	Severe expressive aphasia (nonfluent) 2005	STM	Decreased concentration	Getting lost	Very late (2010)	16	Multiple	Brother (late onset AD), Paternal aunt and Grandfather (dementia). Parents died young.	1. CTE 2. AD (Braak VI/VI)
2	56	Pseudobulbar affect	No	No	Mild word-finding deficits late	Mild STM (late onset)	Mild difficulty with planning/ organizing, problem-solving very late	No	Dysarthria/ dysphagia	5	Multiple	Nil	1. ALS
3	50	Personality-affect flatter; appeared depressed; STM; subtle changes in gait	Yes	1994 MDE, apathy, less empathy, dis-inhibited, agitation/ aggression, anxious, paranoid delusions, hallucinations	Later moderate expression/ comprehension deficits	STM	Decreased concentration late 90s	No	Slower gait, Instability, Tremor, Rigidity, Parkinsonian Gait and RBD, Lost sense of olfaction.	29	Multiple	Sister (PD) Mother & Father (depression)	1. DLBD 2. CTE
4	55	Memory deficits, apathetic, depressed	Yes	Apathetic, agitated, depressed Later paranoid delusions	Word-finding initially then loss of semantic meaning, word substitution	STM	Financial trouble 2009 because of poor judgment	Getting lost	Difficulty walking because of toe amputation	12	Multiple	Vascular dementia paternal grandfather	1. CTE 2. Multiple infarcts
5	64	Memory deficits, irritability	Yes	Aggressive, apathetic, hallucinations, delusions	Word-finding difficulty, increased speech output	STM	Poor judgment early on–let people leave with articles without paying	Getting lost	No	10	Multiple	Mother late onset AD, Father late onset dementia	1. AD
6	48	Motor-slowing; anxious, withdrawn	Yes	Hallucinations; delusions; throwing everything away	Decreased speech output	STM	Loss of judgment, loss of planning/ organizing	Getting lost (late onset)	Dysphagia, Dysarthria, Bradykinesia	15	Multiple	Nil	1. PD

Abbreviations: MDE, major depressive episode; STM, short-term memory; VSP, visuospatial function; PD, Parkinson's disease; AD, Alzheimer's disease; ALS, Amyotrophic Lateral Sclerosis; DLBD, Diffuse Lewy body disease. "Disease Duration" indicates number of years between initial symptoms and death.

RESULTS

OVERVIEW OF CASES

All six participants had been professional football athletes in the CFL, and had played multiple positions including offensive and defensive positions. All participants had histories of multiple concussions, but information about the exact frequency and intensity of head injury could not be determined. Their ages ranged from 61 to 87 years with disease durations of 3–17 years from the onset of first reported neurodegenerative symptoms to death. Additional details are provided in **Table 1**.

CASE FINDINGS

Case 1

Sport history. This patient played football from a young age, continued through university and played professionally in the CFL for 5 years. He played multiple positions, but was predominantly a halfback and kick returner. He had many concussions.

Clinical history. Around age 70, the patient first developed memory impairment, including getting lost, and difficulty concentrating. Apathy was also noted in his early 70s. His hygiene was not impaired, but he rummaged through the family's garbage and pulled out old items. His eating habits changed, as he became bothered by the texture of certain foods, especially meat. He was a restless sleeper, but did not display violent behavior during sleep. He also developed language deficits including word-finding difficulty and semantic paraphasias. By 85 he had developed significant expressive aphasia while his comprehension remained intact until a few weeks before his death. He also showed significant neuropsychiatric symptoms that included increased irritability and agitation. His motor function was preserved until late in his course of illness; he was still walking until age 86 when he became confined to a wheelchair due to unsteadiness. The patient died at age 86 years.

Family history. His family history was significant for a brother who developed AD in his 70's and dementia in his paternal aunt and grandfather. Both his parents died young from unrelated causes.

Neuropathological findings. Neuropathological examination showed a moderately atrophic brain (1290 g) with mild but preferential wasting of the frontal and temporal lobes (**Figure 1**). The ventricles (including the temporal horns of the lateral ventricles) were moderately enlarged. There was cavum septi pellucidi, thinning of the corpus callosum and atrophy of the amygdala and mamillary bodies. The hippocampi appeared normal in size. Examination of the midbrain revealed depigmentation of the substantia nigra (SN) (**Figure 1**).

Microscopically, the brain showed widespread tauopathy. More specifically, hyperphosphorylated-tau staining showed concentration of neurofibrillary tangles (NFTs) predominantly in the superficial layers in the gray matter and depths of sulci (**Figure 2**). There was continuous tau-positive glia in the subpial and patchy areas seen in the grey/white matter junction and around blood vessels. Numerous NFT were also noted in the deeper layers of the cortex as well. Tau distribution was diffuse throughout the brain involving the frontal, temporal (highest populations), and inferior parietal lobes, indusium griseum, and striate and cingulate cortices. There was heavy tau staining in the amygdala and throughout the hippocampus (CA1-4, subiculum and trans-enthorhinal cortex). There were patchy tau-positive inclusions seen throughout the brainstem, as well as in the nucleus basalis of Meynert, the thalamus, hypothalamus, and mammillary bodies. Numerous senile plaques were observed throughout the brain, most notably in the trans-entorhinal cortex. TDP-43 staining was not a feature of this case.

Neuropathological diagnosis. Overall, the pathological patterns of staining showed characteristics of both CTE and severe AD (Braak Stage VI/VI).

Case 2

Sport history. This participant played football, hockey, and rugby from a young age, including 12 years in the CFL playing defense. He had many concussions.

Clinical history. The patient first developed emotional lability and slurred speech at age 56 years, and was subsequently diagnosed with bulbar onset ALS. Over the next few years, he lost his speech and ability to swallow, requiring a feeding tube at age 59 and a tracheotomy at age 61. His limb movements, personality, and cognitive function remained relatively preserved, although there was a mild decline in short memory function at age 60. He died at age 61.

Family history. No family history of a neurodegenerative disease.

Neuropathological findings. Neuropathological examination showed normal brain weight (1540 g) and normal exterior appearance without atrophy (**Figure 1**). Ventricles were of normal size with no cavum septi pellucid. SN showed normal pigmentation.

Microscopic examination revealed loss of neurons in the motor nuclei of multiple cranial nerves—predominantly cranial nerves VII and XII—with TDP-43 positive intracytoplasmic inclusions (**Figure 2**). Some intracytoplasmic TDP-43-positive inclusions and neuronal loss was also noted in the cervical spinal cord involving the lower motor neurons. Inclusions were also noted in the primary motor cortex, and to a lesser extent, in the dentate gyrus. Pathological deposition of hyperphosphorylated tau was very scarce and limited to the trans-entorhinal cortex in the shape of NFTs in neurons. A few beta-amyloid plaques were also noted.

Neuropathological diagnosis. These neuropathological findings were consistent with the diagnosis of amyotrophic lateral sclerosis (ALS).

Case 3

Sport history. This participant retired after a12-year CFL career, playing both offense and defense positions. He had many concussions.

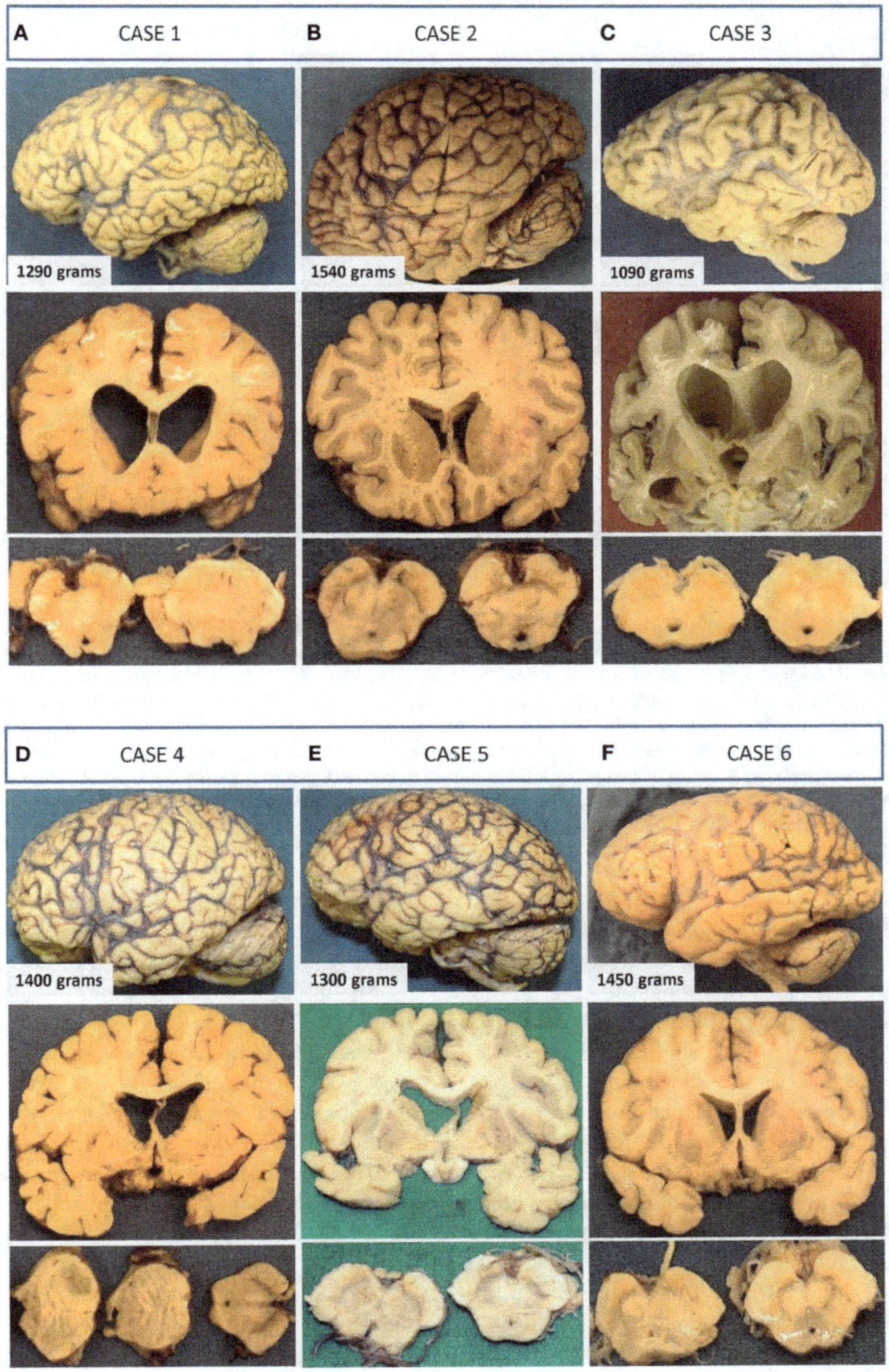

FIGURE 1 | Gross macroscopic findings on neuropathological examination. Selected examples from each case are presented as three vertical panels with lateral views of the unsectioned brain (upper panel), coronal sections through various parts of the cerebrum (middle panel), and axial sections through the brainstem (lower panel). **(A) Case 1:** There is mild-to-moderate atrophy with ventricular enlargement and cavum septi pellucidi. Thinning of the corpus callosum and mild depigmentation of the substantia nigra is also evident. **(B) Case 2:** Unsectioned brain, ventricles, and sections of the midbrain and substantia nigra appear within normal limits with no apparent evidence of neurodegeneration. **(C) Case 3**: Preferential mild-to-moderate atrophy of frontal and temporal lobes with significant enlargement of ventricles seen on coronal sections. A fenestrated septum pellucidum and atrophied amygdala and hippocampus are also seen on this section. The substantia nigra of this patient shows significant loss of pigmentation. **(D) Case 4:** There is mild frontal and temporal lobe atrophy with enlarged ventricles and cavum septi pellucidi. Axial sections of the brainstem show normal appearing substantia nigra and a metastatic lesion in the pons. **(E) Case 5:** Atrophic brain is seen with moderately enlarged ventricles and a normally pigmented substantia nigra. **(F) Case 6:** Minimal atrophy and ventricular enlargement are seen, and there is mild loss in the substantia nigra.

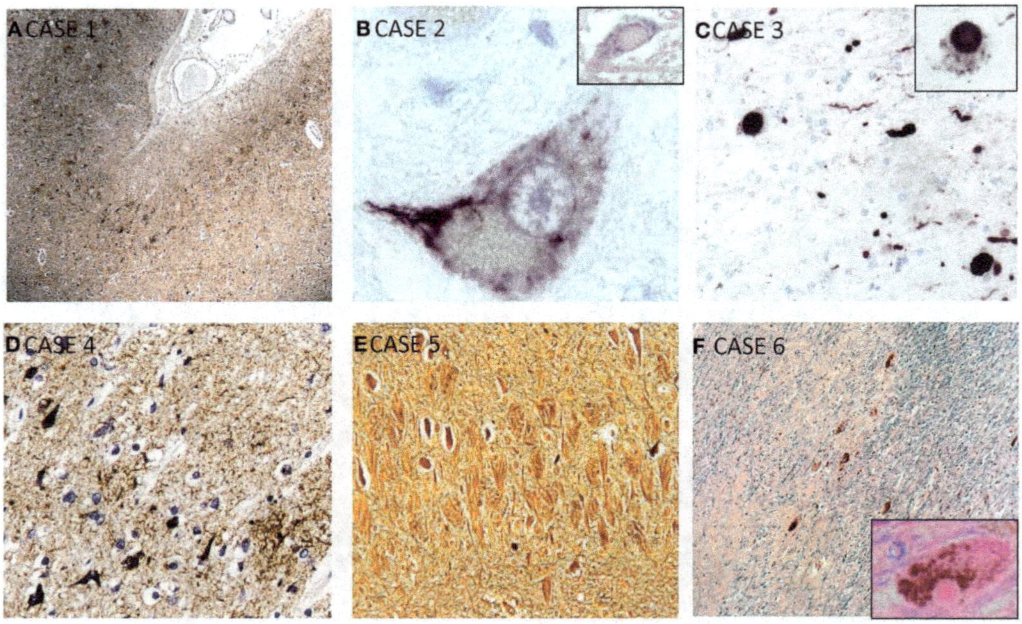

FIGURE 2 | Selected microscopic findings on neuropathological examination. (A) Case 1: High power view of sample of cerebral cortex stained for hyperphosphorylated-tau shows concentration of neurofibrillary tangles predominantly in the superficial layers of the gray matter and in the depths of sulci, which is characteristic of CTE. **(B) Case 2:** Magnified motor neuron in ventral horn of spinal cord shows a representative intracytoplasmic TDP-43 inclusion. Inset shows a hyalin inclusion. **(C) Case 3:** Alpha-synuclein staining showing Lewy bodies and neurites which are seen throughout the cortex, substantia nigra, and locus ceruleus. This patient also had features of CTE (not shown). Inset shows higher power view of cytoplasmic Lewy body. **(D) Case 4:** Immunohistochemisty showing widespread reactivity against tau-positive neurofibrillary and astrocytic tangles in multiple layers. **(E) Case 5:** Bielschowsky silver stain showing numerous neurofibrillary tombstones in the hippocampus. **(F) Case 6:** HandE/LFB and alpha-synuclein staining of representative cortical section showing diffuse Lewy bodies and Lewy neurites. Inset shows Lewy body.

Clinical findings. His wife noticed personality changes, including flat affect and depressed mood, when he was age 50. At age 55, he developed some short-term memory impairment. In his 60s, his family noticed executive deficits in that he could no longer manage his company. At the age of 62, she noticed some subtle changes in his gait. He walked more slowly, and less steadily. He also had a major depressive episode that year and underwent electroconvulsive therapy. He developed a tremor, rigidity, a parkinsonian gait, and rapid eye movement (REM) sleep behavior disorder, and also lost his sense of olfaction. His wife also noted apathy and reduced empathy. In his early 70s, he became disinhibited, had delusions, hallucinations, and episodes of agitation and aggression. He was diagnosed with PD, but the early cognitive changes at the onset of his disease and the subsequent hallucinations were more typical of dementia with Lewy bodies (DLB). The patient died at age 79.

Family history. His sister was reported to have PD. Both his parents suffered from depression.

Neuropathological findings. Neuropathological examination of the brain revealed a moderately atrophic brain with a weight of 1090 g after fixation (**Figure 1**). Moderate volume loss was noted in the frontal, temporal, and parietal lobes, and mild atrophy was noted in the occipital lobe. There was significant ventricular enlargement, thinning of the corpus callosum, and cavum septi pellucidi. Coronal sectioning of the brain revealed significant atrophy of the amygdala and hippocampus. The brainstem examination revealed pallor of the SN (**Figure 1**).

Microscopic examination revealed a widespread tauopathy in the form of neurofibrillary and astrocytic tangles clustering in patches in the superficial layers of most cortical areas in both the sulci and gyral crowns. The primary visual cortex was spared. Tau-immunopositive neurons were most pronounced in the amygdala and hippocampus. There were diffuse astrocytic tangles noted around blood vessels and throughout the parenchyma. Tau-positive inclusions and neurites also populated the subcortical structures including the striatum, globus pallidus, dentate nucleus of the cerebellum, thalamus, subthalamic nucleus, substantia nigra, hypothalamus, septal nuclei, nucleus basalis of Meynert, mammillary bodies, periventricular white matter, locus ceruleus, red nucleus and the nucleus of the third cranial nerve. Localized TDP-43 staining of the amygdala and hippocampus revealed numerous inclusions. Alpha-synuclein staining revealed numerous Lewy bodies and Lewy neurites throughout the cortex, substantia nigra and locus ceruleus suggested advanced Lewy body disease (**Figure 2**). There were senile plaques in the hippocampus and cortical areas that were tau-positive, and stained with Congo red and Gallyas silver. Luxol fast blue stain showed abnormal pallor of the white matter. There was also neuronal loss in the substantia nigra, locus ceruleus, hippocampus, and nucleus basalis of Meynert. Given the extensive neuronal and astrocytic tauopathy, TDP-43 inclusions and synucleinopathy.

Neuropathological diagnosis. This case was diagnosed with combined CTE and diffuse Lewy body disease.

Case 4

Sport history. This participant played football in high school and in the CFL for 6 years. He had many concussions.

Clinical findings. When the patient was 55-years old, his sister noted that he had difficulty with short-term memory and that he was less able to formulate arguments. He subsequently developed visuospatial impairments and was reported to get lost in familiar environments. He developed apathy and agitation, and became very depressed. His loss of judgment led to bankruptcy and at the age of 66, he became a ward of the state. He developed language deficits and exhibited word substitution, and was incoherent at times. He became depressed and had paranoid delusions. His past medical history was unremarkable except for recurrent phlebitis. The patient developed lung cancer and died of its complications at age 67.

Family history. His paternal grandfather had vascular dementia.

Neuropathological findings. Neuropathological examination revealed a brain weight of 1400 g with mild atrophy of the frontal and temporal lobes (**Figure 1**). There were findings consistent with widespread metastatic disease from a lung carcinoma and severe vascular atherosclerotic disease with recent multifocal brain infarctions. There was also thinning of the olfactory tracts and hypothalamus. Coronal sections of the brain showed an enlarged ventricular system, corpus callosum atrophy, and cavum septi pellucidi. Pigmentation of the SN appeared within normal limits (**Figure 1**).

Microscopically, there was mild to moderate neuronal loss and gliosis in CA1, subiculum, entorhinal cortex, amygdala, mammillary bodies, and medial thalamic nuclei. There was granulovacuolar degeneration noted in the CA1 and subiculum area with pronounced subpial gliosis in the trans-entorhinal cortex. Immunohistochemically, there was widespread tau-positive neurofibrillary and astrocytic tangles in multiple layers (superficial > deep) of the cortex, especially in the depths of sulci (**Figure 2**). There were some inclusions noted in the gyral crowns. These inclusions were consistently found in all cortical areas with a predilection for the medial temporal, hippocampus, and amygdala areas. NFTs were also noted in thalamus, peri-ventricular hypothalamic areas extending into the mamillary bodies, the nucleus basalis of Meynert and clustering around blood vessels. Beta-amyloid staining revealed amyloid plaques. TDP-43 and alpha-synuclein staining were unremarkable.

Neuropathological diagnosis. Overall, neuropathological findings and the distribution of tauopathy were compatible with changes seen in CTE. Although there were multiple infarcts noted, they appeared to be relatively recent infarcts and could not fully account for the participant's longer-term dementia.

Case 5

Sport history. This patient played in the CFL for 8 years. He had many concussions.

Clinical findings. At age 64, he began to show behavioral changes, including anger, poor judgment, and irritability. Over the next few years his memory worsened and he began to get lost. He then began having hallucinations of strangers in his home and also developed some misidentification for others and himself. He seemed to no longer recognize himself as he would attack mirrors when he walked in front of them. He developed delusions that people were stealing from him and had episodes of aggression and agitation, as well as impaired motor function. The patient died at age 74.

Family history. His mother had late onset AD and his father had late onset dementia.

Neuropathological findings. His brain was atrophic with a weight of 1300 g after fixation with moderate ventricular enlargement (**Figure 1**). SN showed normal pigmentation.

Microscopic examination revealed numerous NFTs in neurons of the deep cortical layers (**Figure 2**). These were concentrated to the trans-entorhinal cortex, hippocampus, and isocortex with significant extension into the primary visual cortex. There was also significant presence of tangles in nucleus basalis of Meynert, amygdala, substantia nigra, and in the Edinger–Westphal nucleus. Supplementing the tangles were numerous dense-core, beta-amyloid positive plaques. No evident TDP-43 or alpha-synuclein staining was seen.

Neuropathological diagnosis. Overall, findings were consistent with severe AD (Braak Stage VI/VI) without any pathological evidence of CTE.

Case 6

Sport history. He began playing football in high school and played seven years in the CFL. He suffered multiple concussions.

Clinical findings. At age 48, his wife noted that he was becoming withdrawn and then he gradually changed from a confident, assertive, energetic person to an anxious, insecure, and more lethargic person. At age 50, he noted his handwriting had become messier, and also complained of some cramping and numbness in his feet and decreased ability for playing baseball. He also began exhibiting memory deficits, which became progressively worse over the subsequent years. A few years later, his wife noted his speech was slurred and hypophonic and the slowing of his movements became more apparent. He did not have a tremor. At age 54, his wife became concerned about his judgment based on poor business decisions. He became obsessive about bladder incontinence and went to the bathroom multiple times a day, yet seemed incongruously unperturbed when accidents did happen. By age 55, he was having repeated episodes of loss of bladder control. He had vivid dreams that he was convinced were real, but no REM sleep behavior disorder. His judgment continued to deteriorate, and he became less attentive to hygiene. He had delusions and hallucinations, but these stopped with discontinuation of Sinemet therapy. He eventually had episodes of agitation and developed great difficulty ambulating. He had prosopagnosia at age 58. At that time, he began showing difficulty recalling the names of his children. His past medical history was unremarkable. The patient died at age 63.

Family history. No family history of a neurodegenerative disease.

Neuropathological findings. Neuropathological examination showed a brain of normal weight (1450 g) with mild diffuse cortical atrophy. Ventricles were mildly dilated (**Figure 1**).

On microscopic examination, there was diffuse Lewy body disease with Lewy bodies and Lewy neuritis in the cerebral cortex, olfactory bulbs, indusium griseum, SN and limbic system, including the CA2-4 subdivisions of the hippocampus (**Figure 2**). There was extensive neuronal loss in the SN pars compacta, locus ceruleus, dorsal nucleus of CN X and nucleus basalis of Meynert. There was very limited tau labeling in the hippocampus, the amygdala, and peri-amygdala cortex. There was, however, widespread distribution of diffuse amyloid plaques. TDP-43 staining in this case was unremarkable.

Neuropathological diagnosis. Overall, this case showed typical changes of long-term progressive PD. While the tau-deposits in the hippocampal area were age-appropriate Alzheimer-type changes (Braak Stage II/VI), there was no evidence of AD. There was also no pathological evidence consistent with CTE.

DISCUSSION

At present, the diagnosis of CTE requires post-mortem examination. In our case series, a history of participation in professional football and a history of multiple concussions, combined with positive clinical signs and symptoms of progressive neurodegenerative disease, were not inevitably associated in each of the 6 cases with a post-mortem diagnosis of CTE. The neuropathological diagnosis of our six cases comprised: CTE + AD, CTE + diffuse Lewy body disease, CTE + multiple infarcts, AD, ALS, and PD (see **Table 1**). In our case series of professional football athletes, we observed that the reported progressive neurological findings in some athletes participating in contact sports were associated with CTE, while other athletes had more common neurodegenerative conditions, namely AD, PD, and ALS. Moreover, those individuals with post-mortem diagnosis of CTE had co-morbid pathological findings that may also have contributed to the clinical signs and symptoms. Thus, our findings advocate caution in the clinical diagnosis of CTE in patients with histories of contact sports and neurocognitive decline, as other diagnoses of neurodegenerative diseases are also possible. Our findings are consistent with a literature review by Nowak et al. (2009), in which dementia in retired boxers could be explained by pathologies aside from dementia pugilistica (Nowak et al., 2009—see also McKee et al., 2013). In contrast, other previous studies either focused on describing CTE in professional athletes (Omalu et al., 2005, 2006, 2010b,c; McKee et al., 2009, 2010) or found that a majority of professional athletes had CTE (Omalu et al., 2011).

These findings raise questions regarding the relationship between multiple concussions in professional football alumni and CTE, the prevalence of CTE in this population and the risk factors. Previous post-mortem research with larger samples of professional athletes with multiple concussions has suggested a very high incidence rate; however, such studies have been limited by biased samples restricted to clinically symptomatic cases and a lack of medical post-mortem controls with co-morbidities consistent with the professional athlete histories, including comparable medication/substance histories as well as pain disorders, of potential relevance given increasing evidence for the role of neuroinflammatory processes in pain disorders (Davis and Moayedi, 2012).

Our findings cannot address these limitations, but suggest the testable hypothesis that the mapping between multiple concussion history in former professional athletes plus positive progressive clinical findings is not one-to-one with CTE, a hypothesis supported by the expectation that aging professional athletes should be as susceptible as the general aging population to neurodegenerative diseases such as AD, vascular dementia, PD or ALS.

A limitation of our retrospective clinical case series was that historical information was subject to recall bias. The participants' informants could not provide the actual number or severity of the concussions, although there was sufficient information to indicate that each player had sustained multiple concussions throughout their careers. When these players were active participants, concussions were not well recognized, and if recognized, were treated as a minor injury.

CONCLUSION

Our initial experience with this cohort of retired professional football athletes with multiple concussions and progressive neurocognitive decline demonstrates that these cases did not uniformly have neuropathological findings of CTE. Some cases with CTE pathology had concomitant pathologies that could also contribute to cognitive decline. Thus, it is difficult to establish a definitive link between a history of multiple concussions and CTE. Neuropathological examination remains essential for diagnosis of CTE, as other types of brain degeneration may be present in professional athletes with neurocognitive decline. Further research is needed to establish the relationship between multiple concussions and the development of CTE and to examine the prevalence and the risk factors that mediate the relationship between multiple concussions and development of CTE.

ACKNOWLEDGMENTS

We are grateful and would like to thank Dawn Ross, Vicky Proudfoot, Carol Conroy, Joan Toogood, Mary Kuntz, Siobhan Ribbins, Dan Slee, Bill Sokulski, and Tony Gabriel for facilitating the brain donations and for their time and contribution to the subject's histories. We are thankful to Drs. J. H. Jansen, J. Wolfe, J. Michaud, M. C. Guiot, Angela Genge, and C. Petito for their clinical expertise and help with autopsies, and to all the team members of The Canadian Sports Concussion Project. This research was funded by a generous grant from the Physicians' Services Incorporated Foundation to the Canadian Sports Concussion Project.

REFERENCES

Cairns, N. J., Neumann, M., Bigio, E. H., Holm, I. E., Troost, D., Hatanpaa, K. J., et al. (2007). TDP-43 in familial and sporadic frontotemporal lobar degeneration with ubiquitin inclusions. *Am. J. Pathol.* 171, 227–240.

Corsellis, J. A., Bruton, C. J., and Freeman-Browne, D. (1973). The aftermath of boxing. *Psychol. Med.* 3, 270–303.

Davis, K. D., and Moayedi, M. (2012). Central mechanisms of pain revealed through functional and structural MRI. *J. Neuroimmune Pharmacol.* doi: 10.1007/s11481-012-9386-8. [Epub ahead of print].

Dickson, D. (2012). Parkinson's disease and parkinsonism: neuropathology. *Cold Spring Harb. Perspect. Med.* 2:pii: a009258. doi: 10.1101/cshperspect.a009258

Gavett, B. E., Stern, R. A., and McKee, A. C. (2011). Chronic traumatic encephalopathy: a potential late effect of sport-related concussive and subconcussive head trauma. *Clin. Sports Med.* 30, 179–188, xi.

Hyman, B. T., Phelps, C. H., Beach, T. G., Bigio, E. H., Cairns, N. J., Carrillo, M. C., et al. (2012). National Institute on Aging – Alzheimer's Association guidelines for the neuorpathologic assessment of Alzheimer's disease. *Alzheimers Dement.* 8, 1–13.

Martland, H. S. (1928). Punch drunk. *J. Am. Med. Assoc.* 91, 1103–1107.

McKee, A. C., Cantu, R. C., Nowinski, C. J., Hedley-Whyte, E. T., Gavett, B. E., Budson, A. E., et al. (2009). Chronic traumatic encephalopathy in athletes: progressive tauopathy after repetitive head injury. *J. Neuropathol. Exp. Neurol.* 68, 709–735.

McKee, A. C., Gavett, B. E., Stern, R. A., Nowinski, C. J., Cantu, R. C., Kowall, N. W., et al. (2010). TDP-43 proteinopathy and motor neuron disease in chronic traumatic encephalopathy. *J. Neuropathol. Exp. Neurol.* 69, 918–929.

McKee, A. C., Stein, T. D., Nowinski, C., Stern, R. A., Daneshvar, D. H., Alvarez, V. E., et al. (2013). The spectrum of disease in chronic traumatic encephalopathy. *Brain* 136, 46–64.

Mendez, M. F. (1995). The neuropsychiatric aspects of boxing. *Int. J. Psychiatry Med.* 25, 249–262.

Nowak, L. A., Smith, G. G., and Reyes, P. F. (2009). Dementia in a retired world boxing champion: case report and literature review. *Clin. Neuropathol.* 28, 275–280.

Omalu, B., Bailes, J., Hamilton, R. L., Kamboh, M. I., Hammers, J., Case, M., et al. (2011). Emerging histomorphologic phenotypes of chronic traumatic encephalopathy in American athletes. *Neurosurgery* 69, 173–183. discussion: 183.

Omalu, B. I., Bailes, J., Hammers, J. L., and Fitzsimmons, R. P. (2010a). Chronic traumatic encephalopathy, suicides and parasuicides in professional American athletes: the role of the forensic pathologist. *Am. J. Forensic Med. Pathol.* 31, 130–132.

Omalu, B. I., Fitzsimmons, R. P., Hammers, J., and Bailes, J. (2010b). Chronic traumatic encephalopathy in a professional American wrestler. *J. Forensic Nurs.* 6, 130–136.

Omalu, B. I., Dekosky, S. T., Hamilton, R. L., Minster, R. L., Kamboh, M. I., Shakir, A. M., et al. (2006). Chronic traumatic encephalopathy in a national football league player: part II. *Neurosurgery* 59, 1086–1092. discussion: 1092–1093.

Omalu, B. I., Dekosky, S. T., Minster, R. L., Kamboh, M. I., Hamilton, R. L., and Wecht, C. H. (2005). Chronic traumatic encephalopathy in a National Football League player. *Neurosurgery* 57, 128–134. discussion: 128–134.

Omalu, B. I., Hamilton, R. L., Kamboh, M. I., Dekosky, S. T., and Bailes, J. (2010c). Chronic traumatic encephalopathy (CTE) in a National Football League Player: case report and emerging medicolegal practice questions. *J. Forensic Nurs.* 6, 40–46.

Parker, H. L. (1934). Traumatic encephalopathy ('Punch Drunk') of professional pugilists. *J. Neurol. Psychopathol.* 15, 20–28.

Pickett, W., Simpson, K., and Brison, R. J. (2004). Rates and external causes of blunt head trauma in Ontario: analysis and review of Ontario Trauma Registry datasets. *Chronic Dis. Can.* 25, 32–41.

Rishiraj, N., Lloyd-Smith, R., Lorenz, T., Niven, B., and Michel, M. (2009). University men's ice hockey: rates and risk of injuries over 6-years. *J. Sports Med. Phys. Fitness* 49, 159–166.

Stern, R. A., Riley, D. O., Daneshvar, D. H., Nowinski, C. J., Cantu, R. C., and McKee, A. C. (2011). Long-term consequences of repetitive brain trauma: chronic traumatic encephalopathy. *PM R* 3, S460–S467.

11

The utility of age-specific cut-offs for visual rating of medial temporal atrophy in classifying Alzheimer's disease, MCI and cognitively normal elderly subjects

Ranjan Duara[1,2,3,4,5,6]*, David A. Loewenstein[1,3], Qian Shen[1,7], Warren Barker[1], Daniel Varon[1,4], Maria T. Greig[1], Rosie Curiel[3], Joscelyn Agron[1], Isael Santos[1] and Huntington Potter[5†]

[1] Wien Center for Alzheimer's Disease and Memory Disorders, Mount Sinai Medical Center, Miami Beach, FL, USA
[2] Departments of Medicine and Neurology, Miller School of Medicine, University of Miami, Miami, FL, USA
[3] Department of Psychiatry and Behavioral Sciences, Miller School of Medicine, University of Miami, Miami, USA
[4] Department of Neurology, Florida International University College of Medicine, Miami, FL, USA
[5] Departments of Molecular Medicine and Neurology, University of South Florida, Tampa, FL, USA
[6] Johnnie B. Byrd, Sr. Alzheimer's Center and Research Institute, Tampa, FL, USA
[7] Department of Biomedical Engineering, University of Miami, Coral Gables, FL, USA

Edited by:
Manuel Menéndez-González, Hospital Álvarez-Buylla, Spain

Reviewed by:
Katsutoshi Furukawa, Tohoku University, Japan
Elizabeth J. Coulthard, University of Bristol, UK

***Correspondence:**
Ranjan Duara, Mount Sinai Medical Center, Wien AD Research Center, 4300 Alton Road, Miami Beach, FL 33140, USA
e-mail: duara@msmc.com

Background: New research criteria for diagnosing Alzheimer's disease (AD) in the mild cognitive impairment stage (MCI-AD) incorporate biomarkers to assign a level of certainty to the diagnosis. Structural MRI is widely available but greatly under-utilized for assessing atrophy of structures affected in early AD, such as the hippocampus (HP), because the quantification of HP volumes (HP-v) requires special expertise, and normative values have not been established.

Methods: Elderly subjects ($n = 273$) from the Florida ADRC were classified as having no cognitive impairment (cognitively normal, CN), amnestic mild cognitive impairment (aMCI) or AD. Volumes for the hippocampus (HP-v) were measured on structural MRI scans. A validated visual rating system for measuring medial temporal atrophy (VRS-MTA), including hippocampal, entorhinal cortex and perirhinal cortex atrophy was employed. The participants were subdivided into younger (less than or equal to 75 years of age) and older (greater than 75 years of age) subgroups.

Results: Volumetric and VRS-MTA measures were equivalent in predicting classification of CN vs. aMCI for older (area under the receiver operator curves [aROC]: 0.652 vs. 0.723) and younger subjects (aROC: 0.764 vs. 0.736). However, for younger AD subjects, aROC values were significantly higher for VRS-MTA measures (0.920) than for volumetric measures (0.847). Relative to HP-v, VRS-MTA score was significantly more correlated to impairment on a range of memory tests and was more associated with progression of aMCI to AD than HP-v.

Conclusion: Structural MRI with VRS-MTA assessment can serve as a biomarker for supporting the diagnosis of MCI-AD. Age-adjusted VRS-MTA scores are at least as effective as HP-v for distinguishing aMCI and AD from CN and for predicting progression from aMCI to AD. VRS-MTA is convenient for use in the clinic as well as for clinical trials and can readily be incorporated into a standardized radiological report.

Keywords: volumetric measures, hippocampus, visual rating, medial temporal atrophy, aMCI, Alzheimer's disease

INTRODUCTION

Recently revised criteria for diagnosing an early clinical stage of AD ("Mild Cognitive Impairment, or MCI, due to AD"; MCI-AD) (Albert et al., 2011) and "Prodromal AD" (Sperling et al., 2011) incorporate biomarkers to increase the certainty of the diagnosis. One such biomarker, atrophy of the hippocampus (HP) and other medial temporal lobe (MTL) structures on structural MRI, increase the likelihood of a neurodegenerative disorder, such as AD, as the cause of MCI. In spite of the widespread use of MRI scans for the assessment of individuals with various forms of cognitive impairment, this biomarker is used primarily for excluding causes of cognitive impairment other than AD, such as hydrocephalus, vascular and space-occupying lesions. However, MRI can be used to confirm the presence of neurodegenerative pathology among patients presenting with MCI and dementia (Frisoni et al., 2010) and is greatly underutilized for this purpose by clinicians and radiologists. Although prodromal forms of AD are in a continuum with, and may be clinically indistinguishable from what is described as "Probable AD," current diagnostic research standards incorporate a biomarker to support the diagnosis of prodromal AD or MCI-AD It is clear that the diagnosis of both Probable AD and Prodromal AD/MCI-AD would be more secure in the presence of a positive biomarker which provides further evidence of the presence of a neurodegenerative disease (Albert et al., 2011; Sperling et al., 2011).

Neurodegenerative changes such as atrophy which are characteristic of Alzheimer's disease (AD), and occasionally of other dementing diseases, such as Fronto-temporal Lobar Dementia (FTLD) or Hippocampal Sclerosis, may be detected using volumetric analysis or, more conveniently, using visual rating of MRI scans. Nevertheless, the incorporation of MRI for confirming the diagnosis of neurodegenerative disease has yet to receive widespread utility, in part because of (a) lack of awareness of the value and accuracy of MRI for this purpose, (b) automated, quantitative volumetric methods for measuring hippocampal volume are unwieldy, expensive and not easily adapted for routine clinical use, and (c) the lack of widely accepted age-adjusted norms and cut-scores for hippocampal volume (HP-v) and medial temporal atrophy (MTA).

The goal of this study was to evaluate user-friendly methods to evaluate structural MRI scans and to provide appropriate age-adjusted cut scores for both visually rated MTA measures and HP-v structures, which best distinguish normal elderly subjects from those who have AD. Accordingly, we compared hippocampal volumes (HP-v) to a refinement of the semiquantitative visual rating method, initially developed by Scheltens et al. (1995). This new visual rating system for assessing medial temporal atrophy (VRS-MTA) (Duara et al., 2008; Urs et al., 2009) provides a total MTA score by combining atrophy levels in individual medial temporal structures, including the HP, the entorhinal cortex (ERC), and the perirhinal cortex (PRC). We established appropriate age-related cut-offs for both volumetric measures of the HP and VRS-MTA measures, which correctly classified 70–80% of cognitively normal [CN] subjects without cognitive impairment. We chose these levels of specificity because at least 20–30% of CN subjects are known to harbor the pathology of AD on post-mortem evaluation (Morris, 2006). We then compared the accuracy of these two methods for distinguishing CN from subjects with aMCI and AD, the associations of these two measures with neuropsychological measures of cognition and the ability to predict progression from aMCI to dementia.

METHODS

SUBJECT RECRUITMENT

The current sample was recruited from a group of 273 subjects (107 CN, who were enrolled in the Florida Alzheimer's Disease Research Center Clinical Core (FADRC-CC) in Miami Beach FL between 2005 and 2009 (Duara et al., 2010). Subjects were diagnosed as cognitively normal (CN) or having amnestic MCI (aMCI) or dementia. The study was approved by the Institutional Review Board at Mount Sinai Medical Center, Miami Beach, and the University of South Florida, Tampa. All subjects or a legal representative provided informed consent.

EVALUATIONS

The following were completed on all subjects: (1) full clinical history, obtained from a reliable informant; (2) neurological evaluation; (3) psychiatric evaluation, including administration of the Geriatric Depression scale (Sheikh and Yesavage, 1986) and the Neuropsychiatric Inventory (Cummings et al., 1994); (4) Clinical Disease Rating scale (CDR-SB; Morris, 1993); (5) Mini-Mental State Examination (MMSE; Folstein et al., 1975); (6) a neuropsychological test battery, as described below; (7) Unified Parkinson Disease Rating Scale (UPDRS, motor section; Fahn and Elton, 1987) which has been documented as a sensitive tool for quantifying motor dysfunction and parkinsonism in patients with various forms of MCI and dementia.

Cardiovascular Risk (CVR) Score was calculated as the sum of 10 independent risk factors (14) selected from the National Alzheimer's Coordinating Center (NACC) Uniform Data Set (UDS) Subject Health History assessment protocol (Appel et al., 2009).

DIAGNOSTIC PROCEDURES

DETERMINING A CONSENSUS DIAGNOSIS FOR COGNITIVELY NORMAL, DIFFERENT MCI SUBTYPES AND DEMENTIA

The physician assigned a cognitive diagnosis of CN, MCI, or Dementia, as described previously (Duara et al., 2010). Briefly, the PhyDx was based on the subject's entire clinical history and functional status, which was derived from the history itself, CDR rating, functional activity questionnaire, MMSE score and subscores, taking into account the subjects' educational and cultural background, sensory (especially visual and hearing) and motor deficits, language and speech disorders, medical and psychiatric conditions and the perceived reliability of the informant. In addition to the physician's diagnosis, an independent neuropsychological diagnosis was rendered by a neuropsychologist.

NEUROPSYCHOLOGICAL DIAGNOSIS (NPDx)

All neuropsychological tests were administered in the subjects' native language (English or Spanish) and compared to age and education adjusted normative data, as described previously (Loewenstein et al., 2009). The tests included all of those outlined in the NACC protocol (Beekly et al., 2007), as well as additional tests, including the Three Trial Fuld Object Memory Evaluation (FOME; Fuld, 1981), and the Hopkins Verbal Learning Test-Delayed Recall (HVLT; Benedict et al., 1998). Memory measures were: the FOME, HVLT, and Delayed Visual Reproduction of the Wechsler Memory Scale-R (Wechsler, 1987). Non-memory tests included: category fluency (Monsch et al., 1992), letter fluency (language; Monsch et al., 1992), Block Design-WAIS-III (visuospatial; Wechsler, 1997), Trails B (Executive; Army Individual Test Battery, 1944), and Similarities-WAIS-R (Executive; Wechsler, 1997). Neuropsychological classification were made as follows: (a) a test score of 1.5 SD or greater below expected normative values on any single test for MCI syndromes; and (b) 2.0 SD or greater below expected normative values in one memory and one non-memory test for dementia (corresponding to NINCDS-ADRDA criteria; (McKhann et al., 1984). Nomenclature used for NPDx was Normal, Non-Amnestic MCI (naMCI; single or multi-domain), amnestic MCI (aMCI; single or multi-domain) and Dementia.

ALGORITHMIC CONSENSUS COGNITIVE DIAGNOSES (AlgDx)

An algorithmic approach to consensus diagnosis (Duara et al., 2010) combined the PhyDx with the NPDx, as follows: (a) a

PhyDx and a NPDx of Normal received an AlgDx of cognitively normal (CN); (b) a PhyDx diagnosis of MCI and a NPDx of aMCI received an AlgDx of aMCI; (c) a PhyDx of dementia and a NPDx of aMCI or Dementia received an AlgDx of Dementia. Patients diagnosed with aMCI met Petersen criteria for MCI (Petersen et al., 1999). Probable AD was diagnosed according to National Institute of Neurological and Communicative Disorders and Stroke (NINCDS)–Alzheimer's Disease and Related Disorders Association (ADRDA) criteria for AD (McKhann et al., 1984) and the criteria set forth by the National Alzheimer's Coordinating Center.

MRI Scans were acquired using a proprietary 3-D volumetric protocol on a Siemens Symphony, 1.5 Tesla machine (Iselin, NJ) or a GE 1.5 T machine, using proprietary three-dimensional magnetization-prepared rapid-acquisition gradient echo (Siemens) or the three-dimensional spoiled gradient recalled echo (General Electric) sequences; MRI scans were acquired in the coronal plane, and contiguous slices with thickness of 1.5 mm or less were reconstructed.

VOLUMETRIC ANALYSIS OF BRAIN MRIs

Volumetric analysis is performed using Individual Brain Atlas and Statistical Parametric Mapping (IBASPM; Alemán-Gómez et al., 2006). In IBAPSM, the volume of brain regions is calculated after normalization or spatial transformation to Montreal Neurological Institute (MNI; McGill University, 2009) templates. The scans are segmented into three types of tissue in each hemisphere: gray matter, white matter, and cerebrospinal fluid. An individual brain atlas for each subject is created with the transformation matrix obtained from the normalization step, and anatomical automatic labeling (AAL) to specify 116 regions. Hippocampal volume (HP-vol) was calculated as the ratio of the volume of each HP (right and left) to the total intracranial volume (Shen et al., 2011).

VISUAL RATING METHODS ASSESSING BRAIN MRIs

The scope and utility of Scheltens' system was expanded by Duara et al. (2008) and Urs et al. (2009), to provide reliable visual ratings of individual MTL regions, i.e., hippocampus (HPC), ERC, and PRC. Reliability and accuracy were achieved using very thin coronal slices (1.2 to 1.5 mm thickness), perpendicular to the AC-PC line and intersecting the mammillary bodies (Urs et al., 2009). We have previously reported excellent inter-rater reliability for measuring individual MTL structures; kappa values among two raters ranged between 0.75 and 0.94 for inter-rater reliability and 0.87 and 0.93 for intra-rater reliability. (Urs et al., 2009). With VRS-MTA, semi-quantitative assessments of atrophy of the HP, ERC, and PRC were assigned as follows: a score of Grade 0 corresponded to no atrophy, Grade 1 to minimal atrophy, Grade 2 to mild atrophy, Grade 3 to moderate atrophy and Grade 4 to severe atrophy (**Figure 1**). The VRS-MTA program provides a library of drop-down images, depicting the anatomical boundaries of these structures as well as each grade of atrophy for the ERC, HP, and PRC.

ApoE genotype was determined using standard methods (Wenham et al., 1991). ApoEε4 frequencies were subsequently calculated for each diagnostic group.

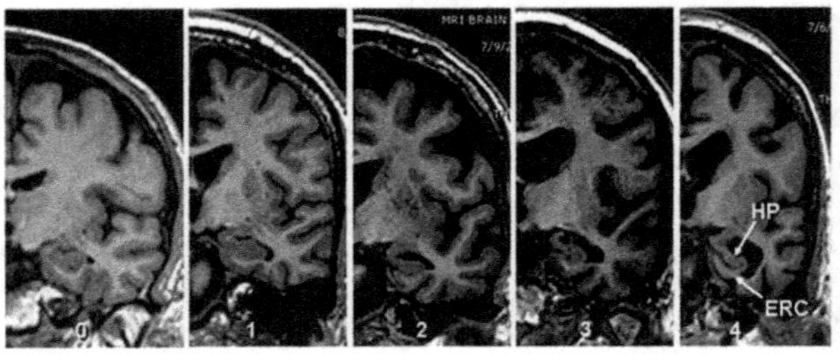

FIGURE 1 | Visual rating scale. Image depicting four degrees of atrophy in Hippocampus and Entorhinal cortex according to visual rating scale where 0 = no atrophy, 1 = minimal atrophy, 2 = mild atrophy, 3 = moderate atrophy and 4 = server atrophy (Score shown corresponds to both structure).

DERIVING CUT-OFFS FOR HP-VOL AND VRS-MTA VALUES FOR DIFFERENT AGE GROUPS AND BOTH BRAIN SIDES

To derive cut-scores for HP-vol (measured as percentage of intracranial volume) for the older CN group we used the scores of 20 subjects, aged 76 years and above (mean age = 79.64 years; $SD = 3.2$ years range = 76–90 years), who had an algorithmic diagnosis of CN. The cut-off scores for the lowest 20% (liberal cut score ≤0.0249%) and 30% (conservative cut score ≤0.0224%) of HP-vol, for each side, which was then used to identify hippocampal atrophy for all diagnostic groups aged 76 or greater. Similarly, we determined the approximate cut score (range of 0–12 points for each side), for highest 20–30% (liberal cut score ≥4) or 30–40% (conservative cut score ≥5) of combined HP, ERC, and PRC ratings on the left and right sides. These cut scores were then used to identify threshold levels of MTA for all diagnostic groups, aged 76 years or greater, separately for the right and left sides in each subject.

To derive a cut-score for the younger CN group, we took the scores of 87 cognitively normal individuals aged 63–75 years (mean age = 68.33 years; $SD = 3.2$ years) and used a similar procedure as for the older CN. The derived cut scores for HP-v (liberal cut score ≤0.027; conservative cut score ≤0.0257) and VRS-MTA ratings (liberal cut score ≥2.0; conservative cut score ≥3) for the right and left sides for each subject. In addition, so as to identify localized atrophy within the medial temporal region on each side, independent of the total VRS-MTA score, we determined the highest VRS scores for the right and left HP and ERC for each subject. For these measures a liberal (≤1.5) and a conservative (≤2.0) cut score were determined that would classify not more than 20 or 33% of both young and old CN group as having abnormal atrophy. These cut scores were also applied to subjects diagnosed with amnestic MCI and dementia.

LONGITUDINAL EVALUATION PROCEDURES

A total of 72 of the 103 subjects had at least one-annual follow-up evaluation (mean = 33.1 months; $SD = 14.1$ months), including neurological, psychiatric and neuropsychological evaluations, and re-diagnosis by the AlgDx. The mean age of this sample was 76.8 ($SD = 5.8$ years) and mean MMSE scores of were 26.1 ($SD = 2.4$) making the sample comparable to the aMCI patients who were originally diagnosed at baseline.

STATISTICAL ANALYSIS

Group comparisons of demographic variables across three study groups were analyzed using analyses of variance (ANOVA) or chi-square tests, as appropriate. *Post-hoc* tests of means were examined by the Tukey-Kramer procedure at $p < 0.05$. Comparative analyses of VRS-MTA and HP-v measures were assessed using receiver operator (ROC) curves. HP-v and MTA-VRS scores were correlated to a broad array of cognitive measures among memory impaired patients. Comparisons between correlation coefficients were tested statistically using SISA binomials (Uitenbroek, 1997). Finally, differences in progression rates across groups were assessed using chi-square procedures.

RESULTS

DEMOGRAPHICS

In the entire sample of subjects (age range = 63–93 years; mean age = 75.0 ± 7.2 years) there were statistically significant demographic differences between CN, aMCI, and AD groups, with regards to age, gender and educational attainment as well as on MMSE scores [$F_{(2,\ 269)} = 172.05$; $p < 0.001$] (**Table 1**). *Post-hoc* tests revealed that CN patients were younger, better educated, had higher MMSE scores and were more frequently female compared to the other two groups. AD subjects were older and had lower MMSE scores than aMCI subjects. There were significant group differences with regards to Spanish vs. English-speaking subjects or percentage of subjects carrying one or more ApoE ϵ4 allele. As indicated in **Table 1**, CN subjects scored higher than aMCI and AD subjects on all neuropsychological measures, and demonstrated less atrophy in comparison to aMCI and AD subjects on VRS-MTA and HP-v scores. AD subjects had more atrophy than aMCI subjects on VRS-MTA and HP-v measures, as well as impairment on all neuropsychological measures, with the exception of the Block Design test, in which there was no difference in scores between AD and aMCI subjects.

PERFORMANCE OF VRS-MTA vs. HP-v

For the discrimination of amnestic MCI from CN, in both the younger and older age groups, there was no difference in the areas under receiver operating curve (aROC) between HP-v measures and VRS-MTA measures ($Z = 1.26$; $p < 0.27$) (**Table 2**). For the discrimination of AD from CN, among the younger age group (63–75 years), VRS-MTA performed better than HP-v (aROC: 0.92 vs. 0.847, $p < 0.046$). The corresponding sensitivity/specificity values for VRS-MAT and HP-v were: 89.2/82.1% and 75.7/82.1% for the more liberal cutoffs described in the methods. There was no difference between the performance of VRS-MTA and HP-v in the older group, for the classification of AD vs. CN. Considering the correct age-associated cut-offs for impairment for the total sample, 63% of those subjects who did not meet criteria for impairment using HP-v, did meet criteria for impairment using VRS-MTA, and conversely, only 30% of those who were VRS-MTA negative were HP-v positive.

CORRELATIONS WITH COGNITIVE MEASURES

In a combined group of aMCI and AD subjects, who had adequate cognitive testing data, both HPv and VRS-MTA measures were strongly correlated with scores on various memory tests and with the category fluency test (a measure of speed of search from semantic lexicon) (**Table 3**). Tests of visuospatial function (block design), processing speed and attention (Trails A) and executive

Table 1 | Demographics and MRI measures.

	CN ($n = 107$)	aMCI ($n = 105$)	AD ($n = 56$)	*f*-value
Age	71.1^c (5.8)	77.9^b (5.3)	79.5^a (6.8)	42.59***
Education	15.0^a (3.2)	12.4^b (3.9)	12.4^b (4.1)	16.71***
Gender (Female)	75.7%	50.0%	53.7%	X^2= 16.93***
Hispanic%	47.4%	48.0%	57.4%	X^2= 1.64***
ApoE%	24.7%	30.6%	42.9%	X^2= 4.13 ***
MMSE	29.0^a (1.1)	25.9^b (2.5)	22.4^c (3.1)	172.05***
Fuld OME	25.7^a (2.0)	18.9^b (4.8)	10.6^c(6.5)	195.35***
HVLT-Total Recall	25.3^a (4.3)	17.4^b (4.5)	13.2^c (4.7)	159.48***
HVLT-DEL	9.2^a (1.7)	3.7^b (2.9)	1.3^c (2.2)	258.75***
Semantic interference test (SIT) score	13.3^a (2.9)	8.2^b (3.2)	3.1^c(3.0)	209.04***
Visual reproduction test-delayed	23.0^a (7.9)	8.3^b (7.2)	3.4^c (5.7)	149.08***
Memory for Passages (Delayed)	11.5^a (3.5)	5.6^b (3.7)	2.2^c (3.0)	149.92***
Two Category Fluency	34.2^a (7.3)	24.1^b (6.2)	17.2^c (5.9)	134.24***
Block Design- WAIS-IV	31.5$_a$ (9.4)	19.11^b (7.9)	18.8^b (7.8)	64.39***
Trails A	35.9^a (11.3)	54.5^b (23.9)	73.5^c (33.5)	55.04***
Trails B	95.1^a (48.2)	199.4^b (88.6)	254.1^c (73.7)	106.58***
HP-v (most impaired side)	0.00275^a (0.0003)	0.00240^b (0.004)	0.00208^c (0.005)	60.3***
VRS-MTA score (most impaired side)	1.7^a (1.8)	4.2^b (2.7)	6.9^c (3.3)	81.31***

*CN, Cognitively normal; aMCI, amnestic cognitive impairment; MMSE, Mini-mental status exam; HVLT, Hopkins verbal learning test; HP-v, Hippocampal volume; VRS-MTA, Visual rating scale-mdial temporal atrophy. ***p < 0.001; means with different superscripts are statistically different at p < 0.05 by the Tukey-Kramer test.*

Table 2 | HP-v and VRS-MTA measures in the classification of subjects with Amnestic MCI and Alzheimer's disease.

Diagnostic comparison and age group	Sensitivity/Specificity (%) for HP-v	aROC for HP-v measure	Sensitivity/Specificity (%) for VRS-MTA	aROC for VRS-MTA measure	Comparison of aROCs for Hp-v and VRS-MTA
AMNESTIC MILD COGNITIVE IMPAIRMENT VERSUS ELDERLY NORMAL					
63–75 years ($n = 60$)	35.0/82.1	0.652 ($SE = 0.06$)	55.0/82.1	0.723 ($SE = 0.06$)	$Z = 1.38$; $p > 0.26$
76+ years ($n = 45$)	60.0/81.6	0.764 ($SE = 0.05$)	51.1 /78.2	0.736 ($SE = 0.05$)	$Z = 0.60$; $p > 0.54$
ALZHEIMER'S DISEASE VERSUS ELDERLY NORMAL					
63–75 years ($n = 37$)	75.7/82.1	0.847 ($SE = 0.05$)	89.2/82.1	0.920 ($SE = 0.03$)	$Z = 2.00$; $p < 0.046$
76+ years ($n = 19$)	63.2/81.6	0.713 ($SE = 0.08$)	68.4/78.2	0.853 ($SE = 0.04$)	$Z = 1.66$; $p < 0.10$

HP-v, hippocampal volume; VRS-MTA, Visual rating system- medial temporal atrophy; aROC, Area under the receiver operating curve; AD, Alzheimer's disease; MCI, amnestic MCI; CN, Cognitively normal.

Table 3 | Comparative correlations between volumetric and VRS-MTA measures among 129 cognitively impaired patients.

	Correlation with HP-v	Correlation with VRS-MTA	Test of difference in correlations coefficients[#]	*p*-value
Fuld object memory evaluation	0.35***	−0.51***	2.33	<0.011
HVLT (Delayed Recall)	0.15	−0.29***	1.91	<0.030
WMS- memory for passages (Delayed Recall)	0.20*	−0.36***	2.27	<0.013
WMS-visual reproduction (Delay Recall)	0.33***	−0.47***	1.96	<0.027
Two word category fluency	0.31***	−0.32***	0.14	446
Trails A	−0.14	0.07	NA	NA
Trails B	−0.05	0.11	NA	NA
Block-design WAIS-II	0.05	−0.09	NA	NA
Similarities WAIS-R	−0.10	0.09	NA	NA

*HP-v, hippocampal volume; VRS-MTA, Visual rating system-medial temporal atrophy. [#]Difference in correlations tested using SISA polynomials (Uitenbroek, 1997)/ *$p < 0.05$, ***$p < 0.001$.*

function (Trails B) were not correlated significantly with HP-v or VRS-MTA imaging measures. In most instances the memory measures (using the Fuld OME, for example) were more strongly correlated with VRS-MTA ($r = -0.51$) than with HP-v ($r = -0.35$) ($t = 2.33$; $p < 0.02$) (**Table 3**).

PROGRESSION FROM aMCI TO AD

Among a sample of aMCI subjects ($n = 72$; mean age $= 76.8 \pm 5.8$ years: educational attainment $= 12.83 \pm 3.6$ years) with adequate follow-up data (mean follow-up period $= 33.1 \pm 14.1$ months) the percentage of progressors vs. non-progressors to AD was predicted using both stringent and liberal VRS-MTA cut-off scores (**Table 4**). Using stringent VRS-MTA criteria, 51% of aMCI subjects scoring at or above the impairment cut-off were found to be progressors, as compared to 21% scoring at or above the impairment cut-off being non-progressors ($\chi^2 = 5.51$; $p = 0.019$). In contrast, for HP-v 41 % of aMCI subjects scoring at or above the impairment cut-off were found to be progressors, as compared to 29% scoring at or above the stringent impairment cut-offs being non-progressors ($\chi^2 = 1.19$; $p = 0.28$).

Table 4 | VRS-MTA score, HP-v and progression from aMCI to AD.

	Progressors to AD	Non-progressors	Chi-square	*p*-value
VRS-MTA score (Conservative criteria)	50.7%	20.6%	5.51	0.019
HP-v (Conservative criteria)	44.1%	28.9%	1.19	0.275

HP-v, hippocampal volume; VRS-MTA, Visual rating system-medial temporal atrophy.

DISCUSSION

In this study, we showed that VRS-MTA is superior to volumetric assessment of the HP (HP-v) for distinguishing aMCI patients and normal elderly controls. When we divided the subjects into "young-old" (63–75 years) and "older-old" (76 years+) subgroups, our previous findings hold true, in much smaller groups of subjects (Duara et al., 2008; Shen et al., 2011). We have also shown that VRS-MTA ratings correlate more strongly than do HP-v with memory measures and CDR ratings (Shen et al., 2011). In this study, we have additionally provided age-corrected cut-scores for HP-v and VRS–MTA scores for classifying subjects with aMCI and AD and have shown that VRS-MTA scores, but not HP-v scores in this cohort, were predictors of progression from aMCI to AD.

The use of structural MRI scans as biomarkers, in association with clinical criteria, for distinguishing CN subjects from those with incipient or Probable AD requires the use of age-adjusted cut- scores for research and for clinical practice. For the first time, to our knowledge, we have shown that specific age-related cut-scores for VRS-MTA and HP-v measures can be used for distinguishing CN from AD subjects. By deriving scores for the most impaired hemisphere, based upon age-related norms, we may have further enhanced the overall sensitivity of VRS-MTA. Indeed, almost two thirds of those subjects who did not meet criteria for impairment using HP-v, did meet criteria for impairment using VRS-MTA, and conversely, less than a third of those who were VRS-MTA negative were HP-v positive. Thus, each measure provides unique information, most notably VRS MTA, which includes independent and additive measures of the HP, ERC, and PRC.

An advantage of using VRS-MTA over HP-v is that regional brain volumes are variable across individuals and need to be normalized by conversion to a ratio of the absolute volume of the HP to intracranial volume, whereas VRS-MTA has built–in normalization and thus avoids multiplicative errors inherent in using ratios of two quantitative variables. From the clinician's vantage point, VRS-MTA has the following additional desirable attributes: (1) measurement and scoring of VRS-MTA is quick and reliable by the clinician, providing a distinct advantage over traditional volumetric techniques; (2) HP-v measurements, as compared to VRS-MTA measurements, require much greater technical stringency in the acquisition of the MRI scans and are far more vulnerable to a variety of measurement errors; (3) HP-v measurements require a technical interface for obtaining quantitative assessment whereas VRS-MTA does not (Duara et al., 2008; Shen et al., 2011). Although volumetric analysis of regional brain atrophy can be performed by a variety of programs which are widely available, they have been used almost exclusively in research applications, and not in clinical practice. Currently, measurement of HP-v is inconvenient and expensive in time and money and technical problems that often occur during the image acquisition protocol may invalidate the use of a substantial proportion of MRI scans performed in the community.

From a biological standpoint it is clear that hippocampal atrophy is non-specific and that the characteristic pathological changes in AD (Braak and Braak, 1985; Braak et al., 2006) begin outside the HP, with development of neurofibrillary tangles in the transentorhinal and entorhinal cortex, spreading subsequently to the subiculum and CA1 regions of the HP. Subsequent spread of pathology occurs to limbic, and ultimately to neocortical regions, such as the precuneus, middle frontal gyrus and posterior cingulate gyrus. The severity of this atrophy, at least in the medial temporal regions, correlates with the severity of underlying AD-related neuropathological changes seen on postmortem (Jack et al., 2002).

The use of VRS-MTA methodology affords a unique perspective, not available to those using quantitative HP-v measures, of the presence and severity of the neurodegenerative process in AD. Atrophy of the entorhinal and perirhinal cortices and the HP, widening of the collateral sulcus and atrophy of the white matter band between the subiculum and the ERC are well known pathological features of AD and are readily visible on appropriately obtained MRI scans acquired or reconstructed in the coronal plane in thin, contiguous brain slices. This information often times serves to confirm the clinical diagnosis, especially in a patient in which non-neurodegenerative causes of cognitive impairment, such as cerebrovascular disease or psychiatric conditions are also under consideration. The absence of confirmatory neurodegenerative findings on the MRI scan alerts the clinician to alternative causes of impaired cognitive performance, such as systemic disorders, attention deficit disorders, sleep-apnea syndrome, depression, anxiety, and cultural or language related factors.

The current investigation has the following advantages over previous studies: (1) Optimal age- related cut-scores for VRS-MTA and HP-v have been derived for normal subjects and then applied to aMCI and AD cases; (2) the importance of frequently-observed asymmetrical atrophy in medial temporal regions and HP-v volumes has been recognized and incorporated into the algorithm for distinguishing CN from aMCI and AD subjects, using either VRS-MTA or HP-v measures (typically, rather than using the most atrophic side in the algorithm, bilateral regions are combined into a single score). Using these methods our results indicate that VRS-MTA is at least as good, and more likely better than using HP-v for distinguishing both younger and older aMCI and AD subjects from CN subjects. VRS-MTA scores are also better correlated than are HP-v measures with memory and functional indices. Finally, VRS-MTA measures are better than HP-v measures in predicting progression to AD or dementia over a defined period of time. This suggests that VRS-MTA may provide a clearer indication of neurodegenerative pathology related to AD than merely HP-v.

Some of the limitations of using VRS-MTA include the fact that ratings are based on assessments performed on a single coronal slice, thereby providing a limited perspective of overall brain pathology (this limitation can be easily overcome by evaluating multiple adjacent coronal slices). In addition, atrophy in the medial temporal regions may not be specific to AD, but in some cases may be indicative of hippocampal sclerosis, frontotemporal lobar dementias, Lewy body dementia, vascular dementia, or cognitive impairment (Jack et al., 2002; Barkhof et al., 2007). Also, a larger and more diverse group of elderly normals will be required to extend age-related cut-off scores further than we have been able to do in this study. Age is a risk factor for AD and other neurodegenerative disorders and up to 30% elderly adults with underlying brain pathology may have sufficient cognitive reserve so that they do not present with cognitive symptoms. Hence, it is likely that among elderly volunteers, who are cognitively normal, substantial AD pathology is present, which may be reflected in their VRS-MTA scores, thereby apparently reducing the specificity of VRS-MTA cut-off scores.

At present, the primary utility of structural MRI, in the diagnosis of disorders causing cognitive impairment, is to rule out specific pathologies such as pathologies as hydrocephalus, vascular, inflammatory or demyelinating, and space-occupying lesions as the cause of the cognitive syndrome, but not for confirming the presence of AD-like pathology and its severity. Our results suggest that VRS-MTA, which could readily be incorporated into the routine assessment of patients presenting with memory symptoms, will likely assist in strengthening the diagnosis of AD or ruling it out, thereby improving both sensitivity and specificity of a clinical diagnosis of probable and prodromal AD. Moreover, VRS-MTA need not be used exclusively for clinical purposes; it could also serve as a research tool, especially in clinical trials when accuracy of the clinical diagnosis is a major requirement.

ACKNOWLEDGMENTS

Research was supported by the National Institute of Aging, NIH 5R01AG020094-03 and NIH 1P50AG025711-03, & Byrd Alzheimer Center and Research Institute grants. Statistical analysis was performed by David A. Loewenstein, Ph.D., University of Miami.

REFERENCES

Albert, M. S., Dekosky, S. T., Dickson, D., Dubois, B., Feldman, H. H., Fox, N. C., et al. (2011). The diagnosis of mild cognitive impairment due to Alzheimer's disease: recommendations from the National Institute on Aging-Alzheimer's Association workgroups on diagnostic guidelines for Alzheimer's disease. *Alzheimers Dement.* 7, 270–279. doi: 10.1016/j.jalz.2011.03.008

Alemán-Gómez, Y., Melie-García, L., and Valdés-Hernandez, P. (2006). "IBASPM: Toolbox for automatic parcellation of brain structures," in *Presented at the 12th Annual Meeting of the Organization for Human Brain Mapping* (Florence). Available on CD-Rom in NeuroImage, Vol. 27, No.1.

Appel, J., Potter, E., Bhatia, N., Shen, Q., Zhao, W., Greig, M. T., et al. (2009). Association of white matter hyperintensity measurements on brain MR imaging with cognitive status, medial temporal atrophy, and cardiovascular risk factors. *AJNR Am. J. Neuroradiol.* 30, 1870–1876. doi: 10.3174/ajnr.A1693

Army Individual Test Battery (1944). *Manual of Directions And Scoring.* Washington, DC: War Department, Adjutant General's Office.

Barkhof, F., Polvikoski, T. M., van Straaten, E. C., Kalaria, R. N., Sulkava, R., Aronen, H. J., et al. (2007). The significance of medial temporal lobe atrophy: a post-mortem MRI study in the very old. *Neurology* 69, 1521–1527. doi: 10.1212/01.wnl.0000277459.83543.99

Beekly, D. L., Ramos, E. M., Lee, W. W., Deitrich, W. D., Jacka, M. E., Wu, J., et al. (2007). NIA Alzheimer's Disease Centers. The National Alzheimer's Coordinating Center (NACC) database: the Uniform Data Set. *Alzheimer Dis. Assoc. Disord.* 21, 249–158. doi: 10.1097/WAD.0b013e318142774e

Benedict, R. H. B., Schretlen, D., Groninger, L., and Brandt, J. (1998). Hopkins verbal learning test-revised: normative data and analysis of inter-form and test-retest reliability. *Clin. Neuropsychol.* 12, 43–55. doi: 10.1076/clin.12.1.43.1726

Braak, H., and Braak, E. (1985). On areas of transition between entorhinal allocortex and temporal isocortex in the human brain. Normal morphology and lamina-specific pathology in Alzheimer's disease. *Acta Neuropathol. (Berl.)* 68, 325–332. doi: 10.1007/BF00690836

Braak, H., Alafuzoff, I., Arzberger, T., Kretzschmar, H., and Del Tredici, K. (2006). Acta Staging of Alzheimer disease-associated neurofibrillary pathology using paraffin sections and immunocytochemistry. *Neuropathol.* 112, 389–404. doi: 10.1007/s00401-006-0127-z

Cummings, J. L., Mega, M., Gray, K., Rosenberg-Thompson, S., Carusi, D. A., and Gornbein, J. (1994). The neuropsychiatric inventory: comprehensive assessment of neuropathology in dementia. *Neurology* 44, 2308–2314. doi: 10.1212/WNL.44.12.2308

Duara, R., Loewenstein, D. A., Greig, M., Acevedo, A., Potter, E., Appel, J., et al. (2010). Reliability and validity of an algorithm for the diagnosis of normal cognition, MCI and dementia: implications for multi-center research studies. *Am. J. Geriatr. Psychiatry.* 18, 363–370. doi: 10.1097/JGP.0b013e3181c534a0

Duara, R., Loewenstein, D. A., Potter, E., Appel, A., Greig, M. T., Urs, R., et al. (2008). Medial temporal lobe atrophy on MRI scans and the diagnosis of Alzheimer disease. *Neurology* 71, 1986–1992. doi: 10.1212/01.wnl.0000336925.79704.9f

Fahn, S., and Elton, R. (1987). "Unified Parkinson's disease rating scale," in *Recent Developments in Parkinson Diseases*, eds S. Fahn, D. Marsden, and D. Calne (London: Macmillan), 153–163.

Folstein, M., Folstein, S., and McHugh, P. (1975). Mini-mental state. A practical method for grading the cognitive state of patients for the physician. *J. Psychiatr. Res.* 12, 189–198. doi: 10.1016/0022-3956(75)90026-6

Frisoni, G. B., Fox, N. C., Jack, C. R. Jr., Scheltens, P., and Thompson, P. M. (2010). The clinical use of structural MRI in Alzheimer disease. *Nat. Rev. Neurol.* 6, 67–77. doi: 10.1038/nrneurol.2009.215

Fuld, P. A. (1981). *Fuld Object-Memory Evaluation.* Illinois, IL: Stoelting Co.

Jack, C. R., Dickson, D. W., Parisin, J. E., Xu, Y. C., Cha, R. H., O'Brien, P. C., et al. (2002). Antemortem MRI findings correlate with hippocampal neuropathology in typical aging and dementia. *Neurology* 58, 750–757. doi: 10.1212/WNL.58.5.750

Loewenstein, D. A., Acevedo, A., Potter, E., Schinka, J. A., Raj, A., Greig, M. T., et al. (2009). Severity of medial temporal atrophy and amnestic mild cognitive impairment: selecting type and number of memory tests. *Am. J. Geriatr. Psychiatry* 17, 1050–1058. doi: 10.1097/JGP.0b013e3181b7ef42

McGill University. (2009). Montreal, QC. Available online at: http://www.bic.mni.mcgill.ca/brainweb/ (Accessed June 12, 2006; July 1, 2009).

McKhann, G., Drachman, D. A., Folstein, M. F., Katzman, R., Price, D. L., and Stadlan, E. (1984). Clinical diagnosis of Alzheimer's disease: report of the NINCDS-ADRDA Work Group under the auspices of the Department of Health and Human Services Task Force on Alzheimer's disease. *Neurology* 34, 939–944. doi: 10.1212/WNL.34.7.939

Monsch, A. Y., Bondi, M. W., Butters, N., Salmon, D. P., Katzman, R., and Thal, L. (1992). Comparison of verbal fluency tasks in the detection of dementia of the Alzheimer's type. *Arch. Neurol.* 49, 1253–1258. doi: 10.1001/archneur.1992.00530360051017

Morris, J. C. (1993). The clinical dementia rating (CDR), Current version and scoring rules. *Neurology* 43, 2412–2414. doi: 10.1212/WNL.43.11.2412-a

Morris, J. C. (2006). Mild cognitive impairment is early-stage Alzheimer disease: time to revise diagnostic criteria. *Arch. Neurol.* 63, 15–16. doi: 10.1001/archneur.63.1.15

Petersen, R. C., Smith, G. E., Waring, S. C., Ivnik, R. J., Tangalos, E. G., and Kokmen, E. (1999). Mild cognitive impairment: clinical characterization and outcome. *Arch. Neurol.* 56, 303–308. doi: 10.1001/archneur.56.3.303

Scheltens, P., Launer, L. J., Barkhof, F., Weinstein, H. C., and van Gool, W. A. (1995). Visual assessment of medial temporal lobe atrophy on magnetic resonance imaging: interobserver reliability. *J. Neurol.* 242, 557–560. doi: 10.1007/BF00868807

Sheikh, J. I., and Yesavage, J. A. (1986). "Geriatric Depression Scale (GDS): recent evidence and development of a shorter version," in *Clinical Gerontology: A Guide to Assessment and Interventions*, ed T. L. Brink (New York, NY: The Haworth Press), 165–173.

Shen, Q., Loewenstein, D., Potter, E., Zhao, W., Appel, J., Greig, M., et al. (2011). Volumetric and visual rating of MRI scans in the diagnosis of amnestic MCI and Alzheimer's Disease. *Alzheimers Dement.* 7, 101–108. doi: 10.1016/j.jalz.2010.07.002

Sperling, R. A., Aisen, P. S., Beckett, L. A., Bennett, D. A., Craft, S., Fagan, A. M., et al. (2011). Toward defining the preclinical stages of Alzheimer's disease: recommendations from the National Institute on Aging-Alzheimer's Association workgroups on diagnostic guidelines for Alzheimer's disease. *Alzheimers Dement.* 7, 280–292. doi: 10.1016/j.jalz.2011.03.003

Urs, R., Potter, E., Barker, W., Appel, J., Loewenstein, D. A., Zhao, W., et al. (2009). Visual rating system (VRS) for assessing magnetic resonance images (MRIs): a tool in the diagnosis of MCI and

Alzheimer's disease. *J. Comput. Assist. Tomogr.* 33, 73–78. doi: 10.1097/RCT.0b013e31816373d8

Uitenbroek, D. G. (1997). *SISA Binomial.* Southampton: D.G. Uitenbroek. Available online at: http://www.quantitativeskills.com/sisa/distributions/binomial.htm (Accessed January 01, 2004)

Wechsler, D. (1987). *The Wechsler Memory Scale-Revised.* San Antonio, TX: The Psychological Corporation.

Wechsler, D. (1997). *The Wechsler Adult Intelligence Scale, 3rd Edn.* San Antonio, TX: The Psychological Corporation.

Wenham, P. R., Price, W. H., and Blandell, G. (1991). Apolipoprotein E genotyping by one-stage PCR. *Lancet* 337, 1158–1159. doi: 10.1016/0140-6736(91)92823-K

12

Methodological considerations in longitudinal morphometry of traumatic brain injury

Junghoon Kim[1]*, Brian Avants[2], John Whyte[1] and James C. Gee[2]

[1] Moss Rehabilitation Research Institute, Elkins Park, PA, USA
[2] Department of Radiology, University of Pennsylvania, Philadelphia, PA, USA

Edited by:
Robin E. A. Green, University of Toronto, Canada

Reviewed by:
Jennie L. Ponsford, Monash University, Australia
Bogdan Draganski, University Lausanne, Switzerland

***Correspondence:**
Junghoon Kim, Moss Rehabilitation Research Institute, 50 Township Line Rd., Elkins Park, PA 19027, USA.
e-mail: kimj@einstein.edu

Traumatic brain injury (TBI) has recently been reconceptualized as a chronic, evolving disease process. This new view necessitates quantitative assessment of post-injury changes in brain structure that may allow more accurate monitoring and prediction of recovery. In particular, TBI is known to trigger neurodegenerative processes and therefore quantifying progression of diffuse atrophy over time is currently of utmost interest. However, there are various methodological issues inherent to longitudinal morphometry in TBI. In this paper, we first overview several of these methodological challenges: lesion evolution, neurosurgical procedures, power, bias, and non-linearity. We then introduce a sensitive, reliable, and unbiased longitudinal multivariate analysis protocol that combines dimensionality reduction and region of interest approaches. This analysis pipeline is demonstrated using a small dataset consisting of four chronic TBI survivors.

Keywords: longitudinal, power, bias, magnetic resonance imaging, sparse canonical correlation analysis

INTRODUCTION

Traumatic brain injury (TBI) triggers a cascade of events that lead to long-term neuropathological and behavioral consequences. Recently, more and more researchers have been conceptualizing TBI as a chronic disease with dynamic and evolving recovery and degeneration processes (e.g., Masel and Dewitt, 2010). Among the post-injury changes in moderate to severe TBI, widespread volume reduction in brain parenchyma, frequently called diffuse atrophy, is probably most prominent and significant (Bigler, 2005; Povlishock and Katz, 2005). An important mechanism of this diffuse change is Wallerian degeneration due to traumatic axonal injury, which may continue months and years after injury. Describing the spatial and temporal characteristics of these degenerative morphological changes may provide important clues for the mechanisms underlying individual differences in functional recovery or decline, ultimately contributing to development of better treatment. In mild TBI, due to limited sensitivity of conventional cross-sectional approach, objective evidence of brain injury has been difficult to obtain. Employing a within-subject longitudinal design, future morphometry studies in this group may reveal evidence of sutle brain changes over time. Ideally, the neural degeneration processes can be tracked longitudinally by conducting repeated assessments using sensitive and reliable *in vivo* non-invasive imaging methods such as structural magnetic resonance imaging (MRI). However, only a handful of studies with a limited number of assessment time points are available to date (e.g., Ross, 2011). Because an increasing number of longitudinal studies are expected in the future, it would be useful to review the methodological challenges inherent in analyzing longitudinal imaging data at the early stage of this area of research. The first goal of this paper is to briefly overview the following methodological considerations in longitudinal morphometry of TBI: lesion evolution (structural changes in lesion over time), neurosurgical procedures (surgery on central nervous system), power (probability to detect changes when they are truly present), bias (directional error in parameter estimation), and non-linearity (relationship that cannot be described by the first degree equations). Another purpose of this article is to introduce a novel method that combines dimensionality reduction and region of interest approaches (Avants et al., 2010a), which intends to serve as an example of sensitive, reliable, and unbiased longitudinal multivariate change detection protocols. This analysis pipeline will be demonstrated and validated using a pilot TBI dataset. We focus on structural MRI measures to quantify neurodegeneration such as volume change and cortical thickness indices. However, the principles and conclusions from this paper may be generalized to data using other imaging modalities and techniques such as diffusion tensor imaging and functional MRI. In addition, the same logic can be applied to quantify neural regeneration.

METHODOLOGICAL CHALLENGES IN LONGITUDINAL MORPHOMETRY OF TBI

LESION EVOLUTION

From the moment of injury, the brain goes through numerous structural changes, both focal and diffuse in nature (Gennarelli and Graham, 2005; Povlishock and Katz, 2005; Kubal, 2012). We here review two types of lesion characteristics that can confound progressive atrophy measurement in a longitudinal imaging study of TBI.

Edema

Posttraumatic edema is accumulation of water in the intracellular and/or extracellular spaces of the brain. The precise time course for human posttraumatic cerebral edema has yet to be determined. If this "brain swelling" is diffuse, it effectively leads to an overestimation of brain volume. Therefore, if the first assessment in a longitudinal study is in the acute phase, researchers must exercise great caution because the changes due to the initial stabilization of the brain are confounded with subsequent atrophy. This results in overestimation of the amount of atrophy over time. If one's primary interest is in the post-acute phase, the first measurement can be done after edema is completely resorbed, e.g., 1–2 months after the injury (e.g., Bendlin et al., 2008; Ng et al., 2008; Sidaros et al., 2009).

Focal encephalomalacia

If the brain suffers from various types of bleeding (hematoma and hemorrhage) or bruises (contusions), local tissue abnormalities appear in the imaging. The size of the lesion in the acute phase is known to evolve (increase or decrease) over time depending on various factors (e.g., Chang et al., 2006). In the post-acute phase, if the cells surviving the acute phase develop atrophy, the size of focal encephalomalacia is likely to grow slowly. Changes in focal lesions over time make it difficult to accurately quantify diffuse atrophy, especially in the perilesional areas. One way to deal with focal abnormalities is to exclude participants with focal injuries or conduct a subgroup analysis by dividing participants into two groups according to the presence of focal lesions. Typically, a lesion volume threshold is employed because it is practically infeasible to exclude the brains with focal lesions of any size. Using different thresholds for cortical and subcortical lesions may make sense considering that smaller lesions in the subcortical regions often have more detrimental functional consequences. However, excluding those with focal lesions will introduce a severity bias. Another way to control the effects of focal lesion is to restrict the analysis only to the areas where no focal lesions are found for all participants. To achieve this, lesion masks are built (typically manually) for each brain and then combined to form a "lesion frequency map" (e.g., Levine et al., 2008; Kim et al., 2010). Recent efforts to develop automatic lesion detection algorithms have shown some success in reducing the burden of manual lesion drawing (e.g., Hillary and Biswal, 2009; Ghosh et al., 2011).

NEUROSURGICAL PROCEDURES

Various neurosurgical procedures, performed to stabilize the injured brain (e.g., evacuation of hematomas/hemorrhages, controlling intra-cranial pressure, etc.), are invasive and cause temporary and/or permanent alterations of the brain. Edema and glial scarring from surgical procedures typically need weeks to months to stabilize, making it challenging to separate the unique effect of surgery and true neural degeneration on longitudinal imaging measures. If neurosurgery leaves focal alterations, they may be dealt with similar methods used for focal encephalomalacia (see section "Focal encephalomalacia"). However, research is lacking in this area. Most neurosurgeries are done during the acute phase. However, procedures such as cranioplasty can be done in the post-acute phase and require careful follow-up. For example, it was recently reported that a significant portion of patients who undergo cranioplasty develop fluid collection underneath the site of operation (Chang et al., 2010; Lee et al., 2011), which may distort brain volume measurement. Even more important is the issue of late cranioplasty and how having skull replaced part-way into a longitudinal study might affect the results.

POWER

Statistical power in structural neuroimaging depends on various factors including effect size, measurement error, method of multiple comparison correction, and sample size. Unfortunately, in longitudinal studies of patients with moderate to severe TBI, sample size is typically small due to participant attrition and numerous exclusion criteria including metal implants, lesion characteristics, and patient movement in the MRI scanner. In mild TBI, while fewer participants' data are lost, the effect size of longitudinal change is expected to be relatively small. Therefore, adopting a sensitive and reliable imaging analysis protocol becomes more crucial to achieve powerful longitudinal change detection. There are various ways to quantify longitudinal changes in the imaging data (e.g., Bosc et al., 2003; Holland et al., 2012). They can be classified into two broad categories: (1) regions-of-interest (ROI) or segmentation based approaches and (2) deformation or registration based methods. Here we briefly discuss these two change detection methods in the context of power.

One way to improve detection power in small imaging datasets is to use a limited number of a priori ROIs and measure longitudinal changes within those ROIs. Typically, ROIs are constructed at each time point for each individual by an "expert" human rater or an automatic segmentation algorithm. The majority of previous longitudinal imaging studies in TBI used this approach (e.g., Ng et al., 2008; Warner et al., 2010; Xu et al., 2010). Assuming that the size and location of the ROIs are on target, this approach is likely to increase statistical power. However, reliable a priori hypotheses are frequently unavailable due to the lack of existing research and thus potentially important changes in unselected regions can be missed. In addition, due to heterogeneous injury mechanisms and lesion characteristics in TBI, using the same set of a priori ROIs across different samples may not be ideal. An important limitation of manually defining ROI is that human raters do not reproduce the same results when measurement is repeated, introducing repeat measurement error. Maintaining high intra- and inter-rater reliability costs a substantial amount of time and effort. Automating ROI construction using computer algorithms is a potential solution. However, automatic segmentation of brain structures, especially when a lesion is present, still remains one of the most challenging tasks.

To overcome some of the limitations of the ROI or segmentation based approach, some researchers have adopted deformation based methods of change detection. These methods do not rely on the researcher to identify specific ROIs and are well-suited to exploratory studies. In deformation or tensor based morphometry (DBM/TBM; e.g., Ashburner et al., 1998; Ashburner and Friston, 2000), one image (e.g., a patient's) is directly warped to the other (e.g., a template) using non-linear deformable spatial registration and the resulting deformation fields are used for quantification of volume differences between the two images. Reliability of this approach is, in general, much higher than manual drawing. Deformation based methods may be used for serial studies as well. To quantify longitudinal changes, a subject's brain at one time point may be directly warped to the same person's brain at later time point (e.g., Sidaros et al., 2009). Directly comparing images effectively bypasses the repeat measurement error issue, offering advantages in terms of statistical power. For TBI, large deformation registration schemes (for an introduction, see Ashburner, 2007) should be used to allow detection of a wide range of volume changes (Kim et al., 2008). Custom or population-specific templates can also help increase detection power (Lepore et al., 2007). Many large deformation algorithms, some of them using diffeomorphisms, are freely available and their performance was recently compared in a large-scale evaluation study (Klein et al., 2009).

More recently, multivariate pattern analysis (MVPA) has been employed to increase detection power over univariate approaches, particularly in fMRI studies (e.g., Haxby et al., 2001). In the last section, we will illustrate an image analysis pipeline that uses MVPA to interrogate longitudinal TBI effects.

BIAS

Bias, a directional error in parameter estimation, can arise in longitudinal morphometry when data from different time points are not treated equivalently. In that sense, avoiding bias in the ROI/segmentation based approach is relatively straightforward because the same system of measurement can be applied to the data at each time point. For example, one can keep the expert raters blinded to the order of measurements or even randomize the images from different time points. In DBM/TBM, however, due to the fact that the images from two or more time points are directly compared, there is a possibility that the images undergo systematically different processing steps.

The issue of bias in longitudinal DBM/TBM has recently become the focus of discussion among researchers investigating the trajectory of atrophy using the Alzheimer's disease Neuroimaging Initiative database (ADNI; www.loni.ucla.edu/ADNI). Partly due to this discussion, several nice summaries on this topic are available in the literature (Holland et al., 2012; Hua et al., 2011; Thompson and Holland, 2011) and they enumerate sources of bias and rules to follow to prevent those biases from affecting the estimate of longitudinal changes. One important issue is designating images at each time point as the source (i.e., image to be warped) or the target (i.e., image to be warped to). Symmetric or inverse-consistent registration methods should be used to avoid bias from asymmetric registration processes. An inverse-consistent or symmetric registration is an algorithm that yields the same correspondences between the images from two time points when the order of them is switched (e.g., Avants et al., 2008). If inverse-consistency cannot be guaranteed by the registration algorithm itself, symmetry may still be achieved by first measuring the changes in both directions independently and then averaging them (Thompson and Holland, 2011). In addition, all images from different time points should undergo the same number of interpolations. For example, Yushkevich and colleagues recently showed that distributing interpolation equally across all of a subject's images is critical for eliminating bias (Yushkevich et al., 2010).

NON-LINEARITY

To our knowledge, most existing longitudinal morphometry studies in TBI have had only two measurement points. As studies with multiple time points emerge, it would be important to consider the potential non-linear nature of the post-injury atrophy. First of all, true biological non-linearity needs to be distinguished from the spurious non-linearity caused by bias. A good example is a controversial study conducted by Hua and colleagues (2010), in which structural atrophy of AD patients was quantified between the baseline and four follow-up scans using TBM. Cumulative atrophy was determined by warping all of the follow-up images to the same baseline image. As a result, the authors found an unexpected non-linearity—i.e., a rapid jump of the atrophy rate between the baseline and the first follow-up point, with more linear increase thereafter. This jump was due to the fact that this study design confounded both interpolation effects and atrophy effects, which have a similar magnitude (approximately 1% change). Subsequent re-analysis studies showed that this trend was replicated even in healthy controls and that a large portion of the bias could be corrected by using inverse-consistent registration methods (Hua et al., 2011; Thompson and Holland, 2011) which interpolate every time point in the same way.

Allowing for the possibility of true biological non-linearity in the atrophy rate after TBI, the next question becomes the exact shape of non-linear degeneration and how much individual variability exists. Growth curve analysis, which is known to be capable of accommodating many mathematical functions, missing data points, variable time intervals, and individual differences, may be a fruitful approach to explore. Mixed effects models have similar advantages.

EXAMPLE OF LONGITUDINAL MULTIVARIATE MORPHOMETRY: A PILOT STUDY

RATIONALE

MVPA has gained acceptance for its ability to combine the benefits of both prior-constrained ROI studies and the exploratory nature of DBM/TBM. This multivariate approach reduces the multiple comparisons problems by clustering regions together in an automated way (known as dimensionality reduction in machine learning) and then allowing hypotheses to be tested on this reduced set of areas. We here hypothesize that, even in a small, heterogeneous TBI sample, there are common areas across individuals that undergo neurodegeneration and that can be detected as regions of correlated white matter (WM) and gray matter (GM) changes (Avants et al., 2010b).

METHOD

In this study, we used best-practice pre-processing to determine two quantitative measures (i.e., cortical thickness and WM volume change) throughout the whole brain in four survivors of diffuse TBI (average age at baseline = 38.3) serial T1 data (**Figure 1**). The average time post-injury at baseline was 6.6 months and the average assessment interval was 15.8 months. We then applied a dimensionality reduction technique, sparse canonical correlation

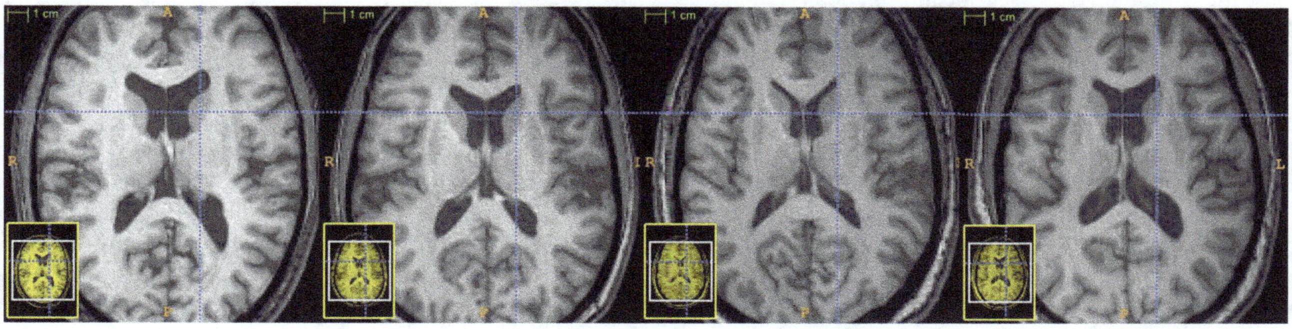

FIGURE 1 | Four TBI survivors' representative axial scans at the baseline.

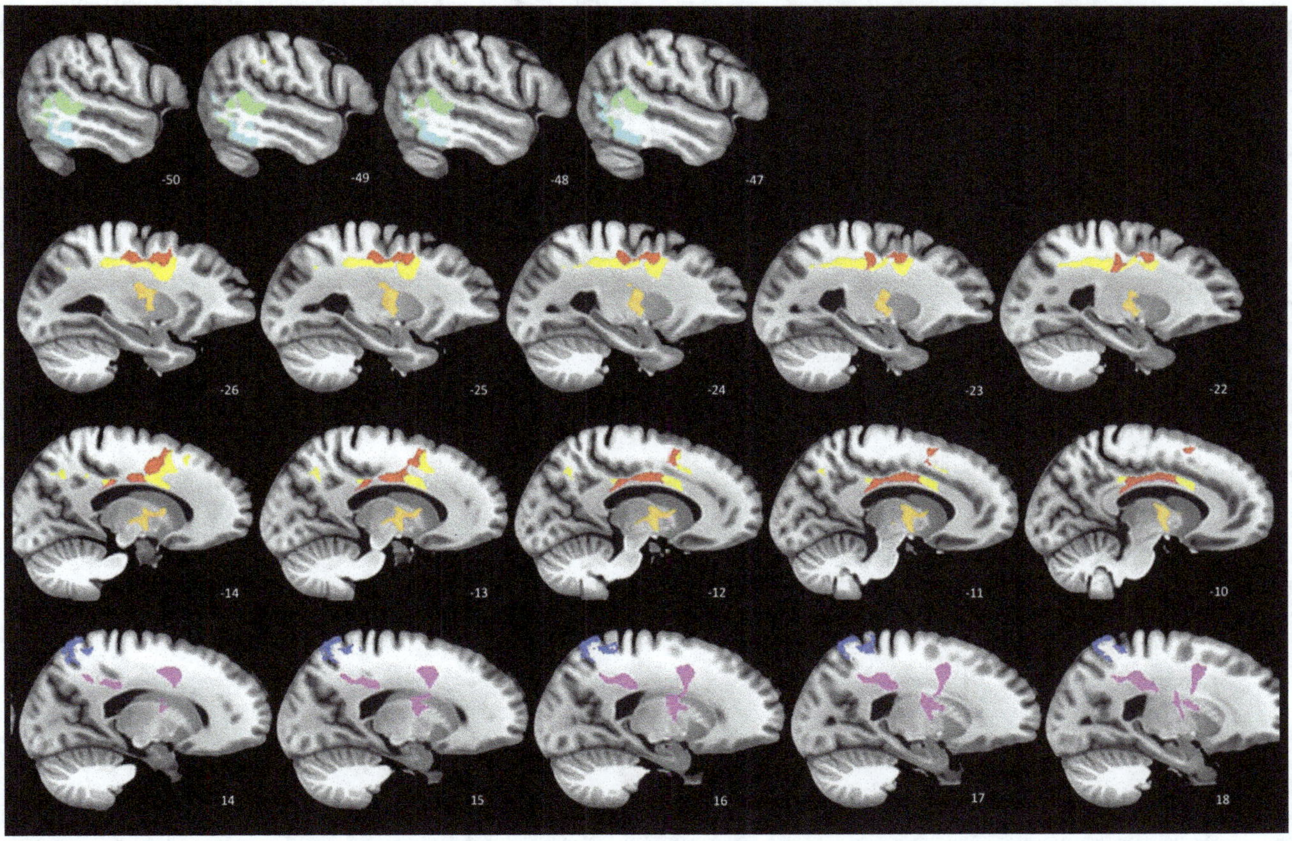

FIGURE 2 | SCCAN reveals multiple cortical and white matter regions of longitudinal atrophy. Cortical areas (cool colors) include posterior temporal lobes, posterior cingulate, and superior parietal lobe. The white matter and deep gray matter (warm colors) regions includes the thalamus (orange, second row), primary motor tract, and the mid- and posterior bodies of the corpus callosum.

analysis for neuroimaging (SCCAN), to obtain a limited number of ROIs that are sensitive and specific to longitudinal change that is related across tissues (Avants et al., 2010a,b). As reviewed above, quantitative longitudinal analyses must be conducted with unbiased techniques if the image-based measurements are to be interpreted physically (Yushkevich et al., 2010). Thus, we used Advanced Normalization Tools (ANTs) and a population-specific template (Avants et al., 2010c; Reuter et al., 2012) to compute the unbiased deformable mapping between each subject's baseline and follow-up image. The resulting diffeomorphic mapping quantifies longitudinal volume changes. We also employed prior-based spatiotemporal maximum a posteriori image segmentation to extract change in the cortical GM over time (Avants et al., 2011) and to identify cortical thickness alterations in each subject. This processing protocol leads to two complementary measures that may be used to assess atrophy—i.e., WM volume change via Jacobian determinant and GM cortical thickness. Thickness is, in general, more sensitive than volumetric measures because it incorporates tissue-specific information (Hutton et al., 2009). Both measures were annualized.

We hypothesized that, in chronic TBI, spatially distinct but covarying atrophy would be observed in both WM and GW and that this atrophy rate would be greater than zero. In summary, the procedure was as follows: (1) Apply the unbiased longitudinal mapping methods (Avants et al., 2010a; Yushkevich et al., 2010); (2) Quantify the annualized volumetric change in WM and the annualized atrophy in GM; (3) Employ SCCAN to identify four localized regions of GM and four correlated and localized regions in WM to be tested for significant atrophy; (4) Use the one-sample t-test with false discovery rate correction (FDR) to determine if the atrophy in SCCAN-identified regions is significant. We arbitrarily limited the number of regions to 4 for WM and 4 for GM considering the small number of participants.

RESULTS AND DISCUSSION

Seven of eight regions (4 WM, 3 GM) were significant at the FDR-corrected $p < 0.1$ level (**Figure 2**). In line with previous TBM studies with larger samples (Kim et al., 2008; Sidaros et al., 2009), these regions included thalamus, corpus callosum, and posterior cingulate (see **Figure 2** legend for the complete list). In the most significant region ($p < 0.015$), the estimated atrophy rates for WM and GM were $7.3 \pm 3.9\%$ and $4.2 \pm 1.8\%$, respectively (mean $\pm$ SD of the amount of atrophy in percentage). FDR-corrected $p < 0.05$ is also achievable if only the most highly correlated regions are tested.

This preliminary study reveals significant longitudinal atrophy patterns after correction for multiple comparisons despite the very few subjects involved. Three main points emerge from this design: (1) significant and localized regions with atrophy may be identified by employing MVPA in longitudinal morphometry of TBI; (2) unbiased approaches are essential for identifying quantitative atrophy measures and retain enough power to be effective in small cohorts; (3) this paradigm is easily extended to include additional modalities and will be more reliable with additional subjects. In addition, future research comparing the current method with alternative approaches are warranted.

ACKNOWLEDGMENTS

This work was funded by grant 5R01NS065980-02 from the NINDS, NIH and a grant with the Pennsylvania Department of Health. The department specifically disclaims responsibility for any analyses, interpretations, or conclusions.

REFERENCES

Ashburner, J. (2007). A fast diffeomorphic image registration algorithm. *Neuroimage* 38, 95–113.

Ashburner, J., and Friston, K. J. (2000). Voxel-based morphometry– the methods. *Neuroimage* 11, 805–821.

Ashburner, J., Hutton, C., Frackowiak, R., Johnsrude, I., Price, C., and Friston, K. (1998). Identifying global anatomical differences: deformation-based morphometry. *Hum. Brain Mapp.* 6, 348–357.

Avants, B., Cook, P. A., McMillan, C., Grossman, M., Tustison, N. J., Zheng, Y., et al. (2010a). Sparse unbiased analysis of anatomical variance in longitudinal imaging. *Med. Image Comput. Comput. Assist. Interv.* 13, 324–331.

Avants, B. B., Cook, P. A., Ungar, L., Gee, J. C., and Grossman, M. (2010b). Dementia induces correlated reductions in white matter integrity and cortical thickness: a multivariate neuroimaging study with sparse canonical correlation analysis. *Neuroimage* 50, 1004–1016.

Avants, B. B., Yushkevich, P., Pluta, J., Minkoff, D., Korczykowski, M., Detre, J., et al. (2010c). The optimal template effect in hippocampus studies of diseased populations. *Neuroimage* 49, 2457–2466.

Avants, B., Epstein, C. L., Grossman, M., and Gee, J. C. (2008). Symmetric diffeomorphic image registration with cross-correlation: evaluating automated labeling of elderly and neurodegenerative brain. *Med. Image Anal.* 12, 26–41.

Avants, B. B., Tustison, N. J., Wu, J., Cook, P. A., and Gee, J. C. (2011). An open source multivariate framework for n-tissue segmentation with evaluation on public data. *Neuroinformatics* 9, 381–400.

Bendlin, B. B., Ries, M. L., Lazar, M., Alexander, A. L., Dempsey, R. J., Rowley, H. A., et al. (2008). Longitudinal changes in patients with traumatic brain injury assessed with diffusion-tensor and volumetric imaging. *Neuroimage* 42, 503–514.

Bigler, E. D. (2005). "Structural imaging," in *Textbook of Traumatic Brain Injury*, eds J. M. Silver, T. W. McAllister, and S. C. Yudofsky (Washington, DC: American Psychiatric Publishing, Inc.), 79–105.

Bosc, M., Heitz, F., Armspach, J. P., Namer, I., Gounot, D., and Rumbach, L. (2003). Automatic change detection in multimodal serial MRI: application to multiple sclerosis lesion evolution. *Neuroimage* 20, 643–656.

Chang, E. F., Meeker, M., and Holland, M. C. (2006). Acute traumatic intraparenchymal hemorrhage: risk factors for progression in the early post-injury period. *Neurosurgery* 58, 647–655. discussion: 655–656.

Chang, V., Hartzfeld, P., Langlois, M., Mahmood, A., and Seyfried, D. (2010). Outcomes of cranial repair after craniectomy. *J. Neurosurg.* 112, 1120–1124.

Gennarelli, T. A., and Graham, D. I. (2005). "Neuropathology," in *Textbook of Traumatic Brain Injury*, eds J. M. Silver, T. W. McAllister, and S. C. Yudofsky (Washington, DC: American Psychiatric Publishing, Inc.), 27–50.

Ghosh, N., Recker, R., Shah, A., Bhanu, B., Ashwal, S., and Obenaus, A. (2011). Automated ischemic lesion detection in a neonatal model of hypoxic ischemic injury. *J. Magn. Reson. Imaging* 33, 772–781.

Haxby, J. V., Gobbini, M. I., Furey, M. L., Ishai, A., Schouten, J. L., and Pietrini, P. (2001). Distributed and overlapping representations of faces and objects in ventral temporal cortex. *Science* 293, 2425–2430.

Hillary, F. G., and Biswal, B. B. (2009). Automated detection and quantification of brain lesions in acute traumatic brain injury using, M. R. I. *Brain Imaging Behav.* 3, 111–122.

Holland, D., McEvoy, L. K., and Dale, A. M. (2012). Unbiased comparison of sample size estimates from longitudinal structural measures in ADNI. *Hum. Brain Mapp.* 33, 2586–2602.

Hua, X., Gutman, B., Boyle, C. P., Rajagopalan, P., Leow, A. D., Yanovsky, I., et al. (2011). Accurate measurement of brain changes in longitudinal MRI scans using tensor-based morphometry. *Neuroimage* 57, 5–14.

Hua, X., Lee, S., Hibar, D. P., Yanovsky, I., Leow, A. D., Toga, A. W., et al. (2010). Mapping Alzheimer's disease progression in 1309 MRI scans: power estimates for different inter-scan intervals. *Neuroimage* 51, 63–75.

Hutton, C., Draganski, B., Ashburner, J., and Weiskopf, N. (2009). A comparison between voxel-based cortical thickness and voxel-based morphometry in normal aging. *Neuroimage* 48, 371–380.

Kim, J., Avants, B., Patel, S., Whyte, J., Coslett, B. H., Pluta, J., et al. (2008). Structural consequences of diffuse traumatic brain injury: a large deformation tensor-based morphometry study. *Neuroimage* 39, 1014–1026.

Kim, J., Whyte, J., Patel, S., Avants, B., Europa, E., Wang, J., et al. (2010). Resting cerebral blood flow alterations in chronic traumatic brain injury: an arterial spin labeling perfusion fMRI study. *J. Neurotrauma* 27, 1399–1411.

Klein, A., Andersson, J., Ardekani, B. A., Ashburner, J., Avants, B., Chiang, M. C., et al. (2009). Evaluation of 14 nonlinear deformation algorithms applied to human brain MRI registration. *Neuroimage* 46, 786–802.

Kubal, W. S. (2012). Updated imaging of traumatic brain injury. *Radiol. Clin. North Am.* 50, 15–41.

Lee, J. W., Kim, J. H., Kang, H. I., Moon, B. G., Lee, S. J., and Kim, J. S. (2011). Epidural fluid collection after cranioplasty: fate and predictive factors. *J. Korean Neurosurg. Soc.* 50, 231–234.

Lepore, N., Brun, C., Pennec, X., Chou, Y. Y., Lopez, O. L., Aizenstein, H. J., et al. (2007). Mean template for tensor-based morphometry using deformation tensors. *Med. Image Comput. Comput. Assist. Interv.* 10, 826–833.

Levine, B., Kovacevic, N., Nica, E. I., Cheung, G., Gao, F., Schwartz, M. L., et al. (2008). The Toronto traumatic brain injury study: injury severity and quantified MRI. *Neurology* 70, 771–778.

Masel, B. E., and Dewitt, D. S. (2010). Traumatic brain injury: a disease process, not an event. *J. Neurotrauma* 27, 1529–1540.

Ng, K., Mikulis, D. J., Glazer, J., Kabani, N., Till, C., Greenberg, G., et al. (2008). Magnetic resonance imaging evidence of progression of subacute brain atrophy in moderate to severe traumatic brain injury. *Arch. Phys. Med. Rehabil.* 89, S35–S44.

Povlishock, J. T., and Katz, D. I. (2005). Update of neuropathology and neurological recovery after traumatic brain injury. *J. Head Trauma Rehabil.* 20, 76–94.

Reuter, M., Schmansky, N. J., Rosas, H. D., and Fischl, B. (2012). Within-subject template estimation for unbiased longitudinal image analysis. *Neuroimage* 61, 1402–1418.

Ross, D. E. (2011). Review of longitudinal studies of MRI brain volumetry in patients with traumatic brain injury. *Brain Inj.* 25, 1271–1278.

Sidaros, A., Skimminge, A., Liptrot, M. G., Sidaros, K., Engberg, A. W., Herning, M., et al. (2009). Long-term global and regional brain volume changes following severe traumatic brain injury: a longitudinal study with clinical correlates. *Neuroimage* 44, 1–8.

Thompson, W. K., and Holland, D. (2011). Bias in tensor based morphometry Stat-ROI measures may result in unrealistic power estimates. *Neuroimage* 57, 1–4. discussion: 5–14.

Warner, M. A., Marquez De La Plata, C., Spence, J., Wang, J. Y., Harper, C., Moore, C., et al. (2010). Assessing spatial relationships between axonal integrity, regional brain volumes, and neuropsychological outcomes after traumatic axonal injury. *J. Neurotrauma* 27, 2121–2130.

Xu, Y., McArthur, D. L., Alger, J. R., Etchepare, M., Hovda, D. A., Glenn, T. C., et al. (2010). Early nonischemic oxidative metabolic dysfunction leads to chronic brain atrophy in traumatic brain injury. *J. Cereb. Blood Flow Metab.* 30, 883–894.

Yushkevich, P. A., Avants, B. B., Das, S. R., Pluta, J., Altinay, M., and Craige, C. (2010). Bias in estimation of hippocampal atrophy using deformation-based morphometry arises from asymmetric global normalization: an illustration in ADNI 3 T MRI data. *Neuroimage* 50, 434–445.

13

Evaluation of annexin A5 as a biomarker for Alzheimer's disease and dementia with lewy bodies

Hitoshi Sohma[1,2]*, Shin-ichi Imai[2], Norio Takei[2], Hirohito Honda[3], Kyoichi Matsumoto[4], Kumiko Utsumi[5], Kayo Matsuki[2], Eri Hashimoto[6], Toshikazu Saito[6] and Yasuo Kokai[2]

[1] *Department of Educational Development, Center for Medical Education, Sapporo Medical University, Sapporo, Japan*
[2] *Department of Biomedical Engineering, School of Medicine, Sapporo Medical University, Sapporo, Japan*
[3] *Mikuri Immunology Laboratory, Inc., Osaka, Japan*
[4] *Sanyo Chemical Industries, Ltd., Kyoto, Japan*
[5] *Department of Neuropsychiatry, Sunagawa City Medical Center, Sunagawa, Japan*
[6] *Department of Neuropsychiatry, School of Medicine, Sapporo Medical University, Sapporo, Japan*

Edited by:
Manuel Menéndez-González, Hospital Álvarez-Buylla, Spain

Reviewed by:
Daniel Ortuño-Sahagun, Centro Universitario de Ciencias Biológicas y Agropecuarias, Mexico
Junming Wang, University of Mississippi Medical Center, USA

****Correspondence:***
Hitoshi Sohma, Department of Educational Development, Center for Medical Education, Sapporo Medical University, South-1, West-17, Chuo-ku, Sapporo 060-8556, Japan.
e-mail: sohma@sapmed.ac.jp

Background: Alzheimer's disease (AD) differs from other forms of dementia in its relation to amyloid beta peptide ($A\beta_{42}$). Using a cell culture model we previously identified annexin A5, a Ca^{2+}, and phospholipid binding protein, as an AD biomarker. Plasma level of annexin A5 was significantly higher in AD patients compared to that in a control group. On the other hand, AD has been identified to share a number of clinical and pathological features with Dementia with Lewy bodies (DLB). The present study was done to examine whether or not plasma annexin A5 is a specific marker for AD, when being compared with the levels of DLB patients. As Apolipoprotein E (ApoE) gene subtype ε4 (ApoE-ε4) has been noticed as the probable genetic factor for AD, we also examined and compared ApoE genotype in both AD and DLB.

Methods: Blood samples were obtained from 150 patients with AD (aged 77.6 ± 6.5 years), 50 patients of DLB (79.4 ± 5.0) and 279 community-dwelling healthy elderly individuals of comparable age and sex (75.6 ± 8.1). All AD patients met NINCDS-ADRDA criteria and all DLB patients were diagnosed as probable DLB according to the latest consensus diagnostic criteria. Quantification was done using the Chemiluminescent Enzyme Immunoassay (CLEIA) Technique (SphereLight assay) using the monoclonal antibodies against annexin A5. DNA genotyping of ApoE was performed by distinguishing unique combinations of Hha1 fragments of PCR-amplified genomic DNA products.

Results: The plasma level of annexin A5 was significantly higher in AD patients than in the healthy individuals (control) ($P < 0.0001$). The plasma annexin A5 level was also significantly higher in DLB patients than in the control group ($P < 0.0001$). From the ROC curves with plasma annexin A5 concentrations, the mean areas under the curve were 0.863 and 0.838 for the AD/control and DLB/control, respectively. The rate of ApoE4 carrier status and the frequency of the ε4 allele were significantly higher in AD or DLB than in control and there was no significant difference between AD and DLB.

Conclusions: These results suggest that both annexin A5 and ApoE4 are common markers for AD and DLB.

Keywords: plasma biomarker, Alzheimer's disease, dementia with lewy bodies, annexin A5, Ca^{2+}-stress, ROC curve, ApoE

INTRODUCTION

The augmented number of dementia patients is remarkable in the aging of society in advanced countries. Alzheimer's disease (AD) accounts for more than half of all dementia, and Dementia with Lewy bodies (DLB) are the second most common, accounting for approximately 15% of cases at autopsy (McKeith et al., 2004), both of which are common forms of neurodegenerative dementia. DLB shares clinical and pathological features with other dementia subtypes such as AD, vascular dementia and Parkinson's disease (PD), which makes it difficult to distinguish in clinical practice. Also, the lack of valid and reliable methods for assessing the core clinical symptoms of both AD and DLB makes its identification even more difficult. The diagnosis of AD is reliant on the use of National Institute of Neurological and Communicative Disorders and Stroke-AD and related Disorders Association (NINCDS-ADRDA) criteria. The NINCDS-ADRDA criteria have high sensitivity (0.93), but low specificity (0.23) in the diagnosis of AD among a group of patients with cortical dementias [AD and frontotemporal dementia (FTD)] (Varma et al., 1999). On the other hand, consensus criteria for DLB were developed in 1996 to assist with the antemortem diagnosis (McKeith et al., 2005). Although the criteria have high specificity (79–100%), the sensitivity is low (20–60%), so that the diagnosis can be missed in many cases during life (Litvan et al., 2003). The revised clinical consensus criteria were published in 2005, which gives greater diagnostic weight to clinical features suggestive of DLB (McKeith et al., 2005). In light of the limited sensitivity of current methods of clinical diagnosis, it is important to establish additional markers that can improve diagnostic accuracy in combination with clinical assessment.

Amyloid β peptide (Aβ), which is a proteolytic product of amyloid precursor protein (APP), accumulates in the brains of AD patients. Its toxicity is thought to cause neural cell death (Mattson, 2004). Amyloid-dependent neurotoxicity is known to perturb Ca^{2+} homeostasis in neuronal cells (LaFerla, 2002). Possibly, Aβ impairs membrane Ca^{2+} pumps and enhances Ca^{2+} influx through voltage-dependent channels and ionotropic glutamate receptors. Focusing on this mechanism, we identified the Ca^{2+}-related protein as a potential biomarker for AD using primary neurons as a cell culture model (Yamaguchi et al., 2010). It was shown that the level of annexin A5 was augmented in both the brain and blood plasma in an AD-model mouse (Tg2576 transgenic mouse), overexpressing mutant human APP (Yamaguchi et al., 2010). In addition, the plasma level of annexin A5 was significantly increased in AD patients compared to that in a control group (p-value of less than 0.0001 in the logistic regression analysis), suggesting that annexin A5 is a favorable marker for AD (Yamaguchi et al., 2010). As annexin A5 binds both Ca^{2+} and lipids, it might have a role to protect against Ca^{2+}-induced damage. A defensive role against apoptosis by annexin A5 is also reported, in that annexin A5 plays a role in interacting with and reducing the toxicity of the amyloidogenic proteins, islet amyloid polypeptides and α-synuclein inclusion (Bedrood et al., 2009).

Apolipoprotein E (ApoE), which is a major component of lipoproteins, is comprised of 299 amino acid residues and plays a role in the metabolism and redistribution of cholesterol. ApoE mediates the uptake of lipoprotein particles in the brain via the low-density lipoprotein (LDL), receptor related protein (LRP), and the very low-density family lipoprotein receptor (VLDL) (Mahley, 1988; Paolo and Kim, 2011). The three major isoforms of ApoE, referred to as ApoE2, E3, and E4, are products of three alleles (ε2, ε3, ε4) at a single gene locus (Mahley, 1988). Three homozygous phenotypes (Apo-E2/2, E3/3, and E4/4) and three heterozygous phenotypes (Apo-E2/3, E3/4, and E2/4) arise from the expression of any two of the three alleles. The ε4 allele of the ApoE gene was identified as the strongest genetic risk factor for AD (Bertram and Tanzi, 2008). Neuropathological studies demonstrated that the frequency of the ApoE gene subtype ε4 (ApoE ε4) allele in DLB is similar to AD and that ApoE4 has also been implicated in the development of DLB (Singletona et al., 2002). We reported that ApoE4 genotypes were similar in AD and DLB, giving further evidence that the ε4 allele is a risk factor for both disorders in Japanese subjects (Kobayashi et al., 2011).

The present study was done to examine whether or not plasma annexin A5 is a specific marker for AD, in comparison with the levels of DLB patients. For that purpose, we analyzed plasma level of DLB patients and compared with those of AD patients and age-matched community dwelling healthy persons as a control. We further discuss taking ApoE4 frequencies into consideration.

MATERIALS AND METHODS

HUMAN BLOOD PLASMA

The Sapporo Medical University Ethics Committee approved human plasma studies on dementia biomarker study in 2007. Informed written consent was obtained from all subjects. All healthy volunteers and patients provided written permission. For patients with impaired cognition we obtained written permission from their family in accordance with the Declaration of Helsinki. Blood samples were obtained from 150 patients with AD (aged 77.6 ± 6.5 years), 50 patients of DLB (aged 79.4 ± 5.0 years), and 279 community-dwelling elderly individuals (healthy volunteers) of comparable age and sex (75.6 ± 8.1 years). All AD patients met NINCDS-ADRDA criteria (McKhann et al., 1984) and DLB patients were diagnosed as probable DLB according to the latest consensus diagnostic criteria (McKeith et al., 2005). The patient's clinical symptoms were evaluated using the revised Hasegawa Dementia scale (HDS-R) (Hasegawa, 1983), Mini-Mental State Examination (MMSE), and clinical dementia rating (CDR). The diagnosis of AD was also confirmed in all patients either by brain magnetic resonance imaging or single photon emission computed tomography. Blood was drawn with Venoject II vacuum tubes containing EDTA-Na (final 4.5 mM) (Terumo, Tokyo, Japan) and the plasma fraction was isolated by centrifugation at 2500 g for 15 min. This was repeated once to avoid possible cell debris in blood. Blood was centrifuged within 6 h after sampling. Plasma fractions were stored at −80°C until use.

QUANTIFICATION OF PLASMA LEVEL OF ANNEXIN A5 USING SANDWICH CLEIA (SPHERELIGHT ASSAY)

Plasma annexin A5 was quantified using the Chemiluminescent Enzyme Immunoassay (CLEIA) Technique (SphereLight assay) as described (Yamaguchi et al., 2010). Briefly, annexin A5 present in the specimen was trapped by a monoclonal antibody (mAb) against annexin A5 (clone No. 23), conjugated to a glass bead and a horseradish peroxidase (HRP)-labeled mAb against annexin A5 (clone No. 49). Unbound materials were removed by washing. The chemiluminescent reagent consists of a luminol solution that includes a phenol-derivative as an enhancer, to which a hydrogen peroxide solution was added. The HRP in the bound conjugate catalyzes the oxidation of the luminol derivative, producing light. The light signals were read by the Olympus SphereLight180 fully automated system (Olympus Optical Co., Ltd., Tokyo, Japan). The amount of HRP conjugate bound was directly proportional to the annexin A5 concentration. The required time and volume of the specimens were 20 min and 40 μl, respectively, for the SphereLight assay. The detection limit proved to be 0.16 ng/ml for annexin A5 and this system was useful to quantify plasma annexin A5 within the range of 0.16–20.0 ng/ml. Reproducible data were obtained by intra-assay and inter-assay (data not shown). Because annexin A5 is present in blood cells (Masuda et al., 2004), if a prolonged period of time has passed (longer than 12 h) after collecting blood until centrifuging, the plasma annexin A5 level increases (data not shown) due to physical damage such as temperature change, osmotic pressure change and so on. To avoid inducible leakage of annexin A5 from blood cells, all the plasma was separated by centrifugation within 6 h of sampling. The detection limit proved to be 0.16 ng/ml of annexin A5 as previously described (Yamaguchi et al., 2010). We also performed a plasma dilution test and reproducibility studies of intra-assay and inter-assay, which confirmed the assay method is reliable (Yamaguchi et al., 2010).

APOLIPOPROTEIN E (ApoE) GENOTYPING

DNA genotyping of ApoE was performed according to the protocol described by Hixson and Vernier (1990). Briefly, using a QIAamp DNA Blood Mini Kit (QIAGEN, Tokyo, Japan), genomic DNA was extracted from the buffy coat after centrifugation of the blood sample according to the manufacturer's instructions. The leukocyte DNA was amplified by PCR using the oligonucleotide primers, Primer 1 (59-TAAGCTTGGCACGGCTGTCCAAGGA-39), and Primer 2 (59-ACAGAATTCGCCCCGGCCTGGTACAC-39) set on common sequence parts of ApoE isoforms. The PCR products were digested with HhaI (New England Biolabs, Japan, Inc., Tokyo, Japan) and the resulting digestion fragments were separated by electrophoresis on polyacrylamide gels (SuperSepTMDNA 15% gel (Wako, Tokyo, Japan)). Each genotype of ApoE was distinguished by unique combinations of Hha1 fragment sizes in all homozygotic and heterozygotic combinations (Hixson and Vernier, 1990). After determining the ApoE genotypes, we investigated the ApoE4 carrier status and the frequency of the ε4 allele in the 279 controls, 150 AD, and 50 DLB cases.

STATISTICAL ANALYSIS

The mean response of each experimental group was compared with its simultaneous control by the unpaired Student's *t*-test. Analysis of variance was used to compare the mean responses of the experimental and control groups. A significant difference was set at $p < 0.05$. Logistic regression modeling was employed to construct receiver operator curves (ROC) by using JMP 9.0.0 (SAS Institute Inc., Cary, NC) to examine the plasma annexin A5 levels in diagnoses of AD and DLB. ROC curve comparisons were based on the area under the curve (AUC), SE, and the associated 95% confidence interval (CI). We subsequently calculated sensitivity of the various models using the predicted probability of each subject by logistic regression modeling with specificity of at least eighty percent. Fisher's exact tests were used to assess the frequencies of the ε4 allele between groups using JMP 9.0.0 (SAS Institute, Cary, NC, USA).

RESULTS

Plasma level of annexin A5 was analyzed using CLEIA Technique (SphereLight assay) as described in Materials and Methods. In this study, we measured 150 samples of AD (age 77.6 ± 6.5), 50 samples of DLB (age 79.4 ± 5.0), and 279 age-matched community dwelling healthy persons (age 75.6 ± 8.1) as a control. When average concentrations of plasma annexin A5 are compared among AD, DLB, and control groups, the values of AD (3.33 ± 1.60) and DLB (3.02 ± 1.08) were significantly higher than healthy control subjects (1.95 ± 0.68) (**Figure 1**). The probability of both AD and DLB can be predicted by a logistic regression model with the plasma level of annexin A5. The ROC analyses revealed good separation of patients with either AD or DLB from healthy control subjects (**Figure 2**). The areas under the curve were 86.3% ($P < 0.0001$) and 83.8% ($P < 0.0001$) for AD and DLB, respectively. That is statistically significant, suggesting that annexin A5 is also a potential biomarker for both AD and DLB. On the other hand, no significant difference was observed between AD and DLB ($p = 0.36$).

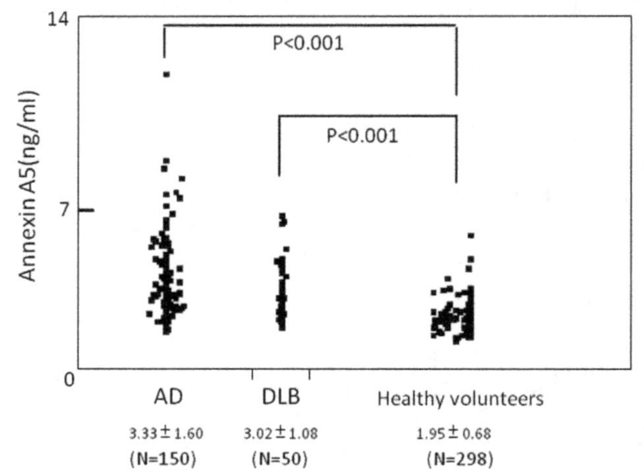

FIGURE 1 | Comparison of plasma levels of annexin A5 in AD, DLB patients, and healthy volunteers (control). For quantitative analysis, we established a chemiluminescent enzyme immunoassay system with monoclonal antibodies against human annexin A5 and measured human plasma annexin A5. Dot blot is shown. Each point represents the plasma annexin A5 concentration of individual. AD, Alzheimer's disease; DLB, dementia with Lewy bodies.

Several risk factors for AD have been suggested such as medical history, life style, environment and genes. Of these, ApoE-ε4 has been noticed as one of the genetic factors. We next identified ApoE gene typing by analyzing the restriction enzyme products of the PCR-amplified ApoE gene as shown in Materials and Methods (**Table 1, Figure 3**). In the control group, 51 out of 279 subjects were ApoE4 carriers (18.3%). Three subjects were homozygous for the ε4 allele (1.1%) and 48 subjects were heterozygous for the e4 allele (17.2%). The total frequency of the ε4 allele was 9.7%. In the AD group, 63 out of 150 subjects were ApoE4 carriers (42.0%). Nine subjects were homozygous for the ε4 allele (6.0%) and 54 subjects were heterozygous for the ε4 allele (36.0%). The total frequency of the ε4 allele was 24.0%. In the DLB group, 21 out of 50 subjects were ApoE4 carriers (42.0%). Three subjects were homozygous for the ε4 allele (6.0%) and 18 subjects were heterozygous for the ε4 allele (36.0%). The total frequency of the ε4 allele was 24.0%. ApoE4 frequencies were compared among AD, DLB, and control groups (Fisher's exact test). ApoE4 carrier status was significantly different between AD and control groups ($p < 0.0001$), and between DLB and control ($p = 0.0004$). Allele frequencies of ApoE ε4 were significantly higher in AD ($p < 0.0001$) and DLB ($p < 0.0001$) than in the control

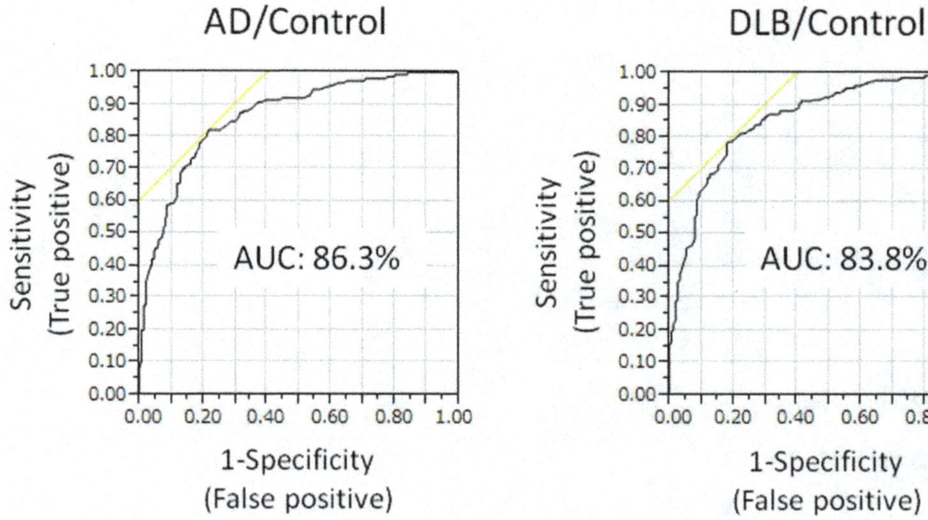

FIGURE 2 | Receiver operating characteristic (ROC) curves showing prediction of either AD or DLB by plasma annexin A5. The probability of either AD or DLB can be predicted by a logistic regression model with the plasma level of annexin A5. The areas under the curve are 86.3 and 83.8% for AD and DLB, respectively. AD, Alzheimer's disease; DLB, dementia with Lewy bodies.

Table 1 | Distribution of ApoE4 carrier status and the frequency of ApoE ε4 allele in the population of AD, DLB, and control groups.

	ApoE4 carrier*		ApoE ε4 allele**	
	Positive	Negative	Positive	Negative
C	51 (18.3%)	228 (81.7%)	57 (10.2%)	501 (89.8%)
AD	63 (42.0%)	87 (58.0%)	72 (24.0%)	228 (76%)
DLB	21 (42.0%)	29 (58.0%)	27 (24.0%)	73 (76.0%)

Numbers in parentheses represent the frequencies of ApoE4 carrier or ApoE ε4 allele. C, control group; AD, Alzheimer's disease group; DLB, dementia with Lewy bodies group.

**Significantly different between AD and control groups ($p < 0.0001$), and between DLB and control ($p = 0.0004$).*

***Significantly higher in AD ($p < 0.0001$) and DLB ($p < 0.0001$) than in the control group. No significant differences in rates of ApoE4 carrier status and the frequencies of the ε4 allele between AD and DLB.*

group. However, there were no significant differences in rates of ApoE4 carrier status ($p = 0.57$) and the frequencies of the ε4 allele ($p = 0.32$) between AD and DLB. These results also indicate the similarity of AD and DLB.

DISCUSSION

SIMILARITY OF AD AND DLB

The toxicity of Aβ is thought to cause neural cell death, which is involved in the pathogenesis AD (Mattson, 2004). Decreased degradation or dyscatabolism of Aβ, presumably related to aging, results in both the accumulation of amyloid beta peptide ($A\beta_{42}$) in the brain and the decreased concentration of $A\beta_{42}$ in CSF. Thus, lowered concentration of CSF $A\beta_{42}$ has been noted as a barometer for AD (Andreasen et al., 2001). AD is the most common neurodegenerative dementia and DLB is the second most common. DLB shares clinical and pathological features with AD, which makes it difficult to distinguish in clinical practice. The CSF levels of $A\beta_{42}$ are similar between AD and DLB (Gomez-Tortosa et al., 2003; Mollenhauer et al., 2005a). Amyloid-dependent neurotoxicity is known to perturb Ca^{2+} homeostasis in neuronal cells (LaFerla, 2002). Possibly, Aβ impairs membrane Ca^{2+} pumps and enhances Ca^{2+} influx through voltage-dependent channels and ionotropic glutamate receptors. Focusing on proteins concerning Ca^{2+} signaling, we identified annexin A5 which is augmented in $A\beta_{42}$ dependent manner and showed it as a potential biomarker for AD (Yamaguchi et al., 2010). Moreover, the plasma level of annexin A5 was shown to be elevated in AD (Yamaguchi et al., 2010). In the present study, plasma level of annexin A5 was shown to be elevated not only in AD but also in DLB.

Genetic factors are increasingly recognized as major risk factors for dementia. Evidence from numerous studies has identified the ApoE gene on chromosome 19 as a major risk factor for AD. ApoE, which is a major component of lipoproteins, is comprised of 299 amino acid residues and plays a role in the metabolism and redistribution of cholesterol (Hatters et al., 2006). Three major common isoforms, designated ApoE2, ApoE3, and ApoE4. ApoE colocalizes with extracellular amyloid deposits, resulting in isoform-specific clearance of Aβ. However, ApoE isoforms differently interact with Aβ isoform specific effects on Aβ-clearance. In ApoE4, domain interaction occurs as a result of a putative salt bridge, leading to tight structural formation. This interaction does not occur to the same extent in ApoE2 and ApoE3 (Dong et al., 1994; Dong and Weisgraber, 1996). ApoE ε4 is associated with an increased risk for AD with an earlier age of disease onset (Kim et al., 2009). On the other hand, findings regarding ApoE polymorphisms in DLB have so far been inconclusive. It was

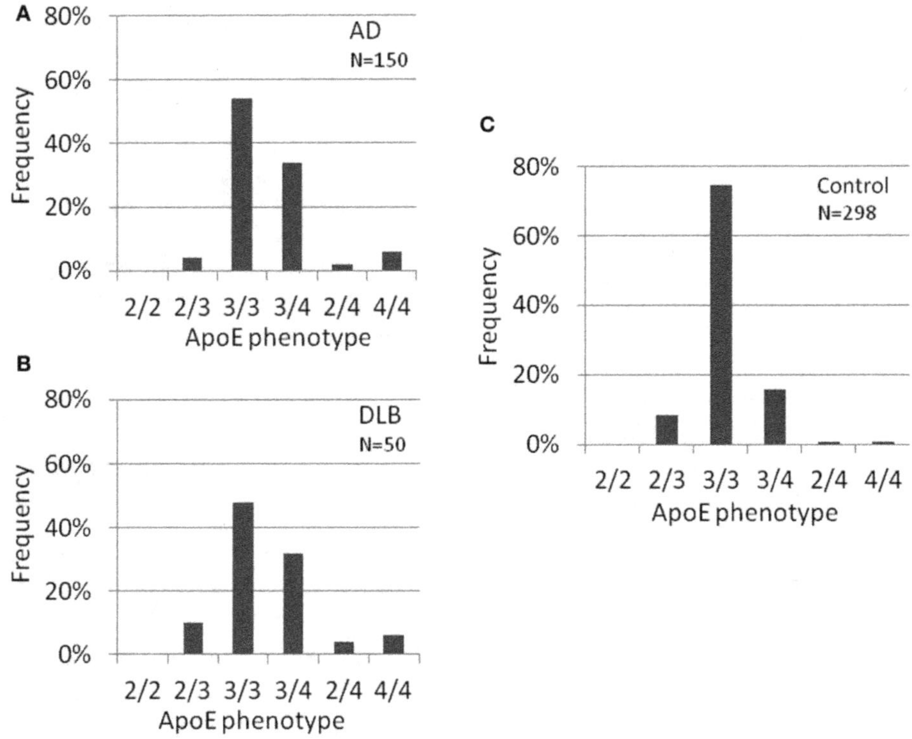

FIGURE 3 | ApoE carrier statuses of AD (A), DLB (B), and healthy volunteers (control) (C). ApoE carrier statuses are significantly different between AD and control, and between DLB and control. However, no significant differences were observed between AD and DLB. ApoE typing was done using pcr and restriction enzyme digestion using genomic DNA. AD, Alzheimer's disease; DLB, dementia with Lewy bodies.

reported that ApoE4 carrier frequency was the highest in AD among AD, DLB, and control groups, and it was higher in DLB than in control groups (Carrillo Garcia et al., 2008). Other findings have shown that ApoE4 carrier and allelic frequencies were comparable for those with AD and DLB [(Kobayashi et al., 2011) and **Table 1**].

Our results for annexin A5 and ApoE4 also revealed similar characteristics for both AD and DLB patients.

DIFFERENCE BETWEEN AD AND DLB

It is apparent that DLB differs from AD in the disease progression and cure response experienced by patients. Accordingly, early differentiation between the two forms of dementia is important for effective and safe management (Aarsland et al., 2008; Sinha et al., 2011). CSF levels of tau protein have been shown to be significantly lower in DLB than in AD, which may help to differentiate between the two diseases (Mollenhauer et al., 2005a,b). On the other hand, another study also suggests that the concentration of phosphorylated tau in CSF, which is highly correlated with total tau levels, may provide a higher specificity to differentiate AD and DLB (Vanderstichele et al., 2006). α-Synuclein is the major constituent of Lewy bodies found in neurons in DLB. As a consequence of increased accumulation of α-synuclein intraneuronally in DLB, several studies have attempted its quantification in CSF. α-Synuclein has been shown to induce disruption of cellular inorganic ion homeostasis such as Ca^{2+}, leading to cell death (Lowe et al., 2004; Danzer et al., 2007; Ying et al., 2011). Whereas some groups show a decrease in the total concentration of CSF α-synuclein in DLB in comparison to other dementias (Mollenhauer et al., 2008; Kasuga et al., 2010), other groups do not find the significant difference for DLB (Spies et al., 1998; Noguchi-Shinohara et al., 2009). Thus, future study on the discrimination of these diseases is expected.

ABOUT BIOMARKERS

One of the main focuses of public health is prevention of disease. Different stages in the disease process can be targeted for preventative action, including prior to development of the disease, during the asymptomatic stage, and following clinical diagnosis. Therefore, three stages of prevention can be recognized (Wright et al., 2009; Weber et al., 2012).

From the CSF proteins identification, and MRI and PET imaging studies, the alteration of both CSF biomarkers ($A\beta_{42}$ and Tau) takes place prior to the appearance of brain structural change or dementia symptoms (Jack et al., 2010). Our *in vitro* data demonstrated that annexin A5 is elevated following the stimulation by $A\beta_{42}$ (Yamaguchi et al., 2010). Thus, onset of the annexin A5 elevation in dementia occurs at the similar time to the deposition of $A\beta_{42}$. Annexin A5 might be expected to be useful in the secondary and tertiary stages. It is conceivable that the appropriate stage for utilizing each biomarker candidate is dependent upon the properties of the biomarker. Therefore, to determine when each biomarker candidate should be utilized it will be necessary to examine the significance of any biological changes that appear at various stages.

Discrimination between neurodegenerative and non-neurodegenerative dementia is another expectation for biomarkers. Shared clinical symptoms between AD and depression in elderly have been reported (Starkstein et al., 2005), which might lead to confusion in medical intervention. Our preliminary data suggest that plasma annexin A5 levels of the six patients with depression was comparable with controls (data not shown), which might implicate annexin A5 as a biomarker for discriminating between neurodegenerative and non-neurodegenerative diseases.

Biomarkers should be reliable, reproducible, non-invasive, simple to perform, and inexpensive. To achieve this role both protein-based and genetic biomarkers have been particularly investigated. Especially plasma biomarker is beneficial by being less invasive in comparison with CSF biomarker. Gene typing is also less invasive since it is available with leukocytes from a blood sample and genetic biomarkers are of great use. ApoE4 ε4 is widely recognized as a potential biomarker for the risk of AD. As we demonstrated in this paper, ApoE ε4 is also a risk factor for DLB, indicating that ApoE ε4 is unable to discriminate between AD and DLB. No applicable genetic marker for such purpose has been reported. Detailed molecular mechanism of the onset of both AD and DLB may be needed to explore genetic factors.

ACKNOWLEDGMENTS

We thank Mr. Kenneth E. Hartman for critical reading of the manuscript. This study was supported by grants from the Ministry of Health, Labor, and Welfare of Japan and from the Ministry of Education, Culture, Sports, Science, and Technology of Japan (grant number 24591686).

REFERENCES

Aarsland, D., Kurz, M., Beyer, M., Bronnick, K., Nore, S. P., and Ballard, C. (2008). Early discriminatory diagnosis of dementia with Lewy bodies. *Dement. Geriatr. Cogn. Disord.* 25, 195–205.

Andreasen, N., Minthon, L., Davidsson, P., Vanmechelen, E., Vanderstichele, H., Winblad, B., et al. (2001). Elevation of CSF-tau and CSF-Aβ42 as diagnostic markers for Alzheimer disease in clinical practice. *Arch. Neurol.* 58, 373–379.

Bedrood, S. S., Jayasinghe, D., Sieburth, M., Chen, S., Erbel, P. C., Butler, R., et al. (2009). Annexin A5 direcly interacts with amyloidogenic proteins and reduces their toxicity. *Biochemistry* 48, 10568–10576.

Bertram, L., and Tanzi, R. E. (2008). Thirty years of Alzheimer's disease genetics: the implications of systematic meta-analysis. *Nat. Rev. Neurosci.* 9, 768–778.

Carrillo Garcia, F., Gil Neciga, E., Alberca, R., Garcia-Solis, D., Millan, J., Rodriguez Uranga, J. J., et al. (2008). Apolipoprotein ε4 in dementia with Lewy bodies. *Neurologia* 23, 152–156.

Danzer, K. M., Haasen, D., Karow, A. R., Moussaud, S., Habeck, M., Giese, A., et al. (2007). Different species of alpha-synuclein oligomers induce calcium influx and seeding. *J. Neurosci.* 27, 9220–9232.

Dong, L.-M., and Weisgraber, K. H. (1996). Human apolipoprotein E4 domain interaction. Arginine 61 and glutamic acid 255 interact to direct the preference for very low density lipoproteins. *J. Biol. Chem.* 271, 19053–19057.

Dong, L.-M., Wilson, C., Wardell, M. R., Simmons, T., Mahley, R. W., Weisgraber, K. H., et al. (1994). Human apolipoprotein E. Role of arginine 61 in mediating the pipoprotein preferences of the E3 and E4 isoforms. *J. Biol. Chem.* 269, 22358–22365.

Gomez-Tortosa, E., Gonzalo, I., Fanjul, S., Sainz, M. J., Cantarero, S., Cemillan, C., et al. (2003). Cerebrospinal fluid markers in dementia with Lewy bodies compared with Alzheimer disease. *Arch. Neurol.* 60, 1218–1222.

Hasegawa, K. (1983). "The clinical assessment of dementia in the aged: a dementia screening scale for grading the cognitive state of patients for clinician," in *Aging in the Eighties and Beyond*, ed M. E. A. Bergener (New York, NY: Springer), 207–218.

Hatters, D. M., Peters-Libeu, C. A., and Weisgraber, K. H. (2006). Apolipoprotein E structure: insights into function. *Trends Biochem. Sci.* 31, 445–454.

Hixson, J. E., and Vernier, D. T. (1990). Restriction isotyping of human apolipoprotein E by gene amplification and cleavage with HhaI. *J. Lipid Res.* 31, 545–548.

Jack, C. R. Jr., Knopman, D. S., Jagust, W. J., Shaw, L. M., Aisen, P. S., Weiner, M. W., et al. (2010). Hypothetical model of dynamic biomarkers of the Alzheimer's pathological cascade. *Lancet Neurol.* 9, 119–128.

Kasuga, K., Tokutake, T., Ishikawa, A., Uchiyama, T., Tokuda, T., Onodera, O., et al. (2010). Differential levels of α-synuclein, β-amyloid42 and tau in CSF between patients with dementia with Lewy bodies and Alzheimer's disease. *J. Neurol. Neurosurg. Psychiatry* 81, 608–610.

Kim, J., Basak, J. M., and Holtzman, D. M. (2009). The role of apolipoprotein E in Alzheimer's disease. *Neuron* 63, 287–303.

Kobayashi, S., Tateno, M., Park, T. W., Utsumi, K., Sohma, H., Ito, Y. M., et al. (2011). Apolipoprotein E4 frequencies in a Japanese population with Alzheimer's disease and dementia with Lewy bodies. *PLoS ONE* 6:e18569. doi: 10.1371/journal.pone.0018569

LaFerla, F. M. (2002). Calcium dyshomeostasis and intracellular signalling in Alzheimer's disease. *Nat. Rev. Neurosci.* 3, 862–872.

Litvan, I., Bhatia, K. P., Burn, D. J., Goetz, C. G., Lang, A. E., McKeith, I., et al. (2003). SIC task force appraisal of clinical diagnostic criteria for Parkinsonian disorders. *Mov. Disord.* 18, 467–486.

Lowe, R., Pountney, D. L., Jensen, P. H., Gai, W. P., and Voelcker, N. (2004). Calcium (II) selectively induces α-synuclein annular oligomers via interaction with the C-terminal domain. *Protein Sci.* 13, 3245–3252.

Mahley, R. W. (1988). Apolipoprotein E: cholesterol transport protein with expanding role in cell biology. *Science* 240, 622–629.

Masuda, J., Takayama, E., Satoh, A., Ida, M., Shinohara, T., Kojima-Aikawa, K., et al. (2004). Levels of annexin IV and V in the plasma of pregnant and postpartum women. *Thromb. Haemost.* 91, 1129–1136.

Mattson, M. P. (2004). Pathways towards and away from Alzheimer's disease. *Nature* 430, 631–639.

McKeith, I., Mintzer, J., Aarsland, D., Burn, D., Chiu, H., Cohen-Mansfield, J., et al. (2004). Dementia with Lewy bodies. *Lancet Neurol.* 3, 19–28.

McKeith, I. G., Dickson, D. W., Lowe, J., Emre, M., O'Brien, J. T., Feldman, H., et al. (2005). Diagnosis and management of dementia with Lewy bodies: third report of the DLB Consortium. *Neurology* 65, 1863–1872.

McKhann, G., Drachman, D., Folstein, M., Katzman, R., Price, D., and Stadlan, E. M. (1984). Clinical diagnosis of Alzheimer's disease: report of the NINCDS-ADRDA work group under the auspices of department of health and human services task force on Alzheimer's disease. *Neurology* 34, 939–944.

Mollenhauer, B., Bibl, M., Trenkwalder, C., Stiens, G., Cepek, L., Steinacker, P., et al. (2005a). Follow-up investigation in cerebrospinal fluid of patients with dementia with Lewy bodies and Alzheimer's disease. *J. Neural Transm.* 112, 933–948.

Mollenhauer, B., Cepek, L., Bibl, M., Wiltfang, J., Schulz-Schaeffer, W. F., Ciesielczyk, B., et al. (2005b). Tau protein, Aβ42 and S-100B protein in cerebrospinal fluid of patients with dementia with Lewy bodies. *Dement. Geriatr. Cogn. Disord.* 19, 164–170.

Mollenhauer, B., Cullen, V., Kahn, I., Krastins, B., Outeiro, T. F., Pepivani, I., et al. (2008). Direct quantification of CSF alpha-synuclein by ELISA and first cross-sectional study in patients with neurodegeneration. *Exp. Neurol.* 213, 315–325.

Noguchi-Shinohara, M., Tokuda, T., Yoshita, M., Kasai, T., Ono, K., Nakagawa, M., et al. (2009). CSF alpha synuclein levels in dementia with Lewy bodies and Alzheimer's disease. *Brain Res.* 1251, 1–6.

Paolo, G. D., and Kim, T.-W. (2011). Linking lipids to Alzheimer's disease: cholesterol and beyond. *Nat. Rev. Neurosci.* 12, 284–296.

Singletona, A. B., Whartona, A., O'Briena, K. K., Walker, M. P., McKeith, I. G., Ballard, C. G., et al. (2002). Clinical and neuropathological correlates of apolipoprotein E genotype in Dementia with Lewy Bodies. *Dement. Geriatr. Cogn. Disord.* 167–175.

Sinha, N., Firbank, M., and O'Brien, J. T. (2011). Biomarkers in dementia with Lewy bodies: a review. *Int. J. Geriatr. Psychiatry* 27, 443–453.

Spies, C. D., Kissner, M., Neumann, T., Blum, S., Voigt, C., Funk, T., et al. (1998). Elevated carbohydrate-deficient transferrin predicts prolonged intensive care unit stay in traumatized men. *Alcohol Alcohol.* 33, 661–669.

Starkstein, S. E., Jorge, R., Mizrahi, R., and Robinson, R. G. (2005). The construct of minor and major depression in Alzheimer's disease. *Am. J. Psychiatry* 162, 2086–2093.

Vanderstichele, H., De Vreese, K., Blennow, K., Andreasen, N., Sindic, C., Ivanoiu, A., et al. (2006). Analytical performance and clinical utility of the INNOTEST PHOSPHO-TAU181P assay for discrimination between Alzheimer's disease and dementia with Lewy bodies. *Clin. Chem. Lab. Med.* 44, 1472–1480.

Varma, A. R., Snowden, J. S., Lloyd, J. J., Talbot, P. R., Mann, D. M. A., and Neary, D. (1999). Evaluation of the NINCDS-ADRDA criteria in the differentiation of Alzheimer's disease and frontotemporal dementia. *J. Neurol. Neurosurg. Psychiatry* 66, 184–188.

Weber, G. F., Warren, J., Sohma, H., Chen, T., Halim, A., and Chakravarty, G. (2012). Biomarkers—a pot of gold or a can of worms? Meeting report from the 2nd World Congress on Biomarkers and Clinical Research, 2011, Baltimore, USA. *Cancer Biol. Ther.* 13, 831–835.

Wright, C. F., Hall, A., Matthews, F. E., and Brayne, C. (2009). Biomarkers, dementia, and public health. *Ann. N.Y. Acad. Sci.* 1180, 11–19.

Yamaguchi, M., Kokai, Y., Imai, S., Utsumi, K., Matsumoto, K., Honda, H., et al. (2010). Investigation of annexin A5 as a biomarker for Alzheimer's disease using neuronal cell culture and mouse model. *J. Neurosci. Res.* 88, 2682–2692.

Ying, Z., Lin, F., Gu, W., Su, Y., Arshad, A., Quuing, H., et al. (2011). α-Synuclein increases U251 cells vulnerability to hydrogen peroxide by disrupting calcium homeostasis. *J. Neural Transm.* 118, 1165–1172.

14

Traumatic brain injury, neuroimaging, and neurodegeneration

Erin D. Bigler[1,2,3,4]*

[1] Department of Psychology, Brigham Young University, Provo, UT, USA
[2] Neuroscience Center, Brigham Young University, Provo, UT, USA
[3] Department of Psychiatry, University of Utah, Salt Lake City, UT, USA
[4] The Brain Institute of Utah, University of Utah, Salt Lake City, UT, USA

Edited by:
Robin E. A. Green, University of Toronto, Canada

Reviewed by:
Robert A. Stern, Boston University School of Medicine, USA
Bogdan Draganski, University Lausanne, Switzerland
Gary Turner, York University, UK

***Correspondence:**
Erin D. Bigler, Department of Psychology, Neuroscience Center, Brigham Young University, 1001 SWKT, Provo, UT 84602, USA
e-mail: erin_bigler@byu.edu

Depending on severity, traumatic brain injury (TBI) induces immediate neuropathological effects that in the mildest form may be transient but as severity increases results in neural damage and degeneration. The first phase of neural degeneration is explainable by the primary acute and secondary neuropathological effects initiated by the injury; however, neuroimaging studies demonstrate a prolonged period of pathological changes that progressively occur even during the chronic phase. This review examines how neuroimaging may be used in TBI to understand (1) the dynamic changes that occur in brain development relevant to understanding the effects of TBI and how these relate to developmental stage when the brain is injured, (2) how TBI interferes with age-typical brain development and the effects of aging thereafter, and (3) how TBI results in greater frontotemporolimbic damage, results in cerebral atrophy, and is more disruptive to white matter neural connectivity. Neuroimaging quantification in TBI demonstrates degenerative effects from brain injury over time. An adverse synergistic influence of TBI with aging may predispose the brain injured individual for the development of neuropsychiatric and neurodegenerative disorders long after surviving the brain injury.

Keywords: traumatic brain injury, TBI, brain development, neuroimaging, neurodegeneration, neuropsychiatric disorders

Neuronal damage from traumatic brain injury (TBI) induces pathophysiological as well as anatomical changes (Blennow et al., 2012) that may set the stage that eventually leads to dementia (Shively et al., 2012). It is well-established and long-known that the damage from a TBI may be severe enough that the cognitive deficits experienced by the individual never return to pre-injury levels; thereby meeting *Diagnostic and Statistical Manual—Fourth Edition—Text Revision* (DSM-IV-TR) criteria for *Dementia Due to Head Trauma* (DSM-IV-TR 294.1x; see Bigler, 2007b, 2009). In the *DSM-5*, this is now classified as *Major Neurocognitive Disorder Due to TBI* (see American Psychiatric Association, 2013). However, accumulating evidence suggests with prior TBI, even in the individual that returns to presumed pre-injury cognitive ability that an increased risk for later in life degeneration occurs increasing the likelihood for a dementing illness (Plassman et al., 2000; Wang et al., 2012). It is this latter aspect of the long term effects of TBI on the aging process that will be the focus of this review. Since the majority of head injuries resulting in TBI occur before middle-age, the basic question examined in this review is the potential role that prior TBI plays in the aging process and the mechanisms whereby prior TBI would adversely influence aging.

When neural tissue is injured and reparative and restorative mechanisms fail to work, cellular morphology changes; this may ultimately result in cell death (Stoica and Faden, 2010). With change in cellular morphology or cell death, either regional or whole brain atrophy results, depending on the severity and type of injury (Pitkanen et al., 1998; Bramlett and Dietrich, 2007; Lifshitz et al., 2007; Tata and Anderson, 2010). In a human post-mortem TBI study of brain volume, Maxwell et al. (2010) examined brain weight of TBI patients who survived several months to years post-injury but were moderately to severely disabled or in a vegetative state. The following brain weights (± standard deviation) were reported: 1442.7 ± 105.0 g for controls, 1329.6 ± 202.9 g for moderately disabled, 1330 ± 140.7 g for severely disabled, and 1275 ± 135.5 g for vegetative state patients. On average moderate-to-severe TBI resulted in approximately a 112 cc of generalized volume loss at post mortem in these relatively young TBI patients (on average 44 years of age at the time of injury and 52 years at the time of death), when compared to age-matched controls who died from non-TBI related causes. While the Maxwell et al. sample was middle age at the time of death, as a group the amount of overall volume loss documented at post-mortem was comparable to that observed in patients 20–30 years older (mean age 71.1 ± 8.3) with various types of dementia at the time of death (see Purohit et al., 2011).

The Maxwell et al. study confirms TBI associated total brain volume (TBV) loss at post-mortem in the patient with chronic brain injury that approximates the degree of brain volume loss in those with brain atrophy from various types of age-related degenerative diseases much later in life. Fortunately, contemporary neuroimaging provides methods for ante-mortem detection of volume loss and its relationship to outcome following TBI, including the prediction of adverse neurological and neuropsychiatric outcome. Having sustained a TBI raises the potential for serious long-term neurobehavioral sequelae (Moretti et al., 2012). Since smaller TBV or brain volume loss from injury, disease or disorder may be a factor associated with a host of neurological and neuropsychiatric disorders (Kempton et al., 2008; Okonkwo et al., 2010; Olesen et al., 2011; Gunther et al., 2012; Skoog et al., 2012), if TBI reduces brain volume, such reductions likely relate to adverse outcome.

For the individual who sustains a TBI and survives the injury, the post-injured brain has to navigate the remainder of life with potentially less resiliency and reserve because of the parenchymal loss (Bigler, 2007b, 2009). Since aging alone—even healthy disease-free aging—is nonetheless associated with brain volume loss, does having TBI-related volume loss accelerate the loss associated with aging? Since less brain volume later in life increases the risk of dementia (Skoog et al., 2012) does brain volume loss from TBI relate to increased dementia and possibly induce further degenerative changes?

TBI induces a number of neuropathological changes like the aggregation of β-amyloid and tau along with neuroinflammatory changes that resemble the pathology of degenerative diseases (Blennow et al., 2012). Do the combination of effects that resemble later in life neurodegenerative changes in the young individual who sustains a TBI become associated with a greater likelihood for transition to a progressive dementing illness later in life?

These questions are addressed in this review which examines volume loss from brain injury, its role in the aging process, and how neuroimaging methods may be used to document such changes.

TBI AND PARENCHYMAL VOLUME LOSS

SIGNIFICANT TBI RESULTS IN BRAIN VOLUME LOSS

Figure 1 is from an adult male who sustained a severe TBI (GCS = 3) but in whom a pre-injury magnetic resonance imaging (MRI) scan had been performed, so pre-injury quantification of ventricular and brain volume could be established. An excellent global measure of brain integrity is the ventricle-to-brain ratio (VBR; Bigler and Tate, 2001), calculated as the total of ventricular volume divided by total brain volume (TBV), multiplied by 100 so that the ratio is reported in whole numbers. Overall, normal VBR for the adult is around 1.5 with a 0.5 standard deviation (Blatter et al., 1995). In cerebral atrophy the reduction in brain volume is accompanied by a passive, compensatory increase in ventricular volume (referred to as hydrocephalus ex vacuo) thereby resulting in increased VBR. Acutely in TBI, presence of cerebral edema results in increased parenchymal volume because of tissue expansion from swelling combined with ventricular compression, reducing the size of the ventricle. In the mildest forms of TBI when edema occurs, this swelling may be transient and brain parenchyma and ventricular volume return to pre-injury levels. If injury is of sufficient severity, however, over time parenchymal degeneration occurs, reflected by brain volume loss in conjunction with hydrocephalus ex vacuo and increased VBR. As seen in this illustration, the pre-injury scan VBR was well within normal limits. However, post-injury computed tomography (CT) findings reflect distinctly reduced VBR, indicative of whole brain edema and ventricular compression, which remained throughout the first week post-injury. However, by 16 weeks post-injury substantial ventricular increase is evident along with a higher VBR score, which continued to increase over the next 2 years post-injury.

Over time, these scans, as shown in **Figure 1**, demonstrate several important points. Compared to the pre-injury brain, post-injury generalized swelling and ventricular compression in the acute and early sub-acute timeframe clearly indicate the non-specific edema and generalized neuroinflammation affects the entirety of the brain. Furthermore, this type of swelling likely compromises overall cerebral perfusion, thereby affecting neural integrity, cellular degradation and apoptosis (Xu et al., 2010) and in rodent TBI models exacerbates hippocampal damage beyond what occurs directly from the TBI (Foley et al., 2013). By the time of the first scan was obtained more than an hour post-injury in the case shown in **Figure 1**, obviously the instantaneous biomechanical shear/strain deformation injuries had occurred and what is primarily being viewed in the first acute scan are the combinations of primary and the initial secondary effects of the injury. By day 7, there is a low density lesion, likely an infarction beginning to evolve adjacent to the caudate, which is particularly evident 2 years post-injury. This demonstrates another TBI principle in that distinctly focal effects, either from shearing and/or vascular effects, may occur within the backdrop of global pathological changes. What is reflected in the scan 2 years post-injury is the summation of all of the pathological effects of TBI—mechanical deformation, axonal shearing resulting in primary axotomy, and likely focal lesion effects as well as the combined effects of secondary axotomy, ischemic damaged from compromised cerebral blood flow and whatever pathological neuroexcitatory effects may have occurred in combination with other neuroinflammatory reactions (Bigler and Maxwell, 2011, 2012). The pathological cascade is complex and as shown in this illustration plays out over an extended period of time. The end-product, however, is a brain reflective of non-specific damage with considerable overall TBV loss.

In a living veteran sample with penetrating brain injury and post-traumatic epilepsy, as a group TBI patients were found to exhibit approximately a 52 cc whole brain volume loss based on neuroimaging findings obtained years post-injury (Raymont et al., 2010). The TBI subjects in the Raymont et al. investigation had sustained injuries not as severe as in the subjects in the Maxwell et al. (2010) investigation and were penetrating in nature, but still exhibited substantial volume loss based on quantitative neuroimaging. Thus, when assessed with *in vivo* neuroimaging methods, TBI may result in substantial volume loss of brain parenchyma, which in turn relates to neurocognitive outcome (Tate et al., 2011), to be reviewed below. Furthermore, *in vivo* quantitative neuroimaging provides methods to examine the course of neurodegenerative changes over time post-injury in those who survive the brain injury.

If the trauma induced volume loss associated with TBI were just the effects of the initial injury, once the acute cascade of degeneration occurred it would be assumed that the injured brain should exhibit no further degeneration. However, if TBI has produced something more than a static brain injury,

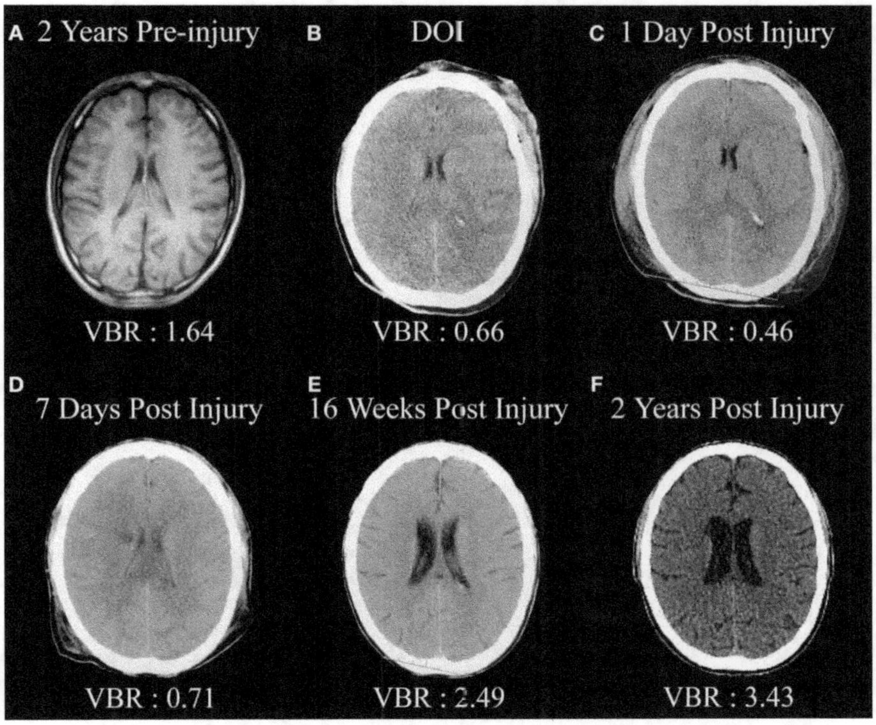

FIGURE 1 | (A) Pre-injury magnetic resonance image (MRI) approximately 2 years prior to a severe traumatic brain injury (TBI). Note the normal size of the ventricular system and ventricle-to-brain (VBR) ratio of 1.64 (normal is approximately 1.5 with a 0.5 standard deviation). **(B)** Day-of-injury initial CT demonstrating brain edema and reduced VBR, which continues to be reflected in **(C,D)**. **(E)** Distinct neurodegeneration has occurred by 16 weeks post-injury, reflected as ventricular dilation and increased VBR, with continued neurodegeneration out to 2 years post-injury as seen in **(F)**.

longitudinal neuroimaging would exhibit progressive changes over time (Greenberg et al., 2008). This would implicate neurodegenerative processes extending well-beyond the point of acute TBI, and the sub-acute timeframe necessary for those initial pathological effects to run their course (Bendlin et al., 2008; Ng et al., 2008; Farbota et al., 2012). Recently, chronic neuroinflammation, particularly involving white matter (WM) has been implicated in some of these progressive changes, including volume loss in the corpus callosum (Johnson et al., 2011, 2013). Since the shear-strain influences of TBI are more likely to damage axons, producing what is referred to as traumatic axonal injury (TAI; see Bigler and Maxwell, 2012) any chronic neuroinflammatory response influencing WM integrity would likely have adverse influences on recovery.

Longer-term pathological effects from TBI, regardless of their nature, would likely interact with the aging process and may set the stage for adverse neuropsychiatric and neurocognitive outcome after injury along with increased risk for age-related neurodegenerative diseases (Lucas et al., 2006; Johnson et al., 2012; Shively et al., 2012). Based on neuroimaging studies of normal brain development over the life span in comparison to the pathological effects of TBI, this review will address three basic issues: (1) dynamic changes in brain volume relate to age, with "normal" age-related reductions in brain volume occurring after the third decade in life, (2) TBI interferes with age-typical brain development depending on the age when injury occurs and while both gray matter (GM) and WM are damaged, trauma selectively damages axons; thereby more disruptive to WM neural connectivity during the aging process post-injury (see Ramlackhansingh et al., 2011), and (3) along with whole-brain, WM and GM volume reductions from TBI, traumatic injury results in more selective frontotemporolimbic damage, atrophic changes identifiable via neuroimaging. Diffuse damage, along with the frontotemporolimbic locus of damage from TBI, pre-disposes the brain injured individual for increased neuropsychiatric morbidity with aging and increased risk for dementia later in life.

DYNAMIC CHANGES IN BRAIN VOLUME OVER THE LIFE SPAN

At birth, TBV is approximately 25% of what it will become in adulthood but the volume increase in brain growth occurs rapidly, where based on magnetic resonance imaging (MRI) volumetric studies by 8 years of age, TBV approximates adulthood (Courchesne et al., 2000). Over the remaining childhood years and throughout adolescence, a dynamic interaction between cellular maturation and pruning along with myelination results in reduced overall GM with increased WM (see **Figure 2**). Knowing the influence of age-typical effects on brain, WM and GM volumes and the fact that all three are in decline later in the aging process (>6th decade of life) indicates their utility as neuroimaging markers of brain parenchymal health earlier in life. Quantitative neuroimaging methods that measure volumetric brain changes demonstrate these effects as shown in **Figure 2**. For

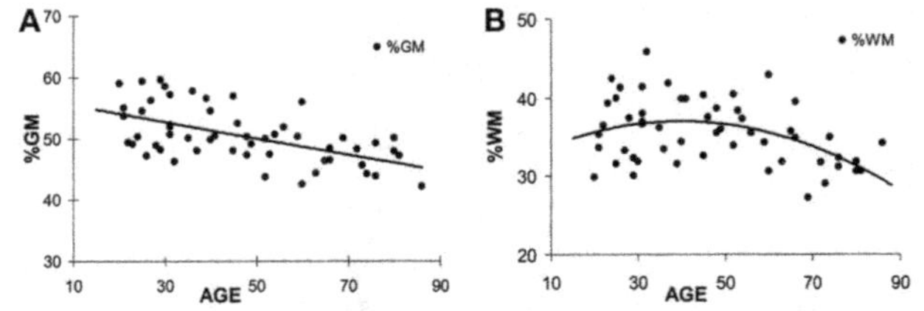

FIGURE 2 | (A,B) These plots are from Ge et al. (2002) and reflect different trajectories of white matter (WM) and gray matter (GM) over the life-span. The percent of GM volume total brain (TBV) volume declines with age whereas the percentage of WM to TBV shows and increase followed by decline later in life. Note that the age at which an individual is injured occurs not in a static brain, but rather in a brain that has age-dependent changes occurring simultaneously with the age when injury occurs. Reproduced with permission from The American Society of Neuroradiology.

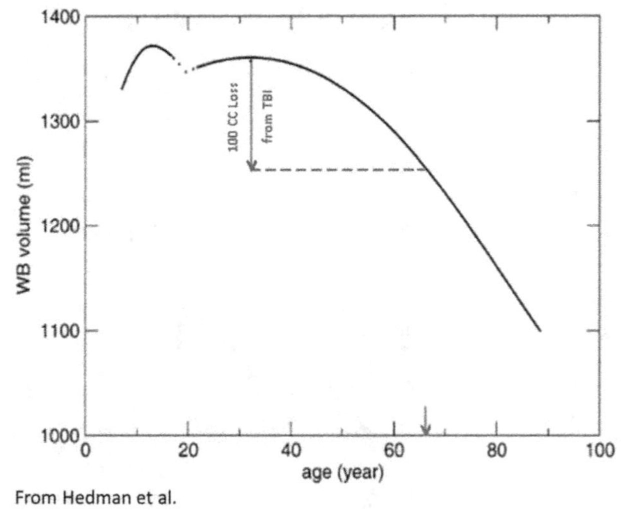

FIGURE 3 | Based on a meta-analysis Hedman et al. (2011) constructed the following TBV plots over the life span from approximately age 4 through 90 years of age. A hypothetical TBI patient injured in their 20's sustaining a volume loss of a 100 cc is depicted with the inference being that although only chronologically a young adult, because of the brain loss, the total reduction of TBV is similar to someone in their 7th decade of life (downward arrow, X-axis). In other words, purely from a TBV perspective, TBI accelerated brain volume loss. Reproduced with permission from Wiley.

example, Ge et al. (2002) plotted the percentage of whole brain WM and GM volume by age from approximately 10 through 90 years, as shown in **Figure 2**. Note that by mid-childhood GM has already started to decrease, which in childhood is thought to reflect normal neuronal pruning, all-the-while WM from late childhood through early adulthood increases and does not peak until early mid-adulthood but thereafter in decline just as GM. Throughout childhood and adolescence TBV reflects several dynamic phases of pruning, modeling and myelination but following peak development in adulthood thereafter a steady decline in TBV occurs as shown in **Figure 3**, adapted from Hedman et al. (2011). The Hedman et al. investigation examined 56 longitudinal MRI studies involving 2211 subjects from four to 88 years of age where they determined that after 35 years of age, a 0.2% per annum volume loss occurred which accelerated to 0.5% per annum after age 60.

Therefore, the early dynamic interplay between GM pruning and increased WM connectivity underlies much of the early ebb-and-flow of overall brain volume within the first three decades of life (see **Figures 2, 3**). However, after stabilization around mid-adulthood, brain volume follows an inexorable decline, which is age dependent. In the developing healthy brain, maturational changes may be measured as volumetric changes, including WM volume; WM connectivity also can be measured with metrics such as fractional anisotropy (FA) based on diffusion tensor imaging (DTI; Shi et al., 2012), MRI structural covariance functions (Zielinski et al., 2010) and functional MRI (fMRI; Rubia, 2012).

Since intracranial volume peaks in mid-childhood, around 8 years of age, and basically remains invariant for the remainder of life (Courchesne et al., 2000), any reduction in TBV is met with increased cerebrospinal fluid (CSF) volume, where notably increasing age results in a linear CSF increase (Inglese and Ge, 2004). Increased whole brain CSF with aging, disease or injury is a reflection of cerebral atrophy (Driscoll et al., 2011). When a significant TBI occurs with resulting volume loss from the injury that injury occurs amidst a developmental backdrop of changing TBV, ventricular and total CSF volume, WM and GM volumes at the time of injury (Tasker, 2006).

Prospective, life-span neuroimaging studies on the effects of TBI have not been done but inferences can be made from longitudinal and childhood developmental studies that have examined TBI patients in the chronic phase post-injury. In child TBI the injury perturbs developmental trajectories which may never return to their pre-injury trajectories (Tasker, 2006; Ewing-Cobbs et al., 2008; Wu et al., 2010; Beauchamp et al., 2011). In adults, any volume loss from brain injury is superimposed on whatever the age-typical volume loss would be, potentially resulting in an acceleration of any age-mediated decline (Bigler, 2007b, 2009). For example, returning to **Figure 3**, if a typical 25-year-old with a pre-injury TBV of 1350 cc (average adult brain volume) lost 100 cc because of a severe TBI (thereby approximating the volume loss for moderately-to-severely disabled individuals with TBI from the Maxwell et al. (2010) study mentioned above) as determined by quantitative neuroimaging several months post-injury that 25-year-old individual would have a TBV equivalent to a 65-year-old (note the point of intercept in **Figure 3** and the down-pointing arrow). Did the brain injury with a 100 cc volume loss impose a 40+ aging effect on the brain in what should be a 25-year-old brain?

Figures 2, 3 are straightforward volumetric markers of brain development, and while they reflect gross anatomy, there are other neuroimaging biomarkers of both WM and GM integrity more sensitive to microstructure and neuronal health that also map onto these volume changes. Such changes show age-related dynamic alterations in energy metabolism including magnetic resonance spectroscopy findings (MRS), magnetization transfer ratios that directly assess WM integrity along with DTI, and resting state fMRI or rs-fMRI (Inglese and Ge, 2004; Rosazza and

Minati, 2011). DTI and rs-fMRI findings in normal development and TBI are particularly important because these neuroimaging tools provide techniques for more directly assessing brain connectivity (Van Den Heuvel and Sporns, 2011; Irimia et al., 2012b). How brain connectivity is either maintained, adapted to or damaged is key to understanding the effects of TBI at any point in the life span as well as normal aging and neurodegenerative disorders (Liu et al., 2013; Steffener et al., 2012; Levin and Smith, 2013; Pandit et al., 2013). Fortunately overall parenchymal volume positively correlates with DTI metrics, especially WM volume (see Harrison et al., 2011, 2013) and thereby TBV and WM volumes likely represent proxies that reflect brain connectivity. Based on the age-dependent volume changes shown in **Figures 2**, **3**, volume measures may be used as biomarkers of underlying brain health, developmental stage and brain connectivity. Reductions in brain volume from TBI would reflect reduced brain connectivity (Palacios et al., 2012, 2013).

As already introduced, the VBR metric represents a simple neuroimaging measurement sensitive to brain parenchymal volume loss as well as changes in CSF that relates to cognitive outcome in TBI (Tate et al., 2011). As rendered from a volume acquisition T1-weighted MRI, **Figure 4** depicts a three-dimensional surface appearance of the brain along with the cerebral ventricles (in blue) in a healthy control compared to a TBI patient with severe brain injury, global cerebral atrophy (note the prominence of the cortical sulci and inter-hemispheric fissure) and increased VBR. What is important about this image of the brain injured patient shown in **Figure 4** is that the TBI occurred when this individual was 12 years of age and the MRI obtained approximately 2 years post-injury. So the distinctly visible atrophic brain is that of a 14-year-old, but the degree of atrophy is similar to an individual seven or eight decades older. The advantage of using the VBR metric is that it automatically adjusts for head size differences due to height, body type and sex differences that influence head and brain size (Lainhart et al., 2006). In typical developing individuals, because normal brain development fills the cranial vault and ventricular size is minimal, VBR findings during childhood are relatively constant after age six and remain so throughout childhood, adolescence and early adulthood. Increases in VBR do occur in normal aging that become overtly notable by middle age but sharply increase after age 65. Chronic VBR changes reflective of generalized atrophy in TBI are directly proportional to the severity of injury (Bigler et al., 2006; Wilde et al., 2006a; Ghosh et al., 2009). Likewise, pathological increases in VBR are found in neurodegenerative disorders (Bigler et al., 2004; Carmichael et al., 2007; Olesen et al., 2011). The VBR in this child was calculated to be 5.55, which in comparison to a "normal" aging VBR would not have occurred until after the 8th decade of life. What will become of this brain as it ages?

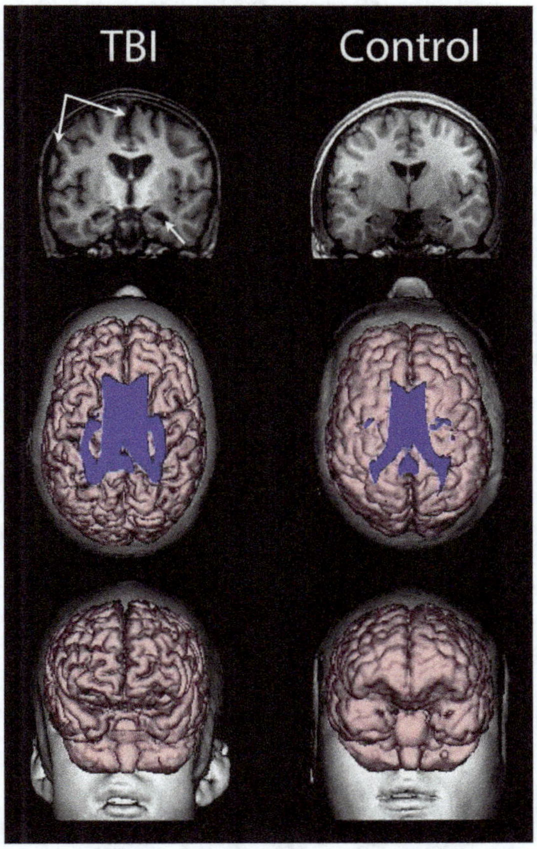

FIGURE 4 | (Top) T1-weighted coronal images of a TBI patient on the left and an age-matched control on the right, both young adolescent males. Upper left-hand arrows point to a prominent interhemispheric fissure and cortical sulci, reflective of whole brain volume loss and generalized cerebral atrophy in the TBI patient. The lower arrow points to an atrophic hippocampus and dilated temporal horn, bilaterally in the TBI patient. **(Middle)** Dorsal view of a 3-D reconstruction of the ventricle in shown in blue superimposed on the flesh-tone brain surface 3-D reconstruction. Calculating whole brain volume and dividing it by total ventricular volume and multiplying by 100 results in a ventricle-to-brain ratio (VBR) of 5.55, which is markedly deviant from normal, which in typical developing controls is generally in the range of 1.5 with a 0.5 standard deviation [see Blatter et al. (1995) and Chang et al. (2005)]. The control subject VBR was 1.45. Frontal view of the 3-D reconstructed brain **(Bottom)** of the individual with TBI showing global frontal atrophy with visibly larger cortical sulci compared to the age-match control subject on the right, again reflective of generalized cerebral atrophy. Increased VBR reflects this type of global brain volume loss, ventricular enlargement, gyral shrinkage and sulcal enlargement.

BRAIN VOLUME REDUCTIONS IN TBI

Presumably, as injury severity increases more numerous and potentially widely distributed pathological effects occur throughout the brain (Adams et al., 2011). This fact likely characterizes the association between injury severity and reduced TBV as reflected by increased VBR. Regardless of how severity is defined (GCS, LOC or PTA) increased severity is associated with increased cerebral atrophy (Bigler et al., 2006), where VBR may triple or more in those with the most severe injury.

Examining VBR changes at different time points post-injury provides insight into the more long-term neurodegenerative effects from sustaining a brain injury. Blatter et al. (1997) examined in a cross-sectional sample VBR at different times post-injury showing dynamic atrophic changes with VBR increases more than 2 years post-injury. The steepest VBR increases post-injury occurred by approximately 3 weeks clearly reflecting the initial neuropathological effects of neuronal death and cellular phagocytosis that results in reduced TBV. However, VBR changes continued to increase in this study beyond 2 years after injury.

Once trauma passes a pathological threshold, *in vitro* studies show that the primary trauma-induced cell loss begins immediately or within hours of injury depending on mechanism of injury, injury severity and the type of induced pathological effects (Cullen et al., 2011). However, as discussed by Bigler and Maxwell (2012) there are any number of potential secondary pathological pathways that could result in more long-term neurodegenerative effects. Confirmation of these long-term effects comes from other investigations as well. For example, Ng et al. (2008) first quantified CSF volume at approximately 4.5 months post-injury, long past the initial sub-acute time frame where Blatter et al. and others (see also Gale et al., 1995) have shown the greatest degree of degenerative change occurs from TBI, continued to show volumetric differences out to 2.5 years post-injury. In severe TBI these visible changes are readily viewed in the individual patient by sequential neuroimaging studies as shown in **Figure 5**. This patient sustained a severe TBI and while significant neurodegenerative effects had occurred by one month post-injury, visible changes progressed over the next 20 months based on scan findings.

In terms of actual volume loss, Sidaros et al. (2009) examined a group of severe TBI patients at approximately 8 weeks post-injury and then again at 12 months. In comparison to controls TBV was reduced by approximately 8.4% within this initial 2-month post-injury timeframe; however, using the patient's 2-month post-acute MRI as the baseline, by 12 months post-injury an additional overall 4% volume loss occurred (range from −0.6 to −9.4%). Translating this into actual brain parenchymal tissue loss (refer to **Figure 3** again), in the typical 1350 cc brain, moderate-to-severe TBI would result on average in more than a 100 cc loss of brain parenchyma. Accordingly, the example given in **Figure 3** actually does reflect a type of reduction in TBV that would occur in the typical young adult sustaining a severe TBI.

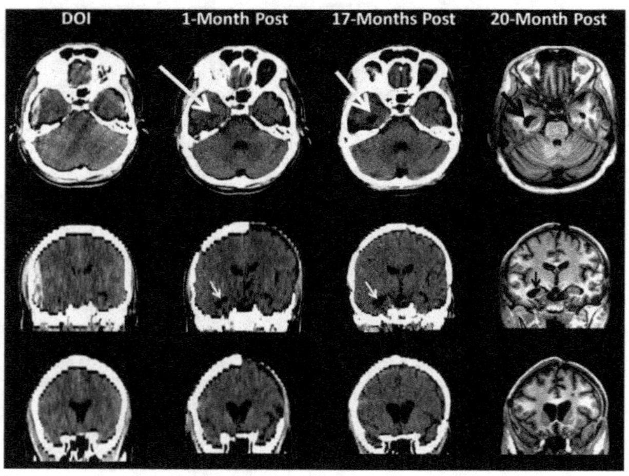

FIGURE 5 | This patient sustained a severe TBI as a consequence of a fall. Note on the day of injury (DOI) the computed tomography (CT) scan demonstrates the presence of a large epidural hematoma with brain displacement. Repeat scanning was performed at 1-month (CT scan), 17 (CT scan) and 20 months (MRI) post-injury. For the CT scans in the middle and bottom rows the coronal sections shown are based on re-sampled axial images with degradation in image resolution but sufficient to depict ventricular changes over time. Note how in the DOI scan the temporal horn is basically undetectable from parenchymal shift from the epidural as well as edema but clearly visible and dilated by 1-Month (white arrow) which increases by 17-months and even more prominent by 20 months as shown in the MRI findings. The bottom coronal images clearly depict increasing dilation of the anterior horns of the lateral ventricular system reflecting brain parenchymal volume loss that progresses from DOI through 20-months post-injury. Note at 1 month the patient still has missing bone-flap from the original craniotomy to treat a contra coup hemorrhagic contusion and subdural hematoma.

From the above discussion of brain volume loss, returning to the Hedman et al. (2011) investigation, given their report of a 0.2–0.5% per annum whole brain volume loss, if severe TBI results in a ~10% volume reduction this far exceeds any per annum "normal" volume loss. In fact that would induce a volume loss that in normal aging would have taken decades to achieve. In adulthood, depending on the age at the time of injury, such a volume loss likely adds to the aging burden on the brain and may accelerate age-effects by several decades. Although overly simplistic, the argument can be made that this volume loss is registered against whatever brain reserve capacity might have been present at the time of the original TBI (Bigler, 2007b), predisposing the individual with TBI to age-mediated neuropsychiatric and neurodegenerative disorders (Bigler, 2009). Traumatic-induced TBV reductions that occur within the first few months post-injury likely occur as a direct effect of the initial pathological response but more long-term TBV reductions would also reflect potential complex interactive age, neuroinflammation and neurodegenerative effects (Amor et al., 2010; Johnson et al., 2013).

In the longest follow-up TBI study to date involving structural neuroimaging, Tomaiuolo et al. (2012) compared patients at one and then 8 years post-injury. **Figure 6** from that study shows progressive changes in the corpus callosum, clearly implicating that further WM degeneration occurs long after the initial active pathological changes within the acute and sub-acute timeframe. Within a year post-injury, as also clearly visible in **Figure 6**, the corpus callosum goes through an initial loss of tracts and overall significant size reduction compared to an age-matched non-TBI control. For comparison, **Figure 6**, at the bottom, also shows normal appearance of DTI-derived fiber tracts involving the corpus callosum and the distinct loss of tracts that may occur in TBI taken from the study by Wilde et al. (2006a). The initial changes within the corpus callosum would mostly be attributable to the acute/sub-acute neuropathological effects including cell death and Wallerian degeneration of WM tracts. However, as shown in the Tomaiuolo et al. study, the continuation of WM degenerative changes from one out to eight years post-injury—as reflected in the continued reduction of the corpus callosum—could not be explained by the initial acute/sub-acute effects and implicates more long-term neurodegenerative sequelae. Tomaiuolo et al. also examined the volume of the hippocampus which interestingly, although significantly smaller than controls in the TBI subjects, did not show additional volume loss out to 8 years post-injury. Such findings are consistent with the progressive yet selective damaging effects of TBI on WM, including long-term neurodegenerative effects which will be discussed next.

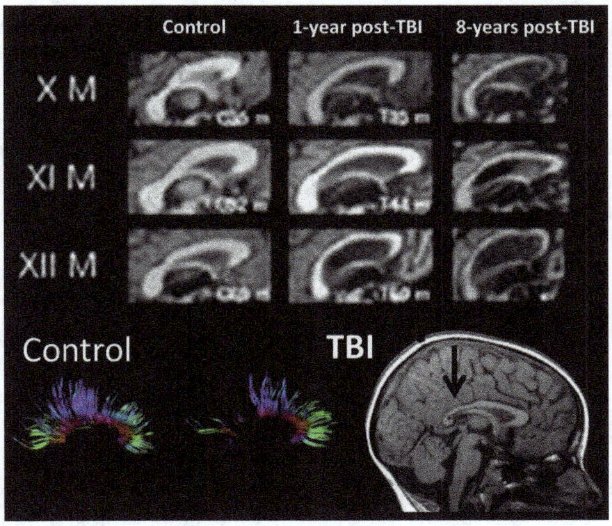

FIGURE 6 | (TOP) Mid-sagittal section through the corpus callosum showing initial atrophy 1-year from TBI, but increasing atrophy within this WM structure expressed over the next 8 years, indicating late neurodegenerative effects on WM. Images reproduced with permission from Tomaiuolo et al. (2012) and Elsevier Science. **(BOTTOM)** Corpus callosum tractography extracted from DTI in a control, compared to a child with severe TBI. The mid-sagittal MRI shows gross thinning of the posterior corpus callosum (dark arrow) but DTI actually demonstrates that this reduced area actually has regions of no DTI-identifiable aggregate WM tracts. Adapted from Wilde et al. (2006b) used with permission from Mary Ann Liebert Publishing.

The vulnerability of the corpus callosum in TBI is of particular interest, because some of the greatest shear/strain effects from trauma occur within the corpus callosum (McAllister et al., 2012; Rowson et al., 2012) and reductions in the size and/or integrity of the corpus callosum, even in mild TBI is well-documented (Aoki et al., 2012). The Tomaiuolo et al. (2012) study demonstrates that whatever initial traumatic effects there are on WM, damage to corpus callosum tracts may progress long after the injury, reflected as corpus callosum volume loss and atrophic changes (see also Tasker, 2006). Furthermore, Galanaud et al. (2012) show that pathological findings on DTI 1 year post-injury predict poor outcome from severe TBI. Interestingly, as already mentioned, Tomaiuolo et al. did not observe progressive changes in the hippocampus. It is very likely that different regions will have different resiliencies and/or vulnerabilities to the effects of injury and aging.

For example, progressive changes in the corpus callosum, long after injury, implicate active degenerative effects that are probably more than just age-mediated degenerative changes specific to WM (Farbota et al., 2012). Given the sensitivity of the DTI technique to detect abnormalities of myelin integrity and gliosis from TBI (Budde et al., 2011; Budde and Frank, 2012), DTI studies of abnormal WM in TBI should be able to document progressive degenerative changes in inter- and intra-hemispheric pathways (see Kim et al., 2008) when prospectively done.

WHITE MATTER VULNERABILITY, DIMINISHED BRAIN CONNECTIVITY OF TBI AND CHANGES OVER TIME

While hemispheric interconnectivity occurs across the corpus callosum, large intra-hemispheric fasciculi connect multiple regions within each hemisphere and likewise, there are long-coursing WM tracts integrating the brainstem and cerebellum with subcortical nuclei and the cerebrum. Shorter U-fibers connect adjacent gyral regions. The previously mentioned study by Bendlin et al., 2008 examined TBI patients (GCS of 13 or below) at 2 months post-injury and followed for more than 1 year post-injury showing longitudinal differences occurred not just within the corpus callosum, but also involving long white matter tracts as well as more short U-fibers. Follow-up with this same cohort out to 4 years post-injury has shown that the degeneration continues years post injury (Farbota et al., 2012). Wang et al. (2011) examined TBI patients earlier in their course of injury (from day-of-injury to within 9 days) and as with Bendlin et al. they followed-up within 14 months post injury and likewise documented ongoing degeneration. Thus, progressive WM degradation has now been documented that extends well into the chronic phase of having sustained a TBI (see also Sidaros et al., 2008, 2009) and Palacios et al. (2012, 2013).

Probably the most salient clinical effect of WM vulnerability is the loss of overall brain connectivity that occurs with TBI (Bonnelle et al., 2012; Caeyenberghs et al., 2012; Irimia et al., 2012a; Palacios et al., 2012). Caeyenberghs et al. (2012) not only showed the presence of disrupted WM integrity in TBI but that this disruption results in diminished cognitive control in those with brain injury. Furthermore, Wang et al. (2011) demonstrated that WM abnormalities both acutely and chronically were predictive of outcome.

The degree of WM integrity inferred directly or indirectly has been the focus of numerous studies in aging and dementia. Given improvements in image quantification the degree of WM lesion burden in the elderly individual is associated with increased levels of dementia and in those where changes in WM are quantified over time, the degree of WM burden predicts transition from mild cognitive impairment (MCI) to Alzheimer's disease (Carlson et al., 2008; Price et al., 2012; Silbert et al., 2012). Silbert et al. (2012), in a longitudinal, prospective neuroimaging study that measured WM volume as well as CSF, identified WM changes 10 years prior to MCI onset. Silbert et al. concluded that "acceleration in WM burden, a common indicator of cerebrovascular disease in the elderly, is a pathological change that emerges early in the presymptomatic phase leading to MCI (p. 741)." In the Silbert et al. investigation, they began neuroimaging studies at age 70, but if the change from 70 to 80 predicts who converts to MCI, what does this mean if baseline WM burden has already been compromised in a TBI patient injured at a much younger age? **Figure 7** shows WM burden in terms of the fluid attenuated inversion recovery or FLAIR signal abnormality and susceptibility weighted imaging (SWI) sequences in TBI patients only one of whom is an adult.

FRONTOTEMPOROLIMBIC LOCUS OF DAMAGE FROM TBI

McAllister (2011) reviews the neuropathological as well as neuroimaging studies that demonstrate a frontotemporolimbic locus

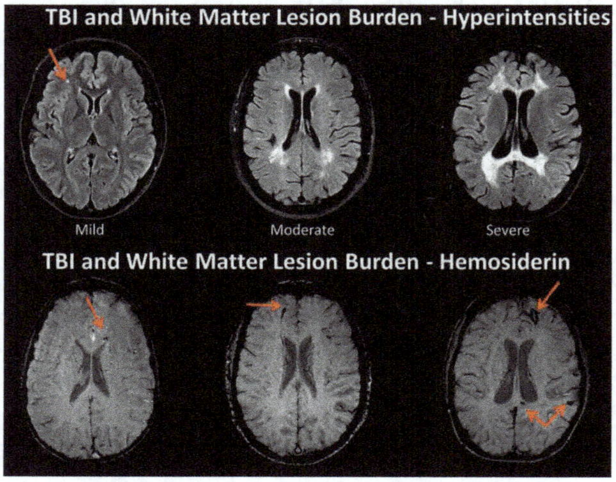

FIGURE 7 | TOP: Fluid attenuated inversion recovery (FLAIR) sequence in three traumatic brain injury (TBI) cases depicting different levels of white matter burden. (Left) a child with mild TBI (mTBI) indicating a solitary, focal white matter hyperintensity (WMH). (Middle) a 62-year-old male with a severe TBI with no white matter abnormalities noted on admission CT. Patient had a GCS of 7 prior to intubation, meeting criteria for severe TBI (Right) 17-year-old injured 2 years prior with an admission GCS of 3. Note the prominent and extensive WMHs widely distributed. **BOTTOM**: The middle and right hand subjects are the same as above, but subject on the left side is a different child with a mild TBI, who did not have a WMH, but did show hemosiderin in the corpus callosum (arrow). Note that both patients with severe injury have some generalized atrophy and ventricular dilation as a reflection of generalized brain volume loss as a consequence of severe TBI along with multiple hemosiderin deposits.

of injury from TBI. Anatomically, Bigler (2007a, 2008) has shown that because of the location of the cranial fossa and dura mater, trauma induced movement of the frontal and temporal lobes creates a mechanical vulnerability for damage to frontotemporolimbic regions of the brain following trauma. Brain deformations involving these structures, in turn increases the likelihood for focal pathology including surface contusions in these regions. Additionally, because of a unique confluence of major WM fasciculi that course through key brain regions in conjunction with network hubs and nodes involving frontotemporolimbic circuitry, even small but strategic WM lesions may have dramatic effects in TBI (Bigler et al., 2010).

The hippocampus has long been recognized as a fundamental limbic system structure. Hippocampal atrophy is a common finding in TBI (Bigler and Maxwell, 2011). As shown in **Figures 3**, **4**, marked bilateral hippocampal atrophy may occur in severe TBI. The selective damage to the hippocampus in TBI is in part related to its positioning within the medial temporal lobe and the above mentioned biomechanical vulnerability of the medial temporal lobe to compression injury, but there are also intrinsic excitotoxic, neurotransmitter and metabolic factors specific to the hippocampus that predispose it to injury as well (see Diaz-Arrastia et al., 2009). Controlled animal experiments show that the hippocampus is particularly sensitive to the effects of trauma, even in mild TBI (Chen et al., 2012), with progressive neuronal death and hippocampal atrophy beyond the acute/sub-acute timeframe (Smith et al., 1997; Immonen et al., 2009). Additionally, given its high metabolic demands combined with over-expression of excitotoxic effects, greater hippocampal damage in TBI is often the outcome (Deng and Xu, 2011; Marquez de la Plata et al., 2011). In children, Wilde et al. (2006b) have shown that hippocampal volume loss from TBI was proportionally the greatest in comparison to all other brain regions examined.

Hippocampal and medial temporal lobe pathology plays a role in many neuropsychiatric and neurodegenerative disorders. For example, obvious pathological changes within the hippocampal formation occur in Alzheimer's disease and related dementias, associated with the memory impairments observed in these disorders (Hodges, 2012). Some level of hippocampal pathology is thought to contribute to major depression that occurs late in life, which also may relate to mild cognitive impairment (MCI; Morra et al., 2009). Additionally, a very complex interplay exists between TBV, aging and hippocampal volume and the transitions from healthy aging to MCI, and from MCI to frank dementia (Apostolova et al., 2012). Successful "aging" of the hippocampal complex and its multimodal efferent and afferent connections is considered a key element of brain plasticity with advancing age (Goh and Park, 2009). Oppositely, any injury to the hippocampus or its afferent/efferent connections such as from TBI likely adds to or advances the aging burden.

Lastly, when the limbic system is viewed in its entirety, it is a complex, highly interconnected system dependent on the integrity of numerous WM pathways. While the hippocampus is central to limbic system integrity, note that functional hippocampal disruption in TBI may occur by lesions quite distal to the hippocampus but occurring within other structures or limbic pathways that either input or output the hippocampus. For example, Wilde et al. (2010) have shown the vulnerability of frontal projections from the anterior cingulum in TBI. Such pathological changes would be a minimum of three synaptic connections from the hippocampus, and while the axonal injury may be specific to the cingulum bundle, it potentially would have some similar effects as if the damage actually had occurred in the hippocampus since part of hippocampal output to frontal cortex projects via the anterior cingulum. More directly, the fornix is vulnerable in TBI (Yallampalli et al., 2013), thereby disrupting the direct output of the hippocampus. Because of the interdependence of the limbic network on each of its constituent parts, intactness at one level does not insure that transfer of information occurs at another. Because of the increased likelihood of hippocampal damage in TBI, even minimal hippocampal damage could be highly disruptive to limbic connectivity and overtime, add to the burden of age effects.

AGING, TBI AND NEURODEGENERATIVE DISORDERS

At the beginning of this discussion it was shown that whole-brain volume is age-dependent, which over time, even in the healthy individual declines. Brain atrophy outside the parameters of that related to normal aging is associated with a host of disease processes and potential adverse age-mediated genetic factors. As such, any environmental condition, such as a TBI that has the potential to influence brain volume loss likely adds to the disease burden that accompanies reduced brain volume during the normal aging process. This is graphically depicted in **Figure 8** when the 14-year-old atrophic brain from a severe TBI is compared side-by-side with the MRI findings from an 86-year-old patient with Alzheimer's disease.

The initial, direct effect of brain injury induces neuroinflammatory reactions that may set the stage for long-term neuroinflammatory effects and neurodegeneration (see Ramlackhansingh et al., 2011; Johnson et al., 2013). The initial direct neurodegenerative changes that occur following TBI are manifested by significant brain atrophy that occurs within the first 6 months post-injury (Gale et al., 1995). While these effects can be accounted for by acute/sub-acute injury mechanisms and their pathological consequences, given the above observations, neuroinflammatory and neurodegenerative processes may extend for years beyond the initial post-injury injury time frame in the TBI patient. These more chronic effects do set the stage for important interactions that occur between the age at the time of injury, aging and age-related vulnerabilities, to later in life neuropsychiatric and progressive neurodegenerative disorders indicating that the lesion in TBI may be much more dynamic (Bigler, 2013). The frontotemporolimbic locus of where TBI induced degenerative changes are most likely to occur in the brain, has a most interesting overlap with brain areas observed in older individuals with increased risk for a variety of age-related neurological and neuropsychiatric disorders. Two examples are given that demonstrate this overlap. Sperling et al. (2011) review the pre-clinical stages of Alzheimer's disease in relationship to key biomarkers that, overtime, increase the likelihood for developing dementia.

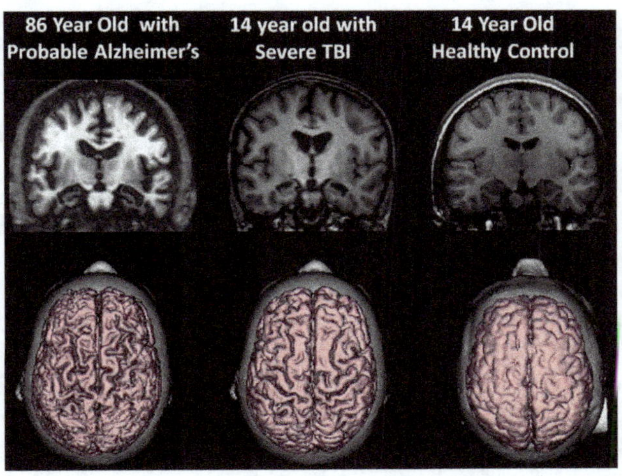

FIGURE 8 | (Top) T1-weighted coronal images approximately at the same level showing hippocampal atrophy in the 86-year-old patient with a clinical diagnosis of Alzheimer's disease and the 14-year-old patient with severe traumatic brain injury (TBI). Note compared to the control coronal image on the right, both the TBI case and the Alzheimer's exhibit hippocampal atrophy, ventricular dilation and sulcal widening. **(Bottom)** All images are 3-D renderings from volume acquisition magnetic resonance imaging (MRI) depicting the dorsal view of the brain in each subject described above. Note the similarity of the diffuse pattern of atrophic change that has occurred in both the patient with Alzheimer's disease and the adolescent who survived severe TBI. Clearly, the elderly patient with Alzheimer's has more severe atrophy but nonetheless the atrophy in the TBI adolescent is substantial, especially when compared to the typical developing adolescent control. Note: The patient with Alzheimer's disease is taken from Jacobson et al. (2009); this patient's clinical findings, including additional neuroimaging and neuropsychological details are described in that publication. Reproduced with permission from John Wiley and Sons.

As in the Jack et al. (2013) review, each of the biomarkers associated with the development of Alzheimer's disease, is also associated with biomarkers relevant to TBI; in particular, the deposition of the amyloid-beta (Aβ), neuroimaging based findings of pathology and presence of cognitive impairment. Aβ, tau pathologies, reduced brain volume, and impaired memory are all part of the pathological and clinical picture of TBI *and* age-associated degenerative diseases (Smith et al., 1999; Emmerling et al., 2000; Ikonomovic et al., 2004; Dekosky et al., 2010), creating the potential association between TBI and Alzheimer's disease and related dementias (Sivanandam and Thakur, 2012). In the Jack et al. review, two individuals are shown at the identical time-point—one with low risk for developing dementia, the other with high risk, for example, a prior history of TBI. Given the associations reviewed above, if the high risk individual were someone with a significant TBI who has recovered to some pre-injury baseline, yet had increased burden because of brain atrophy, mildly reduced cognitive ability and various biomarkers of neuronal injury, given this model the TBI individual would be at higher risk for developing dementia.

Smith (2013) reviewed the long-term consequences of microglial activation associated with TBI and summarized the potential findings as shown in **Figure 9**. This diagram uses the cognitive reserve hypothesis (see Bigler, 2007b) that assumes an inexorable yet normal decline in function with age. Although the brain adapts when injured except in cases of severe catastrophic injuries, the individual may never return to baseline and then as depicted in the illustration the adverse effects may be either synergistic or additive. Regardless of the mechanism, having a brain injury shortens the time for when the dementia threshold would be achieved.

A second example comes from the review by Bozzali et al. (2008) on regional and global atrophy that accompanies cognitive decline in degenerative disease, its frontotemporolimbic distribution and a more direct link between having sustained TBI earlier in life and developing a dementing illness (Plassman et al., 2000; Magnoni and Brody, 2010; Esiri and Chance, 2012; Sivanandam and Thakur, 2012; Wang et al., 2012). The implication from these studies and reviews is that overlapping trauma-induced neurodegenerative effects occur within the same frontotemporolimbic areas associated with age-related neurodegenerative disorders. This association between TBI and later onset of dementia may also relate to the selective WM damage that occurs with TBI and the role that WM pathology plays in the expression of dementia via a breakdown in neural connectivity and networks (Carmichael and Salloway, 2012; Shively et al., 2012; Weinstein et al., 2013).

The above discussion focused mostly on a single event, moderate-to-severe TBI, but since mild TBI (mTBI) constitutes the majority of injuries, if mTBI contributes adversely to the aging process, this could be a major public health concern

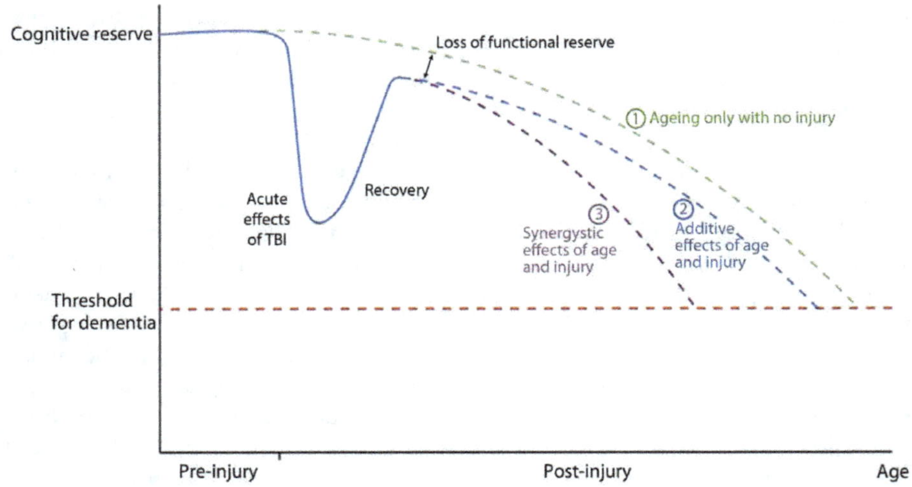

FIGURE 9 | A graphical representation of a postulated cognitive reserve and how head injury may increase the risk of cognitive decline. The broken green line (1) represents the "normal" situation. There is loss of cognitive function with aging until a threshold point is crossed (broken red line) resulting clinically in dementia. After an episode of traumatic brain injury there is a significant decline in cognitive function which recovers, the degree of recovery being dependent on the severity of the head injury. Recovery is, however, not complete resulting in a loss of functional reserve. After this point cognitive decline may be as for normal ageing [broken blue line (2)] with the dementia threshold being crossed earlier due to loss of functional reserve, or there may be a continued synergistic effect of mechanisms initiated by the head injury which accelerates cognitive decline [broken purple line (3)]. Reproduced with permission from John Wiley and Sons and Smith (2013).

(Bazarian et al., 2009). Similarly, multiple concussions or mTBIs are commonplace in some sports (Harmon et al., 2013). Chronic traumatic encephalopathy (CTE) has been demonstrated in athletes with repetitive blows to the head (Victoroff, 2013), yet not necessarily meeting criteria for a clinically diagnosed concussion (McKee et al., 2012). In the largest post-mortem study to date of 85 individuals with CTE, McKee and colleagues have shown that CTE, while it may in some cases be the solitary neuropathological diagnosis, CTE was also associated with cases of Alzheimer's disease, Lewy body disease, frontotemporal lobar degeneration and motor neuron disease. In a subset of American National Football League players who had sustained concussions while playing found that CTE was associated with increased duration of football play and age at time of death. This observation suggests incubation and interactive effect of the prior injury with time and aging effects. McKee et al. (2012) conclude that the association of CTE "... with other neurodegenerative disorders suggests that repetitive brain trauma and hyperphosphorylated tau protein deposition promote the accumulation of other abnormally aggregated proteins including TAR DNA-binding protein 43, amyloid beta protein and alpha-synuclein (p. 43)." Dementia pugilistica has been diagnosed in as high as 20% of retired boxers and may have its onset long after the last boxing match (Kokjohn et al., 2013).

Lehman et al. (2012) found in retired National Football League (NFL) players, a rate of death associated with a neurodegenerative disorder 3 times higher than the general U.S. population. Hart et al. (2013) have also shown in aging, retired NFL players that WM pathology in DTI analyses is related to cognitive dysfunction and depression. While the Plassman et al. (2000) study (which verified presence of TBI in the medical record) reported a positive relationship between prior brain injury and development of dementia, some studies that include self-report of prior TBI do not (Dams-O'Connor et al., 2012). The issue is likely complicated because in the Plassman et al. study, when the mild TBI subjects were assessed independently, as a group they did not have a significantly increased hazard ratio for developing dementia. Returning to the model offered by Jack et al. (2013) and shown in **Figure 8**, those within the mild end of the TBI spectrum with a single head injury would likely have the least risk. Since mTBI constitutes the majority of those with brain injury, the high presence of mTBI with potentially minimal risk factors may be an explanation why some studies do not find an association. Using a retrospective cohort design with documented TBI, Wang et al. (2012) did demonstrate an increased risk for dementia. Sayed et al. (2013) examined a large cohort of individuals with TBI from the National Alzheimer's Coordinating Center Uniform Data set and observed that those with chronic cognitive deficit were those who met criteria for developing dementia. The Sayed et al. study may show that TBI alone may be insufficient to develop dementia, but TBI plus risk factors as outlined in **Figure 9**, reproduced from Smith (2013), such as residual cognitive impairment may be the combination needed for the transition from recovered but not demented to developing dementia post-injury.

Currently, all of the degenerative disorders including CTE require post-mortem confirmation, but ante-mortem neuroimaging studies may provide important insights into how brain injury interacts with the aging process and the development of late neuropathological sequelae. Koerte et al. (2012a,b) have shown DTI changes in athletes, even without symptomatic concussion. What it means to have abnormal

DTI findings in the athlete with a history of concussive or sub-concussive blows to the head is not known at this time, but raises the specter of potential later-in-life reduced brain reserve capacity and increased vulnerability for neuropsychiatric disorder (Bigler et al., 2013).

Recently, Bailey et al. (2012) demonstrated in relatively young professional boxers (~28 years of age) that impaired cerebral hemodynamic function related to history and intensity of sparring and reduced neuropsychological performance. More than three decades after their last concussion, Tremblay et al. (2013) examined athletes with a history of prior concussion compared to those without. Athletes with prior concussions had abnormally enlarged ventricular size, cortical thinning in regions more vulnerable to the aging process and diminished episodic memory and verbal fluency compared to age matched athletes without prior history of concussion, yet demographically matched. Gardner et al. (2012) review the literature on sport-related concussions and DTI showing residuals in terms of WM damage even in this mild end of the TBI spectrum. In a within-subject prospective design, Toth et al. (2013) have shown a statistically significant subtle loss of brain volume by 1 month post injury in mTBI, where TBV was reduced by 1% and ventricular volume increased by 3.4%. However, without pre-injury baseline imaging, what role inflammation may have played in this is not known. These observations indicate that even mild injuries have the potential to initiate a cascade of neuropathological events that influence ageing and the potential to develop a neurodegenerative disorder. Complex genetic (Toth et al., 2013) factors are also likely related to how even mild injury influences outcome and the risk for late in life dementia (Ponsford et al., 2011; Schipper, 2011).

Finally, neuroinflammation specific to WM may play a role in the progression of degenerative brain changes for months to years' post-injury (Smith et al., 2012; Bigler, 2013; Johnson et al., 2013). There may be differential effects of WM inflammatory reactions between child and adult brain injury (Mayer et al., 2012) and DTI may provide a method for *in vivo* tracking of these changes (Voelbel et al., 2012).

SUMMARY

Directly related to the effects of trauma and its severity, TBI may induce widespread neuronal loss and disrupted WM connectivity as part of the primary and secondary effects of the injury along with injury-initiated neuroinflammation and neurodegeneration. Thus, TBI, especially toward the severe end of the spectrum, becomes a major risk factor for untoward effects later in life by reducing brain reserve capacities and diminished neuroplasticity to offset age-mediated decline. In fact, TBI may initiate an adverse synergistic effect with aging to predispose the earlier development of neuropsychiatric symptoms and age-related neurodegenerative diseases in the brain injured individual.

REFERENCES

Adams, J. H., Jennett, B., Murray, L. S., Teasdale, G. M., Gennarelli, T. A., and Graham, D. I. (2011). Neuropathological findings in disabled survivors of a head injury. *J. Neurotrauma* 28, 701–709. doi: 10.1089/neu.2010.1733

American Psychiatric Association. (2013). *Diagnostic and Statistical Manual of Mental Disorders (DSM-5), 5th Edn.* Washington, DC: American Psychiatric Publishing.

Amor, S., Puentes, F., Baker, D., and van der Valk, P. (2010). Inflammation in neurodegenerative diseases. *Immunology* 129, 154–169. doi: 10.1111/j.1365-2567.2009.03225.x

Aoki, Y., Inokuchi, R., Gunshin, M., Yahagi, N., and Suwa, H. (2012). Diffusion tensor imaging studies of mild traumatic brain injury: a meta-analysis. *J. Neurol. Neurosurg. Psychiatry* 83, 870–876. doi: 10.1136/jnnp-2012-302742

Apostolova, L. G., Green, A. E., Babakchanian, S., Hwang, K. S., Chou, Y. Y., Toga, A. W., et al. (2012). Hippocampal atrophy and ventricular enlargement in normal aging, mild cognitive impairment (MCI), and Alzheimer disease. *Alzheimer Dis. Assoc. Disord.* 26, 17–27. doi: 10.1097/WAD.0b013e3182163b62

Bailey, D. M., Jones, D. W., Sinnott, A., Brugniaux, J. V., New, K. J., Hodson, D., et al. (2012). Impaired cerebral haemodynamic function associated with chronic traumatic brain injury in professional boxers. *Clin. Sci. (Lond.)* 124, 177–189. doi: 10.1042/CS20120259

Bazarian, J. J., Cernak, I., Noble-Haeusslein, L., Potolicchio, S., and Temkin, N. (2009). Long-term neurologic outcomes after traumatic brain injury. *J. Head Trauma Rehabil.* 24, 439–451. doi: 10.1097/HTR.0b013e3181c15600

Beauchamp, M. H., Ditchfield, M., Catroppa, C., Kean, M., Godfrey, C., Rosenfeld, J. V., et al. (2011). Focal thinning of the posterior corpus callosum: normal variant or post-traumatic? *Brain Inj.* 25, 950–957. doi: 10.3109/02699052.2011.589791

Bendlin, B. B., Ries, M. L., Lazar, M., Alexander, A. L., Dempsey, R. J., Rowley, H. A., et al. (2008). Longitudinal changes in patients with traumatic brain injury assessed with diffusion-tensor and volumetric imaging. *Neuroimage* 42, 503–514. doi: 10.1016/j.neuroimage.2008.04.254

Bigler, E. D. (2007a). Anterior and middle cranial fossa in traumatic brain injury: relevant neuroanatomy and neuropathology in the study of neuropsychological outcome. *Neuropsychology* 21, 515–531. doi: 10.1037/0894-4105.21.5.515

Bigler, E. D. (2007b). "Traumatic brain injury and cognitive reserve," in *Cognitive Reserve: Theory and Applications*, ed Y. Stern (New York, NY: Taylor and Francis), 85–116.

Bigler, E. D. (2008). Neuropsychology and clinical neuroscience of persistent post-concussive syndrome. *J. Int. Neuropsychol. Soc.* 14, 1–22. doi: 10.1017/S135561770808017X

Bigler, E. D. (2009). "Traumatic brain injury," in *Textbook of Alzheimer Disease and Other Dementias*, eds M. F. Weiner and A. M. Lipton (Washington, DC: The American Psychiatric Publishing, Inc.), 229–246.

Bigler, E. D. (2013). Neuroinflammation and the dynamic lesion in traumatic brain injury. *Brain* 136, 9–11. doi: 10.1093/brain/aws342

Bigler, E. D., Deibert, E., and Filley, C. M. (2013). When is a concussion no longer a concussion? *Neurology* 81, 14–15. doi: 10.1212/WNL.0b013e318299cd0e

Bigler, E. D., and Maxwell, W. L. (2011). Neuroimaging and neuropathology of TBI. *NeuroRehabilitation* 28, 63–74. doi: 10.3233/NRE-2011-0633

Bigler, E. D., and Maxwell, W. L. (2012). Neuropathology of mild traumatic brain injury: relationship to neuroimaging findings. *Brain Imaging Behav.* 6, 108–136. doi: 10.1007/s11682-011-9145-0

Bigler, E. D., McCauley, S. R., Wu, T. C., Yallampalli, R., Shah, S., MacLeod, M., et al. (2010). The temporal stem in traumatic brain injury: preliminary findings. *Brain Imaging Behav.* 4, 270–282. doi: 10.1007/s11682-010-9105-0

Bigler, E. D., Neeley, E. S., Miller, M. J., Tate, D. F., Rice, S. A., Cleavinger, H., et al. (2004). Cerebral volume loss, cognitive deficit and neuropsychological performance: comparative measures of brain atrophy: I. Dementia. *J. Int. Neuropsychol. Soc.* 10, 442–452. doi: 10.1017/S1355617704103111

Bigler, E. D., Ryser, D. K., Gandhi, P., Kimball, J., and Wilde, E. A. (2006). Day-of-injury computerized tomography, rehabilitation status, and development of cerebral atrophy in persons with traumatic brain injury. *Am. J. Phys. Med. Rehabil.* 85, 793–806. doi: 10.1097/01.phm.0000237873.26250.e1

Bigler, E. D., and Tate, D. F. (2001). Brain volume, intracranial volume, and dementia. *Invest. Radiol.* 36, 539–546. doi: 10.1097/00004424-200109000-00006

Blatter, D. D., Bigler, E. D., Gale, S. D., Johnson, S. C., Anderson, C. V., Burnett, B. M., et al. (1995). Quantitative volumetric analysis of brain MR: normative database spanning 5 decades of life. *AJNR Am. J. Neuroradiol.* 16, 241–251.

Blatter, D. D., Bigler, E. D., Gale, S. D., Johnson, S. C., Anderson, C. V., Burnett, B. M., et al. (1997). MR-based brain and cerebrospinal fluid measurement after traumatic brain injury: correlation with neuropsychological outcome. *AJNR Am. J. Neuroradiol.* 18, 1–10.

Blennow, K., Hardy, J., and Zetterberg, H. (2012). The neuropathology and neurobiology of traumatic brain injury. *Neuron* 76, 886–899. doi: 10.1016/j.neuron.2012.11.021

Bonnelle, V., Ham, T. E., Leech, R., Kinnunen, K. M., Mehta, M. A., Greenwood, R. J., et al. (2012). Salience network integrity predicts default mode network function after traumatic brain injury. *Proc. Natl. Acad. Sci. U.S.A.* 109, 4690–4695. doi: 10.1073/pnas.1113455109

Bozzali, M., Cercignani, M., and Caltagirone, C. (2008). Brain volumetrics to investigate aging and the principal forms of degenerative cognitive decline: a brief review. *Magn. Reson. Imaging* 26, 1065–1070. doi: 10.1016/j.mri.2008.01.044

Bramlett, H. M., and Dietrich, W. D. (2007). Progressive damage after brain and spinal cord injury: pathomechanisms and treatment strategies. *Prog. Brain Res.* 161, 125–141. doi: 10.1016/S0079-6123(06)61009-1

Budde, M. D., and Frank, J. A. (2012). Examining brain microstructure using structure tensor analysis of histological sections. *Neuroimage* 63, 1–10. doi: 10.1016/j.neuroimage.2012.06.042

Budde, M. D., Janes, L., Gold, E., Turtzo, L. C., and Frank, J. A. (2011). The contribution of gliosis to diffusion tensor anisotropy and tractography following traumatic brain injury: validation in the rat using Fourier analysis of stained tissue sections. *Brain* 134, 2248–2260. doi: 10.1093/brain/awr161

Caeyenberghs, K., Leemans, A., Heitger, M. H., Leunissen, I., Dhollander, T., Sunaert, S., et al. (2012). Graph analysis of functional brain networks for cognitive control of action in traumatic brain injury. *Brain* 135, 1293–1307. doi: 10.1093/brain/aws048

Carlson, N. E., Moore, M. M., Dame, A., Howieson, D., Silbert, L. C., Quinn, J. F., et al. (2008). Trajectories of brain loss in aging and the development of cognitive impairment. *Neurology* 70, 828–833. doi: 10.1212/01.wnl.0000280577.43413.d9

Carmichael, O. T., Kuller, L. H., Lopez, O. L., Thompson, P. M., Dutton, R. A., Lu, A., et al. (2007). Cerebral ventricular changes associated with transitions between normal cognitive function, mild cognitive impairment, and dementia. *Alzheimer Dis. Assoc. Disord.* 21, 14–24. doi: 10.1097/WAD.0b013e318032d2b1

Carmichael, O. T., and Salloway, S. (2012). Imaging markers of incipient dementia: the white matter matters. *Neurology* 79, 726–727. doi: 10.1212/WNL.0b013e3182662020

Chang, K., Barnea-Goraly, N., Karchemskiy, A., Simeonova, D. I., Barnes, P., Ketter, T., et al. (2005). Cortical magnetic resonance imaging findings in familial pediatric bipolar disorder. *Biol. Psychiatry* 58, 197–203. doi: 10.1016/j.biopsych.2005.03.039

Chen, Z., Leung, L. Y., Mountney, A., Liao, Z., Yang, W., Lu, X. C., et al. (2012). A novel animal model of closed-head concussive-induced mild traumatic brain injury: development, implementation, and characterization. *J. Neurotrauma* 29, 268–280. doi: 10.1089/neu.2011.2057

Courchesne, E., Chisum, H. J., Townsend, J., Cowles, A., Covington, J., Egaas, B., et al. (2000). Normal brain development and aging: quantitative analysis at *in vivo* MR imaging in healthy volunteers. *Radiology* 216, 672–682.

Cullen, D. K., Vernekar, V. N., and Laplaca, M. C. (2011). Trauma-induced plasmalemma disruptions in three-dimensional neural cultures are dependent on strain modality and rate. *J. Neurotrauma* 28, 2219–2233. doi: 10.1089/neu.2011.1841

Dams-O'Connor, K., Gibbons, L. E., Bowen, J. D., McCurry, S. M., Larson, E. B., and Crane, P. K. (2012). Risk for late-life re-injury, dementia and death among individuals with traumatic brain injury: a population-based study. *J. Neurol. Neurosurg. Psychiatry* 84, 177–182. doi: 10.1136/jnnp-2012-303938

Dekosky, S. T., Ikonomovic, M. D., and Gandy, S. (2010). Traumatic brain injury–football, warfare, and long-term effects. *N. Engl. J. Med.* 363, 1293–1296. doi: 10.1056/NEJMp1007051

Deng, P., and Xu, Z. C. (2011). Contribution of Ih to neuronal damage in the hippocampus after traumatic brain injury in rats. *J. Neurotrauma* 28, 1173–1183. doi: 10.1089/neu.2010.1683

Diaz-Arrastia, R., Agostini, M. A., Madden, C. J., and Van Ness, P. C. (2009). Posttraumatic epilepsy: the endophenotypes of a human model of epileptogenesis. *Epilepsia* 50(Suppl. 2), 14–20. doi: 10.1111/j.1528-1167.2008.02006.x

Driscoll, I., Zhou, Y., An, Y., Sojkova, J., Davatzikos, C., Kraut, M. A., et al. (2011). Lack of association between 11C-PiB and longitudinal brain atrophy in non-demented older individuals. *Neurobiol. Aging* 32, 2123–2130. doi: 10.1016/j.neurobiolaging.2009.12.008

Emmerling, M. R., Morganti-Kossmann, M. C., Kossmann, T., Stahel, P. F., Watson, M. D., Evans, L. M., et al. (2000). Traumatic brain injury elevates the Alzheimer's amyloid peptide A beta 42 in human CSF. A possible role for nerve cell injury. *Ann. N.Y. Acad. Sci.* 903, 118–122. doi: 10.1111/j.1749-6632.2000.tb06357.x

Esiri, M. M., and Chance, S. A. (2012). Cognitive reserve, cortical plasticity and resistance to Alzheimer's disease. *Alzheimers Res. Ther.* 4, 7. doi: 10.1186/alzrt105

Ewing-Cobbs, L., Prasad, M. R., Swank, P., Kramer, L., Cox, C. S. Jr., Fletcher, J. M., et al. (2008). Arrested development and disrupted callosal microstructure following pediatric traumatic brain injury: relation to neurobehavioral outcomes. *Neuroimage* 42, 1305–1315. doi: 10.1016/j.neuroimage.2008.06.031

Farbota, K. D., Bendlin, B. B., Alexander, A. L., Rowley, H. A., Dempsey, R. J., and Johnson, S. C. (2012). Longitudinal diffusion tensor imaging and neuropsychological correlates in traumatic brain injury patients. *Front. Hum. Neurosci.* 6:160. doi: 10.3389/fnhum.2012.00160

Foley, L. M., Iqbal O'Meara, A. M., Wisniewski, S. R., Kevin Hitchens, T., Melick, J. A., Ho, C., et al. (2013). MRI assessment of cerebral blood flow after experimental traumatic brain injury combined with hemorrhagic shock in mice. *J. Cereb. Blood Flow Metab.* 33, 129–136. doi: 10.1038/jcbfm.2012.145

Galanaud, D., Perlbarg, V., Gupta, R., Stevens, R. D., Sanchez, P., Tollard, E., et al. (2012). Assessment of white matter injury and outcome in severe brain trauma: a prospective multicenter cohort. *Anesthesiology* 117, 1300–1310. doi: 10.1097/ALN.0b013e3182755558

Gale, S. D., Johnson, S. C., Bigler, E. D., and Blatter, D. D. (1995). Trauma-induced degenerative changes in brain injury: a morphometric analysis of three patients with preinjury and postinjury MR scans. *J. Neurotrauma* 12, 151–158. doi: 10.1089/neu.1995.12.151

Gardner, A., Kay-Lambkin, F., Stanwell, P., Donnelly, J., Williams, W. H., Hiles, A., et al. (2012). A systematic review of diffusion tensor imaging findings in sports-related concussion. *J. Neurotrauma* 29, 2521–2538. doi: 10.1089/neu.2012.2628

Ge, Y., Grossman, R. I., Babb, J. S., Rabin, M. L., Mannon, L. J., and Kolson, D. L. (2002). Age-related total gray matter and white matter changes in normal adult brain. Part I: volumetric MR imaging analysis. *AJNR Am. J. Neuroradiol.* 23, 1327–1333.

Ghosh, A., Wilde, E. A., Hunter, J. V., Bigler, E. D., Chu, Z., Li, X., et al. (2009). The relation between Glasgow Coma Scale score and later cerebral atrophy in paediatric traumatic brain injury. *Brain Inj.* 23, 228–233. doi: 10.1080/02699050802672789

Goh, J. O., and Park, D. C. (2009). Neuroplasticity and cognitive aging: the scaffolding theory of aging and cognition. *Restor. Neurol. Neurosci.* 27, 391–403. doi: 10.3233/RNN-2009-0493

Greenberg, G., Mikulis, D. J., Ng, K., Desouza, D., and Green, R. E. (2008). Use of diffusion tensor imaging to examine subacute white matter injury progression in moderate to severe traumatic brain injury. *Arch. Phys. Med. Rehabil.* 89, S45–S50. doi: 10.1016/j.apmr.2008.08.211

Gunther, M. L., Morandi, A., Krauskopf, E., Pandharipande, P., Girard, T. D., Jackson, J. C., et al. (2012). The association between brain volumes, delirium duration, and cognitive outcomes in intensive care unit survivors: the VISIONS cohort magnetic resonance imaging study*. *Crit. Care Med.* 40, 2022–2032. doi: 10.1097/CCM.0b013e318250acc0

Harmon, K. G., Drezner, J. A., Gammons, M., Guskiewicz, K. M., Halstead, M., Herring, S. A., et al. (2013). American Medical

Society for Sports Medicine position statement: concussion in sport. *Br. J. Sports Med.* 47, 15–26. doi: 10.1136/bjsports-2012-091941

Harrison, D. M., Caffo, B. S., Shiee, N., Farrell, J. A., Bazin, P. L., Farrell, S. K., et al. (2011). Longitudinal changes in diffusion tensor-based quantitative MRI in multiple sclerosis. *Neurology* 76, 179–186. doi: 10.1212/WNL.0b013e318206ca61

Harrison, D. M., Shiee, N., Bazin, P. L., Newsome, S. D., Ratchford, J. N., Pham, D., et al. (2013). Tract-specific quantitative MRI better correlates with disability than conventional MRI in multiple sclerosis. *J. Neurol.* 260, 397–406. doi: 10.1007/s00415-012-6638-8

Hart, J., Kraut, M. A., Womack, K. B., Strain, J., Didehbani, N., Bartz, E., et al. (2013). Neuroimaging of cognitive dysfunction and depression in aging retired National Football League players: a cross-sectional study. *JAMA Neurol.* 70, 326–335. doi: 10.1001/2013.jamaneurol.340

Hedman, A. M., van Haren, N. E., Schnack, H. G., Kahn, R. S., and Hulshoff Pol, H. E. (2011). Human brain changes across the life span: a review of 56 longitudinal magnetic resonance imaging studies. *Hum. Brain Mapp.* 33, 1987–2002. doi: 10.1002/hbm.21334

Hodges, J. R. (2012). Alzheimer's disease and the frontotemporal dementias: contributions to clinico-pathological studies, diagnosis, and cognitive neuroscience. *J. Alzheimers Dis.* 33(Suppl. 1), S211–S217. doi: 10.3233/JAD-2012-129038

Ikonomovic, M. D., Uryu, K., Abrahamson, E. E., Ciallella, J. R., Trojanowski, J. Q., Lee, V. M., et al. (2004). Alzheimer's pathology in human temporal cortex surgically excised after severe brain injury. *Exp. Neurol.* 190, 192–203. doi: 10.1016/j.expneurol.2004.06.011

Immonen, R. J., Kharatishvili, I., Niskanen, J. P., Grohn, H., Pitkanen, A., and Grohn, O. H. (2009). Distinct MRI pattern in lesional and perilesional area after traumatic brain injury in rat–11 months follow-up. *Exp. Neurol.* 215, 29–40. doi: 10.1016/j.expneurol.2008.09.009

Inglese, M., and Ge, Y. (2004). Quantitative MRI: hidden age-related changes in brain tissue. *Top. Magn. Reson. Imaging* 15, 355–363. doi: 10.1097/01.rmr.0000168069.12985.15

Irimia, A., Chambers, M. C., Torgerson, C. M., Filippou, M., Hovda, D. A., Alger, J. R., et al. (2012a). Patient-tailored connectomics visualization for the assessment of white matter atrophy in traumatic brain injury. *Front. Neurol.* 3:10. doi: 10.3389/fneur.2012.00010

Irimia, A., Chambers, M. C., Torgerson, C. M., and Van Horn, J. D. (2012b). Circular representation of human cortical networks for subject and population-level connectomic visualization. *Neuroimage* 60, 1340–1351. doi: 10.1016/j.neuroimage.2012.01.107

Jack, C. R. Jr., Knopman, D. S., Jagust, W. J., Petersen, R. C., Weiner, M. W., Aisen, P. S., et al. (2013). Tracking pathophysiological processes in Alzheimer's disease: an updated hypothetical model of dynamic biomarkers. *Lancet Neurol.* 12, 207–216. doi: 10.1016/S1474-4422(12)70291-0

Jacobson, M. W., Delis, D. C., Peavy, G. M., Wetter, S. R., Bigler, E. D., Abildskov, T. J., et al. (2009). The emergence of cognitive discrepancies in preclinical Alzheimer's disease: a six-year case study. *Neurocase* 15, 278–293. doi: 10.1080/13554790902729465

Johnson, V. E., Stewart, J. E., Begbie, F. D., Trojanowski, J. Q., Smith, D. H., and Stewart, W. (2013). Inflamation and white matter degeneration persist for years after a single traumatic brain injury. *Brain* 136, 28–42.

Johnson, V. E., Stewart, W., and Smith, D. H. (2012). Axonal pathology in traumatic brain injury. *Exp. Neurol.* 246, 35–43. doi: 10.1016/j.expneurol.2012.01.013

Johnson, V. E., Stewart, W., Trojanowski, J. Q., and Smith, D. H. (2011). Acute and chronically increased immunoreactivity to phosphorylation-independent but not pathological TDP-43 after a single traumatic brain injury in humans. *Acta Neuropathol.* 122, 715–726. doi: 10.1007/s00401-011-0909-9

Kempton, M. J., Geddes, J. R., Ettinger, U., Williams, S. C., and Grasby, P. M. (2008). Meta-analysis, database, and meta-regression of 98 structural imaging studies in bipolar disorder. *Arch. Gen. Psychiatry* 65, 1017–1032. doi: 10.1001/archpsyc.65.9.1017

Kim, J., Avants, B., Patel, S., Whyte, J., Coslett, B. H., Pluta, J., et al. (2008). Structural consequences of diffuse traumatic brain injury: a large deformation tensor-based morphometry study. *Neuroimage* 39, 1014–1026. doi: 10.1016/j.neuroimage.2007.10.005

Koerte, I. K., Ertl-Wagner, B., Reiser, M., Zafonte, R., and Shenton, M. E. (2012a). White matter integrity in the brains of professional soccer players without a symptomatic concussion. *JAMA* 308, 1859–1861. doi: 10.1001/jama.2012.13735

Koerte, I. K., Kaufmann, D., Hartl, E., Bouix, S., Pasternak, O., Kubicki, M., et al. (2012b). A prospective study of physician-observed concussion during a varsity university hockey season: white matter integrity in ice hockey players. Part 3 of 4. *Neurosurg. Focus* 33, E3. doi: 10.3171/2012.10.FOCUS12303

Kokjohn, T. A., Maarouf, C. L., Daugs, I. D., Hunter, J. M., Whiteside, C. M., Malek-Ahmadi, M., et al. (2013). Neurochemical profile of dementia pugilistica. *J. Neurotrauma* 30, 981–997. doi: 10.1089/neu.2012.2699

Lainhart, J. E., Bigler, E. D., Bocian, M., Coon, H., Dinh, E., Dawson, G., et al. (2006). Head circumference and height in autism: a study by the Collaborative Program of Excellence in Autism. *Am. J. Med. Genet. A* 140, 2257–2274. doi: 10.1002/ajmg.a.31465

Lehman, E. J., Hein, M. J., Baron, S. L., and Gersic, C. M. (2012). Neurodegenerative causes of death among retired National Football League players. *Neurology* 79, 1970–1974. doi: 10.1212/WNL.0b013e31826daf50

Levin, H., and Smith, D. (2013). Traumatic brain injury: networks and neuropathology. *Lancet Neurol.* 12, 15–16. doi: 10.1016/S1474-4422(12)70300-9

Lifshitz, J., Kelley, B. J., and Povlishock, J. T. (2007). Perisomatic thalamic axotomy after diffuse traumatic brain injury is associated with atrophy rather than cell death. *J. Neuropathol. Exp. Neurol.* 66, 218–229. doi: 10.1097/01.jnen.0000248558.75950.4d

Liu, C. Y., Krishnan, A. P., Yan, L., Smith, R. X., Kilroy, E., Alger, J. R., et al. (2013). Complexity and synchronicity of resting state blood oxygenation level-dependent (BOLD) functional MRI in normal aging and cognitive decline. *J. Magn. Reson. Imaging* 38, 36–45. doi: 10.1002/jmri.23961

Lucas, S. M., Rothwell, N. J., and Gibson, R. M. (2006). The role of inflammation in CNS injury and disease. *Br. J. Pharmacol.* 147(Suppl. 1), S232–S240. doi: 10.1038/sj.bjp.0706400

Magnoni, S., and Brody, D. L. (2010). New perspectives on amyloid-beta dynamics after acute brain injury: moving between experimental approaches and studies in the human brain. *Arch. Neurol.* 67, 1068–1073. doi: 10.1001/archneurol.2010.214

Marquez de la Plata, C. D., Garces, J., Shokri Kojori, E., Grinnan, J., Krishnan, K., Pidikiti, R., et al. (2011). Deficits in functional connectivity of hippocampal and frontal lobe circuits after traumatic axonal injury. *Arch. Neurol.* 68, 74–84. doi: 10.1001/archneurol.2010.342

Maxwell, W. L., MacKinnon, M. A., Stewart, J. E., and Graham, D. I. (2010). Stereology of cerebral cortex after traumatic brain injury matched to the Glasgow outcome score. *Brain* 133, 139–160. doi: 10.1093/brain/awp264

Mayer, A. R., Ling, J. M., Yang, Z., Pena, A., Yeo, R. A., and Klimaj, S. (2012). Diffusion abnormalities in pediatric mild traumatic brain injury. *J. Neurosci.* 32, 17961–17969. doi: 10.1523/JNEUROSCI.3379-12.2012

McAllister, T. W. (2011). Neurobiological consequences of traumatic brain injury. *Dialogues Clin. Neurosci.* 13, 287–300.

McAllister, T. W., Ford, J. C., Ji, S., Beckwith, J. G., Flashman, L. A., Paulsen, K., et al. (2012). Maximum principal strain and strain rate associated with concussion diagnosis correlates with changes in corpus callosum white matter indices. *Ann. Biomed. Eng.* 40, 127–140. doi: 10.1007/s10439-011-0402-6

McKee, A. C., Stein, T. D., Nowinski, C. J., Stern, R. A., Daneshvar, D. H., Alvarez, V. E., et al. (2012). The spectrum of disease in chronic traumatic encephalopathy. *Brain* 136, 43–64.

Moretti, L., Cristofori, I., Weaver, S. M., Chau, A., Portelli, J. N., and Grafman, J. (2012). Cognitive decline in older adults with a history of traumatic brain injury. *Lancet Neurol.* 11, 1103–1112. doi: 10.1016/S1474-4422(12)70226-0

Morra, J. H., Tu, Z., Apostolova, L. G., Green, A. E., Avedissian, C., Madsen, S. K., et al. (2009). Automated 3D mapping of hippocampal atrophy and its clinical correlates in 400 subjects with Alzheimer's disease, mild cognitive impairment, and elderly controls. *Hum. Brain Mapp.* 30, 2766–2788. doi: 10.1002/hbm.20708

Ng, K., Mikulis, D. J., Glazer, J., Kabani, N., Till, C., Greenberg, G., et al. (2008). Magnetic resonance imaging evidence of progression of subacute brain atrophy in moderate to severe traumatic brain injury. *Arch. Phys. Med. Rehabil.* 89,

S35–S44. doi: 10.1016/j.apmr.2008.07.006

Okonkwo, O. C., Alosco, M. L., Jerskey, B. A., Sweet, L. H., Ott, B. R., and Tremont, G. (2010). Cerebral atrophy, apolipoprotein E varepsilon4, and rate of decline in everyday function among patients with amnestic mild cognitive impairment. *Alzheimers Dement.* 6, 404–411. doi: 10.1016/j.jalz.2010.02.003

Olesen, P. J., Guo, X., Gustafson, D., Borjesson-Hanson, A., Sacuiu, S., Eckerstrom, C., et al. (2011). A population-based study on the influence of brain atrophy on 20-year survival after age 85. *Neurology* 76, 879–886. doi: 10.1212/WNL.0b013e31820f2e26

Palacios, E. M., Sala-Llonch, R., Junque, C., Roig, T., Tormos, J. M., Bargallo, N., et al. (2012). White matter integrity related to functional working memory networks in traumatic brain injury. *Neurology* 78, 852–860. doi: 10.1212/WNL.0b013e31824c465a

Palacios, E. M., Sala-Llonch, R., Junque, C., Fernandez-Espejo, D., Roig, T., Tormos, J. M., et al. (2013). Long-term declarative memory deficits in diffuse TBI: correlations with cortical thickness, white matter integrity and hippocampal volume. *Cortex* 49, 646–657. doi: 10.1016/j.cortex.2012.02.011

Pandit, A. S., Expert, P., Lambiotte, R., Bonnelle, V., Leech, R., Turkheimer, F. E., et al. (2013). Traumatic brain injury impairs small-world topology. *Neurology* 80, 1826–1833. doi: 10.1212/WNL.0b013e3182929f38

Pitkanen, A., Tuunanen, J., Kalviainen, R., Partanen, K., and Salmenpera, T. (1998). Amygdala damage in experimental and human temporal lobe epilepsy. *Epilepsy Res.* 32, 233–253. doi: 10.1016/S0920-1211(98)00055-2

Plassman, B. L., Havlik, R. J., Steffens, D. C., Helms, M. J., Newman, T. N., Drosdick, D., et al. (2000). Documented head injury in early adulthood and risk of Alzheimer's disease and other dementias. *Neurology* 55, 1158–1166. doi: 10.1212/WNL.55.8.1158

Ponsford, J., McLaren, A., Schonberger, M., Burke, R., Rudzki, D., Olver, J., et al. (2011). The association between apolipoprotein E and traumatic brain injury severity and functional outcome in a rehabilitation sample. *J. Neurotrauma* 28, 1683–1692. doi: 10.1089/neu.2010.1623

Price, C. C., Mitchell, S. M., Brumback, B., Tanner, J. J., Schmalfuss, I., Lamar, M., et al. (2012). MRI-leukoaraiosis thresholds and the phenotypic expression of dementia. *Neurology* 79, 734–740. doi: 10.1212/WNL.0b013e3182661ef6

Purohit, D. P., Batheja, N. O., Sano, M., Jashnani, K. D., Kalaria, R. N., Karunamurthy, A., et al. (2011). Profiles of Alzheimer's disease-related pathology in an aging urban population sample in India. *J. Alzheimers Dis.* 24, 187–196. doi: 10.3233/JAD-2010-101698

Ramlackhansingh, A. F., Brooks, D. J., Greenwood, R. J., Bose, S. K., Turkheimer, F. E., Kinnunen, K. M., et al. (2011). Inflammation after trauma: microglial activation and traumatic brain injury. *Ann. Neurol.* 70, 374–383. doi: 10.1002/ana.22455

Raymont, V., Salazar, A. M., Lipsky, R., Goldman, D., Tasick, G., and Grafman, J. (2010). Correlates of posttraumatic epilepsy 35 years following combat brain injury. *Neurology* 75, 224–229. doi: 10.1212/WNL.0b013e3181e8e6d0

Rosazza, C., and Minati, L. (2011). Resting-state brain networks: literature review and clinical applications. *Neurol. Sci.* 32, 773–785. doi: 10.1007/s10072-011-0636-y

Rowson, S., Duma, S. M., Beckwith, J. G., Chu, J. J., Greenwald, R. M., Crisco, J. J., et al. (2012). Rotational head kinematics in football impacts: an injury risk function for concussion. *Ann. Biomed. Eng.* 40, 1–13. doi: 10.1007/s10439-011-0392-4

Rubia, K. (2012). Functional brain imaging across development. *Eur. Child Adolesc. Psychiatry.* doi: 10.1007/s00787-012-0291-8. [Epub ahead of print].

Sayed, N., Culver, C., Dams-O'Connor, K., Hammond, F., and Diaz-Arrastia, R. (2013). Clinical phenotype of dementia after traumatic brain injury. *J. Neurotrauma* 30, 1117–1120. doi: 10.1089/neu.2012.2638

Schipper, H. M. (2011). Apolipoprotein E: implications for AD neurobiology, epidemiology and risk assessment. *Neurobiol. Aging* 32, 778–790. doi: 10.1016/j.neurobiolaging.2009.04.021

Shi, Y., Short, S. J., Knickmeyer, R. C., Wang, J., Coe, C. L., Niethammer, M., et al. (2012). Diffusion tensor imaging-based characterization of brain neurodevelopment in primates. *Cereb. Cortex* 23, 36–48. doi: 10.1093/cercor/bhr372

Shively, S., Scher, A. I., Perl, D. P., and Diaz-Arrastia, R. (2012). Dementia resulting from traumatic brain injury: what is the pathology? *Arch. Neurol.* 69, 1245–1251.

Sidaros, A., Engberg, A. W., Sidaros, K., Liptrot, M. G., Herning, M., Petersen, P., et al. (2008). Diffusion tensor imaging during recovery from severe traumatic brain injury and relation to clinical outcome: a longitudinal study. *Brain* 131, 559–572. doi: 10.1093/brain/awm294

Sidaros, A., Skimminge, A., Liptrot, M. G., Sidaros, K., Engberg, A. W., Herning, M., et al. (2009). Long-term global and regional brain volume changes following severe traumatic brain injury: a longitudinal study with clinical correlates. *Neuroimage* 44, 1–8. doi: 10.1016/j.neuroimage.2008.08.030

Silbert, L. C., Dodge, H. H., Perkins, L. G., Sherbakov, L., Lahna, D., Erten-Lyons, D., et al. (2012). Trajectory of white matter hyperintensity burden preceding mild cognitive impairment. *Neurology* 79, 741–747. doi: 10.1212/WNL.0b013e3182661f2b

Sivanandam, T. M., and Thakur, M. K. (2012). Traumatic brain injury: a risk factor for Alzheimer's disease. *Neurosci. Biobehav. Rev.* 36, 1376–1381. doi: 10.1016/j.neubiorev.2012.02.013

Skoog, I., Olesen, P. J., Blennow, K., Palmertz, B., Johnson, S. C., and Bigler, E. D. (2012). Head size may modify the impact of white matter lesions on dementia. *Neurobiol. Aging* 33, 1186–1193. doi: 10.1016/j.neurobiolaging.2011.01.011

Smith, C. (2013). Review: the long-term consequences of microglial activation following acute traumatic brain injury. *Neuropathol. Appl. Neurobiol.* 39, 35–44. doi: 10.1111/nan.12006

Smith, C., Gentleman, S. M., Leclercq, P. D., Murray, L. S., Griffin, W. S., Graham, D. I., et al. (2012). The neuroinflammatory response in humans after traumatic brain injury. *Neuropathol. Appl. Neurobiol.* doi: 10.1111/nan.12008. [Epub ahead of print].

Smith, D. H., Chen, X. H., Nonaka, M., Trojanowski, J. Q., Lee, V. M., Saatman, K. E., et al. (1999). Accumulation of amyloid beta and tau and the formation of neurofilament inclusions following diffuse brain injury in the pig. *J. Neuropathol. Exp. Neurol.* 58, 982–992. doi: 10.1097/00005072-199909000-00008

Smith, D. H., Chen, X. H., Pierce, J. E., Wolf, J. A., Trojanowski, J. Q., Graham, D. I., et al. (1997). Progressive atrophy and neuron death for one year following brain trauma in the rat. *J. Neurotrauma* 14, 715–727. doi: 10.1089/neu.1997.14.715

Sperling, R. A., Aisen, P. S., Beckett, L. A., Bennett, D. A., Craft, S., Fagan, A. M., et al. (2011). Toward defining the preclinical stages of Alzheimer's disease: recommendations from the National Institute on Aging-Alzheimer's Association workgroups on diagnostic guidelines for Alzheimer's disease. *Alzheimers Dement.* 7, 280–292. doi: 10.1016/j.jalz.2011.03.003

Steffener, J., Habeck, C. G., and Stern, Y. (2012). Age-related changes in task related functional network connectivity. *PLoS ONE* 7:e44421. doi: 10.1371/journal.pone.0044421

Stoica, B. A., and Faden, A. I. (2010). Cell death mechanisms and modulation in traumatic brain injury. *Neurotherapeutics* 7, 3–12. doi: 10.1016/j.nurt.2009.10.023

Tasker, R. C. (2006). Changes in white matter late after severe traumatic brain injury in childhood. *Dev. Neurosci.* 28, 302–308. doi: 10.1159/000094156

Tata, D. A., and Anderson, B. J. (2010). The effects of chronic glucocorticoid exposure on dendritic length, synapse numbers and glial volume in animal models: implications for hippocampal volume reductions in depression. *Physiol. Behav.* 99, 186–193. doi: 10.1016/j.physbeh.2009.09.008

Tate, D. F., Khedraki, R., Neeley, E. S., Ryser, D. K., and Bigler, E. D. (2011). Cerebral volume loss, cognitive deficit, and neuropsychological performance: comparative measures of brain atrophy: II. Traumatic brain injury. *J. Int. Neuropsychol. Soc.* 17, 308–316. doi: 10.1017/S1355617710001670

Tomaiuolo, F., Bivona, U., Lerch, J. P., Di Paola, M., Carlesimo, G. A., Ciurli, P., et al. (2012). Memory and anatomical change in severe non missile traumatic brain injury: approximately 1 vs. approximately 8 years follow-up. *Brain Res. Bull.* 87, 373–382. doi: 10.1016/j.brainresbull.2012.01.008

Toth, A., Kovacs, N., Perlaki, G., Orsi, G., Aradi, M., Komaromy, H., et al. (2013). Multi-modal magnetic resonance imaging in the acute and sub-acute phase of mild traumatic brain injury: can we see the difference? *J. Neurotrauma* 30, 2–10. doi: 10.1089/neu.2012.2486

Tremblay, S., De Beaumont, L., Henry, L. C., Boulanger, Y., Evans, A. C., Bourgouin, P., et al. (2013).

Sports concussions and aging: a neuroimaging investigation. *Cereb. Cortex* 23, 1159–1166. doi: 10.1093/cercor/bhs102

Van Den Heuvel, M. P., and Sporns, O. (2011). Rich-club organization of the human connectome. *J. Neurosci.* 31, 15775–15786. doi: 10.1523/JNEUROSCI.3539-11.2011

Victoroff, J. (2013). Traumatic encephalopathy: review and provisional research diagnostic criteria. *NeuroRehabilitation* 32, 211–224.

Voelbel, G. T., Genova, H. M., Chiaravalotti, N. D., and Hoptman, M. J. (2012). Diffusion tensor imaging of traumatic brain injury review: implications for neurorehabilitation. *NeuroRehabilitation* 31, 281–293.

Wang, H. K., Lin, S. H., Sung, P. S., Wu, M. H., Hung, K. W., Wang, L. C., et al. (2012). Population based study on patients with traumatic brain injury suggests increased risk of dementia. *J. Neurol. Neurosurg. Psychiatry* 83, 1080–1085. doi: 10.1136/jnnp-2012-302633

Wang, J. Y., Bakhadirov, K., Abdi, H., Devous, M. D. Sr., Marquez de la Plata, C. D., Moore, C., et al. (2011). Longitudinal changes of structural connectivity in traumatic axonal injury. *Neurology* 77, 818–826. doi: 10.1212/WNL.0b013e31822c61d7

Weinstein, G., Wolf, P. A., Beiser, A. S., Au, R., and Seshadri, S. (2013). Risk estimations, risk factors, and genetic variants associated with Alzheimer's disease in selected publications from the Framingham Heart Study. *J. Alzheimers Dis.* 33(Suppl 1), S439–S445. doi: 10.3233/JAD-2012-129040

Wilde, E. A., Bigler, E. D., Pedroza, C., and Ryser, D. K. (2006a). Post-traumatic amnesia predicts long-term cerebral atrophy in traumatic brain injury. *Brain Inj.* 20, 695–699. doi: 10.1080/02699050600744079

Wilde, E. A., Chu, Z., Bigler, E. D., Hunter, J. V., Fearing, M. A., Hanten, G., et al. (2006b). Diffusion tensor imaging in the corpus callosum in children after moderate to severe traumatic brain injury. *J. Neurotrauma* 23, 1412–1426. doi: 10.1089/neu.2006.23.1412

Wilde, E. A., Ramos, M. A., Yallampalli, R., Bigler, E. D., McCauley, S. R., Chu, Z., et al. (2010). Diffusion tensor imaging of the cingulum bundle in children after traumatic brain injury. *Dev. Neuropsychol.* 35, 333–351. doi: 10.1080/87565641003696940

Wu, T. C., Wilde, E. A., Bigler, E. D., Li, X., Merkley, T. L., Yallampalli, R., et al. (2010). Longitudinal changes in the corpus callosum following pediatric traumatic brain injury. *Dev. Neurosci.* 32, 361–373.

Xu, Y., McArthur, D. L., Alger, J. R., Etchepare, M., Hovda, D. A., Glenn, T. C., et al. (2010). Early nonischemic oxidative metabolic dysfunction leads to chronic brain atrophy in traumatic brain injury. *J. Cereb. Blood Flow Metab.* 30, 883–894. doi: 10.1038/jcbfm.2009.263

Yallampalli, R., Wilde, E. A., Bigler, E. D., McCauley, S. R., Hanten, G., Troyanskaya, M., et al. (2013). Acute white matter differences in the fornix following mild traumatic brain injury using diffusion tensor imaging. *J. Neuroimaging* 23, 224–227. doi: 10.1111/j.1552-6569.2010.00537.x

Zielinski, B. A., Gennatas, E. D., Zhou, J., and Seeley, W. W. (2010). Network-level structural covariance in the developing brain. *Proc. Natl. Acad. Sci. U.S.A.* 107, 18191–18196. doi: 10.1073/pnas.1003109107

15

MTA index: a simple 2D-method for assessing atrophy of the medial temporal lobe using clinically available neuroimaging

Manuel Menéndez-González[1,2,3]*, Alfonso López-Muñiz[2,3], José A. Vega[2], José M. Salas-Pacheco[4] and Oscar Arias-Carrión[5,6]*

[1] Unidad de Neurología, Hospital Álvarez-Buylla, Mieres, Spain
[2] Departamento de Morfología y Biología Celular, Universidad de Oviedo, Oviedo, Spain
[3] Instituto de Neurociencias, Universidad de Oviedo, Oviedo, Spain
[4] Instituto de Investigación Científica, Universidad Juárez del Estado de Durango, Durango, México
[5] Unidad de Trastornos del Movimiento y Sueño (TMS), Hospital General Dr. Manuel Gea González/UNAM, México DF, Mexico
[6] Unidad de Trastornos del Movimiento y Sueño (TMS), Hospital General Ajusco Medio, México DF, Mexico

Edited by:
Gemma Casadesus, Case Western Reserve University, USA

Reviewed by:
Andrea Bozoki, Michigan State University, USA
Eugenia Rota, Ospedale Guglielmo da Saliceto di Piacenza, Italy

****Correspondence:***
Manuel Menéndez-González, Unidad de Neurología, Hospital Álvarez-Buylla, CP 33616, Mieres, Asturias Spain
e-mail: manuelmenendezgonzalez@gmail.com;
Oscar Arias-Carrión, Unidad de Trastornos del Movimiento y Sueno (TMS), Hospital General Dr. Manuel Gea González, Calzada de Tlalpan 4800, Delegación Tlalpan, 14080 México DF, México
e-mail: arias@ciencias.unam.mx

Background and purpose: Despite a strong correlation to severity of AD pathology, the measurement of medial temporal lobe atrophy (MTA) is not being widely used in daily clinical practice as a criterion in the diagnosis of prodromal and probable AD. This is mainly because the methods available to date are sophisticated and difficult to implement for routine use in most hospitals—volumetric methods—or lack objectivity—visual rating scales. In this pilot study we aim to describe a new, simple and objective method for measuring the rate of MTA in relation to the global atrophy using clinically available neuroimaging and describe the rationale behind this method.

Description: This method consists of calculating a ratio with the area of 3 regions traced manually on one single coronal MRI slide at the level of the interpeduncular fossa: (1) the medial temporal lobe (MTL) region (A); (2) the parenchima within the medial temporal region, that includes the hippocampus and the parahippocampal gyrus—the fimbria taenia and plexus choroideus are excluded—(B); and (3) the body of the ipsilateral lateral ventricle (C). Therefrom we can compute the ratio "Medial Temporal Atrophy index" at both sides as follows: $MTAi = (A - B) \times 10/C$.

Conclusions: The MTAi is a simple 2D-method for measuring the relative extent of atrophy in the MTL in relation to the global brain atrophy. This method can be useful for a more accurate diagnosis of AD in routine clinical practice. Further studies are needed to assess the usefulness of MTAi in the diagnosis of early AD, in tracking the progression of AD and in the differential diagnosis of AD with other dementias.

Keywords: medial temporal lobe atrophy, biomarker, Alzheimer, mild cognitive impairment, MRI, neuroimaging, diagnosis

BACKGROUND

Alzheimer's disease's (AD) pathology accumulates for years and may be even decades before it is typically diagnosed (Morris et al., 1996). Sensitive biomarker techniques may be able to pick up signs of neurodegeneration presymptomatically. Recently proposed criteria for research purposes for prodromal AD (Sperling et al., 2011), mild cognitive impairment (MCI) due to AD (Albert et al., 2011), and probable AD dementia (McKhann et al., 2011) incorporate evidence of AD pathology including molecular changes and brain structure and function as supportive biomarkers. MRI-based biomarkers are among the supportive evidence for a diagnosis of early AD and MCI due to AD. By focusing on cortical regions known to be affected in AD dementia, subtle but reliable atrophy is identifiable in asymptomatic individuals nearly a decade before dementia, making this measure a potentially important imaging biomarker of early diagnosis (Dickerson et al., 2011). Volume losses in the medial temporal lobe (MTL) region—composed by the hippocampus and the parahippocampal gyrus—and posterior cingulated and orbitofrontal regions have been observed in AD and confirmed in many studies (Kesslak et al., 1991; Parnetti et al., 1996; Smith and Jobst, 1996; de Leon et al., 1997; Jack et al., 1997; Nagy et al., 1999; Bouwman et al., 2007; Eckerstrom et al., 2010; Jack et al., 2010; Zhang et al., 2010; Apostolova et al., 2012; Ewers et al., 2012; Leung et al., 2013; Heister et al.). This leads to a predictable pattern of brain atrophy that could be very useful to improve diagnosis and follow up and help making a better assessment of the neuroprotective effects of a therapy. The quantification of atrophy in the MTL (MTA) has been attempted using several different neuroimaging measurements, including rating scales, linear measurements, and volumetric methods.

Visual assessment rating scales are quick, and can be performed on large numbers of scans in a clinical setting, the disadvantage being that there is a loss of accuracy compared with objective analysis and are subjected to interrater variability (Westman et al., 2011). Some studies found that visual rating assessment of the MTL gave similar prediction accuracy to multivariate classification and manual hippocampal volumes (Ringman et al., 2010; Duara et al., 2013) while others reported the visual rating assessment failed to detect patients at high risk, such as people carrying mutations of familial AD and also failed to detect progression over time (Ridha et al., 2007; Pereira et al., 2013). In addition, clinical, demographic, and genetic variables can influence the classification of MTA cut-off scores, leading to misdiagnosis in some cases. These variables, in addition to the differential sensitivity and specificity of each cut-off, should be carefully considered when performing visual MTA assessment (Scheltens et al., 1992).

Linear measures of brain regions are easy to take using clinically available neuroimaging. Some studies attempted to define sentinel changes that will allow the use of linear measurements of the hippocampus or the temporal horn to support clinical decision making. These studies have yielded variable results, with sensitivities ranging from 33 to 93% and specificity of approximately 95% (Dahlbeck et al., 1991; Erkinjuntti et al., 1993; Frisoni et al., 2002).

Volumetric analysis provides an accurate and detailed measure of a predetermined circumscribed area or region of interest. For AD, the most used structure is the whole hippocampus. Some indices comparing the extent of atrophy in the hippocampus with the whole brain atrophy are also being described (http://brainatrophyindices.blogspot.com). Manual volumetry is considered the gold standard but it has some drawbacks. First it requires training since the tracer must learn to delineate the hippocampus's boundaries and anterior- and posterior-limits. Then segmentation of the hippocampus takes approximately 20–30 min, depending on user experience (Soininen et al., 1994; Petrella et al., 2003), which limits routine clinical use. Some groups automated segmentation techniques and protocols for multi-atlas driven automatic segmentation of the hippocampus (Morra et al., 2008; Brewer et al., 2009; Kovacevic et al., 2009). Results of a study comparing manual and automated determination of hippocampal volumes in MCI and early AD indicated that these two methods derived highly correlated results with strong agreement (Shen et al., 2010). Albeit homogenization efforts are under development (Frisoni and Jack, 2011; Boccardi et al., 2013), the complexity and diversity of protocols used for volumetry keeps being a limitation today.

In summary, despite convenience and strong correlation to severity of AD pathology, MTA is not being used in daily clinical practice for diagnosing prodromal and probable AD yet, as it is in clinical trials and research studies. This is mainly because the methods already described lack accuracy (visual methods) or are not convenient enough to be routinely used by clinicians in busy departments (volumetric methods).

PURPOSE

In this report we aim to describe a new, objective and simple 2D-method for measuring atrophy of the MTL using clinically available neuroimaging. We also aim to explain the rationale behind this method. However, we do not seek to describe here the validity of this parameter for diagnosing AD since these researches are being conducted currently and results will be addressed in future publications.

PROTOCOL DESCRIPTION

This method consists of measuring the area of 3 brain regions on one single MRI slide and then use these data for calculating a simple ratio. First, we take the coronal slide at the level of the interpeduncular fossa on the TIR sequence. Then, regions are traced manually, simply using the pointer-rule tool of any software for visualizing DICOM images. As guidelines to draw structures and boundaries we followed the atlases by Mai et al. (1997) and Duvernoy (1998). The three areas are: (1) the MTL region (A), defined in a coronal brain slide as the four-sided space bordered in its inferior side by the tentorium cerebelli, in its medial side by the cerebral peduncles, in its upper side by the roof of the temporal horn of the lateral ventricle and in its lateral side by the collateral sulcus and a straight-line linking the collateral sulcus with the lateral edge of the temporal horn of the lateral ventricle; (2) the parenchima within the medial temporal region, that includes the hippocampus and the parahippocampal gyrus—the fimbria taenia and plexus choroideus are excluded—(B); and (3) the body of the ipsilateral lateral ventricle (C) (**Figure 1**). Therefrom, we can compute the ratio "Medial Temporal Atrophy index (MTAi)" at both sides as follows: $MTAi = (A - B) \times 10/C$. An example is shown in **Figure 2**.

If we have two MRI studies from different times (1 = first one, 2 = second one), we can also compute the yearly rate of MTA as follows: $yrMTA = (A2 - B2) - (A1 - B1) \times 120/(\#months\ between\ MRI\ studies)$ and the yearly rate of relative MTA as follows: $(yrMTAr) = (A2 - B2) - (A1 - B1) \times 120/(C2 - C1) \times (\#months\ between\ MRI\ studies)$.

EXPRESSING THE MEDIAL TEMPORAL ATROPHY INDEX

When we compute the MTAi we obtain 2 values, one for each hemisphere. In addition, it is also interesting to compute the median of these 2 values, and the index of asymmetry (IA). We determine the IA using formula $IA = (lMTAi - dMTAi)/(lMTAi + dMTAi) \times 100$. Small positive or negative IA values of magnitude less than $\sim \pm 3\%$ indicate that there is not a significant hemispheric asymmetry and the median MTAi can be used alone as a parameter of the global relative MTA. Higher IA values indicate significant hemispheric asymmetry and the median value should not be used alone since it is not a good representative value of the extent of relative MTA. Thus, the MTAi can be presented directly as the absolute right/left MTAi values or as the median MTAi with the IA (**Table 1**).

RATIONALE BEHIND THE MEDIAL TEMPORAL ATROPHY INDEX

The rationale behind this method is based on two premises: First, AD is a disease affecting the hippocampus, not a disease of the hippocampus. From a neuropathological point of view it is evident that that the characteristic pathological changes in AD begin outside the hippocampus, with development of neurofibrillary tangles in the transentorhinal and entorhinal cortex, spreading subsequently to the subiculum and CA1 regions of the

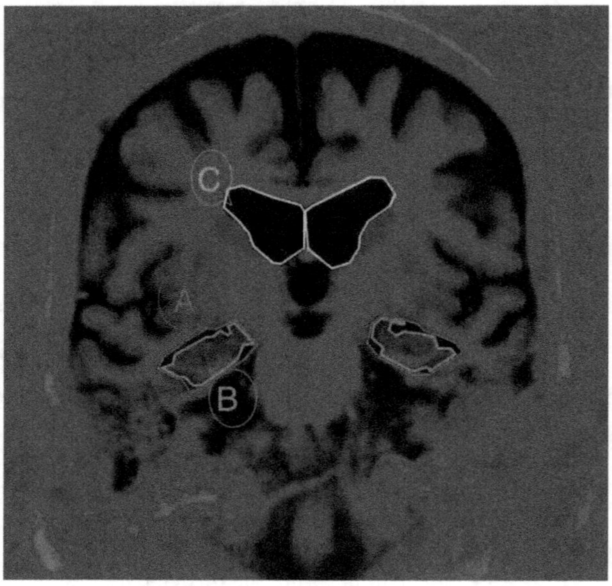

FIGURE 1 | MRI from a patient with MCI with boundaries of the three areas needed for calculating the Medial Temporal Atrophy index (MTAi). The section passes through the interpeduncular fosae. The three areas are: (1) the medial temporal lobe region **(A)**, defined in a coronal brain slide as the space bordered in its inferior side by the tentorium cerebelli, in its medial side by the cerebral peduncles, in its upper side by the roof of the temporal horn of the lateral ventricle and in its lateral side by the colateral sulcus and a straight-line linking the colateral sulcus with the lateral edge of the temporal horn of the lateral ventricle; (2) the parenchima within the medial temporal region, that includes the hippocampus and the parahippocampal girus **(B)**; and (3) the body of the ipsilateral lateral ventricle **(C)**.

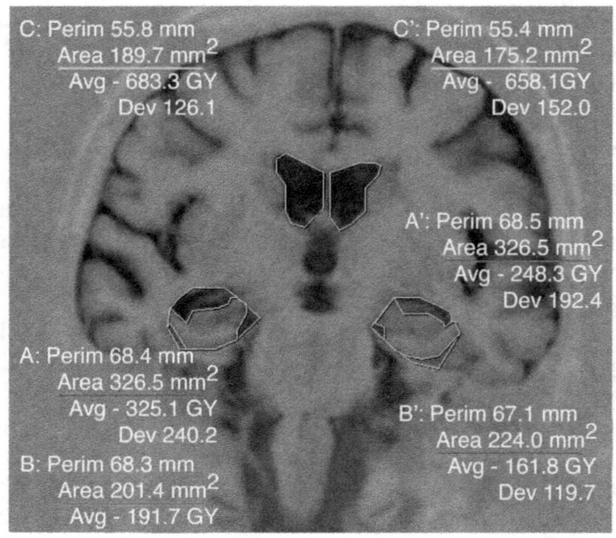

FIGURE 2 | Example of the Medial Temporal Atrophy index (MTAi) in a patient with mild AD. The three areas were traced manually on each hemisphere using the software for visualizing radiological images IMPAX. The data needed to compute the index are displayed automatically. We have underlined the different areas in colors as in **Figure 1**. The MTAi in the right hemisphere is: rMTAi = (326.5 − 201.4) ×10/189.7 = 6.59. The MTAi in the left hemisphere is: lMTAi = (326.5 − 224.0) ×10/175.2 = 5.85. Note how in spite of the coincidence of this case with exactly the same medial temporal region **(A and A')** in both hemispheres, the right MTAi is clearly higher than the left MTAi. Indeed when we calculate the Index of Asymmetry (IA), it is higher than 3: IA = (5, 85 − 6.59)/(5, 85 + 6.59) ×100 = −5, 15%.

hippocampus (Jack et al., 1992; Braak and Braak, 1985; Convit et al., 2000; Kerchner et al., 2010; Lim et al., 2012) and later to limbic, and ultimately to neocortical regions, such as the precuneus, middle frontal gyrus, and posterior cingulate gyrus. The severity of this atrophy, at least in the medial temporal regions, correlates with the severity of underlying neuropathological changes seen on postmortem studies (Echávarri et al., 2011). The second premise is that, despite most volumetric methods focus on the hippocampus and disregard the parahippocampal gyrus, many studies have shown that parahippocampal atrophy is as good indicator of AD as the hippocampus atrophy is (Nestor et al., 2008; Burgmans et al., 2011; Smith et al., 2012; Zarei et al., 2012). Thus, the entorinal cortex, the hippocampus, and the parahippocampal gyrus may be considered as the "epicentrum" of the neurodegenerative process. Therefore, in order to pick up the disease early we do not need to find out the volume of the whole hippocampus but detect atrophy at "the point" where the pathology is visible first.

Table 1 | Mean of the mean Medial Temporal Atrophy index (mMTAi) and Index of Asymmetry (IA) values in short series of patients with MCI (3), mild AD (3), moderate AD (3), severe AD (3), FTLD -not staged- (3), LBD -not staged- (3) and 5 healthy controls. Values are merely illustrative -not informative-.

	Mean mMTAi	Mean AI
Healthy control	2, 4	1, 8
MCI	3, 1	2, 4
Mild AD	4, 6	2, 6
Moderate AD	5, 2	2, 8
Severe AD	5, 8	3, 4
FTLD	3, 8	8, 2
DLB	2, 7	3, 7

THE SLICE SELECTED

Functionally, the hippocampus can be segmented into three distinct anatomical and functional subregions (head, body, and tail), according to the morphology and relative connectivity with prefrontal cortex (PFC), posterior cingulate cortex (PCC), and thalamus, respectively. The AD group show stronger hippocampus–PFC and weaker hippocampus–PCC functional connectivity, the magnitudes of which correlate with cognitive performance (Convit et al., 2000; Dickerson et al., 2011; Libby et al., 2012). In line with this fact and in order to assess the body of the hippocampus we have taken the coronal section passing through the interpeduncular fossa where the body of the hippocampus can be clearly viewed. However, this index might be performed on any other coronal slide where the MTL structures are viewed.

THE AREAS SELECTED

Age-associated differences are detected in the MTL (Parnetti et al., 1996; Jack et al., 1997; Apostolova et al., 2012; Leung et al., 2013) with an acceleration of MTA starting around 72 years of age in healthy people (Jack et al., 1997). However, these changes are modest and their rate of progression over time is relatively slow with a mean rate of about 1.6% per year (Leung et al., 2013). Accelerated MTA is a consistent finding in AD and MCI with rates of about 2.8% in stable MCI, 3.7% in MCI transitioning to AD (MCI progressors), and up to 4.0% in AD (Kesslak et al., 1991; Parnetti et al., 1996; Jack et al., 1997; Bouwman et al., 2007; Eckerstrom et al., 2010; Jack et al., 2010; Apostolova et al., 2012; Ewers et al., 2012; Leung et al., 2013; Heister et al.). Frontotemporal dementia may also lead to MTA, but in a different pattern: frontotemporal dementia and semantic dementia show atrophy in the anterior portion of the hippocampus, and in semantic dementia the atrophy is asymmetrical, with the left hippocampus being affected more severely. No significant hippocampal atrophy is detected in non-fluent progressive aphasia (Barber et al., 1999; Schacter and Wagner, 1999; Chan et al., 2001; van de Pol et al., 2006). Other diseases such as dementia with Lewy bodies do not show MTA or it is much milder (Hashimoto et al., 1998; Whitwell et al., 2007; Chou et al., 2010).

In contrast to MTA, ventricular enlargement (body of lateral ventricles) in old people lacks specificity representing a measure of global brain atrophy due to aging or any neurodegenerative disorder. Global ventricular enlargement correlates with decline in cognitive performance and with cerebrospinal fluid pathologic markers of AD (Thompson et al., 2004; Apostolova et al., 2010). Absolute ventricular volumes and ventricular enlargement are greater in subjects with AD and MCI compared to age-matched controls. Ventricular enlargement also demonstrated sensitivity to disease progression by way of discriminating between subjects with stable MCI and those that progressed to AD (Nestor et al., 2008). However, it is important to note that all these studies were made using absolute ventricular volumes, without differentiation among the different portions of the lateral ventricles, while the lateral (temporal) horns are the portion contributing most to the ventricular enlargement in early AD (Giesel et al., 2006). It is well-known that enlargement of lateral ventricles is a measure of unspecific global brain atrophy since it is strongly associated both with aging in healthy and with neurodegeneration (Apostolova et al., 2012). Almost any neurodegenerative disorder affecting the brain hemispheres leads to some degree of ventricular enlargement, including Parkinson's disease (Meyer et al., 2007; Apostolova et al., 2010; Dalaker et al., 2011), Lewy-Bodies Dementia (Meyer et al., 2007), Frontotemporal Lobe Dementia (Galton et al., 2001; Gordon et al., 2010), and Corticobasal Degeneration (Hauser et al., 1996) and so do some psychiatric conditions (Swayze et al., 1990; Mathalon et al., 2001). Thus, it would be interesting to compare the extent of atrophy in the MTL with the extent of global brain atrophy (**Table 1**).

THE RATIO

This index reflects the rate of atrophy in the MTL—that is a value rather specific of AD since its early stages—in relation to the global unspecific atrophy represented by ventricular enlargement. Thus, it is a measure estimative of the contribution of the atrophy in the MTL to the whole brain atrophy.

ADVANTAGES AND LIMITATIONS OF THE MTA INDEX

From the clinician's point of view, the MTA index has the following advantages over other methods: (1) Measurement and scoring of MTA index is objective and reliable, providing a distinct advantage over visual techniques. (2) Volumetric measurements require the use of special software, and much greater technical stringency in the acquisition of the MRI scans and are far more prone to a variety of measurement errors. Delineating the areas needed for calculating the MTA index is fast and easy; little training is needed. Therefore, it can be implemented for daily clinical practice using basic neuroimaging facilities currently available in most hospitals with busy clinical settings. (3) An additional advantage of using MTA index over volumetric measures is that regional brain volumes are variable across individuals and need to be normalized by conversion to a ratio of the absolute volumes to intracranial volume, whereas the MTA index has built-in normalization and thus avoids multiplicative errors inherent in using ratios of two quantitative variables. (4) The same way, as aging affects both the hippocampus and lateral ventricles independent of AD pathology, aging should be included as covariate in methods providing absolute volumes or scores. The MTA index is an "intra-patient" ratio comparing the MTL and lateral ventricles, so it will probably not need cut-off scores adjusted by age. For the yearly rate of MTA and the yearly rate of relative MTA, normalization is not necessary neither because each subject serves as their own control.

On the other hand, the main limitation of the MTA index is that scoring is based on measurements performed on a single coronal slice, thereby providing a limited perspective of overall brain pathology. It is also expected that other conditions affecting the ventricular morphology, such as hydrocephalus, will probably alter the interpretation of the MTAi in these cases.

This paper is a methodological description only. Cut-off scores have to be calculated and its use as a parameter for diagnosing AD in research and clinical practice has to be validated. Particularly, prospective studies are needed to assess the usefulness of MTA index in the diagnosis of early AD, in tracking the progression of AD and in the differential diagnosis of AD with other dementias.

CONCLUSIONS

We report a new, manual method for assessing medial temporal lobe atrophy (MTA) that is objective and easy to apply using clinically available neuroimaging. It may have some advantages over visual and volumetric methods that still need to be evaluated.

REFERENCES

Albert, M. S., Dekosky, S. T., Dickson, D., Dubois, B., Feldman, H. H., Fox, N. C., et al. (2011). The diagnosis of mild cognitive impairment due to Alzheimer's dis- ease: recommendations from the National Institute on Aging and Alzheimer's Association workgroup. *Alzheimers Dement.* 7, 270–279. doi: 10.1016/j.jalz. 2011.03.008

Apostolova, L. G., Beyer, M., Green, A. E., Hwang, K. S., Morra, J. H., Chou, Y. Y., et al. (2010). Hippocampal, caudate, and ventricular changes in Parkinson's disease with and without dementia. *Mov. Disord.* 25, 687–695. doi: 10.1002/mds.22799

Apostolova, L. G., Green, A. E., Babakchanian, S., Hwang, K. S., Chou, Y. Y., Toga, A. W., et al. (2012). Hippocampal atrophy and ventricular enlarge- ment in normal aging, mild cognitive impairment (MCI), and Alzheimer dis- ease. *Alzheimer Dis. Assoc. Disord.* 26, 17–27. doi: 10.1097/WAD.0b013e31821 63b62

Barber, R., Gholkar, A., Scheltens, P., Ballard, C., McKeith, I. G., and O'Brien, J. T. (1999). Medial temporal lobe atrophy on MRI in demen- tia with Lewy bodies. *Neurology* 52, 1153–1158. doi: 10.1212/WNL.52. 6.1153

Boccardi, M., Bocchetta, M., Apostolova, L. G., Preboske, G., Robitaille, N., Pasqualetti, P., et al. (2013). Establishing magnetic resonance images ori- entation for the EADC-ADNI manual hippocampal segmentation protocol. *J. Neuroimaging.* doi: 10.1111/jon.12065. [Epub ahead of print].

Bouwman, F. H., Schoonenboom, S. N., van der Flier, W. M., van Elk, E. J., Kok, A., Barkhof, F., et al. (2007). CSF biomarkers and medial temporal lobe atrophy predict dementia in mild cognitive impairment. *Neurobiol. Aging* 28, 1070–1074. doi: 10.1016/j.neurobiolaging.2006.05.006

Braak, H., and Braak, E. (1985). On areas of transition between entorhinal allocortex and temporal isocortex in the human brain. Normal morphology and lamina-specific pathology in Alzheimer's disease. *Acta Neuropathol.* 68, 325–332. doi: 10.1007/BF00690836

Brewer, J. B., Magda, S., Airriess, C., and Smith, M. E. (2009). Fully auto- mated quantification of regional brain volumes for improved detection of focal atrophy in Alzheimer disease. *AJNR Am. J. Neuroradiol.* 30, 578–580. doi: 10.3174/ajnr.A1402

Burgmans, S., van Boxtel, M. P., van den Berg, K. E., Gronenschild, E. H., Jacobs, H. I., Jolles, J., et al. (2011). The posterior parahippocampal gyrus is preferentially affected in age-related memory decline. *Neurobiol. Aging* 32, 1572–1578. doi: 10.1016/j.neurobiolaging.2009.09.008

Chan, D., Fox, N. C., Scahill, R. I., Crum, W. R., Whitwell, J. L., Leschziner, G., et al. (2001). Patterns of temporal lobe atrophy in semantic dementia and Alzheimer's disease. *Ann. Neurol.* 49, 433–442. doi: 10.1002/ana.92

Chou, Y. Y., Leporé, N., Saharan, P., Madsen, S. K., Hua, X., Jack, C. R., et al. (2010). Alzheimer's disease neuroimaging initiative. Ventricular maps in 804 ADNI sub- jects: correlations with CSF biomarkers and clinical decline. *Neurobiol. Aging* 31, 1386–1400. doi: 10.1016/j.neurobiolaging.2010.05.001

Convit, A., de Asis, J., de Leon, M. J., Tarshish, C. Y., De Santi, S., and Rusinek, H. (2000). Atrophy of the medial occipitotemporal, inferior, and middle temporal gyri in non-demented elderly predict decline to Alzheimer's disease. *Neurobiol. Aging* 21, 19–26. doi: 10.1016/S0197-4580(99)00107-4

Dahlbeck, J. W., McCluney, K. W., Yeakley, J. W., Fenstermacher, M. J., Bonmati, C., Van Horn, G., et al. (1991). The interuncal distance: a new MR measurement for the hippocampal atrophy of Alzheimer disease. *AJNR Am. J. Neuroradiol.* 12, 931–932.

Dalaker, T. O., Zivadinov, R., Ramasamy, D. P., Beyer, M. K., Alves, G., Bronnick, K. S., et al. (2011). Ventricular enlargement and mild cognitive impairment in early Parkinson's disease. *Mov. Disord.* 26, 297–301. doi: 10.1002/mds.23443

de Leon, M. J., George, A. E., Golomb, J., Tarshish, C., Convit, A., Kluger, A., et al. (1997). Frequency of hippocampal formation atrophy in normal aging and Alzheimer's disease. *Neurobiol. Aging* 18, 1–11. doi: 10.1016/S0197-4580 (96)00213-8

Dickerson, B. C., Stoub, T. R., Shah, R. C., Sperling, R. A., Killiany, R. J., Albert, M. S., et al. (2011). Alzheimer-signature MRI biomarker predicts AD dementia in cognitively normal adults. *Neurology* 76, 1395–1402. doi: 10.1212/WNL.0b013e3182166e96

Duara, R., Loewenstein, D. A., Shen, Q., Barker, W., Varon, D., Greig, M. T., et al. (2013). Volumetric and visual ratings of medical temporal atrophy in AD and MCI: comparison of age-specific cutoffs. *Front. Aging Neurosci.* 5:47. doi: 10.3389/fnagi.2013.00047

Duvernoy, H. M. (1998). *The Human Hippocampus: Functional Anatomy, Vascularization and Serial Sections with MRI.* Berlin: Springer-Verlag. doi: 10.1007/978-3-662-03628-0

Echávarri, C., Aalten, P., Uylings, H. B., Jacobs, H. I., Visser, P. J., Gronenschild, E. H., et al. (2011). Atrophy in the parahippocampal gyrus as an early biomarker of Alzheimer's disease. *Brain Struct. Funct.* 215, 265–271. doi: 10.1007/s00429- 010-0283-8

Eckerstrom, C., Andreasson, U., Olsson, E., Rolstad, S., Blennow, K., Zetterberg, H., et al. (2010). Combination of hippocampal volume and cerebrospinal fluid biomarkers improves predictive value in mild cognitive impairment. *Dement. Geriatr. Cogn. Disord.* 29, 294–300. doi: 10.1159/000289814

Erkinjuntti, T., Lee, D. H., Gao, F., Steenhuis, R., Eliasziw, M., Fry, R., et al. (1993). Temporal lobe atrophy on magnetic resonance imaging in the diagnosis of early Alzheimer's disease. *Arch. Neurol.* 50, 305–310. doi: 10.1001/archneur. 1993.00540030069017

Ewers, M., Walsh, C., Trojanowski, J. Q., Shaw, L. M., Petersen, R. C., Jack, C. R., et al. (2012). Prediction of conversion from mild cognitive impair- ment to Alzheimer's disease dementia based upon biomarkers and neuropsy- chological test performance. *Neurobiol. Aging* 33, 1203–1214. doi: 10.1016/j.neurobiolaging.2010.10.019

Frisoni, G. B., Geroldi, C., Beltramello, A., Bianchetti, A., Binetti, G., Bordiga, G., et al. (2002). Radial width of the temporal horn: a sensitive measure in Alzheimer disease. *AJNR Am. J. Neuroradiol.* 23, 35–47.

Frisoni, G. B., and Jack, C. R. (2011). Harmonization of magnetic resonance- based manual hippocampal segmentation: a mandatory step for wide clinical use. *Alzheimers Dement.* 7, 171–174. doi: 10.1016/j.jalz.2010.0 6.007

Galton, C. J., Gomez-Anson, B., Antoun, N., Scheltens, P., Patterson, K., Graves, M., et al. (2001). Temporal lobe rating scale: application to Alzheimer's disease and frontotemporal dementia. *J. Neurol. Neurosurg. Psychiatr.* 70, 165–173. doi: 10.1136/jnnp.70.2.165

Giesel, F. L., Hahn, H. K., Thomann, P. A., Widjaja, E., Wignall, E., von Tengg- Kobligk, H., et al. (2006). Temporal horn index and volume of medial temporal lobe atrophy using a new semiautomated method for rapid and precise ass- ment. *AJNR Am. J. Neuroradiol.* 27, 1454–1458.

Gordon, E., Rohrer, J. D., Kim, L. G., Omar, R., Rossor, M. N., Fox, N. C., et al. (2010). Measuring disease progression in frontotemporal lobar degeneration: a clinical and MRI study. *Neurology* 74, 666–673. doi: 10.1212/WNL.0b013e3181d1a879

Hashimoto, M., Kitagaki, H., Imamura, T., Hirono, N., Shimomura, T., Kazui, H., et al. (1998). Medial temporal and whole-brain atrophy in dementia with Lewy bodies: a volumetric MRI study. *Neurology* 51, 357–362. doi: 10.1212/WNL.51.2.357

Hauser, R. A., Murtaugh, F. R., Akhter, K., Gold, M., and Olanow, C. W. (1996). Magnetic resonance imaging of corticobasal degeneration. *J. Neuroimaging* 6, 222–226.

Heister, D., Brewer, J. B., Magda, S., Blennow, K., McEvoy, L. K., and Alzheimer's Disease Neuroimaging Initiative. (2011). Predicting MCI outcome with clini- cally available MRI and CSF biomarkers. *Neurology* 77, 1619–1628. doi: 10.1212/WNL.0b013e3182343314

Jack, C. R. Jr., Petersen, R. C., O'Brien, P. C., and Tangalos, E. G. (1992). MR-based hippocampal volumetry in the diagnosis of Alzheimer's disease. *Neurology* 42, 183–188.

Jack, C. R. Jr., Petersen, R. C., Xu, Y. C., Waring, S. C., O'Brien, P. C., Tangalos, E. G., et al. (1997). Medial temporal atrophy on MRI in normal aging and very mild Alzheimer's disease. *Neurology* 49, 786–794. doi: 10.1212/WNL.49.3.786

Jack, C. R. Jr., Wiste, H. J., Vemuri, P., Weigand, S. D., Senjem, M. L., Zeng, G., et al. (2010). Brain beta-amyloid measures and magnetic reso- nance imaging atrophy both predict time-to-progression from mild cognitive impairment to Alzheimer's disease. *Brain* 133, 3336–3348. doi: 10.1093/brain/awq277

Kerchner, G. A., Hess, C. P., Hammond-Rosenbluth, K. E., Xu, D., Rabinovici, G. D., Kelley, D. A., et al. (2010). Hippocampal CA1 apical neuropil atrophy in mild Alzheimer disease visualized with 7-T MRI. *Neurology* 75, 1381–1387. doi: 10.1212/WNL.0b013e3181f736a1

Kesslak, J. P., Nalcioglu, O., and Cotman, C. W. (1991). Quantification of magnetic resonance scans for hippocampal and parahippocampal atrophy in Alzheimer's disease. *Neurology* 41, 51–54. doi: 10.1212/WNL.41.1.51

Kovacevic, S., Rafii, M. S., and Brewer, J. B. (2009). High-throughput, fully automated volumetry for prediction of MMSE and CDR decline in mild cognitive impairment. *Alzheimer Dis. Assoc. Disord.* 23, 139–145. doi: 10.1097/WAD.0b013e318192e745

Leung, K. K., Bartlett, J. W., Barnes, J., Manning, E. N., Ourselin, S., and Fox, N. C. (2013). Azheimer's disease neuroimaging initiative. Cerebral atrophy in mild cognitive impairment and Alzheimer disease: rates and acceleration. *Neurology* 80, 648–654. doi: 10.1212/WNL.0b013e318281ccd3

Libby, L., Ekstrom, A., Ragland, J. D., and Ranganath, C. (2012). Differential con- nectivity of perirhinal and parahippocampal cortices within human hippocam- pal subregions revealed by high-resolution functional imaging. *J. Neurosci.* 32, 6550–6560. doi: 10.1523/JNEUROSCI.3711-11.2012

Lim, H. K., Jung, W. S., Ahn, K. J., Won, W. Y., Hahn, C., Lee, S. Y., et al. (2012). Relationships between hippocampal shape and cognitive performances in drug-naïve patients with Alzheimer's disease. *Neurosci. Lett.* 516, 124–129. doi: 10.1016/j.neulet.2012.03.072

Mai, J. K., Assheuer, J., and Paxinos, G. (1997). *Atlas of the Human Brain.* San Diego, CA: Academic Press.

Mathalon, D. H., Sullivan, E. V., Lim, K. O., and Pfefferbaum, A. (2001). Progressive brain volume changes and the clinical course of Schizophrenia in men: a longi- tudinal magnetic resonance imaging study. *Arch. Gen. Psychiatry* 58, 148–157. doi: 10.1001/archpsyc.58.2.148

McKhann, G. M., Knopman, D. S., Chertkow, H., Hyman, B. T., Jack, C. R. Jr., Kawas, C. H., et al. (2011). The diagnosis of dementia due to Alzheimer's disease: recommendations from the National Institute on Aging-Alzheimer's Association workgroups on diagnostic guidelines for Alzheimer's disease. *Alzheimers Dement.* 7, 263–269. doi: 10.1016/j.jalz.2011.03.005

Meyer, J. S., Huang, J., and Chowdhury, M. H. (2007). MRI confirms mild cognitive impairments prodromal for Alzheimer's, vascular and Parkinson- Lewy body dementias. *J. Neurol. Sci.* 257, 97–104. doi: 10.1016/j.jns.2007.01.016

Morra, J. H., Tu, Z., Apostolova, L. G., Green, A. E., Avedissian, C., Madsen, S. K., et al. (2008). Alzheimer's disease neuroimaging initiative. Validation of a fully automated 3D hippocampal segmentation method using subjects with Alzheimer's disease mild cognitive impairment, and elderly controls. *Neuroimage* 43, 59–68. doi: 10.1016/j.neuroimage.2008.07.003

Morris, J. C., Storandt, M., McKeel, D. W. Jr., Rubin, E. H., Price, J. L., Grant, E. A., et al. (1996). Cerebral amyloid deposition and diffuse plaques in "nor- mal" aging: evidence for presymptomatic and very mild Alzheimer's disease. *Neurology* 46, 707–719. doi: 10.1212/WNL.46.3.707

Nagy, Z., Hindley, N. J., Braak, H., Braak, E., Yilmazer-Hanke, D. M., Schultz, C., et al. (1999). The progression of Alzheimer's disease from limbic regions to the neocortex: clinical, radiological and pathological relationships. *Dement. Geriatr. Cogn. Disord.* 10, 115–120. doi: 10.1159/000017111

Nestor, S. M., Rupsingh, R., Borrie, M., Smith, M., Accomazzi, V., Wells, J. L., et al. (2008). Alzheimer's disease neuroimaging initiative. Ventricular enlarge- ment as a possible measure of Alzheimer's disease progression validated using the Alzheimer's disease neuroimaging initiative database. *Brain* 131, 2443–2454. doi: 10.1093/brain/awn146

Parnetti, L., Lowenthal, D. T., Presciutti, O., Pelliccioli, G. P., Palumbo, R., Gobbi, G., et al. (1996). 1H-MRS, MRI-based hippocampal volumetry, and 99mTc- HMPAO-SPECT in normal aging, age-associated memory impairment, and probable Alzheimer's disease. *J. Am. Geriatr. Soc.* 44, 133–138.

Pereira, J. B., Cavallin, L., Spulber, G., Aguilar, C., Mecocci, P., Vellas, B., et al. (2013). Influence of age, disease onset and ApoE4 on visual medial temporal lobe atrophy cut-offs. *J. Intern. Med.* doi: 10.1111/joim.12148. [Epub ahead of print].

Petrella, J. R., Coleman, R. E., and Doraiswamy, P. M. (2003). Neuroimaging and early diagnosis of Alzheimer disease: a look to the future. *Radiology* 226, 315–336. doi: 10.1148/radiol.2262011600

Ridha, B. H., Barnes, J., van de Pol, L. A., Schott, J. M., Boyes, R. G., Siddique, M. M., et al. (2007). Application of automated medial temporal lobe atrophy scale to Alzheimer disease. *Arch. Neurol.* 64, 849–854. doi: 10.1001/archneur. 64.6.849

Ringman, J. M., Pope, W., and Salamon, N. (2010). Insensitivity of visual assess- ment of hippocampal atrophy in familial Alzheimer's disease. *J. Neurol.* 257, 839–842. doi: 10.1007/s00415-009-5436-4

Schacter, D. L., and Wagner, A. D. (1999). Medial temporal lobe activations in fMRI and PET studies of episodic encoding and retrieval. *Hippocampus* 9, 7–24. doi: 10.1002/(SICI)1098-1063(1999)9:1%3C7::AID-HIPO2%3E3.0.CO;2-K

Scheltens, P., Leys, D., Barkhof, F., Huglo, D., Weinstein, H. C., Vermersch, P., et al. (1992). Atrophy of medial temporal lobes on MRI in "probable" Alzheimer's disease and normal ageing: diagnostic value and neuropsychological correlates. *J. Neurol. Neurosurg. Psychiatr.* 55, 967–972. doi: 10.1136/jnnp.55.10.967

Shen, L., Saykin, A. J., Kim, S., Firpi, H. A., West, J. D., Risacher, S. L., et al. (2010). Comparison of manual and automated determination of hippocampal volumes in MCI and early AD. *Brain Imaging Behav.* 4, 86–95. doi: 10.1007/s11682-010-9088-x

Smith, A. D., and Jobst, K. A. (1996). Use of structural imaging to study the pro- gression of Alzheimer's disease. *Br. Med. Bull.* 52, 575–586. doi: 10.1093/oxford- journals.bmb.a011568

Smith, C. D., Andersen, A. H., and Gold, B. T. (2012). Structural brain alter- ations before mild cognitive impairment in ADNI: validation of volume loss in a predefined antero-temporal region. *J. Alzheimers. Dis.* 31, S49–S58. doi: 10.3233/JAD-2012-120157

Soininen, H. S., Partanen, K., Pitkanen, A., Vainio, P., Hanninen, T., Hallikainen, M., et al. (1994). Volumetric MRI analysis of the amygdala and the hippocam- pus in subjects with age-associated memory impairment: correlation to visual and verbal memory. *Neurology* 44, 1660–1668. doi: 10.1212/WNL.44.9.1660

Sperling, R. A., Aisen, P. S., Beckett, L. A., Bennett, D. A., Craft, S., Fagan, A. M., et al. (2011). Toward defining the preclinical stages of Alzheimer's disease: recommendations from the National Institute on Aging-Alzheimer's Association workgroups on diagnostic guidelines for Alzheimer's disease. *Alzheimers Dement.* 7, 280–292. doi: 10.1016/j.jalz.2011.03.003

Swayze, V. W. II., Andreasen, N. C., Alliger, R. J., Ehrhardt, J. C., and Yuh, W. C. (1990). Structural brain abnormalities in bipolar affective disorder: ventric- ular enlargement and focal signal hyperintensities. *Arch. Gen. Psychiatry* 47, 1054–1059. doi: 10.1001/archpsyc.1990.01810230070011

Thompson, P. M., Hayashi, K. M., De Zubicaray, G. I., Janke, A. L., Rose, S. E., Semple, J., et al. (2004). Mapping hippocampal and ven- tricular change in Alzheimer disease. *Neuroimage* 22, 1754–1766. doi: 10.1016/j.neuroimage.2004.03.040

van de Pol, L. A., Hensel, A., van der Flier, W. M., Visser, P. J., Pijnenburg, Y. A., Barkhof, F., et al. (2006). Hippocampal atrophy on MRI in frontotempo- ral lobar degeneration and Alzheimer's disease. *J. Neurol. Neurosurg. Psychiatr.* 77, 439–442. doi: 10.1136/jnnp.2005.075341

Westman, E., Cavallin, L., Muehlboeck, J. S., Zhang, Y., Mecocci, P., Vellas, B., et al. (2011). AddNeuroMed consortium. Sensitivity and specificity of medial temporal lobe visual ratings and multivariate regional MRI classification in Alzheimer's disease. *PLoS ONE* 6:e22506. doi: 10.1371/journal.pone.0022506

Whitwell, J. L., Weigand, S. D., Shiung, M. M., Boeve, B. F., Ferman, T. J., Smith, G. E., et al. (2007). Focal atrophy in dementia with Lewy bodies on MRI: a distinct pattern from Alzheimer's disease. *Brain* 130(Pt 3), 708–719. doi: 10.1093/brain/awl388

Zarei, M., Beckmann, C. F., Binnewijzend, M. A., Schoonheim, M. M., Oghabian, M. A., Sanz-Arigita, E. J., et al. (2012). Functional segmentation of the hip- pocampus in the healthy human brain and in Alzheimer's disease. *Neuroimage* 66C, 28–35. doi: 10.1016/j.neuroimage.2012.10.071

Zhang, Y., Qiu, C., Lindberg, O., Bronge, L., Aspelin, P., Bäckman, L., et al. (2010). Acceleration of hippocampal atrophy in a non-demented elderly population: the SNAC-K study. *Int. Psychogeriatr.* 22, 14–25. doi: 10.1017/S1041610209991396

16

History of innate immunity in neurodegenerative disorders

Patrick L. McGeer* and Edith G. McGeer

Kinsmen Laboratory of Neurological Research, University of British Columbia, Vancouver, BC, Canada

Edited by:
Roger A. Barker, University of Cambridge and Addenbrooke' Hospital, UK

Reviewed by:
Jason B. Wu, Cedars-Sinai Medical Center, USA
Muzamil Ahmad, Indian Institute of Integrative Medicine, India

****Correspondence:***
Patrick L. McGeer, Kinsmen Laboratory of Neurological Research, University of British Columbia, 2255 Wesbrook Mall, Vancouver, BC, Canada V6T1Z3.
e-mail: mcgeerpl@interchange.ubc.ca

The foundations of innate immunity in neurodegenerative disorders were first laid by Del Rio Hortega (1919). He identified and named microglia, recognizing them as cells of mesodermal origin. Van Furth in 1969 elaborated the monocyte phagocytic system with microglia as the brain representatives. Validation of these concepts did not occur until 1987 when HLA-DR was identified on activated microglia in a spectrum of neurological disorders. HLA-DR had already been established as a definitive marker of immunocompetent cells of mesodermal origin. It was soon determined that the observed inflammatory reaction was an innate immune response. A rapid expansion of the field took place as other markers of an innate immune response were found that were made by neurons, astrocytes, oligodendroglia, and endothelial cells. The molecules included complement proteins and their regulators, inflammatory cytokines, chemokines, acute phase reactants, prostaglandins, proteases, protease inhibitors, coagulation factors, fibrinolytic factors, anaphylatoxins, integrins, free radical generators, and other unidentified neurotoxins. The Nimmerjahn movies demonstrated that resting microglia were constantly active, sampling the surround, and responding rapidly to brain damage. Ways of reducing the neurotoxic innate immune response and stimulating a healing response continue to be sought as a means for ameliorating the pathology in a spectrum of chronic degenerative disorders.

Keywords: HLA-DR, Alzheimer disease, Parkinson disease, complement, neuroinflammation

BACKGROUND

Pio Del Rio Hortega, one of the greatest of all neuroscientists, established the basic foundation of neuroinflammation with his classic 1919 paper "El tercer elemento de los centros nerviosis" (Del Rio Hortega, 1919). He had developed an ammoniacal silver carbonate modification of the Golgi technique. With this new method he was able to identify small spidery cells which he named microglia. He recognized that they were of mesodermal origin, and that they migrated to the brain in late embryonic life. He also recognized their phagocytic capacity by examining their reaction to stab wounds. He categorized their morphology as resting, ameboid, and reactive. By further modifying his technique, he later recognized another type of glial cell which was of epithelial origin and had a sparse cytoplasm. He named these cells oligodendroglia, perhaps because of the difficulty he encountered in staining them.

These two glial cell types made up "the third element" which had baffled Ramon y Cajal. Cajal, Hortega's mentor and employer, had clearly identified astrocytes with his methodology, and knew there were still unclassified glial cells. He thought the cells identified by Hortega might be another astrocytic type that was resistant to staining. He objected to Hortega's desire to publish his results on oligodendroglia, and when Hortega went ahead, believing others would make the same discovery, Cajal dismissed him. Hortega's own account of these travails, which he never published, were obtained after his death, later appearing in part in Haymaker and Adams treatise on the histopathology of the nervous system (Haymaker and Adams, 1980a, pp. 484–485).

Hortega's travails were not limited to his falling out with Cajal. The Madrid laboratory he had set up after his departure from Cajal was bombed out in the Spanish civil war. He moved for a time to Paris, and then to Oxford, but was uncomfortable in these locations. As a Spaniard opposed to Franco, he emigrated to Buenos Aires in 1938 where, in 1945, he died of cancer.

His findings and their interpretation were still being actively challenged long after his death. Some scientists supported his conclusions, others did not. Wilder Penfield was the first prominent investigator to uphold Hortega. He described, in the first issue of the American Journal of Pathology, the various stages of microglia, going from resting to reactive (Penfield, 1925). Numerous others did differing experiments, interpreting microglia cells as being of epithelial origin with unknown function. A detailed account of the continuing controversy, which extended for over six decades, appears in Haymaker and Adams (1980b, Chapter VI). This unjustified controversy may help to explain why Hortega never received a Nobel prize for his epic work.

The next giant step was taken by Ralph van Furth. He elaborated the concept of a monocyte phagocytic system to explain the origin and function of resident phagocytes throughout the body. The Memoranda endorsing the concept, which was introduced at the Conference on Mononuclear Phagocytes held in Lieden in 1969, is available on the web Chttp://www.ncbi.nlm.nih.gov/pmc/articles/PMC2480884/pdf/bullwho00193-0157.pdf. He and his colleagues had studied labeled monocytes and their marrow precursors and followed their appearance as typical macrophages in various organs, including brain (Van Furth and Cohn, 1968). This concept replaced the vague theory of a reticulo-endothelial system introduced by Aschoff (1924) which, despite its shortcomings, had become entrenched in medical teaching.

While van Furth's concept of a monocyte phagocytic system was widely accepted, its relationship to brain microglia was not.

Fujita in particular opposed the idea that microglia were the brain representatives of this system. He injected tritiated thymidine into chick embryos and identified labeled brain cells which he interpreted as glioblasts of subependymal origin (Fujita, 1965). He did later studies of human embryonic brain tissue and reached a similar conclusion, that brain microglia were of epithelial and not mesenchymal origin (Fujita, 1973; Fujita and Kitamura, 1973).

Oemichan et al. (1979) and Wood et al. (1979) also concluded that brain microglia could not be phagocytes of monocytic origin. The reason was that they could not detect the same surface antigens on microglial cells that they were able to detect on peripheral monocytes. The idea became established that inflammation of the brain did not involve microglia, and did not occur unless there was invasion of the brain by peripheral monocytes, which then became transformed into macrophages.

IDENTIFICATION OF HLA-DR POSITIVE MICROGLIA IN HUMAN BRAIN

The entry of our laboratory into the neuroinflammatory field was entirely serendipitous. Several researchers had suggested that AD might result from a herpes infection entering through the nasal passages because of involvement of the rhinencephalon (Ball, 1982). Our effort over some years to detect herpes virus in the CNS had failed, although we were able to detect it in some cases in the trigeminal nucleus, the source of herpes labialis (Walker et al., 1989). We sought the advice of local immunologists regarding what might be a broader indicator of a viral infection, and were counseled to look for HLA-DR since this class II glycoprotein would be responsible for presenting viral epitopes to T-cells. We were even presented with a gift of the HB-104 cell line, known to produce high levels of antibodies against HLA-DR.

The results astonished us. A plethora of cells was visible in AD tissue with a morphology that was completely unfamiliar to us. However we were able to confirm that they were microglia by showing them to the founder of our laboratory, Dr. William Gibson, who had been a student and biographer of Hortega (Prados and Gibson, 1946). The morphology was identical to that published by Del Rio Hortega (1919), permitting us to sense in a very small way the excitement he must have experienced.

As many frustrated investigators well know, peer reviewers, whether evaluating applications for research grants, or papers submitted to journals, are typically well versed in the dogmas of the day. Findings that radically conflict with established views are too often dismissed. Our data conflicted with two dogmas. The first was that microglia were of epithelial origin and were not immunocompetent cells. The second was that brain inflammation was not a characteristic of AD. A pathological journal rejected our initial manuscript, reasoning that the absence of a neuropathologist as an author explained the faulty conclusions. A peer reviewer for a renewal of our grant dismissed it with the comment "the hypothesis is ridiculous." Nevertheless, our first paper appeared as a brief report in Neuroscience Letters (McGeer et al., 1987).

This final validation of Hortega depended on the availability of HB-104, a powerful and highly specific monoclonal antibody. The field of immunohistochemistry had been opened by Cesar Milstein's work on the technique for producing monoclonal antibodies. He was a co-winner of the Nobel prize in 1984 for this accomplishment. Then, as now, the ability to visualize brain biochemistry through the eyes of immunohistochemistry depends on the strength and specificity of the antibodies employed. HB-104 was a particularly good antibody, permitting us to make a clear distinction, which had eluded other investigators, between HLA-DR positive microglia and GFAP positive astrocytes.

We were not the first to report class II staining of brain cells. Lampson and Hickey (1986) had reported class II activity in occasional cell bodies of human brain with the "morphologic appearance of microglia or astrocytes." Similarly deTribolet et al. (1984) reported HLA-DR positive cells in the white matter of normal brain which they interpreted as being astrocytes (deTribolet et al., 1984). Rogers et al. reported HLA-DR positive microglia and astrocytes in AD in an abstract at the Society of Neuroscience meeting in 1986 but, as in our case, formal publication was held up by disbelief in the findings. Their work finally appeared in 1988 (Luber-Narod and Rogers, 1988; Rogers et al., 1988).

These data led to a number of unanswered questions. What was the source of the inflammation in AD? Was it a special phenomenon or a general one that applied to many chronic neurological disorders? If it was a general phenomenon, was it localized to the brain or did it involve the peripheral immune system? Was it helpful or harmful to ongoing degenerative processes? What were the implications for treatment? Exploration of these questions led to the opening up of an important new field of neuroscience, namely neuroinflammation.

ESTABLISHMENT OF NEUROINFLAMMATION AS A DISTINCT FIELD OF NEUROSCIENCE RESEARCH

The question as to whether or not the presence of activated microglia in brain was a special one applying to AD, or a general phenomenon was quickly answered. HLA-DR activated microglia were observed in a variety of degenerative neurological conditions, including Parkinson disease (PD), Pick disease, ALS, Huntington disease, multiple sclerosis, AIDS encephalopathy, parkinsonism dementia of Guam, and the Shy–Drager syndrome (McGeer et al., 1988a). Their phagocytic function was easily demonstrated by melanin being observed within the HLA-DR positive microglia of the SN (McGeer et al., 1988b). Each of these diseases has a differing etiology, so the activated microglial response had to be the consequence of initiating factors in each condition and not the fundamental cause.

At this same time, the laboratory of Kreutzberg in Germany was carrying out work of a more fundamental nature. His team was utilizing the facial nerve axotomy model to examine the CNS reaction to a sterile lesion outside of the CNS. They found activated microglia enveloping damaged neurons of facial nerve cell bodies, with phagocytosis of dead cells taking place. They concluded that microglia might function as antigen presenting cells and thus be the effector cells responsible for recruitment of lymphocytes to the brain resulting in an inflammatory reaction. A review of their results appeared in the first volume of Glia (Streit et al., 1988) and a later review (Kreutzberg, 1996).

Further groundwork was laid by four key papers which appeared in a special issue of Glia in 1993 devoted to microglia. They were by Ling and Wong (1993) describing the origin and nature of microglia; Dickson et al. (1993) detailing cytokines and microglia in Alzheimer disease and AIDS; Banati et al. (1993)

on the cytotoxicity of microglia; and McGeer et al. (1993) on microglia in neurodegenerative diseases generally.

Since our laboratory and that of Joe Rogers, who had founded the Sun Health Research Institute, had identified HLA-DR activated microglia in AD, we joined forces for further investigation of the phenomenon, particularly the role of complement. The name complement was introduced by Paul Ehrlich in the 1890's to explain the heat labile factor in serum which helped antibodies to kill microorganisms. As a result, complement was considered to be a peripherally generated system for assisting the activity of antibodies. It was therefore believed that complement factors would only be found as an accompaniment to immunoglobulin antibodies.

Eikelenboom and Stam (1982) were the first to report the presence of complement factors in AD senile plaques. Previously it had been reported that immunoglobulins were associated with amyloid deposits, which was consistent with prevailing theory (Ishii and Haga, 1975). Our laboratory was able to detect the opsonizing components of the classical complement pathway in association with plaques, and the membrane attack complex in association with dystrophic neurites, consistent with bystander lysis occurring in AD (McGeer et al., 1989).

Working with Joseph Rogers, we were unable to detect immunoglobulins in AD tissue using a host of antibodies. Then Rogers explored the idea that beta amyloid protein itself might be an activator of complement. In a classic paper he and his colleagues demonstrated that immunoglobulin immunostaining did not colocalize with complement, and that beta amyloid protein and its N-terminal fragments bound to C1q directly, thus initiating the complement cascade independently of antibodies (Rogers et al., 1992). But what was the source of the complement proteins? It was soon determined from RNA studies that brain itself was the source (Johnson et al., 1992; Walker and McGeer, 1992). Meanwhile evolutionary studies were underway, establishing that the complement system could be traced back at least as far as horseshoe crabs and that it was the mainstay of innate immunity in most primitive organisms (Zhu et al., 2005). It far predated the antibody producing adaptive immune system which is an invention of higher vertebrates.

Two principles which had broad implications for the developing field of neuroinflammation emerged from this joint endeavor. The first was establishing that complement was part of the innate immune system and further that it had the potential of exacerbating the pathology through formation of the membrane attack complex. The second was showing that the inflammatory reaction in AD did exacerbate the pathology. We decided to explore whether patients on long term anti-inflammatory therapy were relatively spared from AD. We selected rheumatoid arthritic patients because onset of the disease typically appears at an earlier age than AD and involves aggressive anti-inflammatory therapy. The results showed an estimated sixfold sparing of AD in rheumatoid arthritic patients compared with age matched general populations (McGeer et al., 1990). Many subsequent epidemiological studies, in which consumption of NSAIDs in particular were targeted, confirmed these general findings (McGeer and McGeer, 1995).

Rogers was then motivated to establish a Neuroinflammation Working Group of 37 investigators to assemble the rapidly accumulating data on inflammation in AD. The conclusion of the group was that the data represented "a virtual textbook of inflammatory mediators." Included were complement proteins and their regulators, inflammatory cytokines, chemokines, acute phase reactants, prostaglandins, proteases, protease inhibitors, coagulation factors, fibrinolytic factors, integrins, anaphylatoxins, free radical generators, and other unidentified neurotoxins (Akiyama et al., 2000). All are products of the innate immune system of brain, with major contributions coming from neurons, astrocytes, microglia, and endothelial cells.

Parkinson disease was another chronic degenerative disorder where activated microglia were detected in association with the SN lesions (McGeer et al., 1988b). An accidental model of PD provided new insights into the consequences of chronic neuroinflammation. Langston et al. (1984) had identified a group of young drug users who suddenly developed a parkinsonian syndrome. The causative agent (MPP+) was a metabolite of 1-methyl-4-phenyl-1,2,3,6-tetrahydropyridine (MPTP), a contaminant in the street drug they were using. The condition was progressive, and autopsy studies on those who had died from this exposure years previously showed neuroinflammation of the SN similar to that observed in PD (Langston et al., 1999). We found a parallel situation in monkeys. They showed nigral degeneration and activated microglia in the SN 5.5–15 years after systemic exposure to MPTP (McGeer et al., 2003). These findings represent the clearest example of how neuroinflammation, once initiated, can persist, and cause continuing neurodegeneration.

Activated microglia are the pivotal cells. Their functioning *in vivo* has been remarkably demonstrated by the movies of Nimmerjahn et al. (2005). They developed mice transgenic for a green fluorescent protein in microglial cells and used two-photon microscopy through a window in the skull to observe their behavior. Microglial cells in the normal state were found not to be dormant, as implied by their traditional designation as resting, but were extremely active, continuously extending, and retracting their processes to sense their environment. When activated by a laser lesion of a capillary, they surrounded the lesion and phagocytosed the leaking blood.

The innate immune system is the body's first line of defense. As the Nimmerjahn movies demonstrate, it can act immediately. As shown in chronic degenerative diseases, as well as the MPTP model, it can maintain its activity indefinitely without significant engagement of the adaptive immune system. The adaptive immune system is slower to react but more powerful and specific in attacking targets. It depends upon appropriate presentation of epitopes to lymphatic organs so that lymphocytes can be cloned to attack targets where that epitope is exposed. There is a long list of diseases where the adaptive immune system directs self attack on healthy tissues. These conditions are known as autoimmune disorders. They differ from AD and other chronic neurodegenerative disorders where the adaptive immune system does not become significantly engaged. To distinguish between the two, we have suggested that such diseases be described as autotoxic disorders (McGeer and McGeer, 2000).

In theory, the self destruction in autotoxic disorders should be milder and more amenable to therapeutic intervention than the self destruction in autoimmune disorders. The question is how to ameliorate the autotoxic response? Anti-inflammatory and antioxidant approaches have been the most widely utilized to date. But another, and potentially more effective method may be possible. That is to transform microglia from the attack mode, which has been so well characterized, to a healing mode. Such a transformation might result in enhanced phagocytotic activity, coupled with a switch from expressing inflammatory cytokines such as IL-1 and TNF to expressing anti-inflammatory cytokines such as IL-4 and IL-10. In the process the beneficial effects of phagocytosis might be enhanced. For example, suppressing the CD-40/CD 40L interaction in transgenic mice enhances the phagocytic activity of microglia and increase Aβ clearance (Tan et al., 2002). Clearly there is much still to be learned. It can be said that, despite the huge expansion of activity that has taken place in recent years, it is still a field in its infancy.

SUMMARY

Our understanding of the innate immune system in brain commenced with recognition of a single marker, HLA-DR, on a single cell type, microglia, in a single disorder, Alzheimer disease. Twenty five years later, more than a thousand innate immune system markers have been identified which are associated with neurons, astrocytes, oligodendrocytes, and endothelial cells, as well as microglia.

They include, but are not limited to, complement proteins and their regulators, cytokines, chemokines, acute phase reactants, prostaglandins, proteases, protease inhibitors, coagulation factors, fibrinolytic factors, anaphylatoxins, integrins, and free radical generators. They are found in a spectrum of neurological diseases. Some stimulate inflammation, others inhibit it. Shifting the balance from a mode of attack to one of healing holds promise of having significant therapeutic benefit in a spectrum of degenerative diseases. Clearly there is much still to be learned. It can be said that, despite the huge expansion of activity that has taken place in the last 25 years, it is still a field in its infancy.

ACKNOWLEDGMENTS

This work was supported by the Pacific Alzheimer Research Foundation.

REFERENCES

Akiyama, H. Barger, S., Barnum, S., Bradt, B., Bauer, J., Cole, G. M., Cooper, N. R., Eikelenboom, P., Emmerling, M., Fiebich, B. L., Finch, C. E., Frautschy, S., Griffin, W. S., Hampel, H., Hull, M., Landreth, G., Lue, L., Mrak, R., Mackenzie, I. R., McGeer, P. L., O'Banion, M. K., Pachter, J., Pasinetti, G., Plata-Salaman, C., Rogers, J., Rydel, R., Shen, Y., Streit, W., Strohmeyer, R., Tooyoma, I., Van Muiswinkel, F. L., Veerhuis, R., Walker, D., Webster, S., Wegrzyniak, B., Wenk, G., Wyss-Coray, T, and Neuroinflammation Working Group. (2000). Inflammation and Alzheimer's disease. *Neurobiol. Aging* 21, 383–421.

Aschoff, L. (1924). Das reticulo-endotheliale system. *Ergeb. Inn. Med. Kinderheilkd.* 26, 1.

Ball, M. J. (1982). Limbic predilection in Alzheimer dementia: is reactivated herpes virus involved. *Can. J. Neurol. Sci.* 9, 303–306.

Banati, R. B., Gehrmann, J., Schubert, P., and Kreutzberg, G. W. (1993). Cytotoxicity of microglia. *Glia* 7, 111–118.

Del Rio Hortega, P. (1919). El tercer elemento de los centros nerviosis. *Bol. Soc. Esp. Biol.* 9, 69–129.

deTribolet, N., Hamou, M. F., Mach, J.-P., Carrel, S., and Schreyer, M. (1984). Demonstration of HLA-DR antigens in normal human brain. *J. Neurol. Neurosurg. Psychiatr.* 47, 417–418.

Dickson, D. W., Lee, S. C., Mattiace, L. A.,Yen, S. H. C., and Brosnan, C. (1993). Microglia and cytokines in neurological disease, with special reference to AIDS and Alzheimer's disease. *Glia* 7, 75–83.

Eikelenboom, P., and Stam, F. C. (1982). Immunoglobulins and complement factors in senile plaques. *Acta Neuropathol.* 57, 239–242.

Fujita, S. (1965). An autoradiographic study on the origin and fate of the sub-pial glioblast in the embryonic chick spinal cord. *J. Comp. Neurol.* 124, 51–59.

Fujita, S. (1973). Genesis of glioblasts in the human spinal cord as revealed by Feulgen cytophotometry. *J. Comp. Neurol.* 151, 25

Fujita, S., and Kitamura, T. (1973). Origin of brain macrophages and the nature of so-called microglia. *Acta Neuropathol. Suppl.* 6, 291–296.

Haymaker, W., and Adams, R. D. (1980a). *Histology and Histopathology of the Nervous System.* Springfield, IL: C. C. Thomas, 484–485.

Haymaker, W., and Adams, R. D. (1980b). *Histology and Histopathology of the Nervous System,* Chapter VI. Springfield, IL: C. C. Thomas, 481–559.

Ishii, T., and Haga, S. (1975). Identificantion of components of immunoglobulins in senile plaques by means of fluorescent antibody technique. *Acta Neuropathol.* 32, 157–162.

Johnson, S. A., Lampert-Etchells, M., Pasinetti, G. M., Rozovsky, I., and Finch, C. E. (1992). Complement mRNA in the mammalian brain: responses to Alzheimer's disease and experimental brain lesioning. *Neurobiol. Aging* 13, 641–648.

Kreutzberg, G. W. (1996). Microglia: a sensor for pathological events in the CNS. *Trends Neurosci.* 19, 312–318.

Lampson, L. A., and Hickey, W. F. (1986). Monoclonal antibody analysis of MHC expression in human brain biopsies: tissue ranging from "histologically normal" to that showing different levels of glial tumor involvement. *J. Immunol.* 136, 4054–4062.

Langston, J. W., Forno, L. S., and Tetrud, J., Reeves, A. G., Kaplan, J. A., and Karluk, D. (1999). Evidence of active nerve cell degeneration in the substantia nigra of humans years after 1-methyl-4-phenyl-1,2,3,6-tetrahydropyridine exposure. *Ann. Neurol.* 46, 598–605.

Langston, J. W., Irwin, I., Langston, E. B., and Forno, L. S. (1984). 1-Metyl-4-phenylpyridium ion (MPP+): identification of a metabolite of MPTP, a toxin selective to the substantia nigra. *Neurosci. Lett.* 48, 87–92.

Ling, E. A., and Wong, W. C. (1993). The origin and nature of ramified and ameboid microglia – a historical review and current concepts. *Glia* 7, 9–18.

Luber-Narod, J., and Rogers, J. (1988). Immune system associated antigens expressed by cells of the human central nervous system. *Neurosci. Lett.* 94, 17–22.

McGeer, P. L., Akiyama, H., Itagaki, S., and McGeer, E. (1989). Activation of the classical complement pathway in brain tissue of Alzheimer patients. *Neurosci. Lett.* 107, 341–346.

McGeer, P. L., Itagaki, S., and McGeer, E. G. (1988a). Expression of the histocompatibility glycoprotein HLA-DR in neurological disease. *Acta Neuropathol.* 76, 550–557.

McGeer, P. L., Itagaki, S., Akiyama, H., and McGeer, E. G. (1988b). Rate of cell death in parkinsonism indicates active neuropathological process. *Ann. Neurol.* 24, 574–576.

McGeer, P. L., Itagaki, S., Tago, H., and McGeer, E. G. (1987). Reactive microglia in patients with senile dementia of the Alzheimer types are positive for the histocompatibility glycoprotein HLA-DR. *Neurosci. Lett.* 79, 195–200.

McGeer, P. L., Kawamata, T, Walker, D. G., Akiyama, H, Tooyama, I., and McGeer, E. G. (1993). Microglia in degenerative neurological disease. *Glia* 7, 84–92.

McGeer, P. L., and McGeer, E. G. (1995). The inflammatory response system of brain: implications for therapy of Alzheimer and other neurodegenerative disorders. *Brain Res. Rev.* 21, 195–218.

McGeer, P. L., and McGeer, E. G. (2000). Autotoxicity and Alzheimer disease. *Arch. Neurol.* 57, 789–790.

McGeer, P. L., Rogers, J., McGeer, E. G., and Sibley, J. (1990). Does anti-inflammatory treatment protect against Alzheimer disease? *Lancet* 335, 1037.

McGeer, P. L., Schwab, C., Parent, A., and Doudet, D. (2003). Presence of reactive microglia in monkey substantia nigra years after 1-methyl-4-phenyl-1,2,3,6-tetrahydropyridine administration. *Ann. Neurol.* 54, 599–604.

Nimmerjahn, A., Kirchhoff, F., and Helmchen, F. (2005). Resting microglial cells are highly dynamic surveillants of brain parenchyma in vivo. *Science* 308, 1314–1318.

Oemichan, M., Wietholter, H., and Greaves, M. F. (1979). Immunoloical analysis of human microglia: lack of monocytic and lymphoid membrane differentiation antigens. *J. Neuropath. Exp. Neurol.* 38, 99–103.

Penfield, W. (1925). Microglia and the process of phagocytosis in gliomas. *Am. J. Pathol.* 1, 77–89.

Prados, M., and Gibson, W. C. (1946). *Pio del Rio Hortega*, 1882–1945. *J. Neurosurg.* 3, 275–284.

Rogers, J., Cooper, N. R., Webster, S., Schultz, J., McGeer, P. L., Styren, S. D., Civin, W. H., Brachova, L., Bradt, B., Ward, P., and Lieberburg, I. (1992). Complement activation by β-amyloid in Alzheimer disease. *Proc. Natl. Acad. Sci. U.S.A.* 89, 10016–10020.

Rogers, J., Luber-Narod, J., Sturen, C. D., and Civin, W. H. (1988). Expression of immune system-associated antigens by cells of the human central nervous system: relationship to the pathology of Alzheimer's disease. *Neurobiol. Aging* 9, 339–349.

Streit, W. J., Graeber, M. B., and Kreutzberg, G. W. (1988). Functional plasticity of microglia: a review. *Glia* 1, 301–307.

Tan, J., Town, T., Crawford, F., Mori, T., DelleDonne, A., Crescentini, R., Obregan, D., Flavelli, R. A., and Mullan, M. J. (2002). Role of CD40 ligand in amyloidosis in transgenic Alzeheimer's mice. *Nat. Neurosci.* 5, 1288–1293.

Van Furth, R., and Cohn, Z. A. (1968). The origin and kinetics of mononuclear phagocytes. *J. Exp. Med.* 128, 415–435.

Walker, D. G., and McGeer, P. L. (1992). Complement gene expression in human brains: comparison between normal and Alzheimer disease cases. *Brain Res. Mol. Brain Res.* 14, 109–116.

Walker, D. G., O'Kusky, J. R., and McGeer, P. L. (1989). In situ hybridization analysis for herpes simplex virus nucleic acids in Alzheimer disease. *Alzheimer Dis. Assoc. Disord.* 3, 123–131.

Wood, G. W., Gollahon, K. A., Tilzer, S. A., Vats, T., and Morantz, R. A. (1979). The failure of microglia in normal brain to exhibit mononuclear phagocyte markers. *J. Neuropathol. Exp. Neurol.* 38, 369–376.

Zhu, Y., Thangamani, S., and Ho, B. And Ding, J. L. (2005). The ancient origin of the complement system. *EMBO J.* 24, 382–394.

17

Biomarker-based prediction of progression in MCI: comparison of AD signature and hippocampal volume with spinal fluid amyloid-β and tau

Bradford C. Dickerson[1,2,3,4]* and David A. Wolk[5,6,7] for the Alzheimer's Disease Neuroimaging Initiative†

[1] Frontotemporal Dementia Unit, Massachusetts General Hospital and Harvard Medical School, Boston, MA, USA
[2] Department of Neurology, Massachusetts General Hospital and Harvard Medical School, Boston, MA, USA
[3] Massachusetts Alzheimer's Disease Research Center, Massachusetts General Hospital and Harvard Medical School, Boston, MA, USA
[4] Athinoula A. Martinos Center for Biomedical Imaging, Massachusetts General Hospital and Harvard Medical School, Boston, MA, USA
[5] Department of Neurology, University of Pennsylvania, Philadelphia, PA, USA
[6] Alzheimer's Disease Core Center, University of Pennsylvania, Philadelphia, PA, USA
[7] Penn Memory Center, University of Pennsylvania, Philadelphia, PA, USA

Edited by:
Manuel Menéndez-González, Hospital Álvarez-Buylla, Spain

Reviewed by:
Luísa Alves, Universidade Nova de Lisboa and Centro Hospitalar de Lisboa Ocidental, Portugal
Seong An, Gachon University, South Korea

***Correspondence:**
Bradford C. Dickerson, Frontotemporal Dementia Unit, Massachusetts General Hospital and Harvard Medical School, 149, 13th Street, Suite 2691, Charlestown, Boston, MA 02129, USA
e-mail: bradd@nmr.mgh.harvard.edu

†Data used in preparation of this article were obtained from the Alzheimer's Disease Neuroimaging Initiative (ADNI) database (adni.loni.ucla.edu). As such, the investigators within the ADNI contributed to the design and implementation of ADNI and/or provided data but did not participate in analysis or writing of this report. A complete listing of ADNI investigators can be found at: http://adni.loni.ucla.edu/wp-content/uploads/how_to_apply/ADNI_Acknowledgement_List.pdf

Objective: New diagnostic criteria for mild cognitive impairment (MCI) due to Alzheimer's disease (AD) have been developed using biomarkers aiming to establish whether the clinical syndrome is likely due to underlying AD. We investigated the utility of magnetic resonance imaging (MRI) and cerebrospinal fluid (CSF) biomarkers in predicting progression from amnesic MCI to dementia, testing the hypotheses that (1) markers of amyloid and neurodegeneration provide distinct and complementary prognostic information over different time intervals, and that (2) evidence of neurodegeneration in amyloid-negative MCI individuals would be useful prognostically.

Methods: Data were obtained from the ADNI-1 (Alzheimer's Disease Neuroimaging Initiative Phase 1) database on all individuals with a baseline diagnosis of MCI, baseline MRI and CSF data, and at least one follow-up visit. MRI data were processed using a published set of *a priori* regions of interest to derive a measure known as the "AD signature," as well as hippocampal volume. The CSF biomarkers amyloid-β, total tau, and phospho tau were also examined. We performed logistic regression analyses to identify the best baseline biomarker predictors of progression to dementia over 1 or 3 years, and Cox regression models to test the utility of these markers for predicting time-to-dementia.

Results: For prediction of dementia in MCI, the AD signature cortical thickness biomarker performed better than hippocampal volume. Although CSF tau measures were better than CSF amyloid-β at predicting dementia within 1 year, the AD signature was better than all CSF measures at prediction over this relatively short-term interval. CSF amyloid-β was superior to tau and AD signature at predicting dementia over 3 years. When CSF amyloid-β was dichotomized using previously published cutoff values and treated as a categorical variable, a multivariate stepwise Cox regression model indicated that both the AD signature MRI marker and the categorical CSF amyloid-β marker were useful in predicting time-to-event diagnosis of AD dementia.

Conclusion: In amnesic MCI, short-term (1 year) prognosis of progression to dementia relates strongly to baseline markers of neurodegeneration, with the AD signature MRI biomarker of cortical thickness performing the best among MRI and CSF markers studied here. Longer-term (3 year) prognosis in these individuals was better predicted by a marker indicative of brain amyloid. Prediction of time-to-event in a survival model was predicted by the combination of these biomarkers. These results provide further support for emerging models of the temporal relationship of pathophysiologic events in AD and demonstrate the utility of these biomarkers at the prodromal stage of the illness.

Keywords: Alzheimer's disease, MRI, biomarkers, mild cognitive impairment, CSF biomarkers

INTRODUCTION

When insidious in onset and gradually progressive, mild cognitive impairment (MCI) is a clinical syndrome commonly arising as a result of neurodegenerative pathology (Petersen et al., 2006). In living persons, evidence of neurodegenerative pathology is provided by a growing array of imaging and fluid biomarkers. If the goal is to determine whether MCI appears highly likely to be due to underlying Alzheimer pathology, the recently published MCI diagnostic criteria require evidence of (1) cerebral amyloidosis [amyloid positron emission tomography (PET) or cerebrospinal fluid (CSF) amyloid-β] and (2) neurodegeneration [magnetic resonance imaging (MRI)-derived atrophy, fluorodeoxyglucose (FDG)-PET-derived hypometabolism, or CSF tau; Albert et al., 2011]. A number of studies have now shown that, within a group of persons with MCI, the presence and prominence of these biomarkers are predictive of the likelihood of Alzheimer's disease (AD) dementia within a few years (Jack et al., 1999; Hansson et al., 2006; Wang et al., 2006; Vemuri et al., 2009b; Visser et al., 2009; Blennow et al., 2010; De Meyer et al., 2010; Jack et al., 2010; Landau et al., 2010; Buchhave et al., 2012). Despite the importance of observations from these studies, a number of questions remain, particularly when considering how to use biomarkers in the design of clinical trials of putative interventions. Further, as more clinicians are beginning to incorporate these measures into clinical practice, a deeper understanding of the relative implications of these biomarkers is critical.

In persons with MCI, what are the best MRI-derived biomarkers of neurodegeneration with regard to prediction of progression to dementia? One very commonly used measure is hippocampal volume, which has consistently been shown to predict dementia in MCI (Frisoni et al., 2010). We have developed an AD signature cortical thickness marker (Dickerson et al., 2009), and hypothesize that this marker will outperform commonly used MRI-derived biomarkers as an indicator of AD-related neurodegeneration in MCI that is predictive of AD dementia.

Another major question relates to the temporal utility of biomarkers. What are the best markers for short-term vs. longer-term prediction of dementia? Although current clinico-pathologic constructs of AD require evidence of cerebral amyloidosis, data are conflicting as to whether markers of amyloid or neurodegeneration best predict dementia and to our knowledge none have specifically tested hypotheses about the comparative utility of amyloid vs. neurodegenerative markers at different time intervals. We tested two hypothesis here: (1) rapid progression (i.e., over 1 year) from MCI to AD dementia is better predicted by markers of neurodegeneration rather than the presence of amyloid; (2) longer-term progression from MCI to dementia (i.e., 3 years) is best predicted by the presence of abnormal levels of brain amyloid. This prediction follows from the notion that cerebral amyloidosis may be a relatively earlier development in AD pathophysiology compared to evidence of neurodegeneration measured using *in vivo* methods (Jack et al., 2013). Further, neurodegenerative markers appear to be more sensitive to disease state than measures of cerebral amyloid (Jack et al., 2009; Vemuri et al., 2009a). As such, amyloid measures may differentiate individuals who will eventually progress to AD over longer-term follow-up while neurodegenerative markers may indicate an elevated risk for more proximate cognitive decline and dementia.

Finally, the focus of a number of studies of biomarker prediction of AD dementia in amnestic MCI has been on the 50–75% of subjects with evidence of cerebral amyloidosis. What about the other individuals, especially those who may show evidence suggestive of neurodegeneration (Knopman et al., 2012; Petersen et al., 2013)? Are MRI-derived markers useful in predicting dementia in individuals with MCI who do not have evidence of cerebral amyloidosis?

Here we undertook a set of analyses of the Alzheimer's Disease Neuroimaging Initiative (ADNI) dataset to investigate these questions, focusing on the utility of MRI and CSF biomarkers for prognosis in MCI.

MATERIALS AND METHODS

PARTICIPANTS

Data used in the preparation of this article were obtained from the ADNI database[1]. The ADNI was launched in 2003 by the National Institute on Aging (NIA), the National Institute of Biomedical Imaging and Bioengineering (NIBIB), the Food and Drug Administration (FDA), private pharmaceutical companies, and non-profit organizations, as a $60 million, 5-year public–private partnership. The primary goal of ADNI has been to test whether serial MRI, PET, other biological markers, and clinical and neuropsychological assessment can be combined to measure the progression of MCI and early AD. Determination of sensitive and specific markers of very early AD progression is intended to aid researchers and clinicians to develop new treatments and monitor their effectiveness, as well as lessen the time and cost of clinical trials.

The Principal Investigator of this initiative is Michael W. Weiner, MD, VA Medical Center and University of California – San Francisco. ADNI is the result of efforts of many co-investigators from a broad range of academic institutions and private corporations, and subjects have been recruited from over 50 sites across the U.S. and Canada. The initial goal of ADNI was to recruit 800 subjects but ADNI has been followed by ADNI-GO and ADNI-2. To date these three protocols have recruited over 1500 adults, ages 55–90, to participate in the research, consisting of cognitively normal older individuals, people with early or late MCI, and people with early AD. The follow-up duration of each group is specified in the protocols for ADNI-1, ADNI-2, and ADNI-GO. Subjects originally recruited for ADNI-1 and ADNI-GO had the option to be followed in ADNI-2. For up-to-date information, see www.adni-info.org.

For the current analysis, we selected individuals with a baseline diagnosis of MCI who had baseline MRI and CSF data available, and at least 1 year of clinical follow-up ($n = 154$). Detailed diagnostic, inclusion, and exclusion criteria are described on the ADNI website[2].

STANDARD PROTOCOL APPROVALS, REGISTRATIONS, AND PATIENT CONSENTS

Each participant gave written informed consent in accordance with institutional Human Subjects Research Committee guidelines.

MRI IMAGING AND ANALYSIS

Magnetic resonance imaging scans were collected on a 1.5T scanner using a standardized MPRAGE protocol: sagittal plane, TR/TE/TI, 2400/3/1000 ms, flip angle 8°, 24 cm FOV, 192 × 192

[1] www.adni.loni.ucla.edu

[2] http://www.adni-info.org/

in-plane matrix, 1.2 mm slice thickness (Jack et al., 2008). Fully pre-processed scans were downloaded for analysis.

T1 image volumes were examined quantitatively by a cortical surface-based reconstruction and analysis of cortical thickness, using a hypothesis-driven approach as described in multiple previous publications (Bakkour et al., 2009; Dickerson et al., 2009, 2011; Wolk et al., 2010). Briefly, we utilized nine regions of interest (ROIs, see **Figure 1**) previously determined to be associated with AD, the "cortical signature" of AD (Bakkour et al., 2009; Dickerson et al., 2009).

For the purposes of this study, we employed a primary diagnostic biomarker, the single summary "AD signature measure," the average thickness of all nine ROIs. With the goal of adjusting this measure for normal age-related influences on these brain regions, we also measured a set of "Aging signature" ROIs, as previously published (Bakkour et al., 2013). We calculated an "AD signature index" measure by first performing a linear regression in the amyloid-negative control group with the Aging signature as the independent variable and the AD signature as the dependent variable. We then used this equation to calculate the "AD signature index values for each MCI patient." Thus, an individual with a lower AD signature index value has cortical thickness within the AD signature ROIs that is disproportionately smaller than the thickness of the Aging signature ROIs, likely reflecting more specific AD-related neurodegeneration. Alternatively, an individual with a higher AD signature index value has cortical thickness within the AD signature ROIs that is of similar relative magnitude to Aging signature ROIs, possibly reflecting more diffuse effects.

In addition, for comparison purposes, we analyzed hippocampal volume using the measure provided by the automated segmentation procedure from FreeSurfer, divided by total intracranial volume. Our standard procedure is to visually inspect selected coronal slices of each automated segmentation and identify scans with errors in processing of the structure of interest. We also inspect the distribution of the quantitative volumetric data and review scans at either tail of the distribution and outliers in greater detail. In the present analysis, no scans were identified with important errors of hippocampal segmentation.

BASELINE CEREBROSPINAL FLUID MEASURES

We also examined baseline CSF levels of amyloid-β, total tau (t-tau), and phosphorylated tau (p-tau). For the primary analyses, we used the raw values as continuous measures; however, t-tau and p-tau were log-transformed to better approximate normality in distribution. For analyses in which we classified subjects as having CSF amyloid-β values consistent with those of autopsy-proven AD, we used a cutoff value of levels less than 192 (Shaw et al., 2009). Individuals with levels ≥ 192 were considered to be unlikely to have cerebral amyloidosis.

LONGITUDINAL OUTCOMES

Here we used outcomes at 1 or 3 years. The primary outcome measures used in the present analysis were conversion to a diagnosis of AD dementia at 1 or at 3 years.

STATISTICAL ANALYSIS

Tests of group differences were performed using Chi-square analysis (for frequencies) or Analysis of Variance (for continuous measures) with *post hoc* pairwise comparisons where relevant; $a = 0.05$. Since effect sizes were expected to be subtle and strong *a priori* hypotheses were being tested, no multiple comparisons correction procedures were performed. In addition, the impact of biomarkers on clinical outcome was analyzed using separate logistic regression models for each of the two intervals of follow-up, constructed using the dichotomous conversion to dementia outcome measure as the dependent variable. Cox regression models were constructed to investigate the relationship of baseline biomarkers to the likelihood of progression to AD dementia using a more fine-grained time-to-event outcome rather than the two follow-up intervals employed in the other analyses. A multivariate

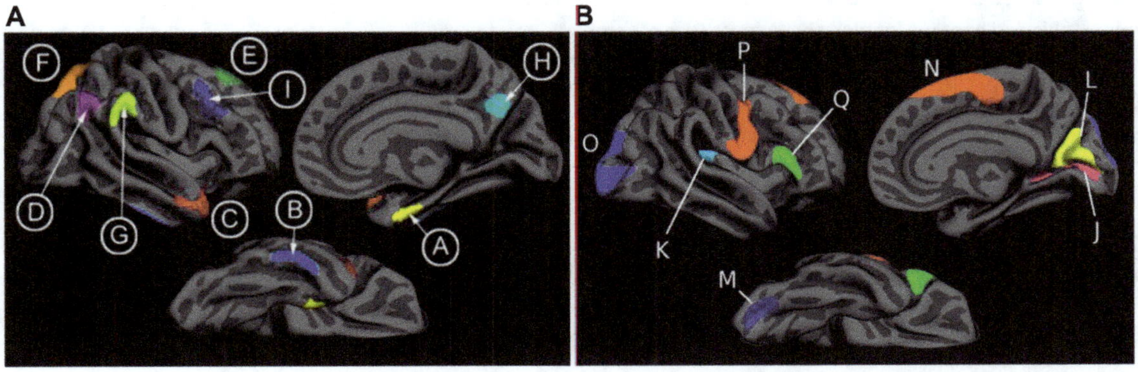

FIGURE 1 | (A) The cortical signature of AD is composed of *a priori* regions of interest in which consistent atrophy has been previously observed in multiple samples of patients with mild AD dementia. **(B)** The cortical signature of normal aging is composed of *a priori* regions of interest in which consistent atrophy has been previously described in healthy cognitively intact older adults compared with younger adults. We calculated the "AD signature index" measure by performing a linear regression with the Aging signature (excluding regions overlapping with AD signature regions; see Figures 1 and 2 of Bakkour et al., 2013) as the independent variable and the AD signature as the dependent variable. The residuals of this regression analysis were then saved as the "AD signature index." Key: A: medial temporal, B: inferior temporal, C: temporal pole, D: Angular, E: superior frontal, F: superior parietal, G: supramarginal, H: precuneus, I: middle frontal, J: calcarine, K: caudal insula, L: cuneus, M: caudal fusiform, N: dorsomedial frontal, O: lateral occipital, P: precentral, Q: inferior frontal.

Cox regression model was then constructed including independent variables that reached a trend-level effect ($p < 0.1$) in the univariate analyses (p-value-to-enter <0.05). Covariates of age, education, and gender were generally not significant in the models and had minimal impact on the findings. Statistical analyses were performed using IBM SPSS 21.0.

RESULTS

Of the 156 MCI participants with baseline MRI and CSF data who were followed for 1 year, 31 (20%) were diagnosed with probable AD dementia. Of the 111 who had 3-year outcome data, 48 (43%) were diagnosed with probable AD dementia. In the subset of MCI participants with baseline CSF evidence of cerebral amyloidosis, 26 of 116 (22%) were diagnosed with probable AD dementia at 1 year and 45 of 83 (54%) at 3 years. In contrast, in the subgroup of MCI participants with normal baseline CSF amyloid-β levels, only 5 of 40 (13%) converted to AD dementia at 1 year and 3 of 27 (11%) at 3 years. See **Table 1** for additional details.

We first sought to determine which of the baseline biomarkers would be useful in prediction of the likelihood of a diagnosis of probable AD dementia in the entire sample of MCI subjects. For the 1-year outcome interval, baseline cortical thickness measured with the AD signature MRI biomarker index was strongly associated with the likelihood of probable AD: a logistic regression model predicting a 1-year AD outcome indicated a nearly threefold increase in the likelihood of AD dementia for each 1 SD thinner cortex [odds ratio (OR) = 2.7, 95% C.I.: [1.7–4.5], $p < 0.0001$). In addition, baseline CSF p-tau levels were predictive of AD dementia, with each 1 SD increase in CSF p-tau levels being associated with a 1.7-fold increase in the likelihood of AD dementia (OR = 1.7, 95% C.I.: [1.09–2.7], $p = 0.02$). None of the other biomarkers demonstrated effects or trend-level effects. In the stepwise multivariate logistic regression model, the AD signature MRI marker entered but CSF p-tau did not, indicating that CSF p-tau did not explain additional variance in outcome beyond that explained by the AD signature MRI marker.

In contrast, 3-year conversion was best predicted by baseline CSF amyloid-β levels, with each 1 SD of reduction indicating a 1.9-fold increase in 3-year likelihood of AD dementia (OR = 1.9, 95% C.I.: [1.2–3.0], $p = 0.003$). A slightly weaker effect was observed for the AD signature index (OR = 1.7, 95% C.I.: [1.12–2.6], $p = 0.01$). Significant effects were also observed for CSF p-tau (OR = 1.8, 95% C.I.: [1.14–2.7], $p = 0.01$) and CSF t-tau (OR = 1.6, 95% C.I.: [1.06–2.5], $p = 0.03$) while hippocampal volume displayed a strong trend (OR = 1.5, 95% C.I.: [1.00–2.29], $p = 0.05$). In the stepwise multivariate model, CSF amyloid-β entered but the other two did not.

Figure 2 depicts the values for the AD signature cortical thickness MRI marker and CSF amyloid-β for each of the three MCI subgroups based on outcome (stable over 3 years, 3-year converters who did not convert by year 1, and 1-year converters). The mean values for CSF amyloid-β are lower in both groups of converters than in stable MCI (1-year: $p < 0.05$; 3-year: $p < 0.01$), but there is no difference based on year of conversion ($p > 0.3$). Alternatively, values for AD signature cortical thickness are lower for both groups of converters than the stable group (1-year: $p < 0.001$; 3-year: $p = 0.05$), but also for the 1-year converters compared to the 3-year converters ($p < 0.05$; all values shown are Z scores derived from the normative values of controls).

We next investigated the utility of biomarkers for prediction of a diagnosis of AD dementia in subgroups of MCI subjects divided on the basis of baseline CSF amyloid-β levels. In the subgroup of MCI subjects with abnormally low baseline CSF amyloid-β levels (consistent with cerebral amyloidosis), 1-year conversion to AD dementia was predicted by the AD signature MRI biomarker (OR = 2.2, 95% C.I.: [1.3–3.8], $p = 0.005$). None of the other biomarkers were predictive in these univariate models. For 3-year prediction, a significant effect for the AD signature MRI biomarker (OR = 1.7, 95% C.I.: [1.1–2.7], $p = 0.03$) and a trend for hippocampal volume (OR = 1.5, 95% C.I.: [0.95–2.5], $p = 0.08$) were observed.

Table 1 | Demographic and baseline biomarker characteristics of sample.

Subject group	1-year outcome (N = 156)		3-year outcome (N = 111)	
N (%) or M (SD)	MCI (N = 125)	AD (N = 31)	MCI (N = 63)	AD (N = 48)
Age (years)	74.9 (7.6)	72.3 (6.90)	74.7 (7.3)	74.3 (7.7)
Gender	84 M: 41 F	17 M: 14 F	47 M: 16 F	30 M: 18 F
Education (years)	15.8 (3.0)	15.1 (3.2)	15.6 (3.0)	15.6 (3.4)
MMSE	27.5 (1.7)	26.7 (1.9)	27.3 (1.8)	26.7 (1.9)
CDR-SB	1.9 (0.8)	2.4 (0.9)*	1.7 (0.6)	2.2 (1.0)*
CSF amyloid-β Z score	−0.73 (1.00)	−0.99 (0.70)	−0.56 (1.12)	−1.15 (0.65)**
CSF Total tau Z score	0.69 (1.07)	1.17 (1.13)	0.74 (1.22)	1.26 (1.13)*
CSF P-tau Z score	0.69 (1.06)	1.20 (0.99)*	0.62 (1.04)	1.12 (0.93)*
AD signature Z score	−0.82 (1.13)	−1.82 (1.27)**	−0.63 (1.12)	−1.26 (1.19)*
Hippo vol Z	−0.94 (1.14)	−1.24 (1.06)	−0.75 (1.05)	−1.15 (1.04)†

*$p < 0.05$, **$p < 0.005$ groups are different from each other.
†$p = 0.05$, groups demonstrate trend-level difference from each other.

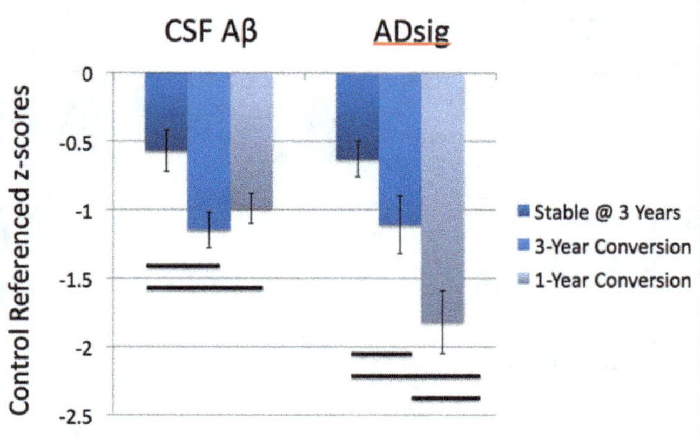

FIGURE 2 | Values for the AD signature cortical thickness and CSF amyloid-β for each of the three MCI subgroups based on outcome (stable over 3 years, 3-year converters, and 1-year converters). The mean values for CSF amyloid-β are lower in both groups of converters than in stable MCI (left), while the values for AD signature index of cortical thickness are lower in the 1-year converters than in the other two groups (right; all values shown are Z scores derived from the normative values of controls and bars represent statistically significant comparisons).

In the subgroup of MCI subjects with normal CSF amyloid-β levels, indicating the likely absence of cerebral amyloidosis, 1-year conversion to AD dementia was best predicted by the AD signature MRI biomarker (OR = 6.4, 95% C.I.: [1.5–27.5], $p = 0.01$), with hippocampal volume showing utility as well (OR = 3.5, 95% C.I.: [1.2–10.7], $p = 0.03$) but not entering the multivariate model. None of the CSF markers demonstrated predictive value. For 3-year prediction, none of the markers were useful although power was extremely low due to the small number of individuals who were diagnosed with AD dementia.

Finally, we performed a survival analysis to investigate the utility of these biomarkers for predicting the time to a diagnosis of AD dementia. Univariate Cox proportional hazards regression models indicated that each of the biomarkers was a predictor of time to diagnosis of AD dementia over the 3-year follow-up period (**Table 2**). In multivariate analysis, a stepwise forward conditional model demonstrated that the AD signature MRI biomarker was the best and only predictor when each independent variable was entered as a continuous variable. However, when CSF amyloid-β was dichotomized using previously published cutoff values (Shaw et al., 2009) and treated as a categorical variable, the multivariate stepwise Cox regression model indicated that both the AD signature MRI marker and the categorical CSF amyloid-β marker were useful in predicting time-to-event diagnosis of AD dementia. Of all the models, this was the model with the overall strongest statistical results ($X^2 = 19.4$, $p < 0.001$). This result is illustrated in **Figure 3** in which the AD signature was also dichotomized to maximize sensitivity and specificity between amyloid-negative controls and amyloid-positive mild AD patients from the ADNI cohort.

Finally, to begin to assess the specificity of the refined AD signature index measure we analyzed the relationships between CSF biomarkers and the raw AD signature measure (in millimeters) and the adjusted AD signature index measure (adjusted for thickness of the Aging signature regions as described in Section "Materials and Methods." The adjusted AD signature index exhibited substantially stronger correlations (**Table 3**) with all CSF biomarkers relative to the raw AD signature, suggesting that this adjustment for "brain age" improves the specificity of this MRI biomarker for AD-related neurodegeneration.

Table 2 | Results of Cox regression analyses of baseline CSF and MRI biomarker measures predicting probable AD diagnosis.

	X^2	HR	95% CI
AD signature	13.7 ($p < 0.001$)**	1.61	1.25–2.08
AD signature dichotomous	12.9 ($p < 0.001$)**	2.28	1.44–3.63
CSF amyloid-β dichotomous	12.2 ($p < 0.001$)**	3.66	1.68–7.99
CSF amyloid-β	7.4 ($p < 0.01$)*	1.42	1.10–1.83
CSF p-tau	9.2 ($p < 0.01$)*	1.47	1.15–1.90
CSF t-tau	5.5 ($p < 0.05$)*	1.33	1.05–1.70
Hippocampal volume	4.8 ($p < 0.05$)*	1.31	1.03–1.67
Combination of CSF dichotomous amyloid-β and AD signature	19.4 ($p < 0.0001$)**	Aβ 3.0 ADsig 1.4	1.38–6.7 1.07–1.77

*$p < 0.05$, **$p < 0.005$.

DISCUSSION

When individuals are diagnosed with MCI, the two most pressing clinical questions relate to etiology and prognosis. We now have a growing armamentarium of biomarkers for AD and other neurodegenerative diseases, and reasonably mature diagnostic criteria for "MCI of the Alzheimer type" (Albert et al., 2011) which hinge on a typical clinical syndrome and the presence of one or more imaging or fluid biomarkers. In this analysis, we used ADNI data to test two major hypotheses in patients with MCI: (1) markers of amyloid and neurodegeneration provide distinct and complementary prognostic information over different time intervals, and that (2) evidence of neurodegeneration in amyloid-negative MCI individuals is useful prognostically. We found compelling support for both hypotheses.

For prediction of AD dementia in MCI, the AD signature cortical thickness biomarker performed better than hippocampal volume. Although CSF tau measures, also putative neurodegenerative biomarkers, were better than CSF amyloid-β at predicting dementia within 1 year, the AD signature was better than all CSF measures at prediction over this relatively short-term interval. CSF amyloid-β was superior to tau and AD signature at predicting dementia over 3 years. In an analysis examining the combined use of CSF and MRI measures, when CSF amyloid-β was dichotomized using previously published cutoff values and treated as a categorical variable, a Cox regression model indicated that both the AD signature MRI marker and the categorical CSF amyloid-β marker were useful in predicting time-to-event diagnosis of AD dementia. These results provide further support for emerging models of the pathophysiology of AD and demonstrate the utility of the combined use of these biomarkers at the prodromal stage of the illness (Jack et al., 2010; Landau et al., 2010; Vemuri et al., 2010).

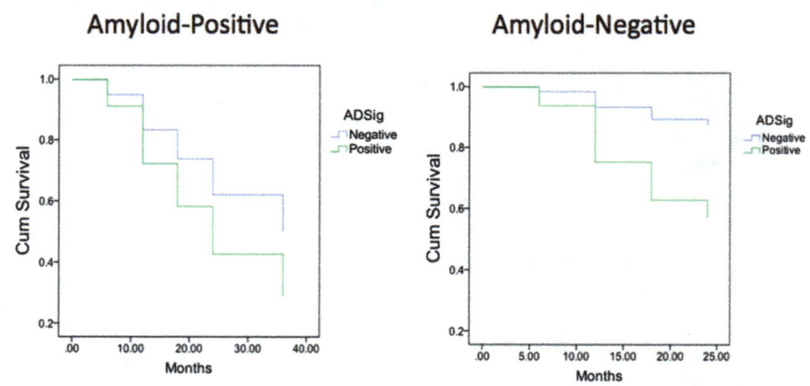

FIGURE 3 | Survival curves in MCI participants who were "amyloid-negative" at baseline (left) vs. those who were "amyloid positive" (right) as a function of baseline AD signature index using dichotomous cutoff.

Table 3 | Relationships of CSF biomarkers to MRI biomarkers.

	Age	CSF t-tau	CSF p-tau	CSF amyloid-β
Aging signature	$r = -0.38$ ($p < 0.001$)	$r = -0.05$ NS	$r = -0.04$ NS	$r = -0.06$ NS
AD signature	$r = -0.30$ ($p < 0.001$)	$r = -0.26$ ($p < 0.01$)	$r = -0.21$ ($p < 0.01$)	$r = -0.09$ NS
Adjusted AD signature	$r = 0.05$ NS	$r = -0.37$ ($p < 0.001$)	$r = -0.35$ ($p < 0.001$)	$r = 0.22$ ($p < 0.01$)
Hippocampal volume	$r = -0.19$ ($p < 0.05$)	$r = -0.04$ NS	$r = -0.03$ NS	$r = 0.05$ NS

A major novel contribution of the present study is the investigation of the prognostic utility of different biomarkers over intervals of varying times after the markers were obtained at baseline. To our knowledge, no prior study has explicitly examined separate follow-up intervals in MCI and measured the differential utility of amyloid vs. structural MRI markers. As we plan clinical trials of pharmacologic and non-pharmacologic interventions in MCI, it is critical not only to consider methods to homogenize the patient population for inclusion (e.g., requiring MCI patients to have cerebral amyloidosis for inclusion); it may also be valuable in some trial designs to use a marker of neurodegeneration to identify patients in whom progression to dementia is likely within a relatively short time interval, such as 1 year. Such a stratified design for inclusion might be valuable in that most such participants would be likely to decline substantially during a reasonable follow-up interval, thereby maximizing power to detect a beneficial effect of the intervention. Of course, it is also possible that in these more "aggressive" cases of prodromal AD a drug might be less efficacious than in more indolent forms of the disease, but that remains an open question.

These considerations are also becoming of greater relevance in clinical practice, particularly in light of recent FDA approval of the amyloid PET ligand florbetapir. Further, with the development of the above-described guidelines for incorporation of biomarkers into the assessment of MCI patients, it is likely that clinicians will be bringing these measures into their clinical practice for prognostication of MCI. The current work emphasizes that these tests may provide somewhat different information, which may have important implications for their value depending on the question that is being addressed. For example, MRI may be more valuable when interested in determining the likelihood of decline in the near future, which could influence life decisions that need to be made within that timeframe whereas the presence of amyloid may more definitively reflect the likelihood of progression, but have less value in predicting the timing.

It seems intuitive, based on current models of biomarkers of AD pathophysiology (Jack et al., 2013), that the presence of cerebral amyloidosis would be valuable for longer-term prognosis while an MRI-derived marker of neurodegeneration would demonstrate utility in shorter-term prognosis. As the individuals with MCI in this study were followed longitudinally, those with baseline cerebral amyloid progressed to dementia at a rate of about 15–20% per year, while only about 10–15% of those without baseline brain amyloid progressed to dementia after 3 years, most doing so within the first year of follow-up. Those who progressed to AD dementia at 3 years had baseline CSF amyloid-β levels that are similarly reduced to those who progressed at 1 year. This is consistent with models that suggest that amyloid deposition is an early feature of the disease that largely plateaus by the symptomatic stage of disease resulting in relatively poor resolution of disease state (i.e., proximity to dementia) at that stage (Villemagne et al., 2013). In contrast, the baseline MRI-derived AD signature measure of cortical thickness was substantially lower in individuals who progressed at 1 year than in those who progressed at 3 years (**Figure 2**). This indicates that once AD-related neurodegenerative cortical atrophy is prominent enough in MCI patients, further cognitive decline and loss of functional independence is imminent. Such a finding demonstrates the greater degree by which markers of neurodegeneration, particularly structural MRI measures, track disease state during symptomatic stages of disease.

The differences described here in temporal prediction and, ultimately, the complementary nature of biomarkers of cerebral amyloidosis with neurodegeneration are quite consistent with a number of recent studies in the literature exploring this issue. For example, Buchhave et al. (2012) recently described that while the presence of low CSF amyloid-β predicted conversion to AD in MCI patients, CSF p-tau status was associated with the timing of this conversion (abnormal: conversion in 0–5 years; normal: conversion in 5–10 years). Another group, also using the ADNI dataset, compared dichotomous measures of hippocampal atrophy, memory testing, and CSF total tau, p-tau, and amyloid-β in prediction of conversion. They found that median survival was generally shorter for neurodegenerative biomarkers while CSF amyloid-β had the longest median time before conversion (Heister et al., 2011). Further, using a FDG-PET "signature" of AD, similar to the structural one applied here, Landau et al. (2010) found that this measure was also superior to CSF amyloid-β for prediction of conversion in MCI patients with mean follow-up under 2 years. This group also described a tighter link between cognitive decline and cerebral amyloidosis, based on amyloid imaging, in asymptomatic individuals, but stronger association of decline with FDG-PET status in MCI (Landau et al., 2012). Thus, the current findings serve as additional support for the leading model of the proposed biomarker cascade (Jack et al., 2013), which has also found additional verification in longitudinal study of asymptomatic dominantly inherited AD mutation carriers (Bateman et al., 2012).

A variety of MRI measures have been proposed as potential biomarkers of neurodegeneration in early AD, both with regard to the identification of presumed atrophy consistent with AD and with regard to monitoring changes over time that indicate progression of neurodegeneration. Hippocampal volume is the most widely employed and discussed measure of this type, and while clearly informative, it is increasingly appearing to be less sensitive and specific than other measures such as regional cortical thickness. We have previously shown using receiver operating characteristic analyses that the AD signature measure is superior to hippocampal volume in discriminating individuals with prodromal AD who progress to dementia within 3 years from those who do not (Bakkour et al., 2009). Here we used logistic and Cox regression models to demonstrate the superiority of the AD signature over hippocampal volume in predicting progression to dementia in both amyloid-positive and amyloid-negative individuals with MCI. Nonetheless, it is worth noting that while not as strongly predictive of conversion as the AD signature, hippocampal volume still had predictive value in most of these analyses consistent with prior work using this measure (for review, see Frisoni et al., 2010). Further, much of the literature has applied cutoff values or categorical groupings of hippocampal volumes in similar analyses to those presented here, which may provide additional predictive power (Jack et al., 1999, 2010; Landau et al., 2010; Heister et al., 2011). Future work should explore optimized cutoffs for the AD signature and other structural measures, allowing for comparison of these measures in both continuous and dichotomous forms.

It is also important to note that we compared CSF molecular biomarkers on an individual basis, as opposed to the combination of these markers. However, it appears that a combination of these measures may further enhance prediction (Shaw et al., 2009; De Meyer et al., 2010). In particular, ratios of t-tau or p-tau to amyloid-β may improve prediction by incorporating both neurodegenerative and amyloid-based measures, akin to our finding that the combination of the AD signature and CSF amyloid-β produced the strongest model in the Cox regression analysis. Nonetheless, the current analysis was developed to specifically compare across these classes of biomarkers and, as such, we chose to keep the CSF measures uncoupled.

In the present study, we employed a novel approach to the calculation of our AD signature measure. In the past, we have generally not adjusted for age-related cortical atrophy, but in some analyses have simply corrected statistically for a participant's chronological age. We recently reported on the cortical signature of normal aging (the "Aging signature"), describing a set of association and sensorimotor regions that undergo the most prominent loss of thickness in cognitively normal elderly adults compared to young adults (Bakkour et al., 2013). In the analyses here, we used the Aging signature set of regions to adjust for the "cortical age" of the individuals, creating an AD signature index, which represents the residual variance of the AD signature after accounting for variations in the Aging signature regional measurements. This corrects for the fact that some individuals may have thinner cortex in at least some of the regions vulnerable to AD simply as a result of more widespread cortical atrophy associated with normal aging, while those with thinner cortex in AD-vulnerable regions who have preserved thickness in Aging-vulnerable regions are much more likely to be exhibiting atrophy associated specifically with AD pathology. To our knowledge, this type of an adjustment of MRI biomarkers has not been performed previously. We are continuing to explore the strengths and weaknesses of this approach.

Finally, our analysis indicated that the MRI-derived AD signature biomarker was useful for predicting progression to dementia within 1 year in MCI participants with baseline CSF amyloid-β levels not low enough to meet typical cutoffs indicating cerebral amyloidosis. Even though the percentage of individuals who progressed to dementia in this subgroup was low (13%), the MRI marker was still useful for prediction in this short time interval. To interpret this finding, we have considered several possibilities. First, it is possible that these individuals have a non-Alzheimer pathology that is associated with atrophy in some of the same structures affected by AD. Although this consideration certainly seems reasonable when the structural MRI measure is of the hippocampus, since pathologies such as hippocampal sclerosis could be playing a role, it seems harder to reconcile with an MRI biomarker measuring a spatially distributed pattern of atrophy. We are currently examining the use of the AD signature marker in differential diagnosis of other neurodegenerative diseases, including frontotemporal dementias and Lewy body dementia; findings from this work will provide important data on the specificity of this marker in other neurodegenerative diseases. It is also possible that these individuals actually have underlying AD pathology but are "below the threshold" of amyloid pathology to meet current CSF cutoffs. This group could also be akin to previously reported cognitively normal and MCI individuals with evidence of AD-like neurodegeneration and negative amyloid status, which has been labeled suspected non-Alzheimer pathology (sNAP; Knopman et al., 2012; Petersen et al., 2013; Prestia et al., 2013). While debate continues regarding the underlying pathology in these individuals, Prestia et al. (2013) also similarly reported that such individuals with an MCI phenotype also had a high rate of conversion to clinical dementia. As they note, it is worth at least considering that these patients may require adaptation of the model of biomarker change used here, as has been recently discussed (Jack et al., 2013). It is also worth noting that the individuals in this group in the present analysis who progressed to dementia were diagnosed clinically with probable AD dementia rather than a non-AD dementia.

Limitations of the present study include the relatively short follow-up period and the small number of individuals who were amyloid-negative at baseline with adequate longitudinal follow-up data. Furthermore, a more broadly representative sample of individuals with MCI might be helpful to better determine whether these findings are generalizable to clinical practice. Nevertheless, we believe the results of the present analysis provide valuable insights about the use of biomarkers in an MCI sample likely to be similar to that considered for clinical trials of putative AD interventions.

ACKNOWLEDGMENTS

Data collection and sharing for this project was funded by the Alzheimer's Disease Neuroimaging Initiative (ADNI; National Institutes of Health Grant U01 AG024904). ADNI is funded by the National Institute on Aging, the National Institute of Biomedical Imaging and Bioengineering, and through generous contributions from the following: Alzheimer's Association; Alzheimer's Drug Discovery Foundation; BioClinica, Inc.; Biogen Idec Inc.; Bristol-Myers Squibb Company; Eisai Inc.; Elan Pharmaceuticals, Inc.; Eli Lilly and Company; F. Hoffmann-La Roche Ltd and its affiliated company Genentech, Inc.; GE Healthcare; Innogenetics, N.V.; IXICO Ltd.; Janssen Alzheimer Immunotherapy Research & Development, LLC.; Johnson & Johnson Pharmaceutical Research & Development LLC.; Medpace, Inc.; Merck & Co., Inc.; Meso Scale Diagnostics, LLC.; NeuroRx Research; Novartis Pharmaceuticals Corporation; Pfizer Inc.; Piramal Imaging; Servier; Synarc Inc.; and Takeda Pharmaceutical Company. The Canadian Institutes of Health Research is providing funds to support ADNI clinical sites in Canada. Private sector contributions are facilitated by the Foundation for the National Institutes of Health (www.fnih.org). The grantee organization is the Northern California Institute for Research and Education, and the study is coordinated by the Alzheimer's Disease Cooperative Study at the University of California, San Diego. ADNI data are disseminated by the Laboratory for Neuro Imaging at the University of California, Los Angeles. This research was also supported by NIH grants P30 AG010129 and K01 AG030514. This research was also supported by NIH grants P30 AG010129, K01 AG030514, and the Dana Foundation. This analysis was also supported by grants from the NIA P50-AG005134, P30AG010124, and the Alzheimer's Association. We thank Michael Brickhouse for his assistance in data management and analysis.

REFERENCES

Albert, M. S., DeKosky, S. T., Dickson, D., Dubois, B., Feldman, H. H., Fox, N. C., et al. (2011). The diagnosis of mild cognitive impairment due to Alzheimer's disease: recommendations from the National Institute on Aging-Alzheimer's Association workgroups on diagnostic guidelines for Alzheimer's disease. *Alzheimers Dement.* 7, 270–279. doi: 10.1016/j.jalz.2011.03.008

Bakkour, A., Morris, J. C., and Dickerson, B. C. (2009). The cortical signature of prodromal AD: regional thinning predicts mild AD dementia. *Neurology* 72, 1048–1055. doi: 10.1212/01.wnl.0000340981.97664.2f

Bakkour, A., Morris, J. C., Wolk, D. A., and Dickerson, B. C. (2013). The effects of aging and Alzheimer's disease on cerebral cortical anatomy: specificity and differential relationships with cognition. *Neuroimage* 76, 332–344. doi: 10.1016/j.neuroimage.2013.02.059

Bateman, R. J., Xiong, C., Benzinger, T. L. S., Fagan, A. M., Goate, A., Fox, N. C., et al. (2012). Clinical and biomarker changes in dominantly inherited Alzheimer's disease. *N. Engl. J. Med.* 367, 795–804. doi: 10.1056/NEJMoa1202753

Blennow, K., Hampel, H., Weiner, M., and Zetterberg, H. (2010). Cerebrospinal fluid and plasma biomarkers in Alzheimer disease. *Nat. Rev. Neurol.* 6, 131–144. doi: 10.1038/nrneurol.2010.4

Buchhave, P., Minthon, L., Zetterberg, H., Wallin, A. K., Blennow, K., and Hansson, O. (2012). Cerebrospinal fluid levels of beta-amyloid 1-42, but not of tau, are fully changed already 5 to 10 years before the onset of Alzheimer dementia. *Arch. Gen. Psychiatry* 69, 98–106. doi: 10.1001/archgenpsychiatry.2011.155

De Meyer, G., Shapiro, F., Vanderstichele, H., Vanmechelen, E., Engelborghs, S., De Deyn, P. P., et al. (2010). Diagnosis-independent Alzheimer disease biomarker signature in cognitively normal elderly people. *Arch. Neurol.* 67, 949–956. doi: 10.1001/archneurol.2010.179

Dickerson, B. C., Bakkour, A., Salat, D. H., Feczko, E., Pacheco, J., Greve, D. N., et al. (2009). The cortical signature of Alzheimer's disease: regionally specific cortical thinning relates to symptom severity in very mild to mild AD dementia and is detectable in asymptomatic amyloid-positive individuals. *Cereb. Cortex* 19, 497–510. doi: 10.1093/cercor/bhn113

Dickerson, B. C., Wolk, D. A., and Alzheimer's Disease Neuroimaging Initiative. (2011) Dysexecutive versus amnesic phenotypes of very mild Alzheimer's disease are associated with distinct clinical, genetic and cortical thinning characteristics. *J. Neurol. Neurosurg. Psychiatry* 82, 45–51. doi: 10.1136/jnnp.2009.199505

Frisoni, G. B., Fox, N. C., Jack, C. R. Jr., Scheltens, P., and Thompson, P. M. (2010). The clinical use of structural MRI in Alzheimer disease. *Nat. Rev. Neurol.* 6, 67–77. doi: 10.1038/nrneurol.2009.215

Hansson, O., Zetterberg, H., Buchhave, P., Londos, E., Blennow, K., and Minthon, L. (2006). Association between CSF biomarkers and incipient Alzheimer's disease in patients with mild cognitive impairment: a follow-up study. *Lancet Neurol.* 5, 228–234. doi: 10.1016/S1474-4422(06)70355-6

Heister, D., Brewer, J. B., Magda, S., Blennow, K., and McEvoy, L. K. (2011). Predicting MCI outcome with clinically available MRI and CSF biomarkers. *Neurology* 77, 1619–1628. doi: 10.1212/WNL.0b013e3182343314

Jack, C. R. Jr., Bernstein, M. A., Fox, N. C., Thompson, P., Alexander, G., Harvey, D., et al. (2008). The Alzheimer's Disease Neuroimaging Initiative (ADNI): MRI methods. *J. Magn. Reson. Imaging* 27, 685–691. doi: 10.1002/jmri.21049

Jack, C. R. Jr., Knopman, D. S., Jagust, W. J., Petersen, R. C., Weiner, M. W., Aisen, P. S., et al. (2013). Tracking pathophysiological processes in Alzheimer's disease: an updated hypothetical model of dynamic biomarkers. *Lancet Neurol.* 12, 207–216. doi: 10.1016/S1474-4422(12)70291-0

Jack, C. R. Jr., Lowe, V. J., Weigand, S. D., Wiste, H. J., Senjem, M. L., Knopman, D. S., et al. (2009). Serial PIB and MRI in normal, mild cognitive impairment and Alzheimer's disease: implications for sequence of pathological events in Alzheimer's disease. *Brain* 132, 1355–1365. doi: 10.1093/brain/awp062

Jack, C. R. Jr., Petersen, R. C., Xu, Y. C., O'Brien, P. C., Smith, G. E., Ivnik, R. J., et al. (1999). Prediction of AD with MRI-based hippocampal volume in mild cognitive impairment. *Neurology* 52, 1397–1403. doi: 10.1212/WNL.52.7.1397

Jack, C. R. Jr., Wiste, H. J., Vemuri, P., Weigand, S. D., Senjem, M. L., Zeng, G., et al. (2010). Brain beta-amyloid measures and magnetic resonance imaging atrophy both predict time-to-progression from mild cognitive impairment to Alzheimer's disease. *Brain* 133, 3336–3348. doi: 10.1093/brain/awq277

Knopman, D. S., Jack, C. R. Jr., Wiste, H. J., Weigand, S. D., Vemuri, P., Lowe, V. J., et al. (2012) Brain injury biomarkers are not dependent on beta-amyloid in normal elderly. *Ann. Neurol.* doi: 10.1002/ana.23816 [Epub ahead of print].

Landau, S. M., Harvey, D., Madison, C. M., Reiman, E. M., Foster, N. L., Aisen, P. S., et al. (2010). Comparing predictors of conversion and decline in mild cognitive impairment. *Neurology* 75, 230–238. doi: 10.1212/WNL.0b013e3181e8e8b8

Landau, S. M., Mintun, M. A., Joshi, A. D., Koeppe, R. A., Petersen, R. C., Aisen, P. S., et al. (2012). Amyloid deposition, hypometabolism, and longitudinal cognitive decline. *Ann. Neurol.* 72, 578–586. doi: 10.1002/ana.23650

Petersen, R. C., Aisen, P., Boeve, B. F., Geda, Y. E., Ivnik, R. J., Knopman, D. S., et al. (2013) Criteria for mild cognitive impairment due to Alzheimer's disease in the community. *Ann. Neurol.* doi: 10.1002/ana.23931 [Epub ahead of print].

Petersen, R. C., Parisi, J. E., Dickson, D. W., Johnson, K. A., Knopman, D. S., Boeve, B. F., et al. (2006). Neuropathologic features of amnestic mild cognitive impairment. *Arch. Neurol.* 63, 665–672. doi: 10.1001/archneur.63.5.665

Prestia, A., Caroli, A., van der Flier, W. M., Ossenkoppele, R., Van Berckel, B., Barkhof, F., et al. (2013). Prediction of dementia in MCI patients based on core diagnostic markers for Alzheimer disease. *Neurology* 80, 1048–1056. doi: 10.1212/WNL.0b013e3182872830

Shaw, L. M., Vanderstichele, H., Knapik-Czajka, M., Clark, C. M., Aisen, P. S., Petersen, R. C., et al. (2009). Cerebrospinal fluid biomarker signature in Alzheimer's disease neuroimaging initiative subjects. *Ann. Neurol.* 65, 403–413. doi: 10.1002/ana.21610

Vemuri, P., Wiste, H. J., Weigand, S. D., Knopman, D. S., Trojanowski, J. Q., Shaw, L. M., et al. (2010). Serial MRI and CSF biomarkers in normal aging, MCI, and AD. *Neurology* 75, 143–151. doi: 10.1212/WNL.0b013e3181e7ca82

Vemuri, P., Wiste, H. J., Weigand, S. D., Shaw, L. M., Trojanowski, J. Q., Weiner, M. W., et al. (2009a). MRI and CSF biomarkers in normal, MCI, and AD subjects: diagnostic discrimination and cognitive correlations. *Neurology* 73, 287–293. doi: 10.1212/WNL.0b013e3181af79e5

Vemuri, P., Wiste, H. J., Weigand, S. D., Shaw, L. M., Trojanowski, J. Q., Weiner, M. W., et al. (2009b). MRI and CSF biomarkers in normal, MCI, and AD subjects: predicting future clinical change. *Neurology* 73, 294–301. doi: 10.1212/WNL.0b013e3181af79fb

Villemagne, V. L., Burnham, S., Bourgeat, P., Brown, B., Ellis, K. A., Salvado, O., et al. (2013). Amyloid beta deposition, neurodegeneration, and cognitive decline in sporadic Alzheimer's disease: a prospective cohort study. *Lancet Neurol.* 12, 357–367. doi: 10.1016/S1474-4422(13)70044-9

Visser, P. J., Verhey, F., Knol, D. L., Scheltens, P., Wahlund, L. O., Freund-Levi, Y., et al. (2009). Prevalence and prognostic value of CSF markers of Alzheimer's disease pathology in patients with subjective cognitive impairment or mild cognitive impairment in the DESCRIPA study: a prospective cohort study. *Lancet Neurol.* 8, 619–627. doi: 10.1016/S1474-4422(09)70139-5

Wang, P. N., Lirng, J. F., Lin, K. N., Chang, F. C., and Liu, H. C. (2006). Prediction of Alzheimer's disease in mild cognitive impairment: a prospective study in Taiwan. *Neurobiol. Aging* 27, 1797–1806. doi: 10.1016/j.neurobiolaging.2005.10.002

Wolk, D. A., Dickerson, B. C., and Alzheimer's Disease Neuroimaging Initiative. (2010). Apolipoprotein E (APOE) genotype has dissociable effects on memory and attentional-executive network function in Alzheimer's disease. *Proc. Natl. Acad. Sci. U.S.A.* 107, 10256–10261. doi: 10.1073/pnas.1001412107

18

Imaging of microglia in patients with neurodegenerative disorders

Marios Politis*, Paul Su and Paola Piccini

Division of Experimental Medicine, Faculty of Medicine, Centre for Neuroscience, Hammersmith Hospital, Imperial College London, London, UK

Edited by:
Roger A. Barker, University of Cambridge and Addenbrooke' Hospital, UK

Reviewed by:
Jason B. Wu, Cedars-Sinai Medical Center, USA
Roger A. Barker, University of Cambridge and Addenbrooke' Hospital, UK

***Correspondence:**
Marios Politis, Hammersmith Hospital, Imperial College London, Cyclotron Building, London W12 0NN, UK.
e-mail: marios.politis@imperial.ac.uk

Microglia constitute the main immune defense in the central nervous system. In response to neuronal injury, microglia become activated, acquire phagocytic properties, and release a wide range of pro-inflammatory mediators that are essential for the annihilation of the neuronal insult. Although the role of microglial activation in acute neuronal damage is well defined, the pathophysiological processes underlying destructive or protective role to neurons following chronic exposure to microglial activation is still a subject of debate. It is likely that chronic exposure induces detrimental effects by promoting neuronal death through the release of neurotoxic factors. Positron emission tomography (PET) imaging with the use of translocator protein (TSPO) radioligands provides an *in vivo* tool for tracking the progression and severity of neuroinflammation in neurodegenerative disease. TSPO expression is correlated to the extent of microglial activation and the measurement of TSPO uptake *in vivo* with PET is a useful indicator of active disease. Although understanding of the interaction between radioligands and TSPO is not completely clear, there is a wide interest in application of TSPO imaging in neurodegenerative disease. In this article, we aim to review the applications of *in vivo* microglia imaging in neurodegenerative disorders such as Parkinson's disease, Huntington's disease, Dementias, and Multiple Sclerosis.

Keywords: dementia, Huntington, microglia, multiple sclerosis, Parkinson, PET, PK11195

INTRODUCTION

Microglia account for approximately 10% of the adult brain cell population and represent the first and main form of immune defense in the central nervous system (CNS; Lawson et al., 1990; Kreutzberg, 1996). Upon CNS injury and disease, microglia become activated and they can be identified and distinguished from their resting phenotype based on a combination of morphological and immunophenotypic changes (Dheen et al., 2007; Ransohoff and Perry, 2009). Microglia initiate immune responses by enhancing the expression of toll-like receptors (TLR) and a wide range of pro-inflammatory mediators such as tumor necrosis factor-alpha (TNFα), interleukin (IL)-1 and IL-6 for the removal of the CNS threat (Suzumura et al., 1996; Hartlage-Rübsamen et al., 1999; Bsibsi et al., 2002; Floden et al., 2005). Microglia may also fulfill a neuroprotective role *via* the release of neurotrophic factors and promotion of neurogenesis for the restoration of normal physiology (Stadelmann et al., 2002). Hence, the acute inflammatory response is generally beneficial, as it tends to minimize injury and promotes tissue repair. However, chronic neuroinflammation is closely related to various neurodegenerative disorders such as Parkinson's disease (PD), Huntington's disease (HD), Dementias, and Multiple sclerosis (MS), although the consequences of sustained microglial activation in these diseases is unclear.

Activated microglia upregulate expression of the 18-kDa translocator protein (TSPO; Chen and Guilarte, 2008; Cosenza-Nashat et al., 2009; Scarf et al., 2009). TSPO are found in abundance throughout the body in peripheral organs (i.e., liver and adrenals), and hematogenous cells, but are present at very low levels in the normal healthy CNS (Banati, 2002). Functionally, TSPO has several biological functions including the control of cholesterol transport and neurosteroid synthesis (Papadopoulos et al., 2006), and may also be involved in the release of pro-inflammatory cytokines during inflammation (Choi et al., 2002; Wilms et al., 2003).

Enhanced TSPO expression can be detected *in vivo* by using positron emission tomography (PET) imaging with the selective TSPO radioligand ^{11}C-PK11195 (Benavides et al., 1988; Pike et al., 1993; Banati et al., 1999), with evidence that increases in ^{11}C-PK11195 binding potential (BP_{ND}) correspond to activation of microglia (Stephenson et al., 1995; Conway et al., 1998; Banati et al., 2000). Although TSPO is also expressed by reactive astrocytes, a ^{11}C-PK11195 PET study of patients with hippocampal sclerosis, a condition histopathologically characterized by marked astrogliosis, did not yield results that were significantly different to healthy normal controls (Banati et al., 1999). This is consistent with the view that reactive astrocytes, *in vivo*, do not significantly contribute to the ^{11}C-PK11195 signal. Therefore, in the absence of invading blood borne cells or severe focal leakage of blood-brain barrier, the increased PK11195 binding is likely to indicate the transition of microglia from a resting to an activated state, and is due to an increase in the number, rather than the affinity, of TSPO (Banati et al., 2000). Hence, the measurement of TSPO uptake using PET provides an *in vivo* tool to monitor progression and severity of neuroinflammation and is a useful indicator of active CNS disease. This article aims to review the use of PET imaging to promote the understanding of activated microglia in neurodegenerative disease.

PARKINSON'S DISEASE AND RELATED DISORDERS

Parkinson's disease is the second most common neurodegenerative disorder of the elderly and is associated with the motor symptoms of tremor, bradykinesia, and rigidity. It is characterized by the extended loss of dopaminergic neurons in the substantia nigra pars compacta, resulting in a deficiency of dopamine in the striatum (Braak et al., 2006), and the presence of alpha-synuclein (α-synuclein)-containing lewy bodies. PD is the most common of a group of parkinsonian movement disorders that also includes Multiple system atrophy (MSA), Corticobasal degeneration (CBD), and Progressive supranuclear palsy (PSP).

The presence of activated microglia close to dopaminergic neurons in post-mortem PD patient brains (McGeer et al., 1988a; Mogi et al., 1994; Langston et al., 1999; Imamura et al., 2003), and PD animal models (Czlonkowska et al., 1996; Kim et al., 2009) suggests a close relationship between neurodegeneration and neuroinflammation in PD. Numerous investigations have proposed a deleterious role of microglial activation in PD based on the vulnerability of dopaminergic neurons to various microglia-derived pro-inflammatory cytokines (Ferrari et al., 2006; Stone et al., 2009; De Lella Ezcurra et al., 2010), while α-synuclein can directly induce activation of microglia (Zhang et al., 2005). However, it seems that the plasticity of microglia must be considered with regards to their contribution in PD, and their role; whether beneficial or detrimental, it may depend on the stimuli present and the stage of disease (Li et al., 2007; Michelucci et al., 2009; Sanchez-Guajardo et al., 2010).

Further clues regarding the role of activated microglia has also come from *in vivo* PET imaging studies (**Table 1**). Significant microglial activation, as reflected by an increase in ^{11}C-PK11195 BP_{ND} was reported in the midbrain and putamen of PD patients when compared to controls, and was found to correlate positively with the motor severity of Parkinsonism (Ouchi et al., 2005; Bartels et al., 2010). These findings suggest that activated microglia has a pathogenic importance in the disease and indicate that the early introduction of a neuroprotective drug to suppress microglial activation could be favorable in PD. Additionally, PD patients exhibited significantly increased ^{11}C-PK11195 BP_{ND} in the basal ganglia, pons, and frontal and temporal cortical regions (Gerhard et al., 2006a). In this study, the increased microglial activation remained unchanged for 2 years, while the patients deteriorated clinically during this period. Hence, it is likely that microglia are activated early in PD, where they remain activated for longer periods and possibly drive progression of the disease (Gerhard et al., 2006a).

Multiple system atrophy is a sporadic neurodegenerative disorder involving a progressive akinetic-rigid syndrome, autonomic failure, and cerebellar dysfunction. It is associated by the appearance of abnormal glial cytoplasmic inclusions (GCI) containing (α-synuclein aggregates and neuronal loss within the nigrostriatal and olivopontocerebellar regions (Lantos and Papp, 1994). The presence of activated microglia is also a prominent feature of MSA (Schwarz et al., 1998). In an *in vivo* PET study of MSA patients, significant ^{11}C-PK11195 BP_{ND} was observed in the putamen, pallidum, pons, substantia nigra pars compacta, and dorsolateral prefrontal cortex, reflecting the known distribution of neuropathological changes in MSA (Gerhard et al., 2003). Although the role of microglia in MSA is inconclusive, microglial activation localization correlated significantly with the locations of GCIs in specific neuroanatomical systems affected in MSA (Ishizawa et al., 2004). A correlation between extent of

Table 1 | Positron emission tomography imaging studies assessing microglia in Parkinsonian disorders.

Study	Disorder	Subjects	PET technique	Main findings
Ouchi et al. (2005)	PD	10 Early PD patients, 10 NC	^{11}C-PK11195	^{11}C-PK11195 BP_{ND} in patients significantly higher than controls Midbrain ^{11}C-PK11195 BP_{ND} values correlated positively with motor disability
Gerhard et al. (2006a)	PD	18 PD patients, 11 NC	^{11}C-PK11195	Significantly increased ^{11}C-PK11195 BP_{ND} in pons, basal ganglia, and frontal and temporal cortical regions ^{11}C-PK11195 signal remained stable for 2 years in subset of patients
Bartels et al. (2010)	PD	14 PD patients, 8 NC	^{11}C-PK11195	Higher contralateral putamen and midbrain ^{11}C-PK11195 BP_{ND} in patients than controls
Gerhard et al. (2003)	MSA	5 MSA patients, 6 NC	^{11}C-PK11195	MSA patients showed significantly increased ^{11}C-PK11195 BP_{ND} in regions reflecting the known distribution of pathologic changes in MSA
Gerhard et al. (2006b)	PSP	4 PSP patients, 7 NC	^{11}C-PK11195	Significantly increased ^{11}C-PK11195 BP_{ND} in basal ganglia, midbrain, frontal lobe, and cerebellum of patients compared to controls Microglial activation remained stable as demonstrated in follow-up scans of two patients
Gerhard et al. (2004)	CBD	4 CBD patients, 5 NC	^{11}C-PK11195	CBD patients had significantly increased ^{11}C-PK11195 BP_{ND} in the cortical regions and basal ganglia that correspond to known distribution of pathological changes in CBD
Henkel et al. (2004)	CBD	1 CBD patient	^{11}C-PK11195	Marked asymmetric microglial activation in corresponding areas of basal ganglia and temporal and parietal cortices

BP_{ND}, binding potential; CBD, corticobasal degeneration; MSA, multiple system atrophy; NC, normal control; PD, Parkinson's disease; PSP, progressive supranuclear palsy.

microglial activation and dopaminergic neurodegeneration has also been reported (Stefanova et al., 2007).

Progressive supranuclear palsy is an adult-onset progressive neurodegenerative disease of unknown cause, characterized by PD-like symptoms such as postural instability and bradykinesia. The pathological hallmark of the disease is neurofibrillary tangles consisting of hyperphosphorylated tau, accompanied by neuronal loss in the thalamus, basal ganglia, and specific brainstem regions (Hauw et al., 1994). Several early studies including immunohistochemical investigations have confirmed the possible involvement of activated microglia in PSP (Kida et al., 1992; Komori et al., 1998; Ishizawa et al., 2000; Ishizawa and Dickson, 2001). ^{11}C-PK11195 PET have also reported significant levels of activated microglia in brain regions known to be affected by the disease process such as the midbrain, cerebellum, pons, frontal lobe, and basal ganglia (Gerhard et al., 2006b). Although these results were unable to support a direct causal contribution to neurodegeneration in PSP, they are at least suggestive of a role of microglia in the disease.

Corticobasal degeneration is a neurodegenerative disorder that affects both cortical and basal ganglial regions, with considerable clinical heterogeneity between patients. Typically, CBD features an asymmetric hypokinetic-rigid syndrome, coupled with alien limb phenomenon and cortical sensory impairment that is unresponsive to dopaminergic therapy (Rebeiz et al., 1968; Gibb et al., 1989). Information on the association of activated microglia in CBD is limited, and mainly coming from immunohistochemical-based assessments (Armstrong et al., 2000; Ishizawa and Dickson, 2001). However, more recent *in vivo* PET investigations have attempted to quantify microglial activation in CBD patients. Increased ^{11}C-PK11195 BP_{ND} was observed in regions such as the caudate nucleus, putamen, substantia nigra pars compacta, pons, and pre- and post central gyrus (Gerhard et al., 2004; Henkel et al., 2004) that correspond to the expected neuropathological changes seen in CBD (Ishizawa and Dickson, 2001; Dickson et al., 2002). These results indicate an involvement of activated microglia in pathogenesis of CBD.

HUNTINGTON'S DISEASE

Huntington's disease is an autosomal, dominant inherited progressive neurodegenerative disorder associated with motor, cognitive, and psychiatric symptoms. It is caused by an abnormal polyglutamine-repeat expansion on the IT15 gene that codes huntingtin, and involves the progressive loss of medium spiny dopaminergic receptor-bearing striatal GABA-ergic neurons (Vonsattel and DiFiglia, 1998). Although the role of chronic neuroinflammation in the HD pathogenesis is not fully understood, post-mortem assessments have reported high levels of activated microglia close to degenerating neurons (McGeer et al., 1988b; Messmer and Reynolds, 1998; Singhrao et al., 1999; Sapp et al., 2001). Upregulated inflammatory cytokines have also been detected in the striatum and plasma, indicative of an inflammatory component in HD (Dalrymple et al., 2007; Björkqvist et al., 2008).

In vivo imaging studies using ^{11}C-PK11195 PET have found increased microglial activation in both premanifest HD gene carriers and manifest HD patients when compared to healthy controls (**Table 2**; Pavese et al., 2006; Tai et al., 2007; Politis et al., 2008, 2011). In premanifest HD patients, significant increases in ^{11}C-PK11195 BP_{ND} in the striatum and hypothalamus was reported, which correlated inversely with neuronal dysfunction as measured by ^{11}C-Raclopride; a marker of dopaminergic D2/D3 receptor availability (Tai et al., 2007; Politis et al., 2008). Interestingly, microglial activation in the striatum, and regions related to cognitive function has been shown to predict the 5-year disease clinical onset in premanifest HD patients (Tai et al., 2007; Politis et al., 2011). These results imply that microglial activation is an early event in the HD disease course, with a possible pathogenic involvement that is associated with a subclinical progression of the disease.

In manifest HD patients, significant ^{11}C-PK11195 BP_{ND} in the striatum, hypothalamus, and various cortical regions was found, that correlated with greater disease burden and higher motor disability (Pavese et al., 2006; Politis et al., 2008, 2011). The cortical

Table 2 | Positron emission tomography imaging studies assessing microglia in Huntington's disease.

Study	Subjects	PET technique	Main findings
Pavese et al. (2006)	11 manifest HD patients, 10 NC	^{11}C-PK11195	Significantly increased ^{11}C-PK11195 BP_{ND} in patients than controls Increased ^{11}C-PK11195 uptake correlated positively with disease severity
Tai et al. (2007)	11 premanifest HD subjects, 10 NC	^{11}C-PK11195	Significantly higher striatal ^{11}C-PK11195 BP_{ND} that correlated inversely with D2 receptor availability Higher striatal uptake correlated with 5 year probability of clinical disease onset
Politis et al. (2008)	10 premanifest HD subjects, 9 manifest HD patients, 10 NC	^{11}C-PK11195	Significantly increased hypothalamic ^{11}C-PK11195 BP_{ND} in both premanifest and manifest subjects compared to controls Inverse correlation between increased hypothalamic ^{11}C-PK11195 BP_{ND} and D2 receptor availability
Politis et al. (2011)	8 premanifest HD subjects, 8 manifest HD patients, 16 NC	^{11}C-PK11195	In premanifest subjects, increased microglial activation in cognitive regions correlated with 5 year probability of clinical disease onset. In manifest HD patients, significantly increased ^{11}C-PK11195 BP_{ND} in globus pallidus, anterior prefrontal cortex, and limbic striatum

BP_{ND}, binding potential; HD, Huntington's disease; NC, normal control.

microglial activation is likely to indicate the involvement of cortical neurons in HD, a well-recognized phenomenon as the disease progresses. Collectively, these findings are consistent with the post-mortem studies (Messmer and Reynolds, 1998; Sapp et al., 2001) and suggest a detrimental microglial contribution to the ongoing neuronal degeneration in HD.

DEMENTIA

Dementias are a group of disorders that are expected to affect more than 100 million people by 2050 raising remarkable financial costs for healthcare (Wimo et al., 2003). AD is the most common cause of dementia and is the most common neurological disorder of the elderly. AD is characterized by the presence of amyloid plaques, neurofibrillary tangles, and activated microglia (for review, see Hardy and Selkoe, 2002). There is a plethora of evidence from post-mortem human AD studies (McGeer et al., 1988a; Venneti et al., 2009) and animal models (Frautschy et al., 1998; Stalder et al., 1999; Leung et al., 2011) reporting a high accumulation of activated microglia in close proximity with the amyloid plaques, and upregulated levels of pro-inflammatory cytokines (Akiyama et al., 2000; Eikelenboom et al., 2002).

Positron emission tomography enables a broad range of functional processes to assess the AD brain *in vivo* (**Table 3**). ^{11}C-PK11195 has been used to demonstrate increased levels of activated microglia in both AD animal models (Venneti et al., 2009) and AD patients (Cagnin et al., 2001; Edison et al., 2008; Yokokura et al., 2011). In AD patients, significant ^{11}C-PK11195 BP_{ND} was consistently observed in the temporal, parietal, and occipital cortices, regions known to be affected by AD pathology (Cagnin et al., 2001; Edison et al., 2008; Yokokura et al., 2011). The increased activated microglia also inversely correlated with the patient Mini-Mental State Examination (MMSE) scores, which is compatible with a role of microglia in neuronal damage (Edison et al., 2008). Interestingly, elevated levels of activated microglia were also detected in patients with amnestic mild cognitive impairment (MCI; Okello et al., 2009a), although this was not observed in another study assessing MCI patients (Wiley et al., 2009). MCI could represent an early precursor stage of AD, since it was found that MCI patients with increased amyloid load were significantly more likely to clinically convert to AD within 3 years (Okello et al., 2009b). Therefore, microglial activation could be an early event in the AD pathogenesis that begins at the MCI stage.

Despite the evidence suggestive of a pathogenic role of activated microglia in AD, it is hypothesized that the accumulation of amyloid plaques is actually due to a failure in microglial clearance mechanisms that would normally remove the protein (Bornemann et al., 2001; DiCarlo et al., 2001; Napoli and Neumann, 2009). This indicates a beneficial, rather than detrimental role of microglia in AD. Notwithstanding the abundance of activated microglia close to senile plaques, they maybe inefficient in the clearance of amyloid, hence, resulting in aggregate formation (Bolmont et al., 2008). It has been shown that in the presence of pro-inflammatory cytokines, phagocytic functions of microglia are compromised (Koenigsknecht-Talboo and Landreth, 2005). Therefore, microglia may confer a dichotomous role in AD, where early microglial activation is possibly neuroprotective involving the removal of amyloid. However, chronic neuroinflammation may downregulate amyloid clearance mechanisms, thus, promoting aggregation and progression of disease.

Frontotemporal lobar degeneration (FTLD) which includes frontotemporal dementia is the name given to a group of pathologically, clinically, and genetically heterogeneous disorders involving focal atrophy of the frontal and temporal lobes, while unlike AD, with sparing of the parietal and occipital regions (Neary et al., 1998). Another important dissimilarity between AD and FTLD pathology is the absence of amyloid plaque formation (Paulus et al., 1993; Mirra and Hyman, 2002). Rather, the key histopathological features of FTLD, depending on subtype,

Table 3 | Positron emission tomography imaging studies assessing microglia in dementias.

Study	Disorder	Subjects	PET technique	Main findings
Cagnin et al. (2001)	AD	8 AD patients, 15 NC	^{11}C-PK11195	AD patients showed significantly increased regional ^{11}C-PK11195 BP_{ND} in the entorhinal, temporoparietal, and cingulate cortex
Edison et al. (2008)	AD	13 AD patients, 10 NC	^{11}C-PK11195	Significant increased ^{11}C-PK11195 BP_{ND} in the cortical regions Inverse correlation between increased cortical microglial activation and MMSE scores
Yokokura et al. (2011)	AD	11 AD patients, 10 NC	^{11}C-PK11195	Significantly increased ^{11}C-PK11195 uptake in the parietotemporal regions of patients than controls Inverse correlation between dementia scores and ^{11}C-PK11195 BP_{ND} values
Wiley et al. (2009)	AD, MCI	6 mild-moderate AD patients, 6 MCI patients, 5 NC	^{11}C-PK11195	No significant differences in brain ^{11}C-PK11195 BP_{ND} between subject groups
Okello et al. (2009a)	MCI	14 MCI patients, 10 NC	^{11}C-PK11195	5 of 13 MCI subjects had increased cortical ^{11}C-PK11195 BP_{ND} compared to controls
Cagnin et al. (2004)	FTLD	5 FTLD patients, 8 NC	^{11}C-PK11195	Significantly increased ^{11}C-PK11195 BP_{ND} in the frontotemporal regions

AD, Alzheimer's disease; BP_{ND}, binding potential; FTLD, frontotemporal lobar degeneration; MCI, mild cognitive impairment; MMSE, mini-mental state examination; NC, normal controls.

includes tau deposition (including Pick bodies) and ubiquitin-positive, tau-negative inclusions (Munoz et al., 2003; Uchihara et al., 2003). *In vivo* PET imaging of FTLD patients detected enhanced microglial activation in the expected frontotemporal regions (Cagnin et al., 2004). In the same study, significant ^{11}C-PK11195 BP_{ND} in the bilateral putamen is also consistent with previous neuropathological data showing the involvement of the basal ganglia in FTLD (Mirra and Hyman, 2002). These observations indicate the presence of an active microglial response that reflects progressive neuronal degeneration. Importantly, the detection of increased microglial activation in affected regions in FTLD suggests that microglial responses occur independently of amyloid deposition, and that neuronal loss alone is enough to induce activation (Cagnin et al., 2004). However, whether this applies to AD pathogenesis requires further investigation.

MULTIPLE SCLEROSIS

Multiple sclerosis is a disease characterized pathologically by inflammatory demyelination and axonal transection, and is the most common cause of non-traumatic disability in young adults (Compston and Coles, 2008).

The involvement of activated microglia has long been proposed in MS (Benveniste, 1997). Post-mortem investigations have detected activated microglia in the cortical GM of MS patients (De Groot et al., 2001; Peterson et al., 2001; Petzold et al., 2002), while histopathological studies have implicated microglia in lesion pathogenesis (for review, see Lassmann, 2008). An observed correlation between neuronal loss and microglial activation was reported in animal experimental MS (Rasmussen et al., 2007). Significant levels of activated microglia was also found in MS patients, especially in the progressive forms of disease that are associated with neurodegeneration (Kutzelnigg et al., 2005; Magliozzi et al., 2010), and selective ablation of parenchymal microglia was able to prevent demyelination and axonal damage (Heppner et al., 2005).

Pathological aspects of MS such as neuroinflammation, demyelination, and neurodegeneration may be explored *in vivo* with PET (for review, see Kiferle et al., 2011). PET with ^{11}C-PK11195 and other tracers has demonstrated inflammatory processes with microglial involvement in MS (**Figure 1**; **Table 4**). In animal experimental MS and human post-mortem brains it has been shown that ^{11}C-PK11195 uptake corresponds to the distribution pattern of activated microglia (Banati et al., 2000). It has also been demonstrated that there is increased ^{11}C-PK11195 BP_{ND} in areas of focal pathology identified by T1- and T2-weighted MRI (Vowinckel et al., 1997; Banati et al., 2000) and in gadolinium-enhanced T1-weighted MRI (Debruyne et al., 2003). Increased ^{11}C-PK11195 BP_{ND} was observed in normal-appearing gray and white anatomical structures (Banati et al., 2000; Debruyne et al., 2003; Versijpt et al., 2005). This is in line with the hypothesis that inflammatory processes initiated by microglia early in MS may constitute the real burden of disease, associated with invisible microglia-mediated damage that occur independently of relapses (Kesselring, 1990; Confavreux et al., 2000). A positive correlation has been suggested between ligand uptake and disease duration, disability, and brain atrophy (Banati et al., 2000; Debruyne et al., 2003; Versijpt et al., 2005), although the correlations were not consistently replicated across the different studies. However, recent

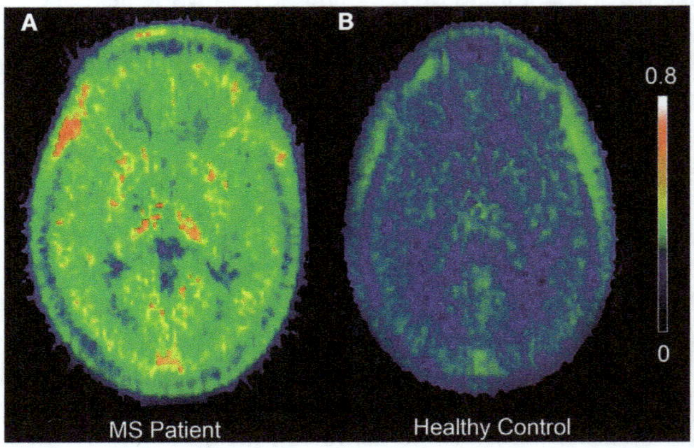

FIGURE 1 | Positron emission tomography images showing increased ^{11}C-PK11195 BP_{ND} in a Multiple Sclerosis patient (A) when compared to a healthy normal control (B). Color bar represents intensity of ^{11}C-PK11195 tracer binding (BP_{ND}). BP_{ND}, binding potential; MS, multiple sclerosis.

data from our group found a significant association between high ^{11}C-PK11195 BP_{ND} in the cortical gray matter and disability in patients with secondary progressive MS, and with higher ^{11}C-PK11195 BP_{ND} in the secondary progressive group than the relapse-remitting MS group (Politis et al., in press). These findings are consistent with a detrimental role of microglia in MS. Enhanced microglial activation in MS has also been detected using the more recently developed TSPO tracers ^{11}C-vinpocetine and ^{11}C-PBR28 (Vas et al., 2008; Oh et al., 2011).

Microglial activation may contribute to the mechanism of axonal injury *via* the release of soluble factors that may either directly or indirectly cause neuronal dysfunction (Peterson et al., 2001; Barnett and Prineas, 2004; Dutta and Trapp, 2006; Zipp et al., 2006; Dal Bianco et al., 2008; Lassmann, 2008; Magliozzi et al., 2010), and consequently result in progressive increase in impairment and disability. However, activated microglia may also exert protective functions with MS through the release of neurotrophic factors (Stadelmann et al., 2002; Napoli and Neumann, 2009), and triggering of remyelination mechanisms (Li et al., 2005; Setzu et al., 2006). This suggests a possible dichromatic role of microglia in MS.

NEW TSPO LIGANDS

^{11}C-PK11195 was the first tracer to be consistently used for the study of activated microglia and neuroinflammation *in vivo*. However, limitations associated with the application of ^{11}C-PK11195 include a high level of non-specific binding (Petit-Taboué et al., 1991), and a poor signal to noise ratio, which complicates its quantification (Boutin et al., 2007). This has prompted the search for novel PET tracers (termed, second generation radioligands) with improved capacities to quantify TSPO expression.

Radioligands such as ^{11}C-PBR28, ^{11}C-DAA1106, ^{18}F-FEDAA1106, and ^{18}F-PBR111 have recently been developed to image TSPO *in vivo* (Gulyás et al., 2002; Ikoma et al., 2007; Fujita et al., 2008; Vas et al., 2008; Yasuno et al., 2008; Oh et al., 2011; for a review, see Chauveau et al., 2008). Published data using the second generation ligands ^{11}C-DAA1106 (Ikoma et al., 2007) and

Table 4 | Positron emission tomography imaging studies assessing microglia in multiple sclerosis.

Study	Subjects	PET technique	Main Findings
Vowinckel et al. (1997)	2 MS patients	^{11}C-PK11195	High ^{11}C-PK11195 BP_{ND} in MRI-defined active MS lesions
Banati et al. (2000)	12 MS patients (RR, SP, PP), 8 NC	^{11}C-PK11195	Increased global and focal (in active MS lesions) ^{11}C-PK11195 BP_{ND} in MS patients
Debruyne et al. (2003)	22 MS patients (RR, SP, PP), 7 NC	^{11}C-PK11195	Increased ^{11}C-PK11195 BP_{ND} in MRI-Gadolinium lesions. Higher uptake in T2 lesions during relapse Positive correlation between ^{11}C-PK11195 BP_{ND} and disease duration
Versijpt et al. (2005)	22 MS patients (RR, SP, PP), 8 NC	^{11}C-PK11195	Significant correlation between brain atrophy and both disease duration and severity For NAWM, ^{11}C-PK11195 BP_{ND} increased with amount of atrophy T2-lesional ^{11}C-PK11195 BP_{ND} values decreased according to increasing atrophy
Vas et al. (2008)	4 MS patients	^{11}C-PK11195, ^{11}C-vinpocetine	Regional uptake values increased in regions of brain damage for both tracers, but markedly higher for ^{11}C-vinpocetine than ^{11}C-PK11195
Oh et al. (2011)	11 MS patients, 7 NC	^{11}C-PBR28	High ^{11}C-PBR28 in MRI-gadolinium lesions in patients Increase in tracer uptake preceded appearance of gadolinium enhancement No difference in global ^{11}C-PBR28 uptake between patients and healthy controls
Politis et al. (in press)	16 MS patients (RR, SP), 8 NC	^{11}C-PK11195	Significant correlation between cortical GM ^{11}C-PK11195 BP_{ND} and disease severity Higher ^{11}C-PK11195 in SP than RR patients

BP_{ND}, binding potential; GM, gray matter; MRI, magnetic resonance image; MS, multiple sclerosis; NAWM, normal-appearing white matter; NC, normal control; PP, primary progressive multiple sclerosis; RR, relapse-remitting multiple sclerosis; SP, secondary progressive multiple sclerosis.

^{18}F-FEDAA1106 (Fujimura et al., 2006) in humans were promising, with both tracers showing significantly higher cerebral uptake than ^{11}C-PK11195. Furthermore, increased ^{11}C-DAA1106 binding was reported in AD patients (Yasuno et al., 2008) that were similar to the previous studies that used ^{11}C-PK11195 (Cagnin et al., 2001).

The only published study using the second generation radioligand ^{11}C-PBR28 found areas of focal increases in radiotracer binding in the brain of MS patients (Oh et al., 2011). Interestingly, the increased focal ^{11}C-PBR28 binding preceded the development of some gadolinium-enhancing lesions. Brain parenchymal ^{11}C-PBR28 binding in MS patients was positively correlated with the duration of the disease, however it was not significantly higher than that of healthy volunteers. Interpretation of these results is limited by the lack of characterization of the binding affinity pattern, which might have significantly affected the comparison between subjects.

It has been recently demonstrated that there are three different affinity patterns for second generation TSPO ligands in healthy volunteers as well as patients with MS, which was evident with all the ligands tested (^{11}C-PBR28; ^{11}C-PBR06; ^{18}F-PBR111; Owen et al., 2010). This presents a methodological problem, as differences in PET signal across subjects cannot be safely interpreted as differences in target density, but may reflect differences in the affinity pattern. A possible approach to solve this problem is based on the use of peripheral binding affinity, which can be characterized to classify subjects into one of the groups, as differences in affinity status between individuals have been shown to be present on peripheral cells as well (Owen et al., 2010).

Interestingly, the difference in binding patterns observed with second generation radioligands was not observed with ^{11}C-PK11195. Also, *in vitro* autoradiography data using ^{11}C-PK11195 suggest a receptor density (B_{MAX}) significantly higher than that found using second generation ligands. It could be speculated that ^{11}C-PK11195 and newer ligands bind to distinct sites within the TSPO molecule.

Although, data obtained from first generation studies have been promising and suggested that ^{11}C-PK11195 could be useful to image acute inflammatory lesions and microglial activation in MS, a conclusive demonstration of the potential of TSPO imaging for the application as disease biomarker, indicative of microglial activation in MS, is still lacking. Furthermore, despite second generation ligands constituting a potential improvement relative to ^{11}C-PK11195 at least from a methodological point of view, a clear advantage in their clinical application as disease biomarkers has not been demonstrated yet.

For these reasons, we aim to characterize a second generation TSPO PET radioligand *in vivo* in humans, and to evaluate its application as a disease biomarker in MS.

Among second generation TSPO tracers, ^{18}F-PBR111 presents different advantages, as there is low difference in its affinity for TSPO between high, medium, low affinity binders. Also, it could be potentially used in clinical applications as it is labeled with fluorine-18. Promising preclinical data, and ongoing studies in neurological patients, suggest it could be a good choice amongst second generation TSPO ligands to progress into studies in MS patients.

CONCLUSION

Inflammation coupled with the presence of activated microglia seems to be a common feature of a wide range of CNS diseases. However, despite a large number of research studies, the exact role of microglia in chronic neurodegenerative diseases remains uncertain. In line with the high plasticity of microglia that allows them to perform numerous CNS functions, microglia are likely to play a dichromatic role in disease, depending on signals present in their microenvironment and the duration of activation. While early microglial activation could represents a beneficial response (i.e., removal of CNS threat, promoting tissue repair and removal of misfolded protein), chronic exposure could induces detrimental effects by promoting neuronal death (i.e., through the sustained release of neurotoxic factors), thus, contributing to progression of disease. PET imaging with the use of TSPO radioligands provides a valuable tool that allows us to track the progression and severity of neuroinflammation in the living brain, and is a useful indicator of active CNS disease. Therefore, the early detection of microglia using PET could offer opportunities for pharmacological interventions to limit the potential disruptive effects of chronic microglial activation. Furthermore, with the development of newer TSPO tracers, the potential for PET imaging research to promote our understanding of activated microglia in CNS disease can only increase.

ACKNOWLEDGMENTS

Our own research is supported by the Michael J Fox Foundation for Parkinson's Research USA, the Parkinson's UK, and the Cure Huntington's Disease Initiative Foundation USA.

REFERENCES

Akiyama, H., Arai, T., Kondo, H., Tanno, E., Haga, C., and Ikeda, K. (2000). Cell mediators of inflammation in the Alzheimer disease brain. *Alzheimer Dis. Assoc. Disord.* 14(Suppl. 1), 47–53.

Armstrong, R. A., Cairns, N. J., and Lantos, P. L. (2000). A quantitative study of the pathological lesions in the neocortex and hippocampus of twelve patients with corticobasal degeneration. *Exp. Neurol.* 163, 348–356.

Banati, R. B., Goerres, G. W., Myers, R., Gunn, R. N., Turkheimer, F. E., Kreutzberg, G. W., Brooks, D. J., Jones, T., and Duncan, J. S. (1999). [11C](R)-PK11195 positron emission tomography imaging of activated microglia in vivo in Rasmussen's encephalitis. *Neurology* 53, 2199–2203.

Banati, R. B., Newcombe, J., Gunn, R. N., Cagnin, A., Turkheimer, F. E., Heppner, F., Price, G., Wegner, F., Giovannoni, G., Miller, D. H., Perkin, G. D., Smith, T., Hewson, A. K., Bydder, G., Kreutzberg, G. W., Jones, T., Cuzner, M. L., and Myers, R. (2000). The peripheral benzodiazepine binding site in the brain in multiple sclerosis: quantitative in vivo imaging of microglia as a measure of disease activity. *Brain* 123(Pt 11), 2321–2337.

Banati, R. B. (2002). Visualizing microglial activation in vivo. *Glia* 40, 206–217.

Barnett, M. H., and Prineas, J. W. (2004). Relapsing and remitting multiple sclerosis: pathology of the newly forming lesion. *Ann. Neurol.* 55, 458–468.

Bartels, A. L., Willemsen, A. T., Doorduin, J., de Vries, E. F., Dierckx, R. A., and Leenders, K. L. (2010). [11C]-PK11195 PET: quantification of neuroinflammation and a monitor of anti-inflammatory treatment in Parkinson's disease? *Parkinsonism Relat. Disord.* 16, 57–59.

Benavides, J., Cornu, P., Dennis, T., Dubois, A., Hauw, J. J., MacKenzie, E. T., Sazdovitch, V., and Scatton, B. (1988). Imaging of human brain lesions with an omega 3 site radioligand. *Ann. Neurol.* 24, 708–712.

Benveniste, E. N. (1997). Role of macrophages/microglia in multiple sclerosis and experimental allergic encephalomyelitis. *J. Mol. Med. (Berl.)* 75, 165–173.

Björkqvist, M., Wild, E. J., Thiele, J., Silvestroni, A., Andre, R., Lahiri, N., Raibon, E., Lee, R. V., Benn, C. L., Soulet, D., Magnusson, A., Woodman, B., Landles, C., Pouladi, M. A., Hayden, M. R., Khalili-Shirazi, A., Lowdell, M. W., Brundin, P., Bates, G. P., Leavitt, B. R., Möller, T., and Tabrizi, S. J. (2008). A novel pathogenic pathway of immune activation detectable before clinical onset in Huntington's disease. *J. Exp. Med.* 205, 1869–1877.

Bolmont, T., Haiss, F., Eicke, D., Radde, R., Mathis, C. A., Klunk, W. E., Kohsaka, S., Jucker, M., and Calhoun, M. E. (2008). Dynamics of the microglial/amyloid interaction indicate a role in plaque maintenance. *J. Neurosci.* 28, 4283–4292.

Bornemann, K. D., Wiederhold, K. H., Pauli, C., Ermini, F., Stalder, M., Schnell, L., Sommer, B., Jucker, M., and Staufenbiel, M. (2001). Abeta-induced inflammatory processes in microglia cells of APP23 transgenic mice. *Am. J. Pathol.* 158, 63–73.

Boutin, H., Chauveau, F., Thominiaux, C., Kuhnast, B., Grégoire, M. C., Jan, S., Trebossen, R., Dollé, F., Tavitian, B., Mattner, F., and Katsifis, A. (2007). In vivo imaging of brain lesions with [(11)C]CLINME, a new PET radioligand of peripheral benzodiazepine receptors. *Glia* 55, 1459–1468.

Braak, H., Rub, U., and Del Tredici, K. (2006). Cognitive decline correlates with neuropathological stage in Parkinson's disease. *J. Neurol. Sci.* 248, 255–258.

Bsibsi, M., Ravid, R., Gveric, D., and van Noort, J. M. (2002). Broad expression of Toll-like receptors in the human central nervous system. *J. Neuropathol. Exp. Neurol.* 61, 1013–1021.

Cagnin, A., Brooks, D. J., Kennedy, A. M., Gunn, R. N., Myers, R., Turkheimer, F. E., Jones, T., and Banati, R. B. (2001). In-vivo measurement of activated microglia in dementia. *Lancet* 358, 461–467.

Cagnin, A., Rossor, M., Sampson, E. L., Mackinnon, T., and Banati, R. B. (2004). In vivo detection of microglial activation in frontotemporal dementia. *Ann. Neurol.* 56, 894–897.

Chauveau, F., Boutin, H., Van Camp, N., Dollé, F., and Tavitian, B. (2008). Nuclear imaging of neuroinflammation: a comprehensive review of [11C]PK11195 challengers. *Eur. J. Nucl. Med. Mol. Imaging* 35, 2304–2319.

Chen, M. K., and Guilarte, T. R. (2008). Translocator protein 18 kDa (TSPO): molecular sensor of brain injury and repair. *Pharmacol. Ther.* 118, 1–17.

Choi, H. B., Khoo, C., Ryu, J. K., van Breemen, E., Kim, S. U., and McLarnon, J. G. (2002). Inhibition of lipopolysaccharide-induced cyclooxygenase-2, tumor necrosis factor-alpha and [Ca2+]i responses in human microglia by the peripheral benzodiazepine receptor ligand PK11195. *J. Neurochem.* 83, 546–555.

Compston, A., and Coles, A. (2008). Multiple sclerosis. *Lancet* 372, 1502–1517.

Confavreux, C., Vukusic, S., Moreau, T., and Adeleine, P. (2000). Relapses and progression of disability in multiple sclerosis. *N. Engl. J. Med.* 343, 1430–1438.

Conway, E. L., Gundlach, A. L., and Craven, J. A. (1998). Temporal changes in glial fibrillary acidic protein messenger RNA and [3H]PK11195 binding in relation to imidazoline-I2-receptor and alpha 2-adrenoceptor binding in the hippocampus following transient global forebrain ischaemia in the rat. *Neuroscience* 82, 805–817.

Cosenza-Nashat, M., Zhao, M. L., Suh, H. S., Morgan, J., Natividad, R., Morgello, S., and Lee, S. C. (2009). Expression of the translocator protein of 18 kDa by microglia, macrophages and astrocytes based on immunohistochemical localization in abnormal human brain. *Neuropathol. Appl. Neurobiol.* 35, 306–328.

Czlonkowska, A., Kohutnicka, M., Kurkowska-Jastrzebska, I., and Czlonkowski, A. (1996). Microglial reaction in MPTP (1-methyl-4-phenyl-1,2,3,6-tetrahydropyridine) induced Parkinson's disease mice model. *Neurodegeneration* 5, 137–143.

Dal Bianco, A., Bradl, M., Frischer, J., Kutzelnigg, A., Jellinger, K., and Lassmann, H. (2008). Multiple sclerosis and Alzheimer's disease. *Ann. Neurol.* 63, 174–183.

Dalrymple, A., Wild, E. J., Joubert, R., Sathasivam, K., Björkqvist, M., Petersén, A., Jackson, G. S., Isaacs, J. D., Kristiansen, M., Bates, G. P., Leavitt, B. R., Keir, G., Ward, M., and Tabrizi, S. J. (2007). Proteomic profiling of plasma in Huntington's disease reveals neuroinflammatory activation and biomarker candidates. *J. Proteome Res.* 6, 2833–2840.

De Groot, C. J., Bergers, E., Kamphorst, W., Ravid, R., Polman, C. H., Barkhof, F., and van der Valk, P. (2001). Post-mortem MRI-guided sampling of multiple sclerosis brain lesions: increased yield of active demyelinating and (p) reactive lesions. *Brain* 124, 1635–1645.

De Lella Ezcurra, A. L., Chertoff, M., Ferrari, C., Graciarena, M., and Pitossi, F. (2010). Chronic expression of low levels of tumor necrosis factor-alpha in the substantia nigra elicits progressive neurodegeneration, delayed motor symptoms and microglia/macrophage activation. *Neurobiol. Dis.* 37, 630–640.

Debruyne, J. C., Versijpt, J., Van Laere, K. J., De Vos, F., Keppens, J., Strijckmans, K., Achten, E., Slegers, G., Dierckx, R. A., Korf, J., and De Reuck, J. L. (2003). PET visualization of microglia in multiple sclerosis patients using [11C]PK11195. *Eur. J. Neurol.* 10, 257–264.

Dheen, S. T., Kaur, C., and Ling, E. A. (2007). Microglial activation, and its implications in the brain diseases. *Curr. Med. Chem.* 14, 1189–1197.

DiCarlo, G., Wilcock, D., Henderson, D., Gordon, M., and Morgan, D. (2001). Intrahippocampal LPS injections reduce Abeta load in APP+PS1 transgenic mice. *Neurobiol. Aging* 22, 1007–1012.

Dickson, D. W., Bergeron, C., Chin, S. S., Duyckaerts, C., Horoupian, D., Ikeda, K., Jellinger, K., Lantos, P. L., Lippa, C. F., Mirra, S. S., Tabaton, M., Vonsattel, J. P., Wakabayashi, K., and Litvan, I. (2002). Office of rare diseases neuropathologic criteria for corticobasal degeneration. *J. Neuropathol. Exp. Neurol.* 61, 935–946.

Dutta, R., and Trapp, B. D. (2006). [Pathology and definition of multiple sclerosis]. *Rev. Prat.* 56, 1293–1298.

Edison, P., Archer, H. A., Gerhard, A., Hinz, R., Pavese, N., Turkheimer, F. E., Hammers, A., Tai, Y. F., Fox, N., Kennedy, A., Rossor, M., and Brooks, D. J. (2008). Microglia, amyloid, and cognition in Alzheimer's disease: an [11C](R)PK11195-PET and [11C]PIB-PET study. *Neurobiol. Dis.* 32, 412–419.

Eikelenboom, P., Bate, C., Van Gool, W. A., Hoozemans, J. J., Rozemuller, J. M., Veerhuis, R., and Williams, A. (2002). Neuroinflammation in Alzheimer's disease and prion disease. *Glia* 40, 232–239.

Ferrari, C. C., Pott Godoy, M. C., Tarelli, R., Chertoff, M., Depino, A. M., and Pitossi, F. J. (2006). Progressive neurodegeneration and motor disabilities induced by chronic expression of IL-1beta in the substantia nigra. *Neurobiol. Dis.* 24, 183–193.

Floden, A. M., Li, S., and Combs, C. K. (2005). Beta-amyloid-stimulated microglia induce neuron death via synergistic stimulation of tumor necrosis factor alpha and NMDA receptors. *J. Neurosci.* 25, 2566–2575.

Frautschy, S. A., Yang, F., Irrizarry, M., Hyman, B., Saido, T. C., Hsiao, K., and Cole, G. M. (1998). Microglial response to amyloid plaques in APPsw transgenic mice. *Am. J. Pathol.* 152, 307–317.

Fujimura, Y., Ikoma, Y., Yasuno, F., Suhara, T., Ota, M., Matsumoto, R., Nozaki, S., Takano, A., Kosaka, J., Zhang, M. R., Nakao, R., Suzuki, K., Kato, N., and Ito, H. (2006). Quantitative analyses of 18F-FEDAA1106 binding to peripheral benzodiazepine receptors in living human brain. *J. Nucl. Med.* 47, 43–50.

Fujita, M., Imaizumi, M., Zoghbi, S. S., Fujimura, Y., Farris, A. G., Suhara, T., Hong, J., Pike, V. W., and Innis, R. B. (2008). Kinetic analysis in healthy humans of a novel positron emission tomography radioligand to image the peripheral benzodiazepine receptor, a potential biomarker for inflammation. *Neuroimage* 40, 43–52.

Gerhard, A., Banati, R. B., Goerres, G. B., Cagnin, A., Myers, R., Gunn, R. N., Turkheimer, F. E., Good, C. D., Mathias, C. J., Quinn, N., Schwarz, J., and Brooks, D. J. (2003). [11C](R)-PK11195 PET imaging of microglial activation in multiple system atrophy. *Neurology* 61, 686–689.

Gerhard, A., Pavese, N., Hotton, G., Turkheimer, F., Es, M., Hammers, A., Eggert, K., Oertel, W., Banati, R. B., and Brooks, D. J. (2006a). In vivo imaging of microglial activation with [11C](R)-PK11195 PET in idiopathic Parkinson's disease. *Neurobiol. Dis.* 21, 404–412.

Gerhard, A., Trender-Gerhard, I., Turkheimer, F., Quinn, N. P., Bhatia, K. P., and Brooks, D. J. (2006b). In vivo imaging of microglial activation with [11C](R)-PK11195 PET in progressive supranuclear palsy. *Mov. Disord.* 21, 89–93.

Gerhard, A., Watts, J., Trender-Gerhard, I., Turkheimer, F., Banati, R. B., Bhatia, K., and Brooks, D. J. (2004). In vivo imaging of microglial activation with [11C](R)-PK11195 PET in corticobasal degeneration. *Mov. Disord.* 19, 1221–1226.

Gibb, W. R., Luthert, P. J., and Marsden, C. D. (1989). Corticobasal degeneration. *Brain* 112, 1171–1192.

Gulyás, B., Halldin, C., Sandell, J., Karlsson, P., Sóvágó, J., Kárpáti, E., Kiss, B., Vas, A., Cselényi, Z., and Farde, L. (2002). PET studies on the brain uptake and regional distribution of [11C]vinpocetine in human subjects. *Acta Neurol. Scand.* 106, 325–332.

Hardy, J., and Selkoe, D. J. (2002). The amyloid hypothesis of Alzheimer's disease: progress and problems on the road to therapeutics. *Science* 297, 353–356.

Hartlage-Rübsamen, M., Lemke, R., and Schliebs, R. (1999). Interleukin-1beta, inducible nitric oxide synthase, and nuclear factor-kappaB are induced in morphologically distinct microglia after rat hippocampal lipopolysaccharide/interferon-gamma injection. *J. Neurosci. Res.* 57, 388–398.

Hauw, J. J., Daniel, S. E., Dickson, D., Horoupian, D. S., Jellinger, K., Lantos, P. L., McKee, A., Tabaton, M., and Litvan, I. (1994). Preliminary NINDS neuropathologic criteria for Steele-Richardson-Olszewski syndrome (progressive supranuclear palsy). *Neurology* 44, 2015–2019.

Henkel, K., Karitzky, J., Schmid, M., Mader, I., Glatting, G., Unger, J. W., Neumaier, B., Ludolph, A. C., Reske, S. N., and Landwehrmeyer, G. B. (2004). Imaging of activated microglia with PET and [11C]PK 11195 in corticobasal degeneration. *Mov. Disord.* 19, 817–821.

Heppner, F. L., Greter, M., Marino, D., Falsig, J., Raivich, G., Hövelmeyer, N., Waisman, A., Rülicke, T., Prinz, M., Priller, J., Becher, B., and Aguzzi, A. (2005). Experimental autoimmune encephalomyelitis repressed by microglial paralysis. *Nat. Med.* 11, 146–152.

Ikoma, Y., Yasuno, F., Ito, H., Suhara, T., Ota, M., Toyama, H., Fujimura, Y., Takano, A., Maeda, J., Zhang, M. R., Nakao, R., and Suzuki, K. (2007). Quantitative analysis for estimating binding potential of the peripheral benzodiazepine receptor with [(11)C]DAA1106. *J. Cereb. Blood Flow Metab.* 27, 173–184.

Imamura, K., Hishikawa, N., Sawada, M., Nagatsu, T., Yoshida, M., and Hashizume, Y. (2003). Distribution of major histocompatibility complex class II-positive microglia and cytokine profile of Parkinson's disease brains. *Acta Neuropathol.* 106, 518–526.

Ishizawa, K., and Dickson, D. W. (2001). Microglial activation parallels system degeneration in progressive supranuclear palsy and corticobasal degeneration. *J. Neuropathol. Exp. Neurol.* 60, 647–657.

Ishizawa, K., Komori, T., Sasaki, S., Arai, N., Mizutani, T., and Hirose, T. (2004). Microglial activation parallels system degeneration in multiple system atrophy. *J. Neuropathol. Exp. Neurol.* 63, 43–52.

Ishizawa, K., Lin, W. L., Tiseo, P., Honer, W. G., Davies, P., and Dickson, D. W. (2000). A qualitative and quantitative study of grumose degeneration in progressive supranuclear palsy. *J. Neuropathol. Exp. Neurol.* 59, 513–524.

Kesselring, J. (1990). The pathogenesis of multiple sclerosis. *Schweiz. Med. Wochenschr.* 120, 1083–1090.

Kida, E., Barcikowska, M., and Niemczewska, M. (1992). Immunohistochemical study of a case with progressive supranuclear palsy without ophthalmoplegia. *Acta Neuropathol.* 83, 328–332.

Kiferle, L., Politis, M., Muraro, P. A., and Piccini, P. (2011). Positron emission tomography imaging in multiple sclerosis-current status and future applications. *Eur. J. Neurol.* 18, 226–231.

Kim, S., Moon, M., and Park, S. (2009). Exendin-4 protects dopaminergic neurons by inhibition of microglial activation and matrix metalloproteinase-3 expression in an animal model of Parkinson's disease. *J. Endocrinol.* 202, 431–439.

Koenigsknecht-Talboo, J., and Landreth, G. E. (2005). Microglial phagocytosis induced by fibrillar beta-amyloid and IgGs are differentially regulated by proinflammatory cytokines. *J. Neurosci.* 25, 8240–8249.

Komori, T., Shibata, N., Kobayashi, M., Sasaki, S., and Iwata, M. (1998). Inducible nitric oxide synthase (iNOS)-like immunoreactivity in argyrophilic, tau-positive astrocytes in progressive supranuclear palsy. *Acta Neuropathol.* 95, 338–344.

Kreutzberg, G. W. (1996). Microglia: a sensor for pathological events in the CNS. *Trends Neurosci.* 19, 312–318.

Kutzelnigg, A., Lucchinetti, C. F., Stadelmann, C., Brück, W., Rauschka, H., Bergmann, M., Schmidbauer, M., Parisi, J. E., and Lassmann, H. (2005). Cortical demyelination and diffuse white matter injury in multiple sclerosis. *Brain* 128, 2705–2712.

Langston, J. W., Forno, L. S., Tetrud, J., Reeves, A. G., Kaplan, J. A., and Karluk, D. (1999). Evidence of active nerve cell degeneration in the substantia nigra of humans years after 1-methyl-4-phenyl-1,2,3,6-tetrahydropyridine exposure. *Ann. Neurol.* 46, 598–605.

Lantos, P. L., and Papp, M. I. (1994). Cellular pathology of multiple system atrophy: a review. *J. Neurol. Neurosurg. Psychiatr.* 57, 129–133.

Lassmann, H. (2008). Mechanisms of inflammation induced tissue injury in multiple sclerosis. *J. Neurol. Sci.* 274, 45–47.

Lawson, L. J., Perry, V. H., Dri, P., and Gordon, S. (1990). Heterogeneity in the distribution and morphology of microglia in the normal adult mouse brain. *Neuroscience* 39, 151–170.

Leung, E., Guo, L., Bu, J., Maloof, M., El Khoury, J., and Geula, C. (2011). Microglia activation mediates fibrillar amyloid-(β toxicity in the aged primate cortex. *Neurobiol. Aging* 32, 387–397.

Li, L., Lu, J., Tay, S. S., Moochhala, S. M., and He, B. P. (2007). The function of microglia, either neuroprotection or neurotoxicity, is determined by the equilibrium among factors released from activated microglia in vitro. *Brain Res.* 1159, 8–17.

Li, W. W., Setzu, A., Zhao, C., and Franklin, R. J. (2005). Minocycline-mediated inhibition of microglia activation impairs oligodendrocyte progenitor cell responses and remyelination in a non-immune model of demyelination. *J. Neuroimmunol.* 158, 58–66.

Magliozzi, R., Howell, O. W., Reeves, C., Roncaroli, F., Nicholas, R., Serafini, B., Aloisi, F., and Reynolds, R. (2010). A Gradient of neuronal loss and meningeal inflammation in multiple sclerosis. *Ann. Neurol.* 68, 477–493.

McGeer, P. L., Itagaki, S., Boyes, B. E., and McGeer, E. G. (1988a). Reactive microglia are positive for HLA-DR in the substantia nigra of Parkinson's and Alzheimer's disease brains. *Neurology* 38, 1285–1291.

McGeer, P. L., Itagaki, S., and McGeer, E. G. (1988b). Expression of the histocompatibility glycoprotein HLA-DR in neurological disease. *Acta Neuropathol.* 76, 550–557.

Messmer, K., and Reynolds, G. P. (1998). Increased peripheral benzodiazepine binding sites in the brain of patients with Huntington's disease. *Neurosci. Lett.* 241, 53–56.

Michelucci, A., Heurtaux, T., Grandbarbe, L., Morga, E., and Heuschling, P. (2009). Characterization of the microglial phenotype under specific pro-inflammatory and anti-inflammatory conditions: effects of oligomeric and fibrillar amyloid-beta. *J. Neuroimmunol.* 210, 3–12.

Mirra, S. S., and Hyman, B. T. (2002). "Aging and dementia," in *Greenfield's Neuropathology*, Vol. 2, eds D. I. Graham and P. L. Lantos (London: Arnold), 195–271.

Mogi, M., Harada, M., Riederer, P., Narabayashi, H., Fujita, K., and Nagatsu, T. (1994). Tumor necrosis factor-alpha (TNF- alpha) increases both in the brain and in the cerebrospinal fluid from parkinsonian patients. *Neurosci. Lett.* 165, 208–210.

Munoz, D. G., Dickson, D. W., Bergeron, C., Mackenzie, I. R., Delacourte, A., and Zhukareva, V. (2003). The neuropathology and biochemistry of frontotemporal dementia. *Ann. Neurol.* 54(Suppl. 15), 24–28.

Napoli, I., and Neumann, H. (2009). Microglial clearance function in health and disease. *Neuroscience* 158, 1030–1038.

Neary, D., Snowden, J. S., Gustafson, L., Passant, U., Stuss, D., Black, S., Freedman, M., Kertesz, A., Robert, P. H., Albert, M., Boone, K., Miller, B. L., Cummings, J., and Benson, D. F. (1998). Frontotemporal lobar degeneration: a consensus on clinical diagnostic criteria. *Neurology* 51, 1546–1554.

Oh, U., Fujita, M., Ikonomidou, V. N., Evangelou, I. E., Matsuura, E., Harberts, E., Fujimura, Y., Richert, N. D., Ohayon, J., Pike, V. W., Zhang, Y., Zoghbi, S. S., Innis, R. B., and Jacobson, S. (2011). Translocator protein PET imaging for glial activation in multiple sclerosis. *J. Neuroimmune Pharmacol.* 6, 354–361.

Okello, A., Edison, P., Archer, H. A., Turkheimer, F. E., Kennedy, J., Bullock, R., Walker, Z., Kennedy, A., Fox, N., Rossor, M., and Brooks, D. J. (2009a). Microglial activation and amyloid deposition in mild cognitive impairment: a PET study. *Neurology* 72, 56–62.

Okello, A., Koivunen, J., Edison, P., Archer, H. A., Turkheimer, F. E., Någren, K., Bullock, R., Walker, Z., Kennedy, A., Fox, N. C., Rossor, M. N., Rinne, J. O., and Brooks, D. J. (2009b). Conversion of amyloid positive and negative MCI to AD over 3 years: an 11C-PIB PET study. *Neurology* 73, 754–760.

Ouchi, Y., Yoshikawa, E., Sekine, Y., Futatsubashi, M., Kanno, T., Ogusu, T., and Torizuka, T. (2005). Microglial activation and dopamine terminal loss in early Parkinson's disease. *Ann. Neurol.* 57, 168–175.

Owen, D. R., Howell, O. W., Tang, S. P., Wells, L. A., Bennacef, I., Bergstrom, M., Gunn, R. N., Rabiner, E. A., Wilkins, M. R., Reynolds, R., Matthews, P. M., and Parker, C. A. (2010). Two binding sites for [3H]PBR28 in human brain: implications for TSPO PET imaging of neuroinflammation. *J. Cereb. Blood Flow Metab.* 30, 1608–1618.

Papadopoulos, V., Baraldi, M., Guilarte, T. R., Knudsen, T. B., Lacapère, J. J., Lindemann, P., Norenberg, M. D., Nutt, D., Weizman, A., Zhang, M. R., and Gavish, M. (2006). Translocator protein (18kDa): new nomenclature for the peripheral-type benzodiazepine receptor based on its structure and molecular function. *Trends Pharmacol. Sci.* 27, 402–409.

Paulus, W., Bancher, C., and Jellinger, K. (1993). Microglial reaction in Pick's disease. *Neurosci. Lett.* 161, 89–92.

Pavese, N., Gerhard, A., Tai, Y. F., Ho, A. K., Turkheimer, F., Barker, R. A., Brooks, D. J., and Piccini, P. (2006). Microglial activation correlates with severity in Huntington disease: a clinical and PET study. *Neurology* 66, 1638–1643.

Peterson, J. W., Bö, L., Mörk, S., Chang, A., and Trapp, B. D. (2001). Transected neurites, apoptotic neurons, and reduced inflammation in cortical multiple sclerosis lesions. *Ann. Neurol.* 50, 389–400.

Petit-Taboué, M. C., Baron, J. C., Barré, L., Travère, J. M., Speckel, D., Camsonne, R., and MacKenzie, E. T. (1991). Brain kinetics and specific binding of [11C]PK 11195 to omega 3 sites in baboons: positron emission tomography study. *Eur. J. Pharmacol.* 200, 347–351.

Petzold, A., Eikelenboom, M. J., Gveric, D., Keir, G., Chapman, M., Lazeron, R. H., Cuzner, M. L., Polman, C. H., Uitdehaag, B. M., Thompson, E. J., and Giovannoni, G. (2002). Markers for different glial cell responses in multiple sclerosis: clinical and pathological correlations. *Brain* 125, 1462–1473.

Pike, V. W., Halldin, C., Crouzel, C., Barré, L., Nutt, D. J., Osman, S., Shah, F., Turton, D. R., and Waters, S. L. (1993). Radioligands for PET studies of central benzodiazepine receptors and PK (peripheral benzodiazepine) binding sites – current status. *Nucl. Med. Biol.* 20, 503–525.

Politis, M., Gianneti, P., Su, P., Turkheimer, F., Keihaninejad, S., Wu, K., Waldman, A., Malik, O., Matthews, P. M., Reynolds, R., Nicholas, R., and Piccini, P. (in press). Increased PK11195 PET binding in the cortex of MS patients correlates with disability. *Neurology.*

Politis, M., Pavese, N., Tai, Y. F., Kiferle, L., Mason, S. L., Brooks, D. J., Tabrizi, S. J., Barker, R. A., and Piccini, P. (2011). Microglial activation in regions related to cognitive function predicts disease onset in Huntington's disease: a multimodal imaging study. *Hum. Brain Mapp.* 32, 258–270.

Politis, M., Pavese, N., Tai, Y. F., Tabrizi, S. J., Barker, R. A., and Piccini, P. (2008). Hypothalamic involvement in Huntington's disease: an in vivo PET study. *Brain* 131(Pt 11), 2860–2869.

Ransohoff, R. M., and Perry, V. H. (2009). Microglial physiology: unique stimuli, specialized responses. *Annu. Rev. Immunol.* 27, 119–145.

Rasmussen, S., Wang, Y., Kivisäkk, P., Bronson, R. T., Meyer, M., Imitola, J., and Khoury, S. J. (2007). Persistent activation of microglia is associated with neuronal dysfunction of callosal projecting pathways and multiple sclerosis-like lesions in relapsing–remitting experimental autoimmune encephalomyelitis. *Brain* 130(Pt 11), 2816–2829.

Rebeiz, J. J., Kolodny, E. H., and Richardson, E. P. Jr. (1968). Corticodentatonigral degeneration with neuronal achromasia. *Arch. Neurol.* 18, 20–33.

Sanchez-Guajardo, V., Febbraro, F., Kirik, D., and Romero-Ramos, M. (2010). Microglia acquire distinct activation profiles depending on the degree of alpha-synuclein neuropathology in a rAAV based model of Parkinson's disease. *PLoS ONE* 5, e8784. doi:10.1371/journal.pone.0008784

Sapp, E., Kegel, K. B., Aronin, N., Hashikawa, T., Uchiyama, Y., Tohyama, K., Bhide, P. G., Vonsattel, J. P., and DiFiglia, M. (2001). Early and progressive accumulation of reactive microglia in the Huntington disease brain. *J. Neuropathol. Exp. Neurol.* 60, 161–172.

Scarf, A. M., Ittner, L. M., and Kassiou, M. (2009). The translocator protein (18 kDa): central nervous system disease and drug design. *J. Med. Chem.* 52, 581–592.

Schwarz, S. C., Seufferlein, T., Liptay, S., Schmid, R. M., Kasischke, K., Foster, O. J., Daniel, S., and Schwarz, J. (1998). Microglial activation in multiple system atrophy: a potential role for NF-kappaB/rel proteins. *Neuroreport* 9, 3029–3032.

Setzu, A., Lathia, J. D., Zhao, C., Wells, K., Rao, M. S., Ffrench-Constant, C., and Franklin, R. J. (2006). Inflammation stimulates myelination by transplanted oligodendrocyte precursor cells. *Glia.* 54, 297–303.

Singhrao, S. K., Neal, J. W., Morgan, B. P., and Gasque, P. (1999). Increased complement biosynthesis by microglia and complement activation on neurons in Huntington's disease. *Exp. Neurol.* 159, 362–376.

Stadelmann, C., Kerschensteiner, M., Misgeld, T., Brück, W., Hohlfeld, R., and Lassmann, H. (2002). BDNF and gp145trkB in multiple sclerosis brain lesions: neuroprotective interactions between immune and neuronal cells? *Brain* 125(Pt 1), 75–85.

Stalder, M., Phinney, A., Probst, A., Sommer, B., Staufenbiel, M., and Jucker, M. (1999). Association of microglia with amyloid plaques in brains of APP23 transgenic mice. *Am. J. Pathol.* 154, 1673–1684.

Stefanova, N., Reindl, M., Neumann, M., Kahle, P. J., Poewe, W., and Wenning, G. K. (2007). Microglial activation mediates neurodegeneration related to oligodendroglial alpha-synucleinopathy: implications for multiple system atrophy. *Mov. Disord.* 22, 2196–2203.

Stephenson, D. T., Schober, D. A., Smalstig, E. B., Mincy, R. E., Gehlert, D. R., and Clemens, J. A. (1995). Peripheral benzodiazepine receptors are colocalized with activated microglia following transient global forebrain ischemia in the rat. *J. Neurosci.* 15(Pt 2), 5263–5274.

Stone, D. K., Reynolds, A. D., Mosley, R. L., and Gendelman, H. E. (2009). Innate and adaptive immunity for the pathobiology of Parkinson's disease. *Antioxid. Redox Signal.* 11, 2151–2166.

Suzumura, A., Sawada, M., and Marunouchi, T. (1996). Selective induction of interleukin-6 in mouse microglia by granulocyte-macrophage colony-stimulating factor. *Brain Res.* 713, 192–198.

Tai, Y. F., Pavese, N., Gerhard, A., Tabrizi, S. J., Barker, R. A., Brooks, D. J., and Piccini, P. (2007). Microglial activation in presymptomatic Huntington's disease gene carriers. *Brain* 130(Pt 7), 1759–1766.

Uchihara, T., Ikeda, K., and Tsuchiya, K. (2003). Pick body disease and Pick syndrome. *Neuropathology* 23, 318–326.

Vas, A., Shchukin, Y., Karrenbauer, V. D., Cselényi, Z., Kostulas, K., Hillert, J., Savic, I., Takano, A., Halldin, C., and Gulyás, B. (2008). Functional neuroimaging in multiple sclerosis with radiolabelled glia markers: preliminary comparative PET studies with [11C]vinpocetine and [11C]PK11195 in patients. *J. Neurol. Sci.* 264, 9–17.

Venneti, S., Lopresti, B. J., Wang, G., Hamilton, R. L., Mathis, C. A., Klunk, W. E., Apte, U. M., and Wiley, C. A. (2009). PK11195 labels activated microglia in Alzheimer's disease and in vivo in a mouse model using PET. *Neurobiol. Aging* 30, 1217–1226.

Versijpt, J., Debruyne, J. C., Van Laere, K. J., De Vos, F., Keppens, J., Strijckmans, K., Achten, E., Slegers, G., Dierckx, R. A., Korf, J., and De Reuck, J. L. (2005). Microglial imaging with positron emission tomography and atrophy measurements with magnetic resonance imaging in multiple sclerosis: a correlative study. *Mult. Scler.* 11, 127–134.

Vonsattel, J. P., and DiFiglia, M. (1998). Huntington disease. *J. Neuropathol. Exp. Neurol.* 57, 369–384.

Vowinckel, E., Reutens, D., Becher, B., Verge, G., Evans, A., Owens, T., and Antel, J. P. (1997). PK11195 binding to the peripheral benzodiazepine receptor as a marker of microglia activation in multiple sclerosis and experimental autoimmune encephalomyelitis. *J. Neurosci. Res.* 50, 345–353.

Wiley, C. A., Lopresti, B. J., Venneti, S., Price, J., Klunk, W. E., DeKosky, S.T., and Mathis, C.A. (2009). Carbon 11-labelled Pittsburgh Compound B and carbon 11-labelled ®-PK11195 positron emission tomographic imaging in Alzheimer disease. *Arch. Neurol.* 66, 60–67.

Wilms, H., Claasen, J., Röhl, C., Sievers, J., Deuschl, G., and Lucius, R. (2003). Involvement of benzodiazepine receptors in neuroinflammatory and neurodegenerative diseases: evidence from activated microglial cells in vitro. *Neurobiol. Dis.* 14, 417–424.

Wimo, A., Winblad, B., Aguero-Torres, H., and von Strauss, E. (2003). The magnitude of dementia occurrence in the world. *Alzheimer Dis. Assoc. Disord.* 17, 63–67.

Yasuno, F., Ota, M., Kosaka, J., Ito, H., Higuchi, M., Doronbekov, T. K., Nozaki, S., Fujimura, Y., Koeda, M., Asada, T., and Suhara, T. (2008). Increased binding of peripheral benzodiazepine receptor in Alzheimer's disease measured by positron emission tomography with [11C]DAA1106. *Biol. Psychiatry* 64, 835–841.

Yokokura, M., Mori, N., Yagi, S., Yoshikawa, E., Kikuchi, M., Yoshihara, Y., Wakuda, T., Sugihara, G., Takebayashi, K., Suda, S., Iwata, Y., Ueki, T., Tsuchiya, K. J., Suzuki, K., Nakamura, K., and Ouchi, Y. (2011). In vivo changes in microglial activation and amyloid deposits in brain regions with hypometabolism in Alzheimer's disease. *Eur. J. Nucl. Med. Mol. Imaging* 38, 343–351.

Zhang, W., Wang, T., Pei, Z., Miller, D. S., Wu, X., Block, M. L., Wilson, B., Zhang, W., Zhou, Y., Hong, J. S., and Zhang, J. (2005). Aggregated alpha-synuclein activates microglia: a process leading to disease progression in Parkinson's disease. *FASEB J.* 19, 533–542.

Zipp, F., Hartung, H. P., Hillert, J., Schimrigk, S., Trebst, C., Stangel, M., Infante-Duarte, C., Jakobs, P., Wolf, C., Sandbrink, R., Pohl, C., Filippi, M., and CCR1 Antagonist Study Group. (2006). Blockade of chemokine signaling in patients with multiple sclerosis. *Neurology* 67, 1880–1883.

Is the subcallosal medial prefrontal cortex a common site of atrophy in Alzheimer's disease and frontotemporal lobar degeneration?

Olof Lindberg[1]*, Eric Westman[1], Sari Karlsson[2], Per Östberg[3], Leif A. Svensson[4], Andrew Simmons[5,6] and Lars-Olof Wahlund[1]

[1] Department of Neurobiology, Care Sciences and Society, Karolinska Institutet, Stockholm, Sweden
[2] Aging Research Centre, Karolinska Institutet, Stockholm, Sweden
[3] Division of Speech and Language Pathology, Department of Clinical Science, Intervention and Technology, Karolinska Institutet, Stockholm, Sweden
[4] Department of Medical Physics, Karolinska University Hospital, Stockholm, Sweden
[5] Institute of Psychiatry, King's College London, London, UK
[6] NIHR Biomedical Research Centre for Mental Health, London, UK

Edited by:
Manuel Menendez Gonzalez, Hospital Álvarez-Buylla, Spain

Reviewed by:
Manuel Menendez Gonzalez, Hospital Álvarez-Buylla, Spain
Sandro M. Krieg, Technical University Munich, Germany

***Correspondence:**
Olof Lindberg, Clinical Geriatrics, Department of Neurobiology, Care Sciences and Society, Karolinska Institutet, Novum, Plan 5, Stockholm SE-141 86, Sweden.
e-mail: olof.lindberg@ki.se

Regions affected late in neurodegenerative disease are thought to be anatomically connected to regions affected earlier. The subcallosal medial prefrontal cortex (SMPC) has connections with the dorsolateral prefrontal cortex (DLPFC), orbitofrontal cortex (OFC), and hippocampus (HC), which are regions that may become atrophic in frontotemporal lobar degeneration (FTLD) and Alzheimer's disease (AD). We hypothesized that the SMPC is a common site of frontal atrophy in the FTLD subtypes and in AD. The volume of the SMPC, DLPFC, OFC, HC, and entorhinal cortex (EC) were manually delineated for 12 subjects with frontotemporal dementia (FTD), 13 with semantic dementia (SD), 9 with progressive nonfluent aphasia (PNFA), 10 AD cases, and 13 controls. Results revealed significant volume loss in the left SMPC in FTD, SD, and PNFA, while the right SMPC was also atrophied in SD and FTD. In AD a non significant tendency of volume loss in the left SMPC was found ($p = 0.08$), with no volume loss on the right side. Results indicated that volume loss reflected the degree of brain connectivity. In SD and AD temporal regions displayed most atrophy. Among the frontal regions, the SMPC (which receives the strongest temporal projections) demonstrated most volume loss, the OFC (which receives less temporal projections) less volume loss, while the DLPFC (which is at multisynaptic distance from the temporal regions) demonstrated no volume loss. In PNFA, the left SMPC was atrophic, possibly reflecting progression from the left anterior insula, while FTD patients may have had SMPC atrophy at the initial stages of the disease. Atrophy of the SMPC may thus be affected by either initial temporal or initial frontal atrophy, making it a common site of frontal atrophy in the dementia subtypes investigated.

Keywords: Alzheimer's disease, frontotemporal dementia, subcallosal medial prefrontal cortex, MRI

INTRODUCTION

In recent years the view that regional atrophy in dementia results from damage to particular brain networks has received increased attention. This view not only relates regional damage to impairment of mental functions, dependent on different brain networks, but also allows inference as to how and where atrophy develops during the course of disease. The assumption is that "later-affected regions bear known anatomical connections with the sites of earlier injury" (Seeley et al., 2009, p. 42). We will refer to this as the "connection hypothesis." The basic mechanism of the connection hypothesis has previously been demonstrated in monkey brain (Woolsey, 1947; Jones and Powell, 1970) and in neuropathological postmortem studies of Alzheimer's disease (AD) (Pearson et al., 1985; De Lacoste and White, 1993).

The underlying mechanism of the connection hypothesis is that molecular pathologies such as β-amyloid, tau, α-synuclein, and TDP-43 aggregate and progress through specific anatomical connections or brain networks (Seeley et al., 2009; Raj et al., 2012). Support for this assumption in both AD and FTLD has been presented in a large study by Seeley et al. (2009). In another study a model of brain connectivity was derived from whole brain tractography on diffusion MRI scans on 14 healthy young controls. On the basis of the strength of connectivity found in this model several networks were proposed that in subsequent analysis was shown to correspond well with Seeley's assumption of network-specific progression of atrophy in FTLD and AD (Raj et al., 2012).

AD and semantic dementia (SD), which is a subtype of frontotemporal lobar degeneration (FTLD), are characterized by severe hippocampal and temporal lobe pathology while the frontal lobes are initially largely spared. This could be interpreted as support for the connection hypothesis because most frontal regions are at a "multisynaptic" distance from the temporal regions first affected. Most regions in the frontal lobe interact with the hippocampus (HC) through the cingulate and posterior parahippocampal gyri and entorhinal cortices (Goldman-Rakic et al., 1984). Disease processes emanating from the temporal cortex must thus progress through a number of synaptic connections to reach the frontal parts of the brain.

Two regions in the frontal lobe, the subcallosal medial prefrontal cortex (SMPC), and to a lesser extent the orbitofrontal cortex (OFC), are exceptions to the multisynaptic communication pattern described above. Studies with retrograde and anterograde tracers on the rhesus monkey brain show that these frontal regions receive direct projections from the hippocampal formation (Goldman-Rakic et al., 1984; Barbas and Blatt, 1995; Carmichael and Price, 1996). Such direct connections also exist in humans (Kahn et al., 2008). The direct projections from the HC to the SMPC and ORB originate mainly from the CA1 field and the subiculum, and contrary to many brain connections, they are strictly ipsilateral and unidirectional (Barbas and Blatt, 1995; Laroche et al., 2000).

Monkey studies suggest that the entorhinal cortex (EC), heavily affected in AD, also projects particularly to the OFC and the SMPC (Ongur and Price, 2000; Munoz and Insausti, 2005; Insausti and Amaral, 2008). There is, however, less convincing evidence for such direct connections between the EC and the SMPC in humans (Kahn et al., 2008).

In addition to the temporal regions, the SMPC has reciprocal connections with several regions in the frontal lobe. Brodmann areas (BA) 9 and 46 in the dorsolateral prefrontal cortex (DLPFC) are connected to BA14 in the SMPC (Carmichael and Price, 1996; Ongur and Price, 2000). It has further been demonstrated that some areas of the SMPC (such as BA25) have reciprocal connections with regions in the OFC, as well as some parts of the anterior agranular insula (Carmichael and Price, 1996; Ongur and Price, 2000).

In accordance with the connection hypothesis it can be assumed that the SMPC and the OFC become pathologically involved in dementia characterized by temporal/hippocampal pathology. This has indeed been shown in both SD (Whitwell and Jack, 2005; Schroeter et al., 2007; Rohrer et al., 2009) and AD (Thompson et al., 2007). According to the connection hypothesis, atrophy might also progress to the SMPC from a number of frontal regions. In the behavioral variant of FTLD called frontotemporal dementia (FTD), the OFC becomes atrophic early (Perry et al., 2006), while the left anterior insula may be the first area to display atrophy in progressive nonfluent aphasia (PNFA) (Rohrer et al., 2009).

The hypothesis of the current study is that the SMPC is a common site of frontal atrophy in all types of FTLD as well as AD because of its anatomical connections with regions suggested to be the first sites of atrophy in these diseases.

To study this we compared the degree of atrophy in the SMPC with atrophy in the EC, the HC, the DLPFC and the OFC in AD and in the three subtypes of FTLD (FTD, PNFA, and SD).

METHODS

PARTICIPANTS

Participants were recruited retrospectively from the Memory Clinic at the Karolinska University Hospital Huddinge, Stockholm, Sweden. All participants went through a standard investigation procedure at the memory clinic. Clinical diagnoses were determined at a multidisciplinary consensus conference with physicians, neuropsychologists, speech-language pathologists, and nurses (Andersson, 2007). FTLD syndromes were diagnosed following international consensus criteria (Neary et al., 1998). Patients with FTLD and AD at different stages of the disease were included. Diagnoses of AD were based on criteria of the ICD-10 International Classification of Diseases, Tenth Revision (ICD-10). The control group (CTL) comprised individuals referred to the memory clinic because of mild subjective forgetfulness in everyday life. Objective cognitive impairment was ruled out through comprehensive neuropsychological assessment (impairment was defined as performance 1.5 SD unit below the age-normal mean on any cognitive test). To further minimize the risk of including participants at the very early stages of neurodegenerative diseases, we included only those participants whose performance did not deteriorate over a minimum of 2-years follow-up. Volumetric MRI data were obtained from 12 FTD, 9 PNFA, 12 SD, and 10 AD patients, as well as 13 CTL subjects.

The study was approved by the Regional Ethical Review Board in Stockholm, Sweden. Demographic and neuropsychological data are presented in **Table 1**. The dementia groups did not differ in age, but all dementia groups had, as expected, significantly lower Mini-Mental State Examination scores (MMSE; Folstein et al., 1975) than the CTL group.

Table 1 | Demographic and neuropsychological characteristics of the investigated groups.

	CTL	FTD	PNFA	SD	AD
Number	13	12	9	13	10
Age (sd)	63.0 (7.4)	61.8 (7.4)	63.9 (6.7)	64.2 (7.3)	64.2 (6.8)
Years of disease (sd)	–	2.50 (2.1)#	3.5 (1.7)	3.9 (1.9)	3.0 (1.3)
MMSE (sd)	29.2 (0.9)	20.8 (6.1)*	16.9 (11.4)*	22.6 (6.9)*	22.4 (6.5)*
Female/male	7/3	9/3	6/3	9/4	7/3

*CTL, controls; FTD, frontotemporal dementia; PNFA, progressive nonfluent aphasia; SD, semantic dementia; AD, Alzheimer's Disease; MMSE, mini mental state examination; sd, standard deviation; *Significantly different from CTL on Kruskal–Wallis test with Mann–Whitney U-test post-hoc. #Significant longer illness duration than FTD in One-Way analysis of variance with a Tukey post-hoc.*

IMAGE ACQUISITION

T1-weighted MR images were acquired on a 1.5T Magnetom Vision Plus scanner (Siemens Medical Systems, Erlangen, Germany). A 3D magnetization-prepared rapid gradient echo pulse sequence (TR, 11.4 ms; TE, 4.4 ms; TI, 300 ms; flip angle, 10°; NEX, 1) was used to obtain 72 contiguous coronal 2.5-mm sections with a 512 × 144 matrix and a 230-mm FOV.

The original images were subsequently interpolated to a 1 × 1 × 1 mm resolution dataset, on which volumetric analyses were performed. Comprehensive quality control was carried out for all MR images as previously described (Simmons et al., 2009, 2011).

CORTICAL PARCELLATION AND VOLUMETRY

The software program MRIcro (Version 1.37; http://www.mricro.com, http://www.mccauslandcenter.sc.edu/mricro/mricron/) was used for parcellation of the cortex. With this software, an image can be viewed in horizontal, sagittal, and coronal directions simultaneously with a reconstruction of the surface of the brain. Measurements were subsequently performed using the HERMES MultiModality software package (Nuclear Diagnostics, Stockholm, Sweden). Regions of interest were traced manually on contiguous coronal sections. The intracranial volume (ICV) was obtained by using a stereologic point-counting technique comprising manual tracing of the ICV on every fourth slice, following landmarks proposed by Eritaia et al. (2000).

The SMPC was traced in the coronal orientation. The anterior border was defined as the first slice in which the callosal white matter connects the two hemispheres (**Figure 1A**) and the posterior border was the last slice in which the inferior part of the corpus callosum could be visualized (**Figure 1B**). Between these landmarks all gray matter on the ventromedial surface was included. Intraclass correlation coefficients (ICCs) were calculated to estimate the reliability of measurements. Tracings of other frontal regions were carried out following Suzuki et al. (2005). For DLPFC we combined the gray matter volume of the superior frontal gyrus with that of the middle frontal gyrus. The reliability of the SMPC measurements was investigated on two occasions and was >0.91 both times. The ICC for other cortical regions has been reported previously (Lindberg et al., 2009), but in short all ICCs were greater than 0.90. All statistical calculations were performed on normalized volume of measured region, derived by dividing the volume of the region by the ICV.

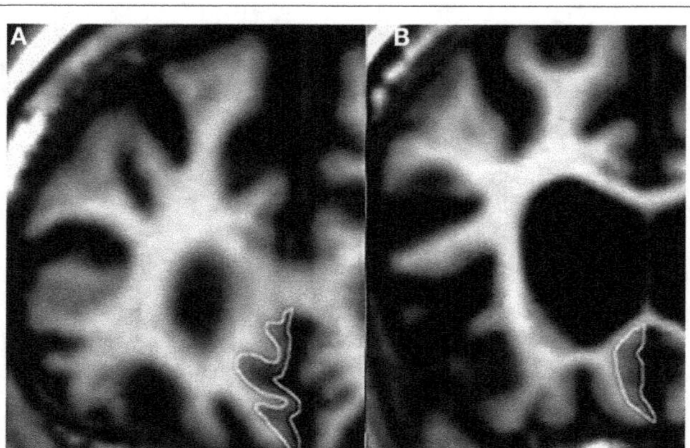

FIGURE 1 | The subcallosal medial prefrontal cortex (SMPC). (A) The anterior border of the delineated region. **(B)** The posterior border of the delineated region.

STATISTICAL ANALYSIS

Volumetric data were analyzed by One-Way analysis of variance with a Fisher LSD *post-hoc* test using Statistica 10 (StatSoft, Inc., 2011). All volumetric data were normalized by ICV by the formula volume of region/ICV. A P value less than 0.05 was considered significant.

CORRELATIONS BETWEEN REGIONAL VOLUMES

To investigate the relationship between frontal and temporal atrophy with atrophy of the SMPC, Pearson's correlation coefficient (r) was calculated for the total normalized volume (left + right side) of each region and the total normalized volume of SMPC.

MULTIVARIATE ANALYSIS

Principle component analysis (PCA) is an unsupervised method which does not use *a priori* information about groups for the analysis. The representations of a multivariate data table X, consisting of rows (observations) and columns (variables) as a low-dimensional plane, is an important feature of PCA. Statistically, PCA reduces the dimensionality and complexity of the data by finding lines and planes in the K-dimensional space (K = number of variables in the model) that approximates the data in the best way possible in the least squares sense. This provides an overview of the data and allows patterns, trends, and outliers to be observed. It is also possible to view relationships between the observations and the variables. A model usually reduces the K-dimensional space to 2–5 dimensions (Eriksson et al., 2006). The results from PCA are visualized by plotting two components in a scatter plot. Components are vectors in the multivariate space along which groups can be separated. These vectors are dominated by the input variables (x). All the components created by the models are, by definition, orthogonal to each other and span the projection plane of the points. Each point in the scatter plot represents one individual subject. Loadings plots illustrate how the original variables influence the new latent variables (components). The PCA model included all five groups (AD, SD, FTD, PNFA, and CTL) and was created to investigate the constellation of clusters that the program uses to separate dementia patients from controls, not to create a model that effectively separated different variants of dementia.

RESULTS

VOLUMETRIC ANALYSIS

The participants with FTD had significantly smaller gray matter volume than the CTL group in all regions studied. The greatest gray matter loss was found in the OFC, SMPC, and HC with a loss of approximately 25% compared to CTL subjects. The EC and right DLPFC regions had approximately 20% volume loss while left DLPFC had 15% loss relative to CTL subjects (**Figure 2**).

Participants with PNFA displayed greater volume loss on the left side. All regions had significant volume loss compared to the

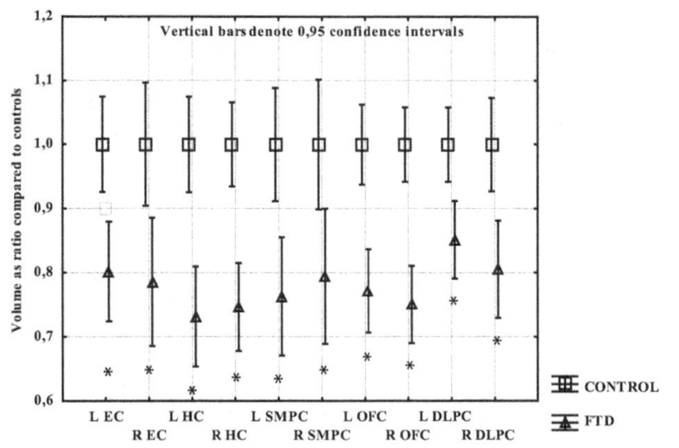

FIGURE 2 | The volume of measured region in FTD expressed as a ratio of CTL volume. CTL volume is set to 1. X-axis denotes the included regions: EC, entorhinal cortex; HC, hippocampus; OFC, orbitofrontal cortex; SMPC, subcallosal medial prefrontal cortex; DLPFC, dorsolateral prefrontal cortex. *$p < 0.01$.

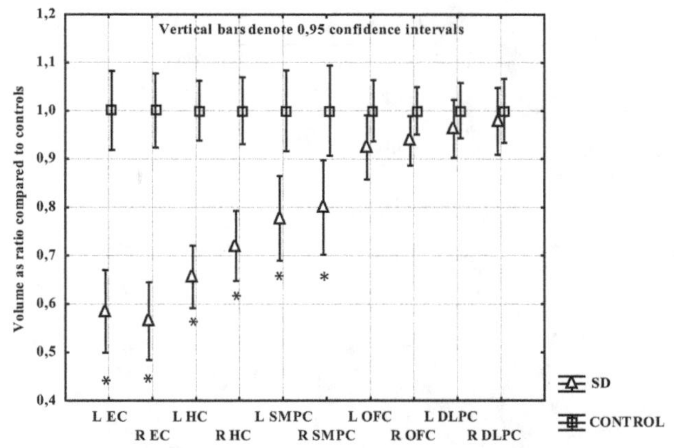

FIGURE 4 | The volume of measured region in SD expressed as a ratio of CTL volume. CTL volume is set to 1. X-axis denotes the included regions: EC, entorhinal cortex; HC, hippocampus; OFC, orbitofrontal cortex; SMPC, subcallosal medial prefrontal cortex; DLPFC, dorsolateral prefrontal cortex. *$p < 0.01$.

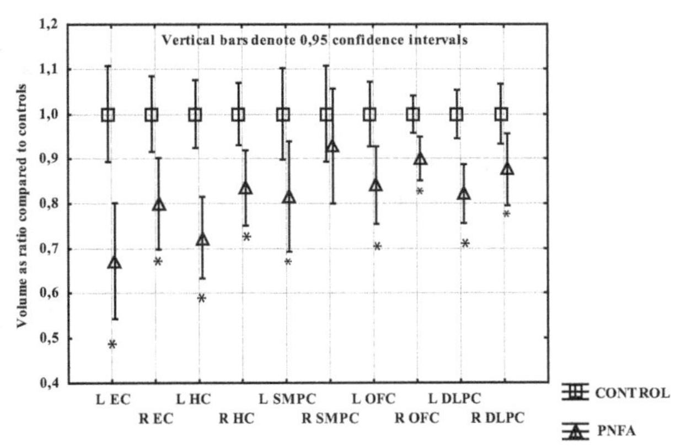

FIGURE 3 | The volume of measured region in PNFA expressed as a ratio of CTL volume. CTL volume is set to 1. X-axis denotes the included regions: EC, entorhinal cortex; HC, hippocampus; OFC, orbitofrontal cortex; SMPC, subcallosal medial prefrontal cortex; DLPFC, dorsolateral prefrontal cortex. *$p < 0.01$.

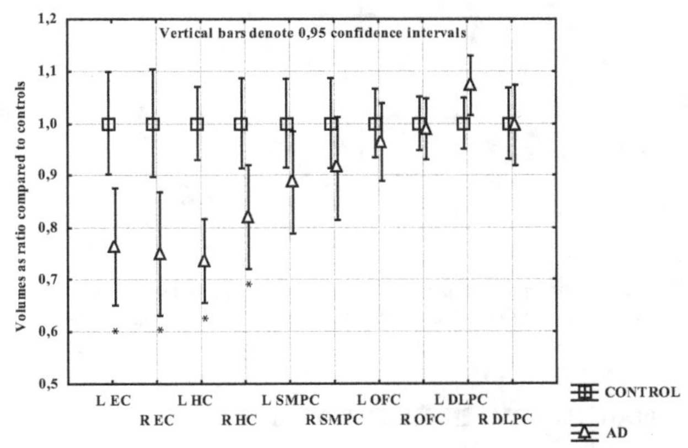

FIGURE 5 | The volume of measured region in AD expressed as a ratio of CTL volume. CTL volume is set to 1. X-axis denotes the included regions: EC, entorhinal cortex; HC, hippocampus; OFC, orbitofrontal cortex; SMPC, subcallosal medial prefrontal cortex; DLPFC, dorsolateral prefrontal cortex. *$p < 0.01$.

CTL group except the right SMPC. The left EC displayed the greatest mean gray matter loss compared to CTL, followed by left HC, left SMPC, and left DLPFC (**Figure 3**).

All temporal regions and the SMPC displayed significant gray matter loss in participants with SD. The EC displayed most loss (around 40%) followed by HC (30%) and then SMPC (25%). No gray matter loss was found in the OFC or DLPFC (**Figure 4**).

In participants with AD only the temporal regions displayed significant gray matter loss. The greatest atrophy was found in EC and left HC (around 25%) followed by right HC (18%). In the left SMPC there was a tendency to volume loss (around 11%; $p = 0.10$), while the right SMPC, left and right OFC and DLPFC did not demonstrate a statistically significant gray matter reduction (**Figure 5**).

PRINCIPAL COMPONENT ANALYSIS (ALL GROUPS)

The PCA model containing all five groups revealed three components, accounting for 70% of the variance of the original data [$R^2(X)$] and its cross-validated predictability, $Q^2(X) = 0.48$. At the extreme left end of the X-axis on the scatter plot (**Figure 6A**), we found the dementia cases that displayed most severe frontal and temporal atrophy, while on the right end we found mostly CTL subjects. The loading plot of the PCA may indicate the relationship between frontal and temporal atrophy and the SMPC (**Figure 6B**). The first component that is plotted along the X-axis can be interpreted as an indicator of general degree of atrophy. The second component (Y-axis) may potentially be interpreted as temporal versus frontal atrophy. Notice that the EC and the HC are plotted relatively close together. The same pattern is observed for DLPFC and OFC.

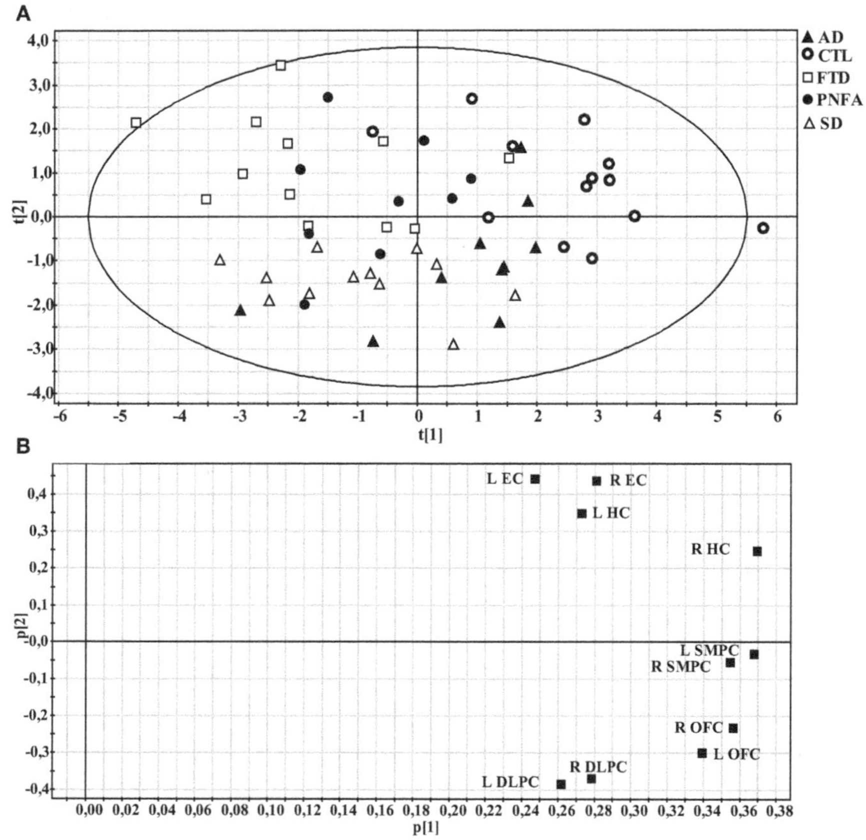

FIGURE 6 | Principal component analysis (PCA) of all subjects. (A) Scatter plot illustrating how individuals are distributed along the first two components. **(B)** Loading plot showing the influence of the regional volumes on the first two components.

CORRELATIONS BETWEEN REGIONAL VOLUMES

In FTD there was a significant correlation between the total normalized volume of OFC and the total normalized volume of SMPC, while no correlation was found between HC and SMPC (**Figures 7A,B**). The SMPC was also correlated with the total volume of DLPFC ($r = 0.76, p = 0.004$).

In SD there was a significant correlation between the total normalized volume of HC and the total normalized volume of SMPC, while no correlation was found between the OFC and SMPC (**Figures 7C,D**).

The total normalized volume of SMPC was not correlated with any other region in AD or in PNFA.

DISCUSSION

This study explored the hypothesis that the SMPC may be particularly vulnerable to atrophy in FTLD and AD because of its anatomical connections with frontal and temporal regions that become atrophic in these diseases. In AD and SD, the EC and the HC have been found to be early sites of atrophy (Braak et al., 1996; Rohrer et al., 2009). The SMPC may receive the densest efferent hippocampal projections in the frontal lobe (Barbas and Blatt, 1995). The OFC receives less dense projections (Munoz and Insausti, 2005) while the DLPFC is at a multiple synaptic distance from the HC. This pattern of connectivity is reflected by the volumetric data. The EC and the HC have most volume loss, followed by the SMPC and the OFC, while the DLPFC has no loss of gray matter volume in AD and SD. As discussed in the introduction, there are some differences between man and monkey in the findings concerning connectivity between the EC and the frontal lobe. If there are direct projections from the EC to the SMPC, then the atrophy of the EC could (as in HC) progress directly to the SMPC. Another possibility is that atrophy of the EC progresses to the HC as these regions are reciprocally connected (Pearson et al., 1985; De Lacoste and White, 1993), and from the HC to the SMPC.

In FTD, volumetric analyses revealed that the OFC and the HC was the most atrophic region compared to CTL. The SMPC has, however, almost as much volume loss. One previous study suggests that the OFC may be the first site of atrophy in FTD (Perry et al., 2006). Another study suggests that the so-called paralimbic network (of which the SMPC is part) becomes atrophic first (Seeley et al., 2008). We found a non-significant difference between the degree of atrophy in the OFC and the SMPC, which potentially could support the view that the SMPC is part of a network that becomes affected first in FTD.

In PNFA, left but not right SMPC was atrophic compared to controls. Volume loss in the left SMPC might reflect a progression from initial atrophy in the left anterior insula.

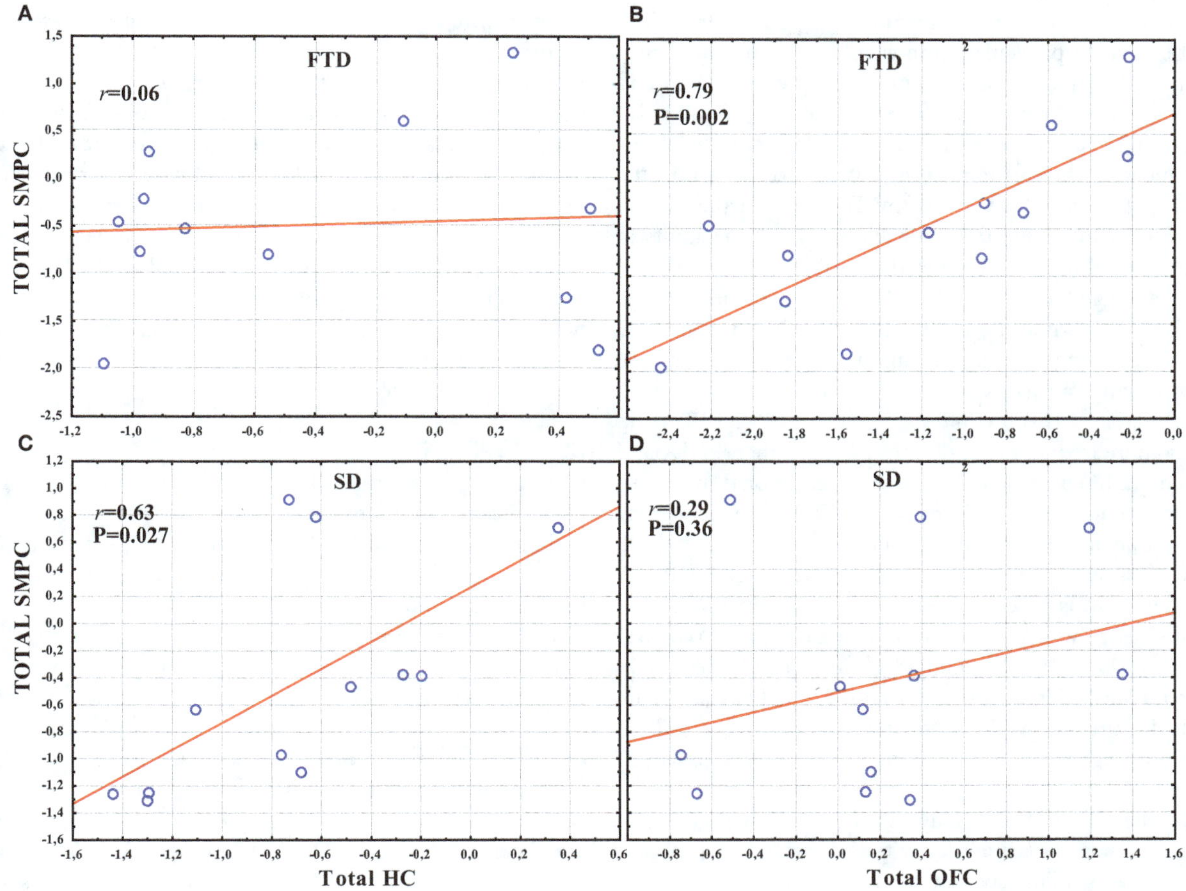

FIGURE 7 | The correlation between the total volume of SMPC, HC and OFC in SD and FTD. (A) The correlation between the total volume of SMPC and HC in FTD. **(B)** The correlation between total volume of SMPC and OFC in FTD. **(C)** The correlation between total volume SMPC and HC in SD. **(D)** The correlation between total volume of SMPC and OFC in SD.

We hypothesized that we also would find atrophy in the SMPC in AD, however only a tendency was found on the left side. The main reason for this was probably the relatively small number of cases included in this dementia group. One reason for not including more AD patients was that we wanted to have approximately the same statistical power for each dementia group. The FTLD group represents almost all patients with this rare diagnosis treated at the memory clinic at Huddinge hospital during a period of 10 years. It should also be noted that the general degree of atrophy was less severe in the AD cases than in the FTLD patients. Another strong indication that HC and SMPC atrophy may be connected is that the ratio of HC volume and SMPC volume is almost identical for AD and SD. Thus the ratio between left HC/Left SMPC is 0.85 in SD and 0.83 in AD, and the ratio between R HC/R SMPC is 0.90 for both SD and AD.

From the discussion above it could be suggested that the development of atrophy in the SMPC may be affected both by frontal as well as temporal atrophy. The results of the PCA may support this finding. As noted in the results section, the EC and the HC as well as the DLPFC and the OFC are closely plotted together in the PCA loading plot. The SMPC is plotted almost in the centre between the EC/HC and the DLPFC/OFC. This could indicate that atrophy of the SMPC may be almost as related to frontal as to temporal atrophy.

This assumption may also be supported by the findings of our correlation analyses. FTD was the dementia subtype that displayed most frontal atrophy (centered in the OFC). In this subtype the total volume of SMPC was correlated with the total volume of OFC, but not with the total volume of HC (**Figures 7A,B**). SD is the subtype that displayed most temporal atrophy centered on HC and EC. Here the total volume of the SMPC was correlated with the total volume of HC, but not with the total volume of OFC (**Figures 7C,D**). Thus the volume of SMPC is correlated to a region with severe frontal atrophy in FTD and to a region with severe temporal atrophy in SD.

Atrophy and laterality of atrophy of the SMPC may also be relevant for behavioral and neuropsychiatric alteration in the variants of dementia included in this investigation. The SMPC is the most posterior part of the ventromedial prefrontal cortex (VMPC). The VMPC has for example been associated with the ability to infer other persons' thoughts and feelings often referred to as "theory of mind" (Gregory et al., 2002), the construct of empathy (Shamay-Tsoory, 2010) and the broad concept of "emotional intelligence," which encompasses a number of social or emotional abilities that enable individuals to smoothly interact in or adapt to a social environment (Bar-On et al., 2003). The right VMPC may be particulary important for certain social abilities, such as theory of mind (Shamay-Tsoory et al., 2005) and empathy (Shamay-Tsoory et al., 2003). Rosen et al. (2005) also found that right SMPC atrophy was associated with disinhibition in dementia, while atrophy of the more anterior parts of the right VMPC was associated with apathy. They have further shown that the right SMPC is important for self-appraisal (the ability to assess one's own abilities) (Rosen et al., 2010).

Our data suggest that the left SMPC may become atrophic in PNFA and AD, while the right side is also involved in FTD and SD. Considering the relative importance of the right side for behavior symptoms (Rosen et al., 2005; Shamay-Tsoory et al., 2005; Rosen et al., 2010) it could be hypothesized that FTD and SD display more frequent alteration of behavior than PNFA and AD. Indeed this has been described in the international consensus criteria for diagnosing the subtypes of FTLD. FTD patients may display "decline in social interpersonal conduct" and SD patients may show "loss of sympathy and empathy" (Neary, 1999). PNFA on the other hand is described as having "early preservation of social skills." For the diagnosis of AD the American Psychiatric Association ([*DSM-IV-TR*], 2000) does not include deficits in social interaction skills, focusing on memory deficits as a core diagnostic feature, in addition to at least one of the following symptoms: aphasia, apraxia, agnosia or defecits in executive functioning.

The fact that the left SMPC may become more involved in AD may potentially also be explained by the connection hypothesis. Several previous studies have found that hippocampal atrophy at initial stages of AD may be more severe on the left side (Shi et al., 2009). Thus pathology may first progress to the left SMPC/VMPC and then as the disease develops to the right temporal lobe and right SMPC/VMPC. Thus the right VMPC may initially be relatively spared in AD and PNFA which may preserve these patients social interaction skills longer than in SD and FTD.

The most important limitation of this study is the lack of longitudinal data to provide direct evidence for how atrophy develops in the brain. The main point of this work is however that brain connectivity in cross-sectional data may provide important clues as to how and where atrophy may develop during the progression of neurodegenerative diseases.

Another limitation is that only structural 3D images were available in this study. Other MRI-techniques such as diffusion tensor imaging (Catani et al., 2012) or resting state MRI (Yi et al., 2012) could potentially reveal signs of pathology in brain networks before atrophy of regions that belong to these networks become detectable.

A third factor that needs to be considered in the interpretation of our results is the characteristics of our control group who sought consultation at the memory clinic because of subjective feelings of forgetfulness. While objective memory deficits were neither found at baseline investigation nor at follow up (with a minimal interval of 2 years), this does not exclude that these individuals may develop a neurodegenerative disorder later than two years after first examination. Differences between the investigated neurodegenerative disease and controls may thus potentially be even larger if subjects without subjective memory complaints had been used as controls.

CONCLUSIONS

Our finding supports the view that the SMPC, owing to its anatomical connections, may become a common site of frontal pathology in AD and FTLD. This supports the assumption that progression of atrophy in dementia may be predicted on the basis of the anatomical connectivity of the first atrophic region. Knowledge of the regional connectivity of the brain may thus help to predict in which regions atrophy will appear in the progression of neurodegenerative diseases.

AUTHOR CONTRIBUTIONS

Olof Lindberg and Eric Westman substantially contributed to conception and design, or acquisition of data, or analysis and interpretation of data. Olof Lindberg, Eric Westman, Sari Karlsson, Per Östberg, Andrew Simmons, Leif A. Svensson, Lars-Olof Wahlund to the drafting of the article or revising it critically for important intellectual content.

ACKNOWLEDGMENTS

This work was supported by Swedish Brain Power, the Strategic Research Programme in Neuroscience at Karolinska Institutet (StratNeuro), Stockholm Medical Image Laboratory and Education (SMILE), the Foundation of: "Gamla tjänarinnor" and the Foundation of: "Ragnhild och Einar Lundströms Minne." Andrew Simmons was supported by funds from NIHR Biomedical Research Centre for Mental Health at the South London and Maudsley NHS Foundation Trust and Institute of Psychiatry, Kings College London, the NIHR Biomedical Research Unit for Dementia at the South London and Maudsley NHS Foundation Trust and Institute of Psychiatry, Kings College London and Alzheimer's Research UK.

REFERENCES

Andersson, C. (2007). *Predictors of Cognitive Decline in Memory Clinic Patients.* Doctoral dissertation. Stockholm: Karolinska Institutet.

Barbas, H., and Blatt, G. J. (1995). Topographically specific hippocampal projections target functionally distinct prefrontal areas in the rhesus monkey. *Hippocampus* 5, 511–533.

Bar-On, R., Tranel, D., Denburg, N. L., and Bechara, A. (2003). Exploring the neurological substrate of emotional and social intelligence. *Brain* 126, 1790–1800.

Braak, H., Braak, E., Yilmazer, D., De Vos, R. A., Jansen, E. N., and Bohl, J. (1996). Pattern of brain destruction in Parkinson's and Alzheimer's diseases. *J. Neural Transm.* 103, 455–490.

Carmichael, S. T., and Price, J. L. (1996). Connectional networks within the orbital and medial prefrontal cortex of macaque monkeys. *J. Comp. Neurol.* 371, 179–207.

Catani, M., dell'Aqua, F., Bizzi, A., Forkel, S., Williams, S., Simmons, A., et al. (2012). Beyond cortical localization in clinico-anatomical correlation. *Cortex* 48, 1262–1287.

De Lacoste, M. C., and White, C. L. 3rd. (1993). The role of cortical connectivity in Alzheimer's disease pathogenesis: a review and model system. *Neurobiol. Aging* 14, 1–16.

Eriksson, L., Jonansson, E., Kettaneh-Wold, N., and Wold, S. (2006). *Multi- and Megavariate Data Analysis Part 1.* Umeå: Umetrics Academy.

Eritaia, J., Wood, S. J., Stuart, G. W., Bridle, N., Dudgeon, P., Maruff, P., et al. (2000). An optimized method for estimating intracranial volume from magnetic resonance images. *Magn. Reson. Med.* 44, 973–977.

Folstein, M. F., Folstein, S. E., and McHugh, P. R. (1975). "Mini-mental state." A practical method for grading the cognitive state of patients for the clinician. *J. Psychiatr. Res.* 12, 189–198.

Goldman-Rakic, P. S., Selemon, L. D., and Schwartz, M. L. (1984). Dual pathways connecting the dorsolateral prefrontal cortex with the hippocampal formation and parahippocampal cortex in the rhesus monkey. *Neuroscience* 12, 719–743.

Gregory, C., Lough, S., Stone, V., Erzinclioglu, S., Martin, L., Baron-Cohen, S., et al. (2002). Theory of mind in patients with frontal variant frontotemporal dementia and Alzheimer's disease: theoretical and practical implications. *Brain* 125, 752–764.

Insausti, R., and Amaral, D. G. (2008). Entorhinal cortex of the monkey: IV. Topographical and laminar organization of cortical afferents. *J. Comp. Neurol.* 509, 608–641.

Jones, E. G., and Powell, T. P. (1970). An anatomical study of converging sensory pathways within the cerebral cortex of the monkey. *Brain* 93, 793–820.

Kahn, I., Andrews-Hanna, J. R., Vincent, J. L., Snyder, A. Z., and Buckner, R. L. (2008). Distinct cortical anatomy linked to subregions of the medial temporal lobe revealed by intrinsic functional connectivity. *J. Neurophysiol.* 100, 129–139.

Laroche, S., Davis, S., and Jay, T. M. (2000). Plasticity at hippocampal to prefrontal cortex synapses: dual roles in working memory and consolidation. *Hippocampus* 10, 438–446.

Lindberg, O., Östberg, P., Zandbelt, B. B., Öberg, J., Zhang, Y., Andersen, C., et al. (2009). Cortical morphometric subclassification of frontotemporal lobar degeneration. *AJNR Am. J. Neuroradiol.* 30, 1233–1239.

Munoz, M., and Insausti, R. (2005). Cortical efferents of the entorhinal cortex and the adjacent parahippocampal region in the monkey (*Macaca fascicularis*). *Eur. J. Neurosci.* 22, 1368–1388.

Neary, D. (1999). Overview of frontotemporal dementias and the consensus applied. *Dement. Geriatr. Cogn. Disord.* 10(Suppl. 1), 6–9.

Neary, D., Snowden, J. S., Gustafson, L., Passant, U., Stuss, D., Black, S., et al. (1998). Frontotemporal lobar degeneration: a consensus on clinical diagnostic criteria. *Neurology* 51, 1546–1554.

Ongur, D., and Price, J. L. (2000). The organization of networks within the orbital and medial prefrontal cortex of rats, monkeys and humans. *Cereb. Cortex* 10, 206–219.

Pearson, R. C., Esiri, M. M., Hiorns, R. W., Wilcock, G. K., and Powell, T. P. (1985). Anatomical correlates of the distribution of the pathological changes in the neocortex in Alzheimer disease. *Proc. Natl. Acad. Sci. U.S.A.* 82, 4531–4534.

Perry, R. J., Graham, A., Williams, G., Rosen, H., Erzinclioglu, S., Weiner, M., et al. (2006). Patterns of frontal lobe atrophy in frontotemporal dementia: a volumetric MRI study. *Dement. Geriatr. Cogn. Disord.* 22, 278–287.

Raj, A., Kuceyeski, A., and Weiner, M. (2012). A network diffusion model of disease progression in dementia. *Neuron* 73, 1204–1215.

Rohrer, J. D., Warren, J. D., Modat, M., Ridgway, G. R., Douiri, A., Rossor, M. N., et al. (2009). Patterns of cortical thinning in the language variants of frontotemporal lobar degeneration. *Neurology* 72, 1562–1569.

Rosen, H. J., Alcantar, O., Rothlind, J., Sturm, V., Kramer, J. H., Weiner, M., et al. (2010). Neuroanatomical correlates of cognitive self-appraisal in neurodegenerative disease. *Neuroimage* 49, 3358–3364.

Rosen, H. J., Allison, S. C., Schauer, G. F., Gorno-Tempini, M. L., Weiner, M. W., and Miller, B. L. (2005). Neuroanatomical correlates of behavioural disorders in dementia. *Brain* 128, 2612–2625.

Schroeter, M. L., Raczka, K., Neumann, J., and Yves Von Cramon, D. (2007). Towards a nosology for frontotemporal lobar degenerations-a meta-analysis involving 267 subjects. *Neuroimage* 36, 497–510.

Seeley, W. W., Crawford, R., Rascovsky, K., Kramer, J. H., Weiner, M., Miller, B. L., et al. (2008). Frontal paralimbic network atrophy in very mild behavioral variant frontotemporal dementia. *Arch. Neurol.* 65, 249–255.

Seeley, W. W., Crawford, R. K., Zhou, J., Miller, B. L., and Greicius, M D. (2009). Neurodegenerative diseases target large-scale human brain networks. *Neuron* 62, 42–52.

Shamay-Tsoory, S. G. (2010). The neural bases for empathy. *Neuroscientist* 17, 18–24.

Shamay-Tsoory, S. G., Tomer, R., Berger, B. D., and Aharon-Peretz, J. (2003). Characterization of empathy deficits following prefrontal brain damage: the role of the right ventromedial prefrontal cortex. *J. Cogn. Neurosci.* 15, 324–337.

Shamay-Tsoory, S. G., Tomer, R., Berger, B. D., Goldsher, D., and Aharon-Peretz, J. (2005). Impaired "affective theory of mind" is associated with right ventromedial prefrontal damage. *Cogn. Behav. Neurol.* 18, 55–67.

Shi, F., Liu, B., Zhou, Y., Yu, C., and Jiang, T. (2009). Hippocampal volume and asymmetry in mild cognitive impairment and Alzheimer's disease: meta-analyses of MRI studies. *Hippocampus* 19, 1055–1064.

Simmons, A., Westman, E., Muehlboeck, S., Mecocci, P., Vellas, B., Tsolaki, M., et al. (2009). MRI measures of Alzheimer's disease and the AddNeuroMed study. *Ann. N.Y. Acad. Sci.* 1180, 47–55.

Simmons, A., Westman, E., Muehlboeck, S., Mecocci, P., Vellas, B., Tsolaki, M., et al. (2011). The AddNeuroMed framework for multi-centre MRI assessment of Alzheimer's disease: experience from the first 24 months. *Int. J. Geriatr. Psychiatry* 26, 75–82.

Suzuki, M., Zhou, S. Y., Takahashi, T., Hagino, H., Kawasaki, Y., Niu, L., et al. (2005). Differential contributions of prefrontal and temporolimbic pathology to mechanisms of psychosis. *Brain* 128, 2109–2122.

Thompson, P. M., Hayashi, K. M., Dutton, R. A., Chiang, M. C., Leow, A. D., Sowell, E. R., et al. (2007). Tracking Alzheimer's disease. *Ann. N.Y. Acad. Sci.* 1097, 183–214.

Whitwell, J. L., and Jack, C. R. Jr. (2005). Comparisons between Alzheimer disease, frontotemporal lobar degeneration, and normal aging with brain mapping. *Top. Magn. Reson. Imaging* 16, 409–425.

Woolsey, C. N. (1947). Patterns of sensory representation in the cerebral cortex. *Fed. Proc.* 6, 437–441.

Yi, L., Wang, J., Jia, L., Zhao, Z., Lu, J., Li, K., et al. (2012). Structural and functional changes in subcortical vascular mild cognitive impairment: a combined voxel-based morphometry and resting-state FMRI study. *PLoS ONE* 7:e44758. doi: 10.1371/journal.pone.0044758

20

Microglial activation – tuning and pruning adult neurogenesis

Christine T. Ekdahl*

Inflammation and Stem Cell Therapy Group, Division of Clinical Neurophysiology, Wallenberg Neuroscience Center, Department of Clinical Sciences, Lund University and Skåne University Hospital, Lund, Sweden

Edited by:
Roger A. Barker, University of Cambridge and Addenbrooke's Hospital, UK

Reviewed by:
Bradley D. Pearce, Emory University School of Medicine, USA
Gerd Kempermann, Center for Regenerative Therapies, Germany

****Correspondence:***
Christine T. Ekdahl, Inflammation and Stem Cell Therapy Group, Division of Clinical Neurophysiology, Wallenberg Neuroscience Center, Department of Clinical Sciences, Lund University and Skåne University Hospital, Sölvegatan 17, SE-221 84 Lund, Sweden.
e-mail: christine.ekdahl_clementson@med.lu.se

New neurons are continuously generated in two adult brain regions: the subgranular zone of the hippocampus and the subependyma by the lateral ventricles, referred to as the neurogenic niches. During their development from neural stem cells to mature functionally integrated neurons numerous choices are made, such as proliferation or quiescence, cell survival or death, migration or establishment, growth or retraction of processes, synaptic assembly or pruning, or tuning of synaptic transmission. The process is altered by physiological stimuli as well as several brain diseases. Microglia are located within the neurogenic niches and have become interesting candidates for modulating neurogenesis in both the healthy and injured brain. They become activated by foreign antigens or changes in the brain homeostasis and transform this innate immunity into an adaptive immune response by recruiting systemic immune cells. Most studies report an acute decrease in the survival of new neurons following this classically activated microglia reaction. The long-term effects are more complex. In neurodegenerative diseases, microglial activation is more heterogeneous and the transformation from a pro- to an anti-inflammatory cytokine profile and the deactivation of microglia is not well defined. The diversity is reflected by numerous reports describing both beneficial and detrimental effects on neurogenesis, primarily on the proliferation, survival, and cell fate. However, relatively few studies have investigated alterations at later stages of neurogenesis including the functional integration. Though likely, it is not established how a fine-tuned cross-talk between microglia and adult-born neurons would work and how it changes upon microglia activation. This review will therefore launch three hypotheses for how microglia might direct synaptic integration of newborn neurons, currently a fast expanding research field.

Keywords: microglia, neurogenesis, synaptic pruning, synaptic transmission, adult-born neurons, subgranular zone, subependyma, neurogenic niche

FROM NEURAL STEM CELLS TO MATURE FUNCTIONALLY INTEGRATED NEURONS – CHOICES TO BE MADE

Neurogenesis persists in two adult brain regions: the subependyma of the lateral ventricles and the subgranular zone (SGZ) of the hippocampal dentate gyrus. In the subependymal layer, multipotential, self-renewing stem cells are the source of newly generated neurons migrating through the rostral migratory stream and incorporating into the olfactory bulb as interneurons (Seaberg and van der Kooy, 2002). New olfactory neurons are thought to participate in both long-term olfactory memory and predator avoidance (Sakamoto et al., 2011; Sultan et al., 2011). From the SGZ, neuronal and glial progenitors with limited self-renewal capacity migrate into the granule cell layer and develop primarily into granule cells, a few becomes interneurons (Seaberg and van der Kooy, 2002; Liu et al., 2003; Livneh and Mizrahi, 2011). The integration of new hippocampal neurons in the adult brain occurs over several months, with an initial tonic GABA-induced depolarization converting into an intermittent GABA-mediated hyperpolarization when the cells are 3 weeks of age (Ge et al., 2008). Mature excitatory synapses are visualized at about 2 months, while spine density increases in the new neurons up to 6 months of age (Zhao et al., 2006). Simultaneously, axons grow and establish either functional glutamatergic synapses with hilar interneurons, mossy cells and CA3 pyramidal neurons (Toni and Sultan, 2011) or occasionally GABAergic inhibitory synapses with granule cells (Liu et al., 2003). The continuous integration of adult-born hippocampal neurons is important for synaptic transmission and bidirectional plasticity in the dentate gyrus. It is suggested to account for an efficient integration of novel incoming information and in memory formation (Dupret et al., 2008; Massa et al., 2011; Sahay et al., 2011), such as pattern separation and pattern integration (Deng et al., 2010).

The development of adult-born neurons may also be described as a continuous decision process. Neural stem cells/progenitors will have to decide whether to proliferate or stay in quiescence. Almost immediately after birth some cells undergo apoptotic death, while others survive. The surviving cells will choose a neuronal or glial fate and thereafter either stay and establish contacts within the SGZ or subependyma, the so-called neurogenic niches, or migrate into other brain regions. The integration of new neurons includes both growth and retraction of dendrites and axons, assembly and pruning of excitatory and inhibitory synapses, and homeostatic tuning of the established synaptic transmission. It becomes evident that in order for the new neurons to make the most appropriate choices for the overall function of the surrounding network, they are dependant on environment cues at most likely all developmental stages.

THE NEUROGENIC NICHE

It is conceivable that the local circuitries within the adult neurogenic niches have region-specific instructive roles in directing neuronal production and stem cell maintenance. It has even been suggested that they may shield ongoing neurogenesis from possible external inhibitory influences (Riquelme et al., 2008). The neurogenic niches consists of several cell types and structures, including: (1) astrocytes that envelop and contact all cell types and structures in the niche, secret diffusible signals, and form a gap junction-dependant syncytium by which they propagate signals and may regulate activation and differentiation of stem cells. They also act as neural stem cells/precursors (Riquelme et al., 2008), (2) ependymal cells by the subependymal layer that regulate the absorption of ions, transport factors from the cerebral spinal fluid into the parenchyma, and act as a source of secreted pro-neurogenic factors like transforming growth factor (TGF)-α and basic fibroblast growth factor (Riquelme et al., 2008), (3) blood vessels that undergo a parallel angiogenesis within the niche and often use common factors with neurogenesis such as vascular endothelial growth factor, nitric oxide and erythropoietin (Riquelme et al., 2008), (4) meningeal projections, extracellular matrix (ECM) proteins, basal lamina, and perivascular cells and fibroblasts, which propagate or modulate signals from the blood vessels and cerebral spinal fluid as well as from surrounding brain parenchyma. Emerging evidence underscore the important interaction between the adult-born neurons and ECM proteins. Cell adhesion to its environment includes matrix components, extracellular proteolytic enzymes, integrins, and non-receptor tyrosine kinases, which influence both gene expression and post-transcriptional signaling cascades (Riquelme et al., 2008; Wojcik-Stanaszek et al., 2011), (5) interneurons and other neighboring mature neurons already highly integrated into the hippocampal network, which may modulate neurogenesis by activity- and signaling-dependent mechanisms (Markwardt et al., 2011; Masiulis et al., 2011; Toni and Sultan, 2011), (6) oligodendrocytes, which are numerous in the subependyma but few in the SGZ. Their interaction with the neural progenitor cells is, however, so far unclear (Morrens et al., 2012), and (7) myeloid cells including microglia and dendritic cells, which are located in close proximity to the newborn neurons, where their activity correlates with the neurogenic response (Ekdahl et al., 2003; Monje et al., 2003; Bulloch et al., 2008; Sierra et al., 2010).

MICROGLIAL ACTIVATION IN THE ADULT BRAIN

A microglia activation profile is constantly modulated by either initiating factors, such as pathogen- or damage-associated molecular patterns (Schratt et al., 2006; Aronica and Crino, 2011) or alterations in electromagnetic fields (Richerson et al., 2005), or intracellular transducing signals, or feed-forward loops amplifying resolution mechanisms, or feed-back loops as counter-regulators (Glass et al., 2010). During brain pathology, the microglial activation is often divided into two phenotypic profiles: the classical M1 and the alternative M2 activation/deactivation state (Gordon, 2003; Mosser, 2003; Michelucci et al., 2009). The classical M1 activation occurs as microglia encounter a foreign antigen. The microglia act as a first line of defense and participate in transforming the innate immunity into an adaptive immune response by recruiting systemic immune cells. The alternative and deactivated M2 phenotype, sometimes called "neuroprotective," is important when switching from a classical inflammatory response to a reduction of pro-inflammatory mediators, an increased production and release of anti-inflammatory cytokines, neurotrophic factors, and a production of cytoactive factors involved in repair and restructuring of the damaged ECM in the brain. However, these M2 phenotypes may also participate in chronic "neuroinflammation" in the brain (Colton, 2009). The heterogeneity becomes evident in for instance neurodegenerative diseases, where the transformation from a pro- to an anti-inflammatory cytokine profile and the deactivation of microglia is neither temporally nor spatially clearly defined. There are even suggestions for a dysfunctional microglia phenotype following long-lasting activation (Graeber, 2010).

In the healthy brain, microglia and/or perivascular cells have been suggested to form an "immunological blood–brain barrier" between the brain parenchyma and the vascular system. However upon activation, by for instance sterile inflammation following trauma, ischemia, or chemical damage, these cells may instead recruit blood-born neutrophils and macrophages and increase the amount of tissue damage (Perry, 2010; Rock et al., 2010; Graeber et al., 2011; Yirmiya and Goshen, 2011). Simultaneously, microglia seems to be able to protect neurons from systemic immune cells by direct engulfment of invading neutrophils (Neumann et al., 2008). Other circulating immune cells are, though, required to maintain and sense brain homeostasis through the choroid plexi, brain meninges and the cerebral blood fluid. For instance, recruitment of systemic circulating T cells specific to CNS antigens can promote the termination of a local neurotoxic inflammatory response together with microglia of a "neuroprotective" phenotype (Ziv et al., 2006; Shechter et al., 2009; Ron-Harel et al., 2011). Taken together, these findings suggest that the activation state of the microglia is closely intermingled with the alertness of systemic immune cells and that there may be a bidirectional cross-talk.

HETEROGENEOUS MICROGLIAL POPULATION WITHIN THE NEUROGENIC NICHES – REGION SPECIFICITY?

Microglial density and phenotype differ between regions of the healthy brain, which could implicate functional differences and sensitivity to the surrounding environment (Lawson et al., 1990; Olah et al., 2011). Also within the subependymal layer of the healthy adult rat brain, microglia constitute a heterogeneous cell population. Here, the vast majority of ionized calcium-binding adapter molecule 1 (Iba1)-immunostained microglia exhibit a ramified or surveying phenotype, followed by an intermediate form with shorter processes, less arborization, and larger soma (Thored et al., 2009). Few express an amoeboid or round morphology (**Figures 1A–D**). There are partly overlapping subpopulations of microglia expressing the phagocytic marker ED1, associated with a pro-inflammatory profile, as well as major histocompatibility complex (MHC) class II, insulin-like growth factor-1 (IGF-1), and triggering receptor expressed on myeloid cells-2, the three latter molecules being associated with alternative or anti-inflammatory microglia activation (Thored et al., 2009; Heldmann et al., 2011). Local proliferation of microglia occurs, but parts of the subependymal microglia population are also blood-born (Thored et al., 2009; Heldmann et al., 2011). Interestingly, following middle cerebral artery occlusion microglia develop different morphological phenotypes within the subependymal layer compared to the striatal peri-infarct area. The differences are evident at least 16 weeks post-injury, including fewer amoeboid and round microglia morphologies and an up-regulation of IGF-1 in the subependyma. This may imply a region-specific, permissive microglia population within the neurogenic niche (Thored et al., 2009). However, a region-specific depletion of parts of the microglia population (expressing CD11b/Mac-1) within the subependyma, early after an ischemic lesion in rats, did not alter the number of newly formed neuroblasts in the striatum or their migratory distance (Heldmann et al., 2011).

In the hippocampal SGZ of rodents housed in an enriched environment, increased number of Iba1+ microglia co-labeled with the anti-inflammatory factors IGF-1 and MHC class II, were found together with T cell recruitment and an increase in neurogenesis. Moreover, T cell deficient mice showed reduced neurogenesis, which could not be overcome by an enriched environment (Ziv et al., 2006). The findings suggest a beneficial role of SGZ microglia possibly instructed by CNS-specific T cells. Conversely, following seizures and in neurodegenerative models of Alzheimer's disease, an increased number of Iba1+ microglia expressing ED1 is evident both acutely and chronically, and primarily cytotoxic for the new neurons (Ekdahl et al., 2003; Bonde et al., 2006; Biscaro, Lindvall, Tesco, Ekdahl, Nitsch, unpublished observation). Taken together, microglia are capable of developing both pro- and anti-inflammatory activation profiles in neurogenic brain areas. Moreover, it is possible that under certain circumstances the temporal and spatial constitution of the activation may even be region-specific.

Apart from the heterogeneous morphology and plethora of immune mediators, the motility and dynamic configurations of the microglia are also likely to reflect different functional aspects. Microglial processes are highly mobile and continuously rebuilt. Two-photon imaging of neocortex has shown active microglia continually surveying their microenvironment even in the normal brain (Nimmerjahn et al., 2005). The motility of microglia and perhaps region-specific features within the neurogenic niches remains to be characterized.

MICROGLIA – BENEFICIAL AND DETRIMENTAL FOR NEUROGENESIS

In the last two decades many studies have implicated a central role for brain parenchymal microglia as well as systemic immune cells during the generation of adult-born neurons (Ekdahl et al., 2009; Whitney et al., 2009; Molina-Holgado and Molina-Holgado, 2010; Russo et al., 2011a). Among the first evidence for a beneficial role of microglia or microglia-released mediators are *in vitro* studies on neural stem cell cultures, where the formation of neuroblasts could be rescued by co-culturing with microglia or conditioned media from microglia (Aarum et al., 2003; Walton et al., 2006). This "pro-neurogenic" function of microglia has since then been further supported by a number of studies from the group of M. Schwartz. Originally, they demonstrated that microglia activated with cytokines related to T cell helper cells promoted neurogenesis *in vitro* (Butovsky et al., 2006) and that CNS-specific T helper cells regulate hippocampal neurogenesis *in vivo* (Ziv et al., 2006). Interestingly, mice devoided of T cells or both T and B cells showed impairments in several hippocampal-dependent spatial learning tests (Kipnis et al., 2004; Brynskikh et al., 2008; Ron-Harel et al., 2008), which could be improved by replenishing T cells or boosting T cell activation by agonist of self-reactive T cells (Kipnis et al., 2004). Even more intriguingly was the finding that cognitive tasks increased the number of T cells located within the meningeal spaces, where T cell depletion induced a pro-inflammatory phenotype of the myeloid cells (Derecki et al., 2010). Since neurogenesis is thought to be important for hippocampal plasticity and memory formation, the health of the systemic immune system could possibly directly or through the interaction with innate non-neuronal cell types, like microglia, continuously shape neuroplasticity in both the healthy and damaged brain. Another recent reports on the beneficial role of microglia for newly formed neurons comes from Bachstetter et al. (2011) who have studied the neuronal transmembrane chemokine fractalkine (FKN)/CX3CL1 and its microglia-expressed receptor, CX3CR1-pathway. Disruption of this pathway in young adult rodents decreased both survival and proliferation of hippocampal neural progenitor cells (Bachstetter et al., 2011). Unchallenged microglia have also been demonstrated to engulf apoptotic bodies of neural progenitors in the SGZ. During normal neurogenesis in the healthy brain, a large proportion of neural progenitors undergo apoptosis within their first days in life. By rapidly removing cell debri, the scavenging properties of microglia could have an important regulator role at the early stages of neurogenesis (Sierra et al., 2010). However, it is not fully clear whether the phagocytosis is beneficial for the surrounding newborn neurons by reducing pro-inflammatory mediators, or may be detrimental by further inducing apoptotic neuronal death (Magnus et al., 2001; Neher et al., 2011).

The first studies suggesting an acute detrimental role of activated microglia for neurogenesis were performed in rats following intraparenchymal lipopolysaccharide (LPS) injections (Ekdahl et al., 2003; Monje et al., 2003). LPS-induced microglial activation led to a dramatic decrease in the survival of newly formed hippocampal neurons. The pivotal role of microglial activation was further substantiated following both epileptic seizures and irradiation, where hippocampal neurogenesis could be rescued by inhibiting microglia activation through either administration of the anti-inflammatory agent minocycline or non-steroidal anti-inflammatory drugs (Ekdahl et al., 2003; Monje et al., 2003). Pro-inflammatory cytokines like interleukin (IL)-1, IL-6, and tumor necrosis factor (TNF), released acutely by activated microglia, have been suggested as important mediators between the microglia and the new neurons (Monje et al., 2003;

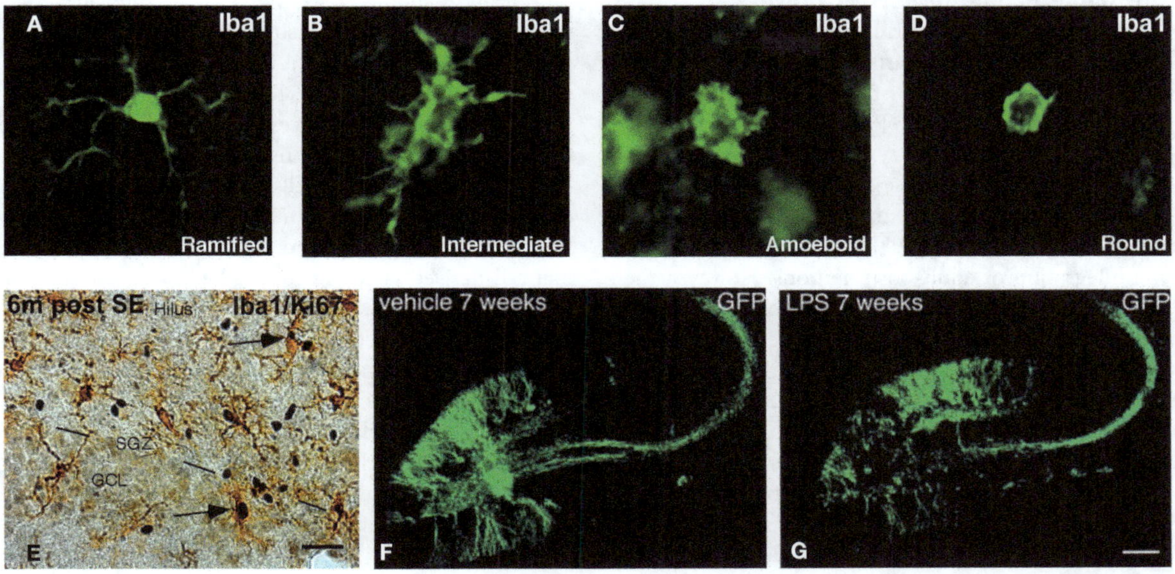

FIGURE 1 | Microglia and newly generated neurons in the neurogenic niche of the adult rat brain. (A–D) Photomicrographs showing four distinct phenotypes of Iba1+ microglia. **(E)** Image of Iba1+ microglia within the subgranular zone (SGZ) of the hippocampal dentate gyrus 6 months after electrically induced status epilepticus. Arrows mark microglia that express Ki-67, which implicate an ongoing proliferation. **(F,G)** Retroviral-GFP vector labeling of 7-week-old adult-born neurons in the hippocampus following vehicle or LPS-induced microglial activation. The cell bodies of the newly generated neurons are located in the SGZ and granule cell layer of the dentate gyrus. Their dendritic trees are visible throughout the molecular layer and their axons extend into the dentate hilus and the CA3 region. Modified from Bonde et al. (2006), Jakubs et al. (2008), and Thored et al. (2009).

Iosif et al., 2006; Yirmiya and Goshen, 2011). Also prostaglandins released by the microglia may negatively regulate different steps of neurogenesis. In support, mice lacking cyclooxygenase-1 lack both the acute LPS-induced decrease in proliferation, survival, and differentiation of new hippocampal neurons (Russo et al., 2011b).

When the initiating agent for microglia activation is no longer present and the acute pro-inflammatory phase is over, an anti-inflammatory cytokine profile may develop, as shown after LPS-stimulation (Cacci et al., 2008). This profile may be beneficial for the newly formed neurons, since for instance administration of anti-inflammatory cytokines like TGF-β, has provided beneficial effects on neurogenesis in the subependyma (Mathieu et al., 2010a). However, if the microglia are continuously activated, they may partly sustain their release of oxidative stressors, which could be neurotoxic (Glass et al., 2010; Nathan and Ding, 2010; Polazzi and Monti, 2010). The result may be disease-specific interaction between microglia and the newborn neurons (Graeber et al., 2011). Microglia are, though, important for terminating immune/immune-like responses, by, i.e., recruitment of systemic immune cells (Frank-Cannon et al., 2009; Shechter et al., 2009; Polazzi and Monti, 2010; Rivest, 2011; Ron-Harel et al., 2011), and may thereby protect new neurons and even recruit neural progenitors for repair (Czeh et al., 2010; Mathieu et al., 2010b). The correlation between seizure-induced microglial activation and neurogenesis is a typical example of this complexity. A severe seizure insult induces a strong transient increase in hippocampal neurogenesis (Parent et al., 1997), followed by a chronic decrease below control levels (Hattiangady and Shetty, 2010). In the acute phase, microglia activation is prominent within the SGZ and has been suggested to compromise the early survival of the new neurons (Ekdahl et al., 2003). Six months later, the microglial activation is decreased but still present (Bonde et al., 2006; **Figure 1E**). This may imply also a long-term negative correlation between the production of new neurons and the chronically activated microglia. However, the newly formed neurons generated directly after the seizure insult, that survived the acute post-seizure environment, are still present 6 months later. They have even been estimated to comprise about 10% of the total dentate granule cell layer. These adult-born neurons are surrounded by the chronically activated microglia, which may instead favor a possible supportive role of the chronically activated microglia (Bonde et al., 2006). Because the initial seizure insult is followed by additional spontaneous seizures throughout the life of the animals, there is a possibility for recurrent triggering of the microglial activation. Whether subpopulations of microglia with either detrimental or beneficial effect on the surrounding newborn neurons co-exist within the neurogenic niche is not known and may be directly depending on the number of spontaneous seizures. The initial severity of the seizure insult is directly correlated to both the number of activated microglia as well as the neurogenic response (Mohapel et al., 2004). In addition, parts of the newly generated neurons migrate aberrantly out into the dentate hilus, which may perhaps be due to the well-known seizure-induced death of hilar interneurons and the prominent population of activated hilar microglia. Collectively, these findings support a primarily beneficial interaction between microglia and new neurons in the intact brain. However, the cross-talk is complex and probably double-edged in pathological conditions, especially following long-term microglial activation.

THE ROLE OF MICROGLIA DURING FUNCTIONAL INTEGRATION OF ADULT-BORN NEURONS – AN EQUALIZER AMPLIFYING AND FILTERING SYNAPTIC SIGNALING?

Until now, most studies on the cross-talk between microglia and adult-born neurons have focused on the effect on the early stages of neurogenesis, such as proliferation, survival, and neuronal fate. The role of microglia at later stages of neurogenesis, i.e., during synaptic assembly, stability, and transmission is less characterized. Today, there is no direct evidence that microglia could regulate synaptic integration of adult-born neurons. However, there is some evidence and several suggestions that microglia regulate synaptic pruning and transmission in mature neurons, currently a fast expanding research area. Three main working hypotheses can be put forward for how microglia may also regulate synaptic integration of adult-born neurons: (1) involvement of microglia in synaptogenesis and pruning, (2) modulation of perisynaptic structures, and (3) spine structure and synaptic transmission.

MICROGLIA MAY BE INVOLVED IN SYNAPTOGENESIS AND PRUNING OF SYNAPSES ON ADULT-BORN NEURONS

This hypothesis is based on recent studies describing how microglia may be involved in synaptic elimination/stripping/pruning by phagocytic engulfment of synapses on mature neurons in the healthy brain (Paolicelli et al., 2011; Tremblay and Majewska, 2011). By electron microscopy and two-photon *in vivo* imaging of the primary visual cortex of juvenile mice during visual manipulations, subtle changes in the behavior of quiescent microglia were observed. This included geometric regulation of perisynaptic extracellular spaces, contact with subsets of structurally dynamic and transient dendritic spines, and phagocytic engulfment of intact synapses (Tremblay et al., 2010; Tremblay and Majewska, 2011). The findings were further substantiated by Paolicelli et al. (2011) proposing synaptic pruning by microglia during postnatal development in mice. Mice lacking microglia expressing the chemokine FKN receptor CX3CR1, exhibited a transient reduction in microglia number correlated with a delayed synaptic pruning. This resulted in an excess of dendritic spines and immature electrophysiological properties of CA1 pyramidal neurons at P13 and P16 in the CX3CR1 knockout mice (Paolicelli et al., 2011). The occurrence of synaptic pruning has also been correlated with the duration of the microglia-synaptic contacts. *In vivo* imaging studies of the ischemic brain, suggest more persistent contacts between microglia processes and dendritic spines and axon terminals, compared to the transient 4–5 min of normal contacts observed in the healthy brain. Following longer interactions in the pathological environment, these contacted synapses often disappeared (Wake et al., 2009; Kettenmann et al., 2011). In several brain pathologies, such as following axonal lesions or immune mediated-cortical lesions, pruning of synapses from the perikaryon and dendrites is evident. The suggested consequence of synaptic pruning during these conditions has been neuroprotection (Cullheim and Thams, 2007; Trapp et al., 2007; Kettenmann et al., 2011).

An interesting possible signaling pathway between the microglia and the synaptic structures on the new neurons is the complement cascade. Since the complements are involved in opsonization and cytolysis, they have become attractive possible candidates for executing synaptic pruning in both the healthy and injured brain. Mice deficient in the initiating protein in the classical complement cascade, C1q, exhibit large sustained defects in synapse elimination, excessive excitatory synapses and axon terminals in mature neurons (Stevens et al., 2007; Chu et al., 2010). Neural progenitor cells and immature neurons express the receptors for complement fragments C3a and C5a. C3a stimulates neuronal migration and differentiation, by modulating stromal cell-derived factor-1a-induced extracellular-signal-regulated kinases phosphorylation. Mice lacking C3 signaling (including C3a and C5a) have reduced basal neurogenesis as well as decreased survival of ischemia-generated new striatal neurons (Rahpeymai et al., 2006; Shinjyo et al., 2009). Also complement receptor 2 (Cr2) is expressed in adult neural progenitor cells from the dentate gyrus, though, Cr2 knockout mice exhibit increased hippocampal neurogenesis (Moriyama et al., 2011). Together these results suggest a fundamental role of the complements for neurogenesis, including proper synaptic pruning and integration of newly formed neurons. However, in a mouse model of glaucoma, unwanted synapses may be tagged by complement for elimination, which suggests that complement-mediated synaptic pruning can become aberrantly reactivated in neurodegenerative disease (Stevens et al., 2007). In human temporal lobe epilepsy with hippocampal sclerosis, the complements factors are expressed in both astrocytes, mature neurons and microglia, but particularly in microglia (Aronica et al., 2007). Whether it is really the microglia that eliminate the complement-tagged neuronal synaptic terminals on either mature or newly formed neurons, in the intact and the damaged brain, is not yet shown (Perry and O'Connor, 2008; Tremblay and Majewska, 2011). Another suggested pathway between microglia and newborn neurons is the MHC class I and its related receptors, which is expressed in both microglia and in neurospheres and the subependymal layer (Popa et al., 2011). MHC class I molecules have been shown to influence both the strength and pattern of synaptic elimination (Cullheim and Thams, 2007; Kettenmann et al., 2011).

MICROGLIA MAY MODULATE THE PERISYNAPTIC STRUCTURE OF SYNAPSES ON ADULT-BORN NEURONS

Microglia might affect synaptic transmission though proteolytic modification of the perisynaptic environment (Tremblay and Majewska, 2011). This would include inactivation, degradation, and/or activation of the ECM, leading to compartmentalization of proteases, ions, cytokines, and neurotransmitters within individual synapses. One interesting possible pathway is through the matrix metalloproteases (MMP), such as MMP-9, shown already to be involved in the migration and differentiation of adult neural progenitor cells in the subependymal layer (Barkho et al., 2008) Another candidate is via a disintegrin and metalloproteases (ADAMs), implicated in dopamine-induced release of epidermal growth factor from stem cells in the subventricular zone (O'Keeffe and Barker, 2011). Proteolytic remodeling of the ECM by MMPs may convert trophic factors to their biologically active forms (i.e., vascular endothelial growth factor and TGF-β) and thereby influence synaptic integration. ECM ligands, such as integrin receptors, provide outside-in signals for cells to sense their microenvironment. This leads to modulation of receptor tyrosine kinases, which closely cooperate with growth factors (Wojcik-Stanaszek et al., 2011).

MICROGLIA MAY MODULATE THE STRUCTURE OF DENDRITIC SPINES AND SYNAPTIC TRANSMISSION IN ADULT-BORN NEURONS

Another mechanism by which microglia may regulate neuronal activity is through remodeling of dendritic spine morphology, including size, shape, and motility (Tremblay and Majewska, 2011), as well as synaptic adhesion and transmission. The dendritic structure is closely associated with its synaptic activity and activity-driven changes in synaptic efficacy may modulate spine morphology due to alterations in the underlying actin cytoskeleton (Fortin et al., 2011).

There are also several immune mediators involved in synaptic remodeling of mature neurons. For instance, in cultured hippocampal neurons, TNF receptor-associated protein 1 knockdown modulated the morphology of dendritic spines (Kubota et al., 2009). TNF deficient mice displayed also smaller dendritic trees in the hippocampus (McCoy and Tansey, 2008). Furthermore, mice lacking IL-1β receptor had reduced dendritic spine size (Goshen et al., 2009) and IL-6 over-expression in cerebellar granule cells caused impairments in granule cell adhesion, migration, and increased formation of excitatory synapses on granule cells (Wei et al., 2011). MicroRNAs, which may control the expression of hundreds of genes (Schratt et al., 2006), were recently suggested to be interacting with immune mediators. Knocking down miR-132 in PC12 cells resulted in an increased expression of especially pro-inflammatory molecules. Interestingly, retroviral knockdown of miR-132 impaired the integration of newborn neurons in the adult hippocampus. (Luikart et al., 2011). However, whether or not the structural synaptic changes in either mature or newly formed neurons directly depend on cytokines released by the microglia is not clear.

When synapses have been established, microglia might fine-tune the synaptic strength to ensure proper synaptic transmission and plasticity (Beique et al., 2011). Mice lacking CX3CR1 show alterations in both hippocampal long-term potentiation (LTP) and long-term depression (LTD), supporting a microglia-driven neuronal plasticity during development and in mature neurons (Bachstetter et al., 2011; Maggi et al., 2011; Paolicelli et al., 2011). In addition, LPS-activated microglia in acute mice hippocampal slices enhance the frequencies of excitatory postsynaptic currents in mature neurons. This effect was abolished by applying purinergic antagonists, especially against the P2Y1 receptor, which is only expressed on interneurons and astrocytes in the hippocampus. By producing ATP, microglia may thereby act on astrocytes through purinergic signaling, which could amplify the ATP production, release glutamate, and act on mature neuronal glutamatergic receptors (Tremblay et al., 2011). Moreover, prolonged changes in electrical activity may lead to uniform adjustments in the strength of all synapses, called homeostatic synaptic scaling/tuning (Stellwagen and Malenka, 2006). Synaptic scaling in response to prolonged blockade of neuronal activity *in vitro* can be mediated by TNF-α from glial cells (astrocytes and/or microglia; Stellwagen and Malenka, 2006). Also, TNF-α may increase the expression of AMPA receptors on synapses (Pickering et al., 2005), resulting in excitatory synaptic scaling, and decrease GABAA receptor expression (McCoy and Tansey, 2008). When adult-born hippocampal neurons integrate into a pathological environment, hosting either seizure- (Jakubs et al., 2006) or LPS-induced microglial activation (Jakubs et al., 2008; **Figures 1F,G**), they possess an increased inhibitory synaptic drive onto their afferent synapses, compared to new neurons formed in healthy conditions. Conversely, in a less severe seizure-environment, without a prominent microglial activation, this increase is lacking (Wood et al., 2011). How or whether it is really the microglial activation that account for these changes observed in the synaptic transmission of newborn neurons needs further investigations, though, it is a tempting speculation.

Microglia may also regulate synaptic transmission in newly formed neurons by directly targeting synaptic adhesion molecules. Seizure-induced microglial activation is associated with structural changes in dendrite spine formation (Murphy et al., 2011), as well as altered expression of synaptic adhesion molecules and scaffolding proteins on newly formed hippocampal neurons (Jackson, Chugh, Nilsson, Karlström, Lindvall, Ekdahl, unpublished observation). In support, several adhesion molecules have been shown to modulate synaptic integration of newborn neurons. One of the most studied adhesion molecules is the polysialated neural cell adhesion molecule (NCAM), which is specifically expressed on new neurons (Gascon et al., 2010). Another interesting pathway is the N-cadherin/beta-catenin/neurogenin signaling cascade, which has been shown to modulate adhesion, neuronal differentiation, and neurite outgrowth in neurospheres (Chen et al., 2006). Also the adhesion molecules neuroligin 3 and 4 are involved in presynaptic differentiation and synapse formation in human induced pluripotent stem cell-derived neurons (Kim et al., 2011). The adhesion molecules may be regulated by immune mediators released by microglia, such as TNF. A recent report described reduced expression of the N-cadherin by TNF receptor-associated protein 1 knockdown in cultured hippocampal neurons (Kubota et al., 2009).

CONCLUDING REMARKS

Various brain pathologies and physiological stimulations modify neurogenesis (Zhao et al., 2008). Two of the strongest modulators include epileptic seizures involving the SGZ of the dentate gyrus (Bengzon et al., 1997; Parent et al., 1997; Jakubs et al., 2006) and ischemia close to the subependymal layer (Arvidsson et al., 2002). Understanding the signaling pathways between the new neurons and the environment within the neurogenic niches in pathological conditions, may yield new targets for therapeutic interventions. Several drugs are currently studied in order to increase the neuroprotective functions of microglia or to shift the microglial phenotype toward neuroprotection (Polazzi and Monti, 2010). However, microglia in particular may exhibit strong compensatory mechanisms upon external modulation and quickly rearrange their proliferation capacity and phenotypic characteristics. The heterogeneity of the microglial activation makes predictions of the outcome from immune-modulating therapies very difficult (Rivest, 2011). Future studies on the impact of more subtle tunings of the cross-talk between microglia and the newly formed neurons may perhaps ease these interventions.

REFERENCES

Aarum, J., Sandberg, K., Haeberlein, S. L., and Persson, M. A. (2003). Migration and differentiation of neural precursor cells can be directed by microglia. *Proc. Natl. Acad. Sci. U.S.A.* 100, 15983–15988.

Aronica, E., Boer, K., van Vliet, E. A., Redeker, S., Baayen, J. C., Spliet, W. G., van Rijen, P. C., Troost, D., da Silva, F. H., Wadman, W. J., and Gorter, J. A. (2007). Complement activation in experimental and human temporal lobe epilepsy. *Neurobiol. Dis.* 26, 497–511.

Aronica, E., and Crino, P. B. (2011). Inflammation in epilepsy: clinical observations. *Epilepsia* 52(Suppl. 3), 26–32.

Arvidsson, A., Collin, T., Kirik, D., Kokaia, Z., and Lindvall, O. (2002). Neuronal replacement from endogenous precursors in the adult brain after stroke. *Nat. Med.* 8, 963–970.

Bachstetter, A. D., Morganti, J. M., Jernberg, J., Schlunk, A., Mitchell, S. H., Brewster, K. W., Hudson, C. E., Cole, M. J., Harrison, J. K., Bickford, P. C., and Gemma, C. (2011). Fractalkine and CX 3 CR1 regulate hippocampal neurogenesis in adult and aged rats. *Neurobiol. Aging* 32, 2030–2044.

Barkho, B. Z., Munoz, A. E., Li, X., Li, L., Cunningham, L. A., and Zhao, X. (2008). Endogenous matrix metalloproteinase (MMP)-3 and MMP-9 promote the differentiation and migration of adult neural progenitor cells in response to chemokines. *Stem Cells* 26, 3139–3149.

Beique, J. C., Na, Y., Kuhl, D., Worley, P. F., and Huganir, R. L. (2011). Arc-dependent synapse-specific homeostatic plasticity. *Proc. Natl. Acad. Sci. U.S.A.* 108, 816–821.

Bengzon, J., Kokaia, Z., Elmer, E., Nanobashvili, A., Kokaia, M., and Lindvall, O. (1997). Apoptosis and proliferation of dentate gyrus neurons after single and intermittent limbic seizures. *Proc. Natl. Acad. Sci. U.S.A.* 94, 10432–10437.

Bonde, S., Ekdahl, C. T., and Lindvall, O. (2006). Long-term neuronal replacement in adult rat hippocampus after status epilepticus despite chronic inflammation. *Eur. J. Neurosci.* 23, 965–974.

Brynskikh, A., Warren, T., Zhu, J., and Kipnis, J. (2008). Adaptive immunity affects learning behavior in mice. *Brain Behav. Immun.* 22, 861–869.

Bulloch, K., Miller, M. M., Gal-Toth, J., Milner, T. A., Gottfried-Blackmore, A., Waters, E. M., Kaunzner, U. W., Liu, K., Lindquist, R., Nussenzweig, M. C., Steinman, R. M., and McEwen, B. S. (2008). CD11c/EYFP transgene illuminates a discrete network of dendritic cells within the embryonic, neonatal, adult, and injured mouse brain. *J. Comp. Neurol.* 508, 687–710.

Butovsky, O., Ziv, Y., Schwartz, A., Landa, G., Talpalar, A. E., Pluchino, S., Martino, G., and Schwartz, M. (2006). Microglia activated by IL-4 or IFN-gamma differentially induce neurogenesis and oligodendrogenesis from adult stem/progenitor cells. *Mol. Cell. Neurosci.* 31, 149–160.

Cacci, E., Ajmone-Cat, M. A., Anelli, T., Biagioni, S., and Minghetti, L. (2008). In vitro neuronal and glial differentiation from embryonic or adult neural precursor cells are differently affected by chronic or acute activation of microglia. *Glia* 56, 412–425.

Chen, J., Zacharek, A., Li, Y., Li, A., Wang, L., Katakowski, M., Roberts, C., Lu, M., and Chopp, M. (2006). N-cadherin mediates nitric oxide-induced neurogenesis in young and retired breeder neurospheres. *Neuroscience* 140, 377–388.

Chu, Y., Jin, X., Parada, I., Pesic, A., Stevens, B., Barres, B., and Prince, D. A. (2010). Enhanced synaptic connectivity and epilepsy in C1q knockout mice. *Proc. Natl. Acad. Sci. U.S.A.* 107, 7975–7980.

Colton, C. A. (2009). Heterogeneity of microglial activation in the innate immune response in the brain. *J. Neuroimmune Pharmacol.* 4, 399–418.

Cullheim, S., and Thams, S. (2007). The microglial networks of the brain and their role in neuronal network plasticity after lesion. *Brain Res. Rev.* 55, 89–96.

Czeh, M., Gressens, P., and Kaindl, A. M. (2010). The yin and yang of microglia. *Dev. Neurosci.* 33, 199–209.

Deng, W., Aimone, J. B., and Gage, F. H. (2010). New neurons and new memories: how does adult hippocampal neurogenesis affect learning and memory? *Nat. Rev. Neurosci.* 11, 339–350.

Derecki, N. C., Cardani, A. N., Hui Yang, C., Quinnies, K. M., Crihfield, A., Lynch, K. L., and Kipnis, J. (2010). Regulation of learning and memory by meningeal immunity: a key role for IL-4. *J. Exp. Med.* 207, 1067–1080.

Dupret, D., Revest, J. M., Koehl, M., Ichas, F., De Giorgi, F., Costet, P., Abrous, D. N., and Piazza, P. V. (2008). Spatial relational memory requires hippocampal adult neurogenesis. *PLoS ONE* 3, e1959. doi:10.1371/journal.pone.0001959

Ekdahl, C. T., Claasen, J. H., Bonde, S., Kokaia, Z., and Lindvall, O. (2003). Inflammation is detrimental for neurogenesis in adult brain. *Proc. Natl. Acad. Sci. U.S.A.* 100, 13632–13637.

Ekdahl, C. T., Kokaia, Z., and Lindvall, O. (2009). Brain inflammation and adult neurogenesis: the dual role of microglia. *Neuroscience* 158, 1021–1029.

Fortin, D. A., Srivastava, T., and Soderling, T. R. (2011). Structural modulation of dendritic spines during synaptic plasticity. *Neuroscientist.* doi:10.1177/1073858411407206 [Epub ahead of print].

Frank-Cannon, T. C., Alto, L. T., McAlpine, F. E., and Tansey, M. G. (2009). Does neuroinflammation fan the flame in neurodegenerative diseases? *Mol. Neurodegener.* 4, 47.

Gascon, E., Vutskits, L., and Kiss, J. Z. (2010). The role of PSA-NCAM in adult neurogenesis. *Adv. Exp. Med. Biol.* 663, 127–136.

Ge, S., Sailor, K. A., Ming, G. L., and Song, H. (2008). Synaptic integration and plasticity of new neurons in the adult hippocampus. *J. Physiol.* 586, 3759–3765.

Glass, C. K., Saijo, K., Winner, B., Marchetto, M. C., and Gage, F. H. (2010). Mechanisms underlying inflammation in neurodegeneration. *Cell* 140, 918–934.

Gordon, S. (2003). Alternative activation of macrophages. *Nat. Rev. Immunol.* 3, 23–35.

Goshen, I., Avital, A., Kreisel, T., Licht, T., Segal, M., and Yirmiya, R. (2009). Environmental enrichment restores memory functioning in mice with impaired IL-1 signaling via reinstatement of long-term potentiation and spine size enlargement. *J. Neurosci.* 29, 3395–3403.

Graeber, M. B. (2010). Changing face of microglia. *Science* 330, 783–788.

Graeber, M. B., Li, W., and Rodriguez, M. L. (2011). Role of microglia in CNS inflammation. *FEBS Lett.* 585, 3798–3805.

Hattiangady, B., and Shetty, A. K. (2010). Decreased neuronal differentiation of newly generated cells underlies reduced hippocampal neurogenesis in chronic temporal lobe epilepsy. *Hippocampus* 20, 97–112.

Heldmann, U., Mine, Y., Kokaia, Z., Ekdahl, C. T., and Lindvall, O. (2011). Selective depletion of Mac-1-expressing microglia in rat subventricular zone does not alter neurogenic response early after stroke. *Exp. Neurol.* 229, 391–398.

Iosif, R. E., Ekdahl, C. T., Ahlenius, H., Pronk, C. J., Bonde, S., Kokaia, Z., Jacobsen, S. E., and Lindvall, O. (2006). Tumor necrosis factor receptor 1 is a negative regulator of progenitor proliferation in adult hippocampal neurogenesis. *J. Neurosci.* 26, 9703–9712.

Jakubs, K., Bonde, S., Iosif, R. E., Ekdahl, C. T., Kokaia, Z., Kokaia, M., and Lindvall, O. (2008). Inflammation regulates functional integration of neurons born in adult brain. *J. Neurosci.* 28, 12477–12488.

Jakubs, K., Nanobashvili, A., Bonde, S., Ekdahl, C. T., Kokaia, Z., Kokaia, M., and Lindvall, O. (2006). Environment matters: synaptic properties of neurons born in the epileptic adult brain develop to reduce excitability. *Neuron* 52, 1047–1059.

Kettenmann, H., Hanisch, U. K., Noda, M., and Verkhratsky, A. (2011). Physiology of microglia. *Physiol. Rev.* 91, 461–553.

Kim, J. E., O'Sullivan, M. L., Sanchez, C. A., Hwang, M., Israel, M. A., Brennand, K., Deerinck, T. J., Goldstein, L. S., Gage, F. H., Ellisman, M. H., and Ghosh, A. (2011). Investigating synapse formation and function using human pluripotent stem cell-derived neurons. *Proc. Natl. Acad. Sci. U.S.A.* 108, 3005–3010.

Kipnis, J., Cohen, H., Cardon, M., Ziv, Y., and Schwartz, M. (2004). T cell deficiency leads to cognitive dysfunction: implications for therapeutic vaccination for schizophrenia and other psychiatric conditions. *Proc. Natl. Acad. Sci. U.S.A.* 101, 8180–8185.

Kubota, K., Inoue, K., Hashimoto, R., Kumamoto, N., Kosuga, A., Tatsumi, M., Kamijima, K., Kunugi, H., Iwata, N., Ozaki, N., Takeda, M., and Tohyama, M. (2009). Tumor necrosis factor receptor-associated protein 1 regulates cell adhesion and synaptic morphology via modulation of N-cadherin expression. *J. Neurochem.* 110, 496–508.

Lawson, L. J., Perry, V. H., Dri, P., and Gordon, S. (1990). Heterogeneity in the distribution and morphology of microglia in the normal adult mouse brain. *Neuroscience* 39, 151–170.

Liu, S., Wang, J., Zhu, D., Fu, Y., Lukowiak, K., and Lu, Y. M. (2003). Generation of functional inhibitory neurons in the adult rat hippocampus. *J. Neurosci.* 23, 732–736.

Livneh, Y., and Mizrahi, A. (2011). Long-term changes in the morphology and synaptic distributions of adult-born neurons. *J. Comp. Neurol.* 519, 2212–2224.

Luikart, B. W., Bensen, A. L., Washburn, E. K., Perederiy, J. V., Su, K. G., Li, Y., Kernie, S. G., Parada, L. F., and Westbrook, G. L. (2011). miR-132 mediates the integration of newborn neurons into the adult dentate gyrus. *PLoS ONE* 6, e19077. doi:10.1371/journal.pone.0019077

Maggi, L., Scianni, M., Branchi, I., D'Andrea, I., Lauro, C., and Limatola, C. (2011). CX3CR1 deficiency alters hippocampal-dependent plasticity phenomena blunting the effects of enriched environment. *Front. Cell. Neurosci.* 5:22. doi:10.3389/fncel.2011.00022

Magnus, T., Chan, A., Grauer, O., Toyka, K. V., and Gold, R. (2001). Microglial phagocytosis of apoptotic inflammatory T cells leads to down-regulation of microglial immune activation. *J. Immunol.* 167, 5004–5010.

Markwardt, S. J., Dieni, C. V., Wadiche, J. I., and Overstreet-Wadiche, L. (2011). Ivy/neurogliaform interneurons coordinate activity in the neurogenic niche. *Nat. Neurosci.* 14, 1407–1409.

Masiulis, I., Yun, S., and Eisch, A. J. (2011). The interesting interplay between interneurons and adult hippocampal neurogenesis. *Mol. Neurobiol.* 44, 287–302.

Massa, F., Koehl, M., Wiesner, T., Grosjean, N., Revest, J. M., Piazza, P. V., Abrous, D. N., and Oliet, S. H. (2011). Conditional reduction of adult neurogenesis impairs bidirectional hippocampal synaptic plasticity. *Proc. Natl. Acad. Sci. U.S.A.* 108, 6644–6649.

Mathieu, P., Piantanida, A. P., and Pitossi, F. (2010a). Chronic expression of transforming growth factor-beta enhances adult neurogenesis. *Neuroimmunomodulation* 17, 200–201.

Mathieu, P., Battista, D., Depino, A., Roca, V., Graciarena, M., and Pitossi, F. (2010b). The more you have, the less you get: the functional role of inflammation on neuronal differentiation of endogenous and transplanted neural stem cells in the adult brain. *J. Neurochem.* 112, 1368–1385.

McCoy, M. K., and Tansey, M. G. (2008). TNF signaling inhibition in the CNS: implications for normal brain function and neurodegenerative disease. *J. Neuroinflammation* 5, 45.

Michelucci, A., Heurtaux, T., Grandbarbe, L., Morga, E., and Heuschling, P. (2009). Characterization of the microglial phenotype under specific pro-inflammatory and anti-inflammatory conditions: effects of oligomeric and fibrillar amyloid-beta. *J. Neuroimmunol.* 210, 3–12.

Mohapel, P., Ekdahl, C. T., and Lindvall, O. (2004). Status epilepticus severity influences the long-term outcome of neurogenesis in the adult dentate gyrus. *Neurobiol. Dis.* 15, 196–205.

Molina-Holgado, E., and Molina-Holgado, F. (2010). Mending the broken brain: neuroimmune interactions in neurogenesis. *J. Neurochem.* 114, 1277–1290.

Monje, M. L., Toda, H., and Palmer, T. D. (2003). Inflammatory blockade restores adult hippocampal neurogenesis. *Science* 302, 1760–1765.

Moriyama, M., Fukuhara, T., Britschgi, M., He, Y., Narasimhan, R., Villeda, S., Molina, H., Huber, B. T., Holers M., and Wyss-Coray, T. (2011) Complement receptor 2 is expressed in neural progenitor cells and regulates adult hippocampal neurogenesis. *J. Neurosci.* 31, 3981–3989.

Morrens, J., Van Den Broeck, W., and Kempermann, G. (2012). Glial cells in adult neurogenesis. *Glia* 60, 159–174.

Mosser, D. M. (2003). The many faces of macrophage activation. *J. Leukoc. Biol.* 73, 209–212.

Murphy, B. L., Pun, R. Y., Yin, H., Faulkner, C. R., Loepke, A. W., and Danzer, S. C. (2011). Heterogeneous integration of adult-generated granule cells into the epileptic brain. *J. Neurosci.* 31, 105–117.

Nathan, C., and Ding, A. (2010). Nonresolving inflammation. *Cell* 140, 871–882.

Neher, J. J., Neniskyte, U., Zhao, J. W., Bal-Price, A., Tolkovsky, A. M , and Brown, G. C. (2011). Inhibition of microglial phagocytosis is sufficient to prevent inflammatory neuronal death. *J. Immunol.* 186, 4973–4983.

Neumann, J., Sauerzweig, S., Ronicke, R., Gunzer, F., Dinkel, K., Ullrich, O., Gunzer, M., and Reymann, K. G. (2008). Microglia cells protect neurons by direct engulfment of invading neutrophil granulocytes: a new mechanism of CNS immune privilege. *J. Neurosci.* 28, 5965–5975.

Nimmerjahn, A., Kirchhoff, F., and Helmchen, F. (2005). Resting microglial cells are highly dynamic surveillants of brain parenchyma in vivo. *Science* 308, 1314–1318.

O'Keeffe, G. C., and Barker, R. A. (2011). Dopamine stimulates epidermal growth factor release from adult neural precursor cells derived from the subventricular zone by a disintegrin and metalloprotease. *Neuroreport* 22, 956–958

Olah, M., Biber, K., Vinet, J., and Boddeke, H. W. (2011). Microglia phenotype diversity. *CNS Neurol. Disord. Drug Targets* 10, 108–118.

Paolicelli, R. C., Bolasco, G., Pagani, F., Maggi, L., Scianni, M., Panzanelli, P., Giustetto, M., Ferreira, T. A., Guiducci, E., Dumas, L., Ragozzino, D., and Gross, C. T. (2011). Synaptic pruning by microglia is necessary for normal brain development. *Science* 333, 1456–1458.

Parent, J. M., Yu, T. W., Leibowitz, R. T., Geschwind, D. H., Sloviter, R. S., and Lowenstein, D. H. (1997). Dentate granule cell neurogenesis is increased by seizures and contributes to aberrant network reorganization in the adult rat hippocampus. *J. Neurosci.* 17, 3727–3738.

Perry, V. H. (2010). Contribution of systemic inflammation to chronic neurodegeneration. *Acta Neuropathol.* 120, 277–286.

Perry, V. H., and O'Connor, V. (2008). C1q: the perfect complement for a synaptic feast? *Nat. Rev. Neurosci.* 9, 807–811.

Pickering, M., Cumiskey, D., and O'Connor, J. J. (2005). Actions of TNF-alpha on glutamatergic synaptic transmission in the central nervous system. *Exp. Physiol.* 90, 663–670.

Polazzi, E., and Monti, B. (2010). Microglia and neuroprotection: from in vitro studies to therapeutic applications. *Prog. Neurobiol.* 92, 293–315.

Popa, N., Cedile, O., Pollet-Villard, X., Bagnis, C., Durbec, P., and Boucraut, J. (2011). RAE-1 is expressed in the adult subventricular zone and controls cell proliferation of neurospheres. *Glia* 59, 35–44.

Rahpeymai, Y., Hietala, M. A., Wilhelmsson, U., Fotheringham, A., Davies, I., Nilsson, A. K., Zwirner, J., Wetsel, R. A., Gerard, C., Pekny, M., and Pekna, M. (2006). Complement: a novel factor in basal and ischemia-induced neurogenesis. *EMBO J.* 25, 1364–1374.

Richerson, S., Ingram, M., Perry, D., and Stecker, M. M. (2005). Classification of the extracellular fields produced by activated neural structures. *Biomed. Eng. Online* 4, 53. doi:10.1186/1475-925X-4-53

Riquelme, P. A., Drapeau, E., and Doetsch, F. (2008). Brain micro-ecologies: neural stem cell niches in the adult mammalian brain. *Philos. Trans. R. Soc. Lond. B Biol. Sci.* 363, 123–137.

Rivest, S. (2011). The promise of anti-inflammatory therapies for CNS injuries and diseases. *Expert Rev. Neurother.* 11, 783–786.

Rock, K. L., Latz, E., Ontiveros, F., and Kono, H. (2010). The sterile inflammatory response. *Annu. Rev. Immunol.* 28, 321–342.

Ron-Harel, N., Cardon, M., and Schwartz, M. (2011). Brain homeostasis is maintained by "danger" signals stimulating a supportive immune response within the brain's borders. *Brain Behav. Immun.* 25, 1036–1043.

Ron-Harel, N., Segev, Y., Lewitus, G. M., Cardon, M., Ziv, Y., Netanely, D., Jacob-Hirsch, J., Amariglio, N., Rechavi, G., Domany, E., and Schwartz, M. (2008). Age-dependent spatial memory loss can be partially restored by immune activation. *Rejuvenation Res.* 11, 903–913.

Russo, I., Barlati, S., and Bosetti, F. (2011a). Effects of neuroinflammation on the regenerative capacity of brain stem cells. *J. Neurochem.* 116, 947–956.

Russo, I., Amornphimoltham, P., Weigert, R., Barlati, S., and Bosetti, F. (2011b). Cyclooxygenase-1 is involved in the inhibition of hippocampal neurogenesis after lipopolysaccharide-induced neuroinflammation. *Cell Cycle* 10, 2568–2573.

Sahay, A., Scobie, K. N., Hill, A. S., O'Carroll, C. M., Kheirbek, M. A., Burghardt, N. S., Fenton, A. A., Dranovsky, A., and Hen, R. (2011). Increasing adult hippocampal neurogenesis is sufficient to improve pattern separation. *Nature* 472, 466–470.

Sakamoto, M., Imayoshi, I., Ohtsuka, T., Yamaguchi, M., Mori, K., and Kageyama, R. (2011). Continuous neurogenesis in the adult forebrain is required for innate olfactory responses. *Proc. Natl. Acad. Sci. U.S.A.* 108, 8479–8484.

Schratt, G. M., Tuebing, F., Nigh, E. A., Kane, C. G., Sabatini, M. E., Kiebler, M., and Greenberg, M. E. (2006). A brain-specific microRNA regulates dendritic spine development. *Nature* 439, 283–289.

Seaberg, R. M., and van der Kooy, D. (2002). Adult rodent neurogenic regions: the ventricular subependyma contains neural stem cells, but the dentate gyrus contains restricted progenitors. *J. Neurosci.* 22, 1784–1793.

Shechter, R., London, A., Varol, C., Raposo, C., Cusimano, M., Yovel, G., Rolls, A., Mack, M., Pluchino, S., Martino, G., Jung, S., and Schwartz, M. (2009). Infiltrating blood-derived macrophages are vital cells playing an anti-inflammatory role in recovery from spinal cord injury in mice. *PLoS Med.* 6, e1000113. doi:10.1371/journal.pmed.1000113

Shinjyo, N., Stahlberg, A., Dragunow, M., Pekny, M., and Pekna, M. (2009). Complement-derived anaphylatoxin C3a regulates in vitro differentiation and migration of neural progenitor cells. *Stem Cells* 27, 2824–2832.

Sierra, A., Encinas, J. M., Deudero, J. J., Chancey, J. H., Enikolopov, G., Overstreet-Wadiche, L. S., Tsirka, S. E., and Maletic-Savatic, M. (2010). Microglia shape adult hippocampal neurogenesis through apoptosis-coupled phagocytosis. *Cell Stem Cell* 7, 483–495.

Stellwagen, D., and Malenka, R. C. (2006). Synaptic scaling mediated by glial TNF-alpha. *Nature* 440, 1054–1059.

Stevens, B., Allen, N. J., Vazquez, L. E., Howell, G. R., Christopherson, K. S., Nouri, N., Micheva, K. D., Mehalow, A. K., Huberman, A. D., Stafford, B., Sher, A., Litke, A. M., Lambris, J. D., Smith, S. J., John, S. W., and Barres, B. A. (2007). The classical complement cascade mediates CNS synapse elimination. *Cell* 131, 1164–1178.

Sultan, S., Rey, N., Sacquet, J., Mandairon, N., and Didier, A. (2011). Newborn neurons in the olfactory bulb selected for long-term survival through olfactory learning are prematurely suppressed when the olfactory memory is erased. *J. Neurosci.* 31, 14893–14898.

Thored, P., Heldmann, U., Gomes-Leal, W., Gisler, R., Darsalia, V., Taneera, J., Nygren, J. M., Jacobsen, S. E., Ekdahl, C. T., Kokaia, Z., and Lindvall, O. (2009). Long-term accumulation of microglia with proneurogenic phenotype concomitant with persistent neurogenesis in adult subventricular zone after stroke. *Glia* 57, 835–849.

Toni, N., and Sultan, S. (2011). Synapse formation on adult-born hippocampal neurons. *Eur. J. Neurosci.* 33, 1062–1068.

Trapp, B. D., Wujek, J. R., Criste, G. A., Jalabi, W., Yin, X., Kidd, G. J., Stohlman, S., and Ransohoff, R. (2007). Evidence for synaptic stripping by cortical microglia. *Glia* 55, 360–368.

Tremblay, M. E., Lowery, R. L., and Majewska, A. K. (2010). Microglial interactions with synapses are modulated by visual experience. *PLoS Biol.* 8, e1000527. doi:10.1371/journal.pbio.1000527

Tremblay, M. E., and Majewska, A. K. (2011). A role for microglia in synaptic plasticity? *Commun. Integr. Biol.* 4, 220–222.

Tremblay, M. E., Stevens, B., Sierra, A., Wake, H., Bessis, A., and Nimmerjahn, A. (2011). The role of microglia in the healthy brain. *J. Neurosci.* 31, 16064–16069.

Wake, H., Moorhouse, A. J., Jinno, S., Kohsaka, S., and Nabekura, J. (2009). Resting microglia directly monitor the functional state of synapses in vivo and determine the fate of ischemic terminals. *J. Neurosci.* 29, 3974–3980.

Walton, N. M., Sutter, B. M., Laywell, E. D., Levkoff, L. H., Kearns, S. M., Marshall, G. P. II, Scheffler, B., and Steindler, D. A. (2006). Microglia instruct subventricular zone neurogenesis. *Glia* 54, 815–825.

Wei, H., Zou, H., Sheikh, A. M., Malik, M., Dobkin, C., Brown, W. T., and Li, X. (2011). IL-6 is increased in the cerebellum of autistic brain and alters neural cell adhesion, migration and synaptic formation. *J. Neuroinflammation* 8, 52.

Whitney, N. P., Eidem, T. M., Peng, H., Huang, Y., and Zheng, J. C. (2009). Inflammation mediates varying effects in neurogenesis: relevance to the pathogenesis of brain injury and neurodegenerative disorders. *J. Neurochem.* 108, 1343–1359.

Wojcik-Stanaszek, L., Gregor, A., and Zalewska, T. (2011). Regulation of neurogenesis by extracellular matrix and integrins. *Acta Neurobiol. Exp. (Wars)* 71, 103–112.

Wood, J. C., Jackson, J. S., Jakubs, K., Chapman, K. Z., Ekdahl, C. T., Kokaia, Z., Kokaia, M., and Lindvall, O. (2011). Functional integration of new hippocampal neurons following insults to the adult brain is determined by characteristics of pathological environment. *Exp. Neurol.* 229, 484–493.

Yirmiya, R., and Goshen, I. (2011). Immune modulation of learning, memory, neural plasticity and neurogenesis. *Brain Behav. Immun.* 25, 181–213.

Zhao, C., Deng, W., and Gage, F. H. (2008). Mechanisms and functional implications of adult neurogenesis. *Cell* 132, 645–660.

Zhao, C., Teng, E. M., Summers, R. G. Jr., Ming, G. L., and Gage, F. H. (2006). Distinct morphological stages of dentate granule neuron maturation in the adult mouse hippocampus. *J. Neurosci.* 26, 3–11.

Ziv, Y., Ron, N., Butovsky, O., Landa, G., Sudai, E., Greenberg, N., Cohen, H., Kipnis, J., and Schwartz, M. (2006). Immune cells contribute to the maintenance of neurogenesis and spatial learning abilities in adulthood. *Nat. Neurosci.* 9, 268–275.

21

Longitudinal diffusion tensor imaging and neuropsychological correlates in traumatic brain injury patients

Kimberly D. Farbota[1,2], Barbara B. Bendlin[1,3], Andrew L. Alexander[4], Howard A. Rowley[5], Robert J. Dempsey[6] and Sterling C. Johnson[1,3]*

[1] Geriatric Research and Education Clinical Center, William S. Middleton Memorial Veterans Hospital, Madison, WI, USA
[2] University of Wisconsin Neuroscience Training Program, Madison, WI, USA
[3] Department of Medicine, University of Wisconsin School of Medicine and Public Health, Madison, WI, USA
[4] Department of Medical Physics, University of Wisconsin School of Medicine and Public Health, Madison, WI, USA
[5] Department of Radiology, University of Wisconsin School of Medicine and Public Health, Madison, WI, USA
[6] Department of Neurological Surgery, University of Wisconsin School of Medicine and Public Health, Madison, WI, USA

Edited by:
Robin E. A. Green, University of Toronto, Canada

Reviewed by:
Fernando Maestú, Complutense University, Spain
David M. Schnyer, University of Texas, USA

***Correspondence:**
Sterling C. Johnson, Department of Medicine, William S. Middleton Memorial VA Hospital, University of Wisconsin, 2500 Overlook Terrace, Madison, WI 53705, USA.
e-mail: scj@medicine.wisc.edu

Traumatic brain injury (TBI) often involves focal cortical injury and white matter (WM) damage that can be measured shortly after injury. Additionally, slowly evolving WM change can be observed but there is a paucity of research on the duration and spatial pattern of long-term changes several years post-injury. The current study utilized diffusion tensor imaging to identify regional WM changes in 12 TBI patients and nine healthy controls at three time points over a four year period. Neuropsychological testing was also administered to each participant at each time point. Results indicate that TBI patients exhibit longitudinal changes to WM indexed by reductions in fractional anisotropy (FA) in the corpus callosum, as well as FA increases in bilateral regions of the superior longitudinal fasciculus (SLF) and portions of the optic radiation (OR). FA changes appear to be driven by changes in radial (not axial) diffusivity, suggesting that observed longitudinal FA changes may be related to changes in myelin rather than to axons. Neuropsychological correlations indicate that regional FA values in the corpus callosum and sagittal stratum (SS) correlate with performance on finger tapping and visuomotor speed tasks (respectively) in TBI patients, and that longitudinal increases in FA in the SS, SLF, and OR correlate with improved performance on the visuomotor speed (SS) task as well as a derived measure of cognitive control (SLF, OR). The results of this study showing progressive WM deterioration for several years post-injury contribute to a growing literature supporting the hypothesis that TBI should be viewed not as an isolated incident but as a prolonged disease state. The observations of long-term neurological and functional improvement provide evidence that some ameliorative change may be occurring concurrently with progressive degeneration.

Keywords: traumatic brain injury, diffusion tensor imaging, longitudinal, neuropsychology, recovery, DTI, TBI

INTRODUCTION

Traumatic brain injury (TBI) affects more than 1.4 million people every year in the United States (CDC, 2006). These injuries are the most common source of neurological impairment among young and middle-aged adults, and can produce long-term cognitive deficits that hinder patients' ability to function independently, lower their quality of life and increase the risk of developing co-morbid neurological disorders (Anderson et al., 1995; Kiraly and Kiraly, 2007; Bombardier et al., 2010; Malec et al., 2010; Risdall and Menon, 2010; Sharp and Ham, 2011). Previous research has shown that the progression of structural pathology in the first year following injury includes decreased white matter (WM) integrity throughout the brain (Povlishock and Christman, 1995; Trivedi et al., 2007; Xu et al., 2007; Marquez de la Plata et al., 2008; Sidaros et al., 2008; Lin et al., 2010), but little is known about WM changes that occur after this first year. Concomitant to slowly occurring atrophy and WM degradation, TBI patients typically demonstrate measurable cognitive and motor improvements in the first and subsequent years post-injury. This study aims to identify long-term patterns of WM change following TBI, as well as how variations in WM integrity correlate with both neuropsychological test performance and change in test performance over time (Levin, 2003; Staudt, 2010).

Diffusion tensor imaging (DTI) is sensitive to WM damage immediately following TBI and useful in monitoring longitudinal changes (Filippi et al., 2001; Xu et al., 2007; Bendlin et al., 2008). DTI, which is based on the principle that water molecule movement is restricted by barriers to diffusion that vary in the brain depending on tissue type or pathology, [for review see Le Bihan (1991)], is sensitive to changes in the microstructure of WM.

Several studies have shown that DTI accurately detects damage in tissue that may appear normal when measured with conventional MRI (Arfanakis et al., 2002; Chan et al., 2003) and that DTI can be of clinical importance when tracing recovery (Filippi et al., 2001; Arfanakis et al., 2002; Field et al., 2003). These capabilities make DTI well suited for assessing WM damage caused by TBI and for tracking how WM changes progress longitudinally following injury.

The current study is an extension of a prior study conducted on this same cohort of TBI patients. The previous paper (Bendlin et al., 2008), included whole-brain DTI and volumetric analyses of patients at two months and one year post-injury. Results showed gray and WM alterations over time in TBI compared to control. Regions of reduced WM integrity included corpus callosum, forceps major and minor, anterior corona radiata, external capsule, cerebral peduncle, superior longitudinal fasciculus (SFL), uncinate fasciculus, and corticopontine tract. The current study extends the previous work with the addition of a third time point approximately four years post-injury. Furthermore, the current study includes axial and radial diffusivity analyses (which may allow inference concerning the cause of WM changes), and increases the power to detect group-wise effects by restricting analyses to the WM.

The primary metric used to assess WM integrity in this study is fractional anisotropy (FA). FA describes the extent to which a diffusion process is anisotropic or directionally constrained. In brain WM, higher FA is associated with greater WM integrity (Alexander et al., 2007). As noted above, we also employed two secondary metrics: axial diffusivity and radial diffusivity. Axial diffusivity refers to the movement of water along the principle axis of a WM tract. Animal studies have demonstrated that high axial diffusivity is associated with healthy axons, and low axial diffusivity is associated with axonal damage (Song et al., 2002, 2003). Radial diffusivity refers to the movement of water perpendicular to the principle axis of a WM tract. Animal studies have demonstrated that low radial diffusivity is associated with healthy myelin, and high radial diffusivity is associated with myelin damage (Wheeler-Kingshott and Cercignani, 2009). Investigating how these secondary metrics change over time in brain regions demonstrating longitudinal differences in FA can provide additional insight into the processes underlying WM change.

The first major goal of the current study was to characterize longitudinal changes in regional brain WM microstructure using DTI in conjunction with neuropsychological testing. Due to previous reports of volume loss and WM decline in the corpus callosum, as well as the emergent theory of TBI as the initiation of a disease state, we predicted that this structure would demonstrate continued decline throughout the duration of the study within the TBI group (Gale et al., 1995; Bigler et al., 1996; Kim et al., 2008; Kumar et al., 2010; Masel and DeWitt, 2010; Matsukawa et al., 2011; Ljungqvist et al., 2011). While decline in many regions is likely, patients typically continue to improve cognitively; thus we also sought to determine whether FA increases may occur in other regions, which may suggest consolidation or remodeling of WM tracts associated with recovery. Candidate regions include corticospinal tract regions (cerebral peduncle, internal capsule) and longitudinal tracts (superior and inferior longitudinal faciculi) due to previous research indicating improvements in certain diffusion metrics in a subset of these regions (Sidaros et al., 2008) and the presence of damage in these regions observed in cross-sectional studies done close to the time of injury but not in those done several years post-TBI (Kraus et al., 2007; Bendlin et al., 2008).

The second major goal of this study was to identify correlations between FA and neuropsychological task performance cross-sectionally at each time point studied, as well as determine whether changes in task performance over time correlated with changes in FA longitudinally. Due to previous research indicating that higher corpus callosum FA is associated with better performance on manual motor tasks in brain injury patients, we predicted that scores on a fine motor finger tapping task employed in this study would correlate with FA in this region among TBI patients (Caeyenberghs et al., 2011a,b). Furthermore, we predicted that increases in FA within the longitudinal tracts would correlate with improved performance on the more complex neuropsychological tasks such as the Cognitive Oral Word Association Test (COWAT), or the cognitive component of the Trail Making Test. Finally, we expected patients who had sustained more severe injuries, as measured by the 24 h post-resuscitation Glasgow Coma Score (GCS), to demonstrate a greater degree of initial microstructural damage and longitudinal WM change than patients who sustained less severe injuries.

METHODS

TBI PATIENTS

Forty-six TBI patients participated in an initial MRI scan, thirty-six returned for a second visit, and twenty returned for a third visit. DTI was acquired in sixteen individuals at all three time points (three were subsequently excluded due to excessive motion, and one more was excluded due to a second head injury sustained in a motor vehicle accident between visits 2 and 3). The mean age of the final group of twelve patients (ten males and two females) was 35.00 ± 12.76 years at the beginning of the study; mean education was 13.17 ± 1.75 years. The majority of the patients received acute treatment at the University of Wisconsin Hospital and Clinics level 1 trauma center and were referred from the departments of Neurosurgery, Trauma and/or Rehabilitation. The inclusion criteria for TBI consisted of involvement in a rapid impact injury to the brain (such as a motor vehicle accident or fall) causing a loss of consciousness. Evidence of brain injury included admittance for emergency medical attention following loss of consciousness in the field, a GCS score either at the emergency room (ER) or upon hospital admission of less than or equal to 13, and a post-resuscitation GCS score of 5 or above. All patients had day of injury CT scans that were positive for visible brain injury. All TBI patients were less than three months post-injury at their first visit, and most were studied between eight and twelve weeks post-injury depending on their availability and other medical issues related to the injury. Exclusion criteria consisted of current major Axis I psychiatric disease or history of major medical condition (e.g., cancer, diabetes, or diagnosed neurological condition), as well as any previous diagnosis of substance dependence, or an undiagnosed pattern of behavior demonstrating longstanding maladaptive use of alcohol or other drugs. All patients gave informed written consent under a protocol approved by the University of Wisconsin Health Sciences Institutional Review Board.

HEALTHY CONTROLS

Thirty-six control participants were recruited from the community and from the University of Wisconsin Madison campus via advertisement. Twenty of these participants returned for two additional visits. Acquisition errors resulted in the loss of four participants who did not have adequate DTI at all three time points; and in seven cases DTI was not acquired at one of the visits due to time constraints; DTI scans acquired from nine participants at all three time points were used in the final analysis. The mean age of the final group of nine healthy controls (four males, five females) was 31.44 ± 12.38 years at the beginning of the study; education was 14.77 ± 2.22 years. Exclusion criteria were identical to the TBI group (with the exception of head injury also being exclusionary for controls). MR scanning of control participants occurred on approximately the same schedule as that of TBI patients. All participants gave informed written consent under a protocol approved by the University of Wisconsin Health Sciences Institutional Review Board.

PROCEDURES

Volunteers participated in three testing sessions, each consisting of MR imaging and neuropsychological testing. TBI patients were tested at three visits, Visit 1, acquired approximately two months (mean = 63 days) post-injury (ranging from 28 to 81 days), Visit 2, approximately one year (mean = 318 days) after Visit 1 (ranging from 226 to 381 days) and Visit 3, approximately three years (mean = 1187 days) after Visit 2 (ranging from 956 to 1651 days). Controls also participated in three visits with approximately one year (mean = 286 days) between Visit 1 and 2 (ranging from 74 to 374 days) and three years (mean = 1096 days) between Visit 2 and 3 (ranging from 778 to 2011 days).

NEUROPSYCHOLOGICAL EXAMINATION

On the day of each scan, a neuropsychological battery that included: COWAT, WRAT-III (Wide Range Achievement Test-reading subtest, an approximation of pre-morbid intelligence), Finger Tapping (during which participants tapped a lever for 10 s as fast as possible for three trials and the average was used), Digit Span (a measure of working memory) and Trail Making Tests A (a visual-motor speed task) and B (a combination task requiring both visual-motor skill and rapid cognitive set shifting) was administered to each participant. These tests were selected based on previous research in our laboratory suggesting their probable relevance to TBI induced behavioral changes. Some of our analyses also included Trails B cognitive component scores which were calculated by subtracting each subject's Trails A score (visuomotor) from his or her Trails B score (visuomotor and cognitive) to isolate the cognitive component of the Trails B task. Statistical analysis of neuropsychological test results was performed as follows: for each test, a general linear model repeated measures test was carried out in SPSS 20.0. From these models, main effects of group and time as well as a group by time interaction were derived. Simple effects analyses were performed by using independent samples one-tailed t-tests to assess between-groups differences in task performance at each time point, and by using paired samples one-tailed t-tests to assess within groups changes in task performance across time points.

MAGNETIC RESONANCE IMAGING

All participants underwent magnetic resonance on a General Electric 3.0 T (Waukesha, WI) MRI system with a quadrature birdcage head coil. Structural scans included an axial T1-weighted inversion recovery-prepped spoiled gradient echo scan (inversion time = 600 ms, repetition time (TR)/echo time (TE)/flip angle = 9 ms/1.8 ms/20°; acquisition matrix = 256 × 192 interpolated to 256 × 256; field of view (FOV) = 240 mm; and 124 slices 1.2 mm thick). Diffusion tensor imaging was performed using a cardiac-gated, diffusion-weighted sequence with the following parameters: 12 directions with diffusion weighting of 1114 s/mm^2 and a non-diffusion-weighted reference image (B0); TR = 10–15 s; TE = 78.2 ms; number of averages: 3; acquisition matrix = 120 × 120 interpolated to 256 × 256; FOV = 240 mm; 39 contiguous 3 mm thick axial slices. The scan resulted in 0.9375 × 0.9375 × 3 mm voxels. Prior to the diffusion-weighted scan, high order shimming was performed to minimize EPI distortions. A neuroradiologist (HR) reviewed all structural MRI images to identify the location and extent of lesions associated with the TBI and to identify non-injury related brain abnormalities that might exclude participants from the statistical analyses. Additionally, a high resolution 2D axial T2* gradient echo sequence sensitive to both DAI and contusions was collected for evaluation by a neuroradiologist who confirmed the presence of brain injury. Imaging parameters were as follows: gradient echo read-out with TR = 325 ms, TE = 20 ms; flip angle = 15°; acquisition matrix = 256 × 192 interpolated to 256 × 256; FOV = 240 mm; 22 5 mm thick axial slices, with a 1 mm skip between slices; and receiver bandwidth = ±15.83 kHz.

DIFFUSION TENSOR IMAGE PROCESSING

Image distortions in the DTI-data caused by eddy currents were corrected using a 2D affine co-registration function, align linear, in the Automated Image Registration software package (http://www.loni.ucla.edu/Software/AIR). Non-linear image distortion from static field (B0) inhomogeneities was corrected using the acquired field map and implemented in the prelude (Phase Region Expanding Labeller for Unwrapping Discrete Estimates) and fugue (FMRIB's Utility for Geometrically Unwarping EPIs) tools from the FSL software suite (Smith et al., 2004). After distortion corrections, 3D maps of the diffusion tensor and derived measures, FA, axial diffusivity (determined using the principle eigenvalue, L1) and radial diffusivity (determined using the average of the secondary and tertiary eigenvalues, L2 and L3), were calculated. For each subject, the FA, radial diffusivity, and axial diffusivity maps from Visits 2 and 3 were then co-registered to the corresponding maps from Visit 1 using flirt (FSL) 12-parameter affine co-registration. Normalization was then performed using fNIRT in FSL. Normalization of the Visit 1 maps to the FSL FMRIB58_FA_1 mm template was performed for each subject. The transformation derived from this normalization was then applied to the co-registered maps acquired during Visits 2 and 3. The maps from each time point for each measure were visually checked for alignment to each other and the template.

STATISTICAL ANALYSIS

Primary statistical analyses were performed on FA maps using factorial ANOVA statistical modules in SPM8. Gender was used as a covariate in all analyses. Because this study focused only on WM change, all SPM analyses were restricted to regions within a WM mask to increase our power to detect longitudinal change. The WM mask was created by applying a threshold of 0.5 (**Figure 1**) to the mean FA map of all subjects, and then binarizing the resulting image using fslmaths (FMRIB Software Library). To determine whether there were overall group differences in longitudinal FA change, we tested for an interaction between group and time within the factorial model. The hypothesis that there would be longitudinal change within the TBI group was tested using simple effects analyses, also within the factorial model framework.

Secondary statistical analyses using axial and radial diffusivity maps were also performed using factorial ANOVA statistical modules in SPM8. Because these analyses were employed to further examine the causes of FA change, axial, and radial diffusivity analyses were restricted to regions where significant FA results were observed. We hypothesized that increases in FA would be driven by decreased radial diffusivity and/or increased axial diffusivity, and also conversely that decreases in FA would be driven by increased radial diffusivity and/or increased axial diffusivity.

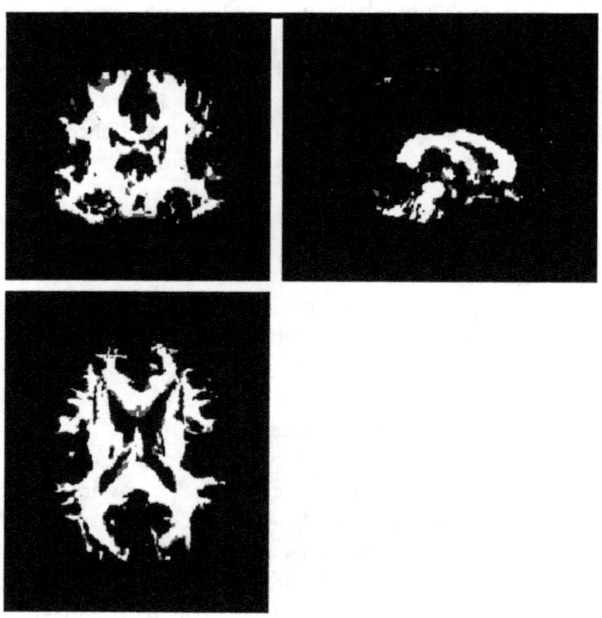

FIGURE 1 | Because this study focused only on white matter change, all SPM analyses were restricted to regions within a white matter mask to increase our power to detect longitudinal change. The white matter mask was created by applying a threshold of 0.5 to the mean FA map of all subjects, and then binarizing the resulting image. This figure shows the white matter mask in three orthogonal directions. The left side of the mask is patient left and the right is patient right.

Correlations with neuropsychological test scores were assessed using linear regression implemented in SPM8, where test scores were independent variables and FA maps were the dependent variables. We hypothesized that we would see positive regional correlations between FA and task performance. In addition to direct correlations between neuropsychological test scores and FA values, we also tested hypotheses concerning how changes in FA and changes in neuropsychological performance might correlate. In these cases, differences in neuropsychological test scores between two time points were calculated for each subject, as were differences in FA during the same interval. FA differences were determined by subtracting the later maps from the earlier maps for each subject. Correlations between FA change maps and changes in neuropsychological test scores were also assessed using linear regression implemented in SPM8, where changes in test scores were independent variables and FA change maps were the dependent variables. All correlation analyses of neuropsychological measures were limited to regions within the WM mask used in general FA analyses.

STATISTICAL THRESHOLD

A voxel-level threshold of $\alpha = 0.001$ (uncorrected) was used for all contrasts. Multiple-comparison correction for FA analyses was performed using estimates from a Monte-Carlo simulation performed with AlphaSim to achieve a corrected cluster-level threshold of $\alpha = 0.05$ (Forman et al., 1995). The Monte-Carlo simulation determined based on randomly computed images that a cluster with 581 voxels with the same dimensions, voxel probability threshold, and smoothness parameters as FA images inputted for analysis would be unlikely (at the $\alpha = 0.05$ cluster-level corrected threshold) to be significant only by chance. Thus, a cluster-level threshold of 581 voxels was used in all FA analyses. For secondary factorial analyses of axial and radial diffusivity and regression analyses used to test neuropsychological correlations cluster-levels were determined individually for each SPM at the significance levels noted above.

RESULTS

DEMOGRAPHIC AND BEHAVIORAL RESULTS

There were no significant differences in age ($t = -1.131$, df $= 19$, two-tailed $p = 0.272$) or years of education ($t = -1.861$, df $= 19$, two-tailed $p = 0.078$) between the TBI and control groups. There were significantly more males in the TBI group compared to the control group ($\chi^2_{(1,\ 12)} = 4.535$, $p = 0.033$). Demographic results are shown in **Table 1**. Repeated measures analyses of neuropsychological test results indicated a main effect of group in the DSPAN, Trails B, and COWAT tasks, as well as a group by time interaction for the COWAT task (**Table 2**). Simple effects analyses of neuropsychological tests performance indicated that TBI patients' performance was significantly worse than that of controls on Digit Span, Trails A and B at Visits 1, 2, and 3. TBI patients also differed from controls on the COWAT at Visits 1 and 2. No significant group differences were seen in WRAT-III or Finger Tapping. TBI patients demonstrated

Table 1 | Individual level subject demographics for patients and controls and select patient injury characteristics.

Subject	Age	Education	Sex	GCSadmit	GCS24	Hrs15	Injury notes
PATIENTS							
1	19	12	M	3T	7	334	DAI
2	49	12	M	15	15	0	DAI, subarachnoid hemorrhage, CC damage
3	19	14	F	3T	11	91	Subarachnoid hemorrhage, subdural hematoma
4	24	14	M	3	7	662	DAI, contusions, epidural hematoma, subarachnoid hemorrhage
5	39	10	M	3T	6	835	Extensive contusions, subdural hematoma
6	45	12	M	3T	14	270	Skull fracture, frontal contusion, CC damage
7	29	13	M	3	14	179	DAI, contusions, skull fracture
8	52	16	F	11	13	97	Skull fracture, subarachnoid hemorrhage, subdural hematoma,
9	51	12	M	7	7	726	Depressed skull fracture, subdural and epidural hematomas
10	19	13	M	3T	5	49	Extensive hemorrhages, CC shearing
11	37	14	M	9	7	116	DAI, subarachnoid hemorrhage, subdural hematoma, shearing
Mean (SD)	35.0 (12.8)	13.2 (1.5)	83% M	5.7 (4.2)	9.6(3.8)	305.4(297.8)	
CONTROLS							
12	22	19	F				
13	22	15	M				
14	29	13	F				
15	27	16	F				
16	25	12	F				
17	19	16	F				
18	36	16	M				
19	24	13	M				
20	51	13	M				
Mean (SD)	29.2 (9.7)	14.8 (2.2)	44% M				
p	0.272	0.078	0.033				

Age of participants indicates the mean age of participants at the start of the study. P-values are based on the results of two-tailed independent-samples t-tests for age and education and a chi-squares test for gender proportions. Abbreviations are as follows: GCSadmit = Glasgow Coma Scale score at hospital admission, GCS24 = Glasgow Coma Scale score 24 h post-injury, 15 h = Number of hours before patient reached a GCS score of 15, DAI = Diffuse axonal injury, CC = corpus callosum, T = Patient was intubated at the time of GCS assessment.

significant improvements on the DSPAN, Trails A, B, and COWAT tests between Visit 1 and 2, and also showed significant improvement on the Trails A, B and COWAT tests between Visit 1 and 3. Controls demonstrated significant improvement on the Trails A and B tasks between Visit 1 and 2. All neurological test results are shown in **Table 2**.

DTI RESULTS

The FA factorial analysis revealed a group by time interaction in the genu of the corpus callosum (**Figure 2**). Analyses of the secondary metrics (using separate factorial models for axial diffusivity and radial diffusivity maps) demonstrated that there was also a group by time interaction in this region in the radial diffusivity model, but not the axial diffusivity model (**Figure 2**). Together these analyses indicate that the group by time interaction observed in the genu in the FA analysis was driven by changes in radial (not axial) diffusivity.

A main effect of time was observed throughout the corpus callosum in the primary FA analysis (**Figure 3**). A corresponding main effect of time was observed in this region in the radial, but not the axial, diffusivity analysis (**Figure 3**). A main effect of group was observed in WM tracts throughout the brain, including the cerebral peduncle, inferior and superior longitudinal fascicule (ILF and SLF), internal and external capsule, inferior fronto-occipital fasciculus, sagittal stratum (SS), corpus callosum, fornix, optic radiations (ORs), thalamic radiations, uncinate fasciculus, and corona radiata (**Figure 4**). Axial and radial diffusivity analyses revealed a main effect of group in genu, fornix, and ILF in the axial model and a main effect of group throughout the corpus callosum, as well as in the fornix, ILF, ORs, and thalamic radiations in the radial model (**Figure 4**).

Simple effects analyses within the FA factorial model demonstrated that TBI subjects exhibited a significant decrease in FA throughout the corpus callosum between the first and third visits (**Figure 5A**). We hypothesized that this change would be driven either by a decrease in axial diffusivity, an increase in radial diffusivity, or some combination of the two. Analyses of the secondary metrics limited to this corpus callosum region were used to test this hypothesis. Results showed that TBI subjects did not demonstrate any decreases in axial diffusivity in this region, while they did exhibit significant increases in radial diffusivity in both the genu and isthmus of the corpus callosum (**Figure 5A**). Controls did not demonstrate significant longitudinal FA decreases in any brain regions.

Table 2 | Neuropsychological test results.

Task	Time 1 n, Mean (SD)	Time 2 n, Mean (SD)	Time 3 n, Mean (SD)
TBI GROUP RESULTS			
WRAT-III	12, **44.7** (6.5)	12, **44.5** (12.3)	11, **45.6** (5.7)
DSPAN[a]	12, **14.3*****† (3.6)	12, **15.6*** (3.7)	11, **15.6*** (4.6)
Trails A	12, **42.0***† (21.5)	12, **30.8*** (6.4)	12, **28.7*****† (7.1)
Trails B[a]	11, **101.3***† (29.0)	12, **78.6*** (20.9)	12, **68.8***† (36.4)
COWAT[b]	12, **21.2***††† (10.2)	12, **33.8*** (10.6)	12, **39.6**†† (12.4)
FT	10, **44.1** (14.7)	12, **45.9** (7.6)	12, **45.7** (6.9
CONTROL GROUP RESULTS			
WRAT-III	8, **50.0** (5.1)	7, **50.0** (6.1)	9, **55.7** (5.2)
DSPAN	8, **20.1** (3.4)	7, **20.6** (3.9)	9, **20.4** (5.2)
Trails A	8, **25.1** (6.9)	7, **24.6**†† (5.4)	9, **20.3** (4.5)
Trails B	8, **55.0** (25.6)	7, **51.5**† (20.4)	9, **38.6** (7.1)
COWAT	8, **41.8** (7.8)	7, **44.6** (8.9)	9, **45.9** (11.9)
FT	6, **45.6** (10.8)	7, **48.9** (6.9)	9, **48.3** (6.8)

*Test abbreviations are as follows: WRAT-III = Wide Range Achievement Test (reading subtest), DSPAN = Digit Span Test, Trails A = Trail Making Test A (motor), Trails B = Trail Making Test B (motor and cognitive), COWAT = Cognitive Oral Word Association Test, FT DOM = Dominant Hand Finger Tapping Test. Means are of raw scores. Repeated measures analyses based on general linear models were carried out for each neuropsychological test and significant results ($p < 0.05$) are noted next to task names in the following manner: [a]indicates a main effect of group and [b]indicates a group by time interaction. None of the models demonstrated a significant effect of time. Between-groups differences were calculated using independent samples one-tailed t-tests, and significance levels are denoted as follows: *$p < 0.05$, **$p < 0.01$, ***$p < 0.001$. Between groups differences are noted by the patient average scores only. Within-groups differences were calculated using paired samples one-tailed t-tests, and significance levels are denoted as follows: †$p < 0.05$, ††$p < 0.01$, †††$p < 0.001$. Differences between time 1 and 2 are noted by the first time point average, differences between time 2 and 3 are noted by the second time point average, and differences between time 1 and 3 are noted by the third time point average.*

In order to determine whether the decrease in FA in the corpus callosum within the TBI group between the first and third visits was driven primarily by early changes during the first interval or late changes during the second interval, each interval was assessed individually within the FA factorial model. These secondary analyses were limited to the corpus callosum region where a change had been observed between the first and third time points. Results demonstrated that significant changes could be seen in the genu and body of the corpus callosum during the first interval (**Figure 5B**), but no significant clusters were identified during the second interval. Axial and radial diffusivity analyses within this region indicated that an increase in radial diffusivity was present in the genu during the first interval among TBI subjects (**Figure 5B**), however, no accompanying decrease in axial diffusivity was observed.

Simple effects analyses within the FA factorial model also demonstrated that TBI subjects exhibited significant FA increases in bilateral regions of the SLF as well as in an OR region on the left side of the brain between the first and third visits (**Figure 6**). Again, we hypothesized that changes observed among TBI patients would be driven either by decreases in axial diffusivity, increases in radial diffusivity, or some combination of the two. Analyses of the secondary metrics limited to these regions were used to test this hypothesis. Results showed that TBI subjects did not demonstrate any increases in axial diffusivity in these regions between the first and third visits, however, significant decreases in radial diffusivity were observed in all regions tested (**Figure 6**). Controls did not exhibit significant longitudinal FA increases in any brain regions.

In order to determine whether the increases in FA in the bilateral SLF and left OR within the TBI group between the first and third visits were driven primarily by early changes during the first interval or late changes during the second interval, each interval was assessed individually within the FA factorial model. These secondary FA increase analyses were limited to the regions where a change had been observed between the first and third time points. No significant clusters were identified during either the first or second intervals individually, suggesting that the observed change occurred gradually over the four year study duration.

Between-groups simple effects analyses demonstrated that the TBI group had reduced FA compared to the control group in the cerebral peduncle, ILF, SLF, internal and external capsule, inferior fronto-occipital fasciculus, SS, corpus callosum, fornix, ORs, thalamic radiations, uncinate fasciculus, and corona radiata at all three visits. There were no regions in which the TBI group had greater FA than the control group at any of the three time points. We hypothesized that FA reductions would be driven by a combination of reduced axial and increased radial diffusivity. Secondary analyses confirmed this hypothesis, demonstrating that the TBI group had reduced axial diffusivity compared to controls in parts of the cerebral peduncle, external capsule, internal capsule, OR, fornix, SLF, and ILF at all three time points. Increased radial diffusivity among TBI patients was observed in all regions in which group differences in FA were observed at all three time points.

NEUROPSYCHOLOGICAL CORRELATIONS

Contrary to our hypothesis, we did not observe any correlations between an individual's GCS score and regional WM FA at any of the three time points. Of the seven neuropsychological measures tested for correlation with FA, two tests, Trails A and dominant hand finger tapping, were significantly correlated with regional FA values among the TBI subjects. No significant correlations were observed between FA and neuropsychological test performance among control subjects. Finger tapping scores correlated positively with FA in the splenium of the corpus callosum at the second time point (**Figure 7**). A lowered statistical threshold $\alpha = 0.01$ enabled observation of smaller splenium clusters when the equivalent correlational tests were run for the first and third time points, however, only the second time point result surpassed significance levels employed in this study. Trails A performance correlated positively with FA in bilateral regions of the SS at the first time point, and a unilateral region in the left SS at the second time point (**Figure 8A**).

Correlations between FA changes and changes in neuropsychological measures over time were also significant for two neuropsychological measures, Trails A and B cognitive component. No equivalent correlations were observed among controls for any measure. There was a positive correlation between change in the

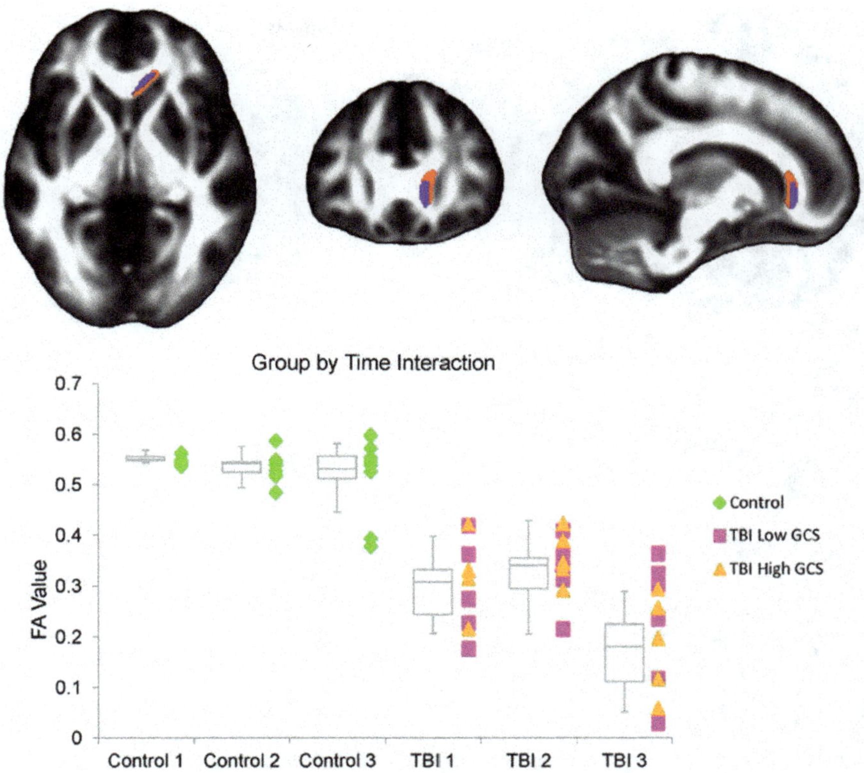

FIGURE 2 | (Top) A significant interaction between group and interval was observed within the FA factorial model. There were inter-interval dissimilarities in group-wise patterns of FA change in the genu of the corpus callosum (red). Axial and radial diffusivity analyses were restricted to regions demonstrating an FA effect. Within this region, a significant interaction was also observed in the radial diffusivity factorial model (overlapping blue region), but not the axial diffusivity factorial model. The left side of the statistical map is patient left and right is patient right. **(Bottom)** This graph shows the average FA value for each subject at each of the three time points within the corpus callosum cluster demonstrating an FA effect. Controls are marked as green diamonds, TBI patients with a 24 h GCS score of 7 or lower are marked as pink squares, and patients with a 24 h GCS score of 10 or higher are marked as orange triangles. Box plots indicate the 75th percentile, median, and 25th percentile FA values of each group at each time point, and whiskers indicate 1.5 times inter-quartile ranges.

Trails A score between the first and third time points and change in FA over the same duration (where an increase in FA was associated with a reduction in time to complete Trails A) in the right SS (**Figure 8B**). No significant correlations were observed between change in Trails A score and change in FA during either sub-interval of the study (from time one to time two or from time two to time three). A positive correlation between FA change and change in the Trails B cognitive component between time one and time three was observed in the left superior SLF and the right OR (**Figure 9**). Analysis of this correlation during each of the sub-intervals did not reveal any regions of significant clusters between the first and second time point, but a significant cluster was observed in the right posterior SLF between the second and third time points (**Figure 9**).

DISCUSSION

Longitudinal brain changes following TBI are sparsely documented. In this study we examined TBI patients over a period of four years and found that rather than showing a circumscribed period of brain degeneration following injury, TBI involves a protracted period of brain change that continues for several years. The results of this study suggest that studying alterations in brain WM may provide clues to neuropsychological function following TBI, and potentially inform upon the clinical course of patients following injury.

In our study, we found significant effects in the corpus callosum, which is commonly injured in TBI. The group by time interaction observed in the FA factorial model combined with the simple effects analyses indicates that the TBI subjects demonstrated a significantly greater reduction in FA in the genu of the corpus callosum during the first year post-injury than during the subsequent three years of the total follow-up period. This result is commensurate with previous work on a different subset of individuals in this cohort indicating FA reductions in this region during the first year post-injury (Bendlin et al., 2008), as well as other previous studies that have also found longitudinal WM decline in this region during the first year (Xu et al., 2007; Wu et al., 2010). Our results also demonstrated that the observed FA effect was driven by increased radial, rather than decreased axial, diffusivity, which is consistent with previous observations (Sidaros et al., 2008; Kumar et al., 2010). Other recent research has indicated that initial injury to the genu is highly predictive of patient outcome (in terms of general disability), however, we did not

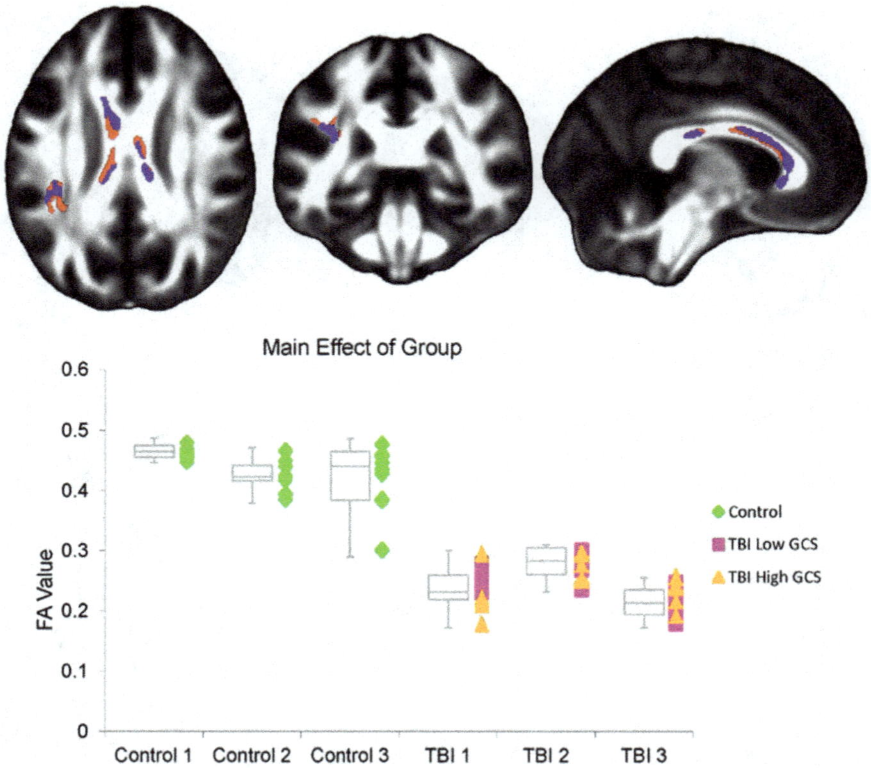

FIGURE 3 | (Top) A significant effect of time was observed throughout the corpus callosum as well as in the left SLF within the FA factorial model (red). Axial and radial diffusivity analyses were restricted to regions demonstrating an FA effect. Within this region, a significant effect of time was also observed within the radial diffusivity factorial model (overlapping blue region), but not the axial diffusivity factorial model. The left side of the statistical map is patient left and right is patient right. (**Bottom**) This graph shows the average FA value for each subject at each of the three time points within the corpus callosum cluster demonstrating an FA effect. Controls are marked as green diamonds, TBI patients with a 24 h GCS score of 7 or lower are marked as pink squares, and patients with a 24 h GCS score of 10 or higher are marked as orange triangles. Box plots indicate the 75th percentile, median, and 25th percentile FA values of each group at each time point, and whiskers indicate 1.5 times inter-quartile ranges.

observe correlations between FA change in this region over time and change in neuropsychological task performance (Matsukawa et al., 2011).

The main effect of time combined with simple effects analyses indicate that TBI patients experienced a continued decline in FA throughout the corpus callosum that continued throughout the duration of the four year period studied, and that this decrease was driven by increases in radial diffusivity. It has been suggested that initial tearing, shearing, and misalignment of axons initiates an inflammatory cascade that leads to further WM damage, myelin loss, and gliosis, and we expect that these processes were critical to the gradual, long-term FA reductions observed here (Povlishock, 2000).

The main effect of group combined with between-groups simple effects analyses indicate that TBI subjects exhibited reduced FA in several major tracts, that this difference was persistent for at least four years post-injury, and that a combination of reduced axial and increased radial diffusivity gave rise to these FA differences. These results collectively demonstrate that in several major tracts there is reduced directional coherence of WM among our TBI subjects that is both widespread and long-lasting. These between-groups differences are consistent with cross-sectional observations (Chan et al., 2003; Nakayama et al., 2006; Kiraly and Kiraly, 2007; Xu et al., 2007; Bendlin et al., 2008; Sidaros et al., 2008; Wang et al., 2011).

Our simple effects results also demonstrate that TBI subjects demonstrated increases in FA in the SLF bilaterally as well as in a portion of the OR during the course of the study, potentially signifying improvement of WM integrity or alternatively showing loss of crossing fibers in these brain regions. No previous study that we are aware of has demonstrated longitudinal increases in FA among TBI patients. This is likely because no previous study that we are aware of followed patients for four years as the current study did, and the FA increases we observed appear to have taken place gradually during the four year study duration. Previous research has, however, identified apparent improvements in FA in animal models of TBI (Rubovitch et al., 2011), and in either axial or radial diffusivity among human TBI patients (Sidaros et al., 2008; Kumar et al., 2010), indicating that our present finding is potentially replicable. This evidence of subtle neurological recovery merits further investigation, particularly in clinical settings. The secondary result indicating that this increase in FA was driven by a longitudinal decrease in radial diffusivity (rather than an increase in axial diffusivity) could suggest improved myelin integrity within the tract, however, it is equally plausible that progressive loss of damaged axons that is observed in animal models

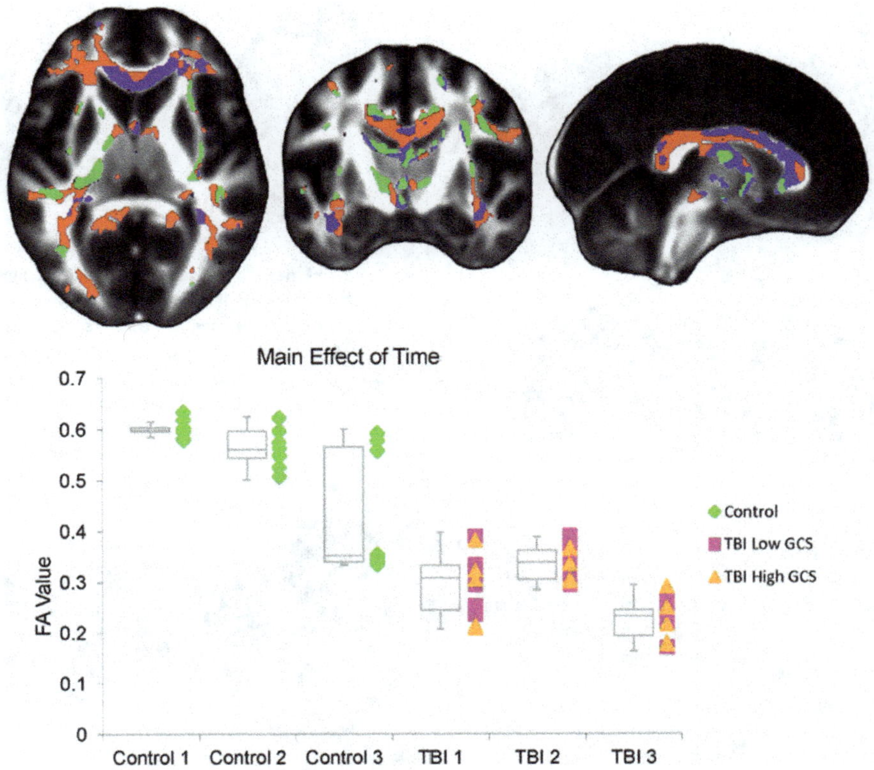

FIGURE 4 | (Top) A significant effect of group was observed within the FA factorial model in several white matter tracts throughout the brain, including the cerebral peduncle, inferior and superior longitudinal fascicule (ILF and SLF), internal and external capsule, inferior fronto-occipital fasciculus, sagittal stratum, corpus callosum, fornix, optic radiations, thalamic radiations, uncinate fasciculus, and corona radiata (red). Axial and radial diffusivity analyses were restricted to regions demonstrating an FA effect. Within this set of regions, a significant effect of group was also observed within the radial diffusivity factorial model (overlapping blue regions), as well as the axial diffusivity factorial model (overlapping green yellow regions). Regions in which a significant effect was seen in the FA, radial diffusivity, and axial diffusivity models are shown in green. The left side of the statistical map is patient left and right is patient right. **(Bottom)** This graph shows the average FA value for each subject at each of the three time points within the regions demonstrating an FA effect. Controls are marked as green diamonds, TBI patients with a 24 h GCS score of 7 or lower are marked as pink squares, and patients with a 24 h GCS score of 10 or higher are marked as orange triangles. Box plots indicate the 75th percentile, median, and 25th percentile FA values of each group at each time point, and whiskers indicate 1.5 times inter-quartile ranges.

of TBI (Creed et al., 2011) may underlie the observed FA changes in our TBI cohort.

The fact that longitudinal changes in radial (rather than axial) diffusivity were found in the same regions where FA changes were found warrants further attention. In the literature, findings concerning radial diffusivity and TBI tend to be relatively consistent across studies, whereas findings relating to axial diffusivity are inconsistent. Many studies have reported longitudinal increases in radial diffusivity in the absence of changes in axial diffusivity and like in the current study these changes have frequently been localized to the corpus callosum (Mac Donald et al., 2007; Newcombe et al., 2007; Ewing-Cobbs et al., 2008; Tasker et al., 2010). Differences in axial diffusivity, however, have been inconsistent, with some groups finding increases (Sidaros et al., 2008; Tasker et al., 2010), decreases (Li et al., 2011) or no change (Mac Donald et al., 2007) in both the corpus callosum and other regions. These inconsistencies may be due to differences in how long after injury patient scans were obtained. While FA variations may be related to myelin change, axonal change, or differences in directional coherence of fibers (e.g., presence of absence of crossing fibers), changes in axial diffusivity are thought to be associated primarily with axonal changes while changes in radial diffusivity are thought to relate to myelin changes (Song et al., 2002; Alexander et al., 2007; Xie et al., 2010). These findings indicate that progressive FA loss observed among our subjects was likely driven by progressive myelin pathology, possibly due to persistent inflammation (Ramlackhansingh et al., 2011). While progressive FA increases observed could have been driven by improvements in myelin integrity, the removal of axons with damaged myelin by phagocytotic processes likely also contributed to our result.

While it is not plausible to determine why some regions showed FA increases while others showed decreases with imaging data alone, it is nonetheless instructive to speculate on this matter. One likely contributing factor is the specific injuries sustained by this cohort of TBI patients. The corpus callosum is frequently that center of severe damage during TBI, and the subjects in this cohort were no exception. Several subjects' initial radiology notes included mentions of corpus callosal damage, but none mentioned other tracts specifically. It is possible, therefore,

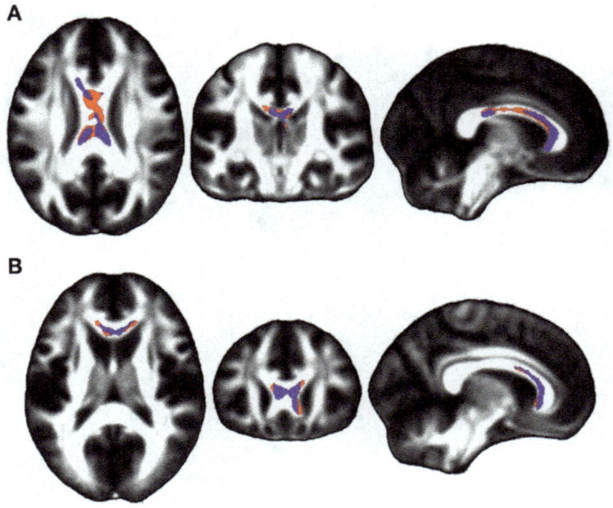

FIGURE 5 | (A) Simple effects analysis within the FA factorial model revealed a significant region of the corpus callosum in which TBI subjects exhibited greater FA at the first time point compared to the third time point (red), indicating a longitudinal FA reduction during the four year study duration. The equivalent test in controls did not produce any significant clusters. Secondary axial and radial diffusivity analyses were renstricted to regions demonstrating an FA effect. Axial and radial diffusivity analyses demonstrated that in this region there was a significant increase in radial diffusivity, but no decrease in axial diffusivity, during the four year study (overlapping blue region). **(B)** Analysis of this region during the two sub-intervals revealed that there was a significant FA reduction between the first and second time points in the genu of the corpus callosum among TBI subjects (red), but no clusters between the second and third time points. Secondary axial and radial diffusivity analyses were restricted to regions demonstrating an FA effect. Axial and radial diffusivity analyses demonstrated that in this region there was a significant increase in radial diffusivity, but no decrease in axial diffusivity, between the first and second time points (overlapping blue region). The left side of the statistical map is patient left and right is patient right.

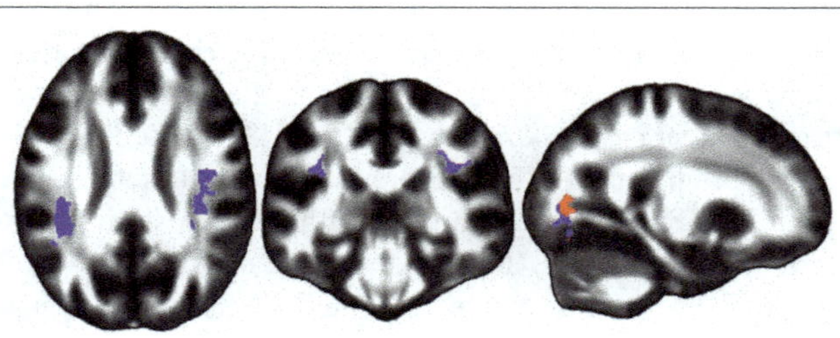

FIGURE 6 | Simple effects analysis within the FA factorial model revealed significant regions in the bilateral SLF in which TBI subjects exhibited greater FA at the third time point compared to the first time point (red), indicating a longitudinal FA increase during the four year study duration. The equivalent test in controls did not produce any significant clusters. Secondary axial and radial diffusivity analyses were restricted to this region demonstrating an FA effect. Axial and radial diffusivity analyses demonstrated that in this region there was a significant decrease in radial diffusivity during the four year study period (overlapping blue region), but no accompanying increase in axial diffusivity. The left side of the statistical map is patient left and right is patient right.

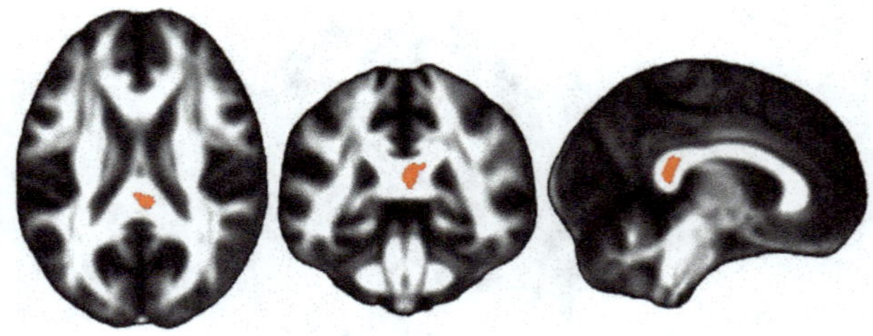

FIGURE 7 | Linear regression analyses, in which neuropsychological test scores were the independent variables and FA maps were the dependent variables, demonstrated a significant correlation between performance on a finger tapping task and FA in the splenium of the corpus callosum among TBI patients at the second time point (red). The left side of the statistical map is patient left and right is patient right.

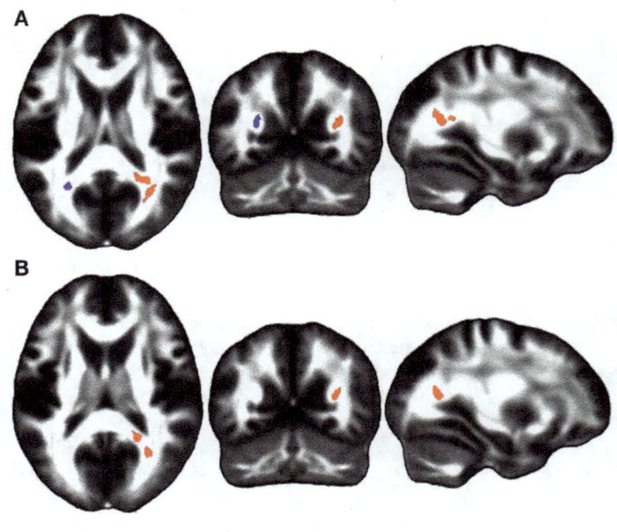

FIGURE 8 | (A) Linear regression analyses demonstrated a significant positive correlation between TBI patients' performance on the Trails A visuomotor speed task and FA in bilateral regions of the sagittal stratum at the first time point (red), and in a unilateral region of the left sagittal stratum at the second time point (overlapping blue region). **(B)** A positive correlation was also observed between change in Trails A score between the first and third time points and change in sagittal stratum FA over the same four year study duration (red). The left side of the statistical map is patient left and right is patient right.

the continued deterioration was observed in regions with greater initial damage. Another complementary possibility is that differential tract properties promote different responses to insult. Research with animal models has demonstrated that astrocytic proliferation can occur in responses to focal injury, but only certain subclasses of neurons are capable of this type of structural remodeling (Blizzard et al., 2011). Further research, most likely in animal models, is necessary to determine why certain regions continue to deteriorate post-injury while others remain static or even improve.

GCS score and WM integrity were not correlated in TBI patients, likely due to the heterogeneity of patients' injuries. It is probable that more severely injured individuals had greater WM

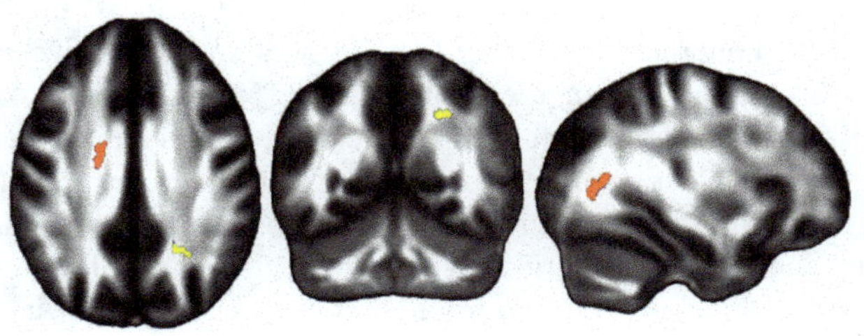

FIGURE 9 | Linear regression analyses revealed a significant positive correlation between change in the cognitive component of the Trails B score between time one and time three and FA change in the left superior SLF and right optic radiation over the same four year study duration (red). Analyses of sub-intervals revealed there was also a significant positive correlation between change in the Trails B cognitive component between the first and second time points, and FA change in the right posterior SLF over the same one year first interval duration (yellow). The left side of the statistical map is patient left and right is patient right.

damage near impact sites, but variable injury locations across subjects precluded group-wise identification of these differences. The neuropsychological correlations we observed were consistent with our hypothesis that FA and neuropsychological task performance would correlate positively. In TBI patients, damage to the splenium indexed by lower FA was associated with slower finger tapping speed, consistent with previous studies linking corpus callosum to manual motor tasks (Muetzel et al., 2008; Caeyenberghs et al., 2011a,b).

Faster performance on the Trails A test was associated with higher FA in the SS, an interesting finding given that this tract is known to be implicated in visuomotor functions. Individuals with greater damage to this tract likely had more difficulty completing the task (Makris et al., 2005; Hao et al., 2011). Over time, this relationship held, with a subset of TBI patients showing longitudinal improvements in Trails A completion speed between the first and third time points and a corresponding increase in FA in the SS over the same interval.

Correlations were also observed between change in the Trails B cognitive component score over time and change in FA values among TBI patients. A correlation was observed between the first and third time points in the left SLF and the right OR, as well as in the right SLF between the second and third time points. Previous work has demonstrated that FA in the SLF is is associated with complex functions such as attentiveness, working memory and reading skills (Karlsgodt et al., 2008; Frye et al., 2010). The SLF subserves a wide variety of connective functions, and the longitudinal improvements in directional coherence of fibers within this tract among TBI patients in this study may have contributed to improved scores on the Trails B cognitive component measure. Interestingly, we also found a relationship in the OR (a tract relevant to the relay of visual information from the lateral geniculate nucleus to the visual cortex); this may suggest that subtracting Trails A scores from Trails B scores does not entirely remove the visuomotor element of the task, or possibly that this tract is important for subserving the cognitive component of a visuomotor task. Overall, our neuropsychological correlations demonstrate that the differences in FA observed in our study do indeed have an impact on cognitive and motor function, and that subtle increases in FA over time reflect WM change that is related to improved functionality in patients. While it should be noted that the neuropsychological correlations reported in the current study may be specific to the set of patients included and their particular patterns of WM damage, it is nonetheless informative to identify functional relevancies of WM change.

In addition to the primary analyses and results presented in this paper, we also conducted an investigatory simple effects analysis of whole-brain radial diffusivity changes within our patients. This analysis was carried out within the radial diffusivity factorial model used in our primary analysis, but the search was not restricted to regions demonstrating FA change. The results of this analysis, which used the same statistical parameters as our primary FA analysis, indicated that within our cohort longitudinal decreases in radial diffusivity (approximating improvements in myelin integrity) were found in regions throughout the brain during the four year study duration. Regions included superior and inferior longitudinal fasiculi, internal and external capsules, the descending corticospinal tract, and forceps major and minor (**Figure A1**). While this analysis is beyond the planned scope and goals of the current study, it is provocative and may be informative to future research.

The results of this study likely have significant clinical relevance. Specifically, it is notable that we observed WM changes occurring for several years post-injury because the continued malleability of the injured brain holds promise for the effectiveness of treatments well beyond the three to six month window in which treatments are typically prescribed. The FA increase observed in this study has particular relevance to treatment options, as it reflects plasticity and represents a potential physiological basis of rehabilitation. In order to truly assess the relevance of these results to clinical applications, a clinical trial study would be necessary. In such a study, DTI would be used as an outcome measure with the expectation that patients undergoing treatment would exhibit less deterioration or greater improvement in regional brain WM integrity. A positive result would underscore the clinical relevance of our findings.

The current study has methodological limitations that should be considered. Firstly, the results of our study may be limited by methodological limitations imposed by performing a patient and control comparison. For example, it is possible that preprocessing of imaging data and even MR signal of interest can be affected differentially by group. Voxel-wise comparisons of brain images are dependent upon accurate alignment to a template; in order to minimize error, all FA maps were visually inspected for within-subject tract alignment to the template and alignment across all participants. Another potential limitation concerns the greater ratio of women to men in the control group compared to the TBI group. Due to this, we used gender as a covariate in all analyses. In this study we were not able to account for the intensity or duration of rehabilitations programs in which some of our patients participated. Future clinical trials are critical to understanding how rehabilitation programs impact neurological recovery.

Concurrent volume loss exhibited by TBI patients could also have confounded our results. Volume loss following injury is well established in the TBI literature (Levine et al., 2008; Merkley et al., 2008; Sidaros et al., 2009), and has also been observed in this particular cohort of patients (Bendlin et al., 2008). While any DTI study done on this patient population will have results obtained in the context of volume loss, it is nonetheless important to acknowledge that tissue contraction, in addition to microstructural reorganization, may contribute to observed changes in DTI metrics. To ensure that our results were not due solely to volumetric changes, we conducted a native space region of interest analysis on the genu of the corpus callosum. The genu was selected because it is a functionally relevant region and is easily identifiable. FA values were extracted from 3 mm spherical ROIs placed in the center of the genu in each participant's native space DTI images from Visits 1, 2, and 3. Independent samples two-tailed t-tests showed that TBI patients had reduced FA compared to controls at all three time points (Visit 1: Controls-$m = 0.77$, TBIs-$m = 0.67$, $p = 0.005$; Visit 2: Controls-$m = 0.79$, TBIs-$m = 0.63$, $p = 0.0003$; Visit 3: Controls-$m = 0.79$, TBIs-$m = 0.61$, $p = 0.001$). Paired samples two-tailed t-tests showed that TBI patients demonstrated a reduction in FA between Visits 1 and 2 ($p = 0.01$) as well as between visits 1 and 3 ($p = 0.04$). Paired samples t-tests showed no longitudinal changes within the control group. These results mirror the observations made in our whole-brain analysis, and partially allay concerns about the confounding effects of concurrent volume change.

Finally, the results of this study may be limited by the small number of participants that were followed through all three time points. The TBI population and college aged controls are both itinerant populations, and therefore, difficult to track for long periods of time. Notwithstanding this limitation, follow-up of TBI patients over three time points makes this an extremely valuable sample. Furthermore, we did not find significant differences in age, education or injury severity within either group between those who dropped out of the study and those who completed all three visits, suggesting that selective drop-out did not bias the results.

In this study, we show that TBI patients exhibit longitudinal WM changes that continue for at least four years post-injury. These changes include both progressive reductions in FA (observed in the corpus callosum) as well as progressive FA increases (observed in the bilateral SLF). Within the regions where FA changes were found, radial diffusivity alterations were present—suggesting myelin changes continued to occur throughout the period studied. Furthermore, neuropsychological correlations indicate that diffusion metrics are related to cognitive and motor abilities, and that improved directional coherence within tracts is relevant to improved task performance in certain brain regions among TBI patients. The fact that changes continued to develop for several years post-injury provides support for the hypothesis that TBI is not merely an event but rather the initiation of a prolonged disease state with potentially lifelong systemic impacts. FA increases are of particular note due to the unprecedented nature of these findings. TBI is generally conceptualized as strictly a degenerative condition and evidence of what might be long-term neurological improvement could be of significant clinical importance. We strive to continue to improve our understanding of these long-term effects following traumatic injury. An important area of work going forward will be to capitalize on signs of gradual long-term neurological and functional improvement observed in TBI, and to further understand the brain correlates of ameliorative change, which likely occurs alongside progressive degeneration.

ACKNOWLEDGMENTS

This study was supported by a Merit Review Grant from the Department of Veterans Affairs, the NIH MH65723 (SCJ), NIH AG000213 and by the facilities and resources of the William S. Middleton Memorial Veterans Hospital. The assistance of Lisa Newman, Amy Hawley, Donald McLaren, and Erik Kastman is greatly appreciated. We would also like to acknowledge the support of researchers and staff at the Waisman Center, University of Wisconsin, Madison, where MR imaging took place. Finally, we thank all the patients who took part in this study. The contents of this report do not necessarily represent the views of the Department of Veterans Affairs or the United States Government.

REFERENCES

Alexander, A. L., Lee, J. E., Lazar, M., and Field, A. S. (2007). Diffusion tensor imaging of the brain. *Neurotherapeutics* 4, 316–329.

Anderson, C. V., Bigler, E. D., and Blatter, D. D. (1995). Frontal lobe lesions, diffuse damage, and neuropsychological functioning in traumatic brain-injured patients. *J. Clin. Exp. Neuropsychol.* 17, 900–908.

Arfanakis, K., Haughton, V. M., Carew, J. D., Rogers, B. P., Dempsey, R. J., and Meyerand, M. E. (2002). Diffusion tensor MR imaging in diffuse axonal injury. *AJNR Am. J. Neuroradiol.* 23, 794–802.

Bendlin, B. B., Ries, M. L., Lazar, M., Alexander, A. L., Dempsey, R. J., Rowley, H. A., Sherman, J. E., and Johnson, S. C. (2008). Longitudinal changes in patients with traumatic brain injury assessed with diffusion-tensor and volumetric imaging. *Neuroimage* 42, 503–514.

Bigler, E. D., Blatter, D. D., Johnson, S. C., Anderson, C. V., Russo, A. A., Gale, S. D., Ryser, D. K., MacNamara, S. E., and Bailey, B. J. (1996). Traumatic brain injury, alcohol and quantitative neuroimaging: preliminary findings. *Brain Inj.* 10, 197–206.

Blizzard, C. A., Chuckowree, J. A., King, A. E., Hosie, K. A., McCormack, G. H., Chapman, J. A., Vickers, J. C., and Dickson, T. C. (2011). Focal damage to the adult rat neocortex induces wound healing accompanied by axonal sprouting and dendritic structural plasticity. *Cereb. Cortex* 21, 281–291.

Bombardier, C. H., Fann, J. R., Temkin, N. R., Esselman, P. C., Barber, J., and Dikmen, S. S. (2010). Rates of major depressive disorder and clinical outcomes following traumatic brain injury. *JAMA* 303, 1938–1945.

Caeyenberghs, K., Leemans, A., Coxon, J., Leunissen, I., Drijkoningen, D., Geurts, M., Gooijers, J., Michiels, K., Sunaert, S., and Swinnen, S. P. (2011a). Bimanual coordination and corpus callosum microstructure in young adults with traumatic brain injury: a diffusion tensor imaging study. *J. Neurotrauma* 28, 897–913.

Caeyenberghs, K., Leemans, A., Geurts, M., Linden, C. V., Smits-Engelsman, B. C., Sunaert, S., and Swinnen, S. P. (2011b). Correlations between white matter integrity and motor function in traumatic brain injury patients. *Neurorehabil. Neural Repair* 25, 492–502.

Chan, J. H., Tsui, E. Y., Peh, W. C., Fong, D., Fok, K. F., Leung, K. M., Yuen, M. K., and Fung, K. K. (2003). Diffuse axonal injury: detection of changes in anisotropy of water diffusion by diffusion-weighted imaging. *Neuroradiology* 45, 34–38.

Creed, J. A., DiLeonardi, A. M., Fox, D. P., Tessler, A. R., and Raghupathi, R. (2011). Concussive brain trauma in the mouse results in acute cognitive deficits and sustained impairment of axonal function. *J. Neurotrauma* 28, 547–563.

Ewing-Cobbs, L., Prasad, M. R., Swank, P., Kramer, L., Cox, C. S. Jr., Fletcher, J. M., Barnes, M., Zhang, X., and Hasan, K. M. (2008). Arrested development and disrupted callosal microstructure following pediatric traumatic brain injury: relation to neurobehavioral outcomes. *Neuroimage* 42, 1305–1315.

Field, A. S., Hasan, K., Jellison, B. J., Arfanakis, K., and Alexander, A. L. (2003). Diffusion tensor imaging in an infant with traumatic brain swelling. *AJNR Am. J. Neuroradiol.* 24, 1461–1464.

Filippi, C. G., Ulug, A. M., Ryan, E., Ferrando, S. J., and van Gorp, W. (2001). Diffusion tensor imaging of patients with HIV and normal-appearing white matter on MR images of the brain. *AJNR Am. J. Neuroradiol.* 22, 277–283.

Forman, S. D., Cohen, J. D., Fitzgerald, M., Eddy, W. F., Mintun, M. A., and Noll, D. C. (1995). Improved assessment of significant activation in functional magnetic resonance imaging (fMRI): use of a cluster-size threshold. *Magn. Reson. Med.* 33, 636–647.

Frye, R. E., Hasan, K., Malmberg, B., Desouza, L., Swank, P., Smith, K., and Landry, S. (2010). Superior longitudinal fasciculus and cognitive dysfunction in adolescents born preterm and at term. *Dev. Med. Child Neurol.* 52, 760–766.

Gale, S. D., Johnson, S. C., Bigler, E. D., and Blatter, D. D. (1995). Nonspecific white matter degeneration following traumatic brain injury. *J. Int. Neuropsychol. Soc.* 1, 17–28.

Hao, X., Xu, D., Bansal, R., Dong, Z., Liu, J., Wang, Z., Kangarlu, A., Liu, F., Duan, Y., Shova, S., Gerber, A. J., and Peterson, B. S. (2011). Multimodal magnetic resonance imaging: the coordinated use of multiple, mutually informative probes to understand brain structure and function. *Hum. Brain Mapp.* doi: 10.1002/hbm.21440. [Epub ahead of print].

Karlsgodt, K. H., van Erp, T. G., Poldrack, R. A., Bearden, C. E., Nuechterlein, K. H., and Cannon, T. D. (2008). Diffusion tensor imaging of the superior longitudinal fasciculus and working memory in recent-onset schizophrenia. *Biol. Psychiatry* 63, 512–518.

Kim, J., Avants, B., Patel, S., Whyte, J., Coslett, B. H., Pluta, J., Detre, J. A., and Gee, J. C. (2008). Structural consequences of diffuse traumatic brain injury: a large deformation tensor-based morphometry study. *Neuroimage* 39, 1014–1026.

Kiraly, M., and Kiraly, S. J. (2007). Traumatic brain injury and delayed sequelae: a review–traumatic brain injury and mild traumatic brain injury (concussion) are precursors to later-onset brain disorders, including early-onset dementia. *ScientificWorldJournal* 7, 1768–1776.

Kraus, M. F., Susmaras, T., Caughlin, B. P., Walker, C. J., Sweeney, J. A., and Little, D. M. (2007). White matter integrity and cognition in chronic traumatic brain injury: a diffusion tensor imaging study. *Brain* 130(Pt 10), 2508–2519.

Kumar, R., Saksena, S., Husain, M., Srivastava, A., Rathore, R. K., Agarwal, S., and Gupta, R. K. (2010). Serial changes in diffusion tensor imaging metrics of corpus callosum in moderate traumatic brain injury patients and their correlation with neuropsychometric tests: a 2-year follow-up study. *J. Head Trauma Rehabil.* 25, 31–42.

Le Bihan, D. (1991). Molecular diffusion nuclear magnetic resonance imaging. *Magn. Reson. Q.* 7, 1–30.

Levin, H. S. (2003). Neuroplasticity following non-penetrating traumatic brain injury. *Brain Inj.* 17, 665–674.

Levine, B., Kovacevic, N., Nica, E. I., Cheung, G., Gao, F., Schwartz, M. L., and Black, S. E. (2008). The Toronto traumatic brain injury study: injury severity and quantified MRI. *Neurology* 70, 771–778.

Li, J., Li, X. Y., Feng, D. F., and Gu, L. (2011). Quantitative evaluation of microscopic injury with diffusion tensor imaging in a rat model of diffuse axonal injury. *Eur. J. Neurosci.* 33, 933–945.

Lin, M. R., Chiu, W. T., Chen, Y. J., Yu, W. Y., Huang, S. J., and Tsai, M. D. (2010). Longitudinal changes in the health-related quality of life during the first year after traumatic brain injury. *Arch. Phys. Med. Rehabil.* 91, 474–480.

Ljungqvist, J., Nilsson, D., Ljungberg, M., Sorbo, A., Esbjornsson, E., Eriksson-Ritzen, C., and Skoglund, T. (2011). Longitudinal study of the diffusion tensor imaging properties of the corpus callosum in acute and chronic diffuse axonal injury. *Brain Inj.* 25, 370–378.

Mac Donald, C. L., Dikranian, K., Bayly, P., Holtzman, D., and Brody, D. (2007). Diffusion tensor imaging reliably detects experimental traumatic axonal injury and indicates approximate time of injury. *J. Neurosci.* 27, 11869–11876.

Makris, N., Kennedy, D. N., McInerney, S., Sorensen, A. G., Wang, R., Caviness, V. S. Jr., and Pandya, D. N. (2005). Segmentation of subcomponents within the superior longitudinal fascicle in humans: a quantitative, *in vivo*, DT-MRI study. *Cereb. Cortex* 15, 854–869.

Malec, J. F., Brown, A. W., Moessner, A. M., Stump, T. E., and Monahan, P. (2010). A preliminary model for posttraumatic brain injury depression. *Arch. Phys. Med. Rehabil.* 91, 1087–1097.

Marquez de la Plata, C. D., Hart, T., Hammond, F. M., Frol, A. B., Hudak, A., Harper, C. R., O'Neil-Pirozzi, T. M., Whyte, J., Carlile, M., and Diaz-Arrastia, R. (2008). Impact of age on long-term recovery from traumatic brain injury. *Arch. Phys. Med. Rehabil.* 89, 896–903.

Masel, B. E., and DeWitt, D. S. (2010). Traumatic brain injury: a disease process, not an event. *J. Neurotrauma* 27, 1529–1540.

Matsukawa, H., Shinoda, M., Fujii, M., Takahashi, O., Yamamoto, D., Murakata, A., and Ishikawa, R. (2011). Genu of corpus callosum in diffuse axonal injury induces a worse 1-year outcome in patients with traumatic brain injury. *Acta Neurochir. (Wien)* 153, 1687–1693. discussion 1693–1694.

Merkley, T. L., Bigler, E. D., Wilde, E. A., McCauley, S. R., Hunter, J. V., and Levin, H. S. (2008). Diffuse changes in cortical thickness in pediatric moderate-to-severe traumatic brain injury. *J. Neurotrauma* 25, 1343–1345.

Muetzel, R. L., Collins, P. F., Mueller, B. A. M., Schissel, A., Lim, K. O., and Luciana, M. (2008). The development of corpus callosum microstructure and associations with bimanual task performance in healthy adolescents. *Neuroimage* 39, 1918–1925.

Nakayama, N., Okumura, A., Shinoda, J., Yasokawa, Y. T., Miwa, K., Yoshimura, S. I., and Iwama, T. (2006). Evidence for white matter disruption in traumatic brain injury without macroscopic lesions. *J. Neurol. Neurosurg. Psychiatry* 77, 850–855.

Newcombe, V. F., Williams, G. B., Nortje, J., Bradley, P. G., Harding, S. G., Smielewski, P., Coles, J. P., Maiya, B., Gillard, J. H., Hutchinson, P. J., Pickard, J. D., Carpenter, T. A., and Menon, D. K. (2007). Analysis of acute traumatic axonal injury using diffusion tensor imaging. *Br. J. Neurosurg.* 21, 340–348.

Povlishock, J. T. (2000). Pathophysiology of neural injury: therapeutic opportunities and challenges. *Clin. Neurosurg.* 46, 113–126.

Povlishock, J. T., and Christman, C. W. (1995). The pathobiology of traumatically induced axonal injury in animals and humans: a review of current thoughts. *J. Neurotrauma* 12, 555–564.

Ramlackhansingh, A. F., Brooks, D. J., Greenwood, R. J., Bose, S. K., Turkheimer, F. E., Kinnunen, K. M., Gentleman, S., Heckemann, R. A., Gunanayagam, K., Gelosa, G., and Sharp, D. J. (2011). Inflammation after trauma: microglial activation and traumatic brain injury. *Ann. Neurol.* 70, 374–383.

Risdall, J. E., and Menon, D. K. (2010). Traumatic brain injury. *Philos. Trans. R. Soc. Lond. B Biol. Sci.* 366, 241–250.

Rubovitch, V., Ten-Bosch, M., Zohar, O., Harrison, C. R., Tempel-Brami, C., Stein, E., Hoffer, B. J., Balaban, C. D., Schreiber, S., Chiu, W. T., and Pick, C. G. (2011). A mouse model of blast-induced mild traumatic brain injury. *Exp. Neurol.* 232, 280–289.

Sharp, D. J., and Ham, T. E. (2011). Investigating white matter injury after mild traumatic brain injury. *Curr. Opin. Neurol.* 24, 558–563.

Sidaros, A., Engberg, A. W., Sidaros, K., Liptrot, M. G., Herning, M., Petersen, P., Paulson, O. B., Jernigan, T. L., and Rostrup, E. (2008). Diffusion tensor imaging during recovery from severe traumatic brain injury and relation to clinical outcome: a longitudinal study. *Brain* 131(Pt 2), 559–572.

Sidaros, A., Skimminge, A., Liptrot, M. G., Sidaros, K., Engberg, A. W., Herning, M., Paulson, O. B., Jernigan, T. L., and Rostrup, E. (2009). Long-term global and regional brain volume changes following severe traumatic brain injury: a longitudinal study with clinical correlates. *Neuroimage* 44, 1–8.

Smith, S. M., Jenkinson, M., Woolrich, M. W., Beckmann, C. F., Behrens, T. E., Johansen-Berg, H., Bannister, P. R., De Luca, M., Drobnjak, I., Flitney, D. E., Niazy, R. K., Saunders, J., Vickers, J., Zhang, Y., De Stefano, N., Brady, J. M., and Matthews, P. M. (2004). Advances in functional and structural MR image analysis and implementation as FSL. *Neuroimage* 23(Suppl. 1), S208–S219.

Song, S. K., Sun, S. W., Ju, W. K., Lin, S. J., Cross, A. H., and Neufeld, A. H. (2003). Diffusion tensor imaging detects and differentiates axon and myelin degeneration in mouse optic nerve after retinal ischemia. *Neuroimage* 20, 1714–1722.

Song, S. K., Sun, S. W., Ramsbottom, M. J., Chang, C., Russell, J., and Cross, A. H. (2002). Dysmyelination revealed through MRI as increased radial (but unchanged axial) diffusion of water. *Neuroimage* 17, 1429–1436.

Staudt, M. (2010). Brain plasticity following early life brain injury: insights from neuroimaging. *Semin. Perinatol.* 34, 87–92.

Tasker, R. C., Westland, A. G., White, D. K., and Williams, G. B. (2010). Corpus callosum and inferior forebrain white matter microstructure are related to functional outcome from raised intracranial pressure in child traumatic brain injury. *Dev. Neurosci.* 32, 374–384.

Trivedi, M. A., Ward, M. A., Hess, T. M., Gale, S. D., Dempsey, R. J., Rowley, H. A., and Johnson, S. C. (2007). Longitudinal changes in global brain volume between 79 and 409 days after traumatic brain injury: relationship with duration of coma. *J. Neurotrauma* 24, 766–771.

Wang, J. Y., Bakhadirov, K., Abdi, H., Devous, M. D. Sr., Marquez de la Plata, C. D., Moore, C., Madden, C. J., and Diaz-Arrastia, R. (2011). Longitudinal changes of structural connectivity in traumatic axonal injury. *Neurology* 77, 818–826.

Wheeler-Kingshott, C. A., and Cercignani, M. (2009). About "axial" and "radial" diffusivities. *Magn. Reson. Med.* 61, 1255–1260.

Wu, T. C., Wilde, E. A., Bigler, E. D., Li, X., Merkley, T. L., Yallampalli, R., McCauley, S. R., Schnelle, K. P., Vasquez, A. C., Chu, Z., Hanten, G., Hunter, J. V., and Levin, H. S. (2010). Longitudinal changes in the corpus callosum following pediatric traumatic brain injury. *Dev. Neurosci.* 32, 361–373.

Xie, M., Tobin, J. E., Budde, M. D., Chen, C. I., Trinkaus, K., Cross, A. H., McDaniel, D. P., Song, S. K., and Armstrong, R. C. (2010). Rostrocaudal analysis of corpus callosum demyelination and axon damage across disease stages refines diffusion tensor imaging correlations with pathological features. *J. Neuropathol. Exp. Neurol.* 69, 704–716.

Xu, J., Rasmussen, I. A., Lagopoulos, J., and Haberg, A. (2007). Diffuse axonal injury in severe traumatic brain injury visualized using high-resolution diffusion tensor imaging. *J. Neurotrauma* 24, 753–765.

The role of apolipoprotein E (*APOE*) genotype in early mild cognitive impairment (E-MCI)

Shannon L. Risacher[1], Sungeun Kim[1,2], Li Shen[1,2], Kwangsik Nho[1], Tatiana Foroud[3], Robert C. Green[4], Ronald C. Petersen[5], Clifford R. Jack Jr.[6], Paul S. Aisen[7], Robert A. Koeppe[8], William J. Jagust[9], Leslie M. Shaw[10], John Q. Trojanowski[10], Michael W. Weiner[11,12] and Andrew J. Saykin[1,2,3]*, for the Alzheimer's Disease Neuroimaging Initiative (ADNI)[†]

[1] Department of Radiology and Imaging Sciences, Center for Neuroimaging, Indiana University School of Medicine, Indianapolis, IN, USA
[2] Center for Computational Biology and Bioinformatics, Indiana University School of Medicine, Indianapolis, IN, USA
[3] Department of Medical and Molecular Genetics, Indiana University School of Medicine, Indianapolis, IN, USA
[4] Division of Genetics, Department of Medicine, Brigham and Women's Hospital and Harvard Medical School, Boston, MA, USA
[5] Department of Neurology, Mayo Clinic, Rochester, MN, USA
[6] Department of Radiology, Mayo Clinic, Rochester, MN, USA
[7] Department of Neurology, University of California, San Diego, San Diego, CA, USA
[8] Department of Radiology, University of Michigan, Ann Arbor, MI, USA
[9] Department of Neurology, University of California, Berkeley, Berkeley, CA, USA
[10] Department of Pathology and Laboratory Medicine, University of Pennsylvania School of Medicine, Philadelphia, PA, USA
[11] Departments of Radiology, Medicine, and Psychiatry, University of California, San Francisco, San Francisco, CA, USA
[12] Department of Veterans Affairs Medical Center, San Francisco, CA, USA

[†] Data used in preparation of this article were obtained from the Alzheimer's Disease Neuroimaging Initiative (ADNI) database (adni.loni.ucla.edu). As such, the investigators within the ADNI contributed to the design and implementation of ADNI and/or provided data but did not participate in analysis or writing of this report. A complete listing of ADNI investigators can be found at: http://adni.loni.ucla.edu/wp-content/uploads/how_to_apply/ADNI_Acknowledgement_List.pdf

Edited by:
Manuel Menéndez-González, Hospital Álvarez-Buylla, Spain

Reviewed by:
Gregory A. Jicha, University of Kentucky, USA
Maria S. M. Palomo, Centro de Especialidades de la Avenida de Portugal y guardias de Neurología, Spain
Marwan N. Sabbagh, Banner Sun Health Research Institute, USA

***Correspondence:**
Andrew J. Saykin, Department of Radiology and Imaging Sciences, Center for Neuroimaging, Indiana University School of Medicine, IU Health Neuroscience Center, Suite 4100, 355 West 16th Street, Indianapolis, IN 46202, USA.
e-mail: asaykin@iupui.edu.

Objective: Our goal was to evaluate the association of *APOE* with amyloid deposition, cerebrospinal fluid levels (CSF) of Aβ, tau, and p-tau, brain atrophy, cognition and cognitive complaints in E-MCI patients and cognitively healthy older adults (HC) in the ADNI-2 cohort.

Methods: Two-hundred and nine E-MCI and 123 HC participants from the ADNI-2 cohort were included. We evaluated the impact of diagnostic status (E-MCI vs. HC) and *APOE* ε4 status (ε4 positive vs. ε4 negative) on cortical amyloid deposition (AV-45/Florbetapir SUVR PET scans), brain atrophy (structural MRI scans processed using voxel-based morphometry and Freesurfer version 5.1), CSF levels of Aβ, tau, and p-tau, and cognitive performance and complaints.

Results: E-MCI participants showed significantly impaired cognition, higher levels of cognitive complaints, greater levels of tau and p-tau, and subcortical and cortical atrophy relative to HC participants ($p < 0.05$). Cortical amyloid deposition and CSF levels of Aβ were significantly associated with *APOE* ε4 status but not E-MCI diagnosis, with ε4 positive participants showing more amyloid deposition and lower levels of CSF Aβ than ε4 negative participants. Other effects of *APOE* ε4 status on cognition and CSF tau levels were also observed.

Conclusions: *APOE* ε4 status is associated with amyloid accumulation and lower CSF Aβ, as well as increased CSF tau levels in early prodromal stages of AD (E-MCI) and HC. Alternatively, neurodegeneration, cognitive impairment, and increased complaints are primarily associated with a diagnosis of E-MCI. These findings underscore the importance of considering *APOE* genotype when evaluating biomarkers in early stages of disease.

Keywords: apolipoprotein E (APOE), early mild cognitive impairment (E-MCI), Florbetapir/AV-45/Amyvid, positron emission tomography (PET), magnetic resonance imaging (MRI), cerebrospinal fluid (CSF), Alzheimer's disease neuroimaging initiative (ADNI)

INTRODUCTION

Alzheimer's disease (AD) is the most common age-related neurodegenerative disease, featuring cognitive decline, accumulation of amyloid plaques and neurofibrillary tangles, and extensive neurodegeneration (Alzheimer's Association, 2011; McKhann et al., 2011). The most commonly accepted prodromal AD stage is mild cognitive impairment (MCI), which is characterized by clinically-relevant cognitive dysfunction in the absence of significant interference with daily functioning (Petersen et al., 1999; Albert et al., 2011). Amnestic MCI features marked memory impairments which are predictive of progression to clinical AD. Recently, MCI patients have been classified into two forms based on severity: early MCI (E-MCI) and late MCI (L-MCI). Relative to an age-appropriate normative level, E-MCI patients show an approximately 1–1.5 standard deviation (SD) decline in memory, while L-MCI patients show a 1.5 SD or greater decline. These designated cut-offs for E-MCI and L-MCI have not been fully explored to date. However, the identification of participants with a 1–1.5 SD deficit in memory as E-MCI may be more sensitive for identifying participants in the earliest stages of cognitive decline. However, the specificity of these diagnostic criteria has yet to be determined and may be lower than the L-MCI cut-offs, allowing participants with more diverse causal factors of cognitive decline (other than prodromal AD) to be included in this diagnostic category. Future studies examining these clinical criteria and clinical and pathological outcomes of identified E-MCI patients relative to L-MCI patients will be important for understanding the cognitive changes observed in these patients. Importantly, these new guidelines provide an opportunity to evaluate the role of AD biomarkers and other potential disease-causing factors in a very early clinical stage. In fact, a recent study demonstrated increased amyloid binding measured using [^{18}F]Florbetapir positron emission tomography (PET) in patients with E-MCI relative to HC, but no alterations in metabolism as assessed using [^{18}F]FDG PET (Wu et al., 2012).

The most common genetic variant associated with late-onset AD is the apolipoprotein E (*APOE*) ε4 allele (Corder et al., 1993; Bertram et al., 2010). The presence of an ε4 allele confers a significantly higher likelihood of developing AD. *APOE* genotype is also associated with AD biomarkers, with the presence of an *APOE* ε4 allele associated with greater amyloid deposition (Drzezga et al., 2009; Morris et al., 2010; Fleisher et al., 2011), a higher degree and faster rate of neurodegeneration (Moffat et al., 2000; Caroli and Frisoni, 2010), alterations in brain function and glucose metabolism (Bookheimer et al., 2000; Bondi et al., 2005; Langbaum et al., 2009), changes in cerebrospinal fluid (CSF) measures of amyloid and tau (Vemuri et al., 2010; Tosun et al., 2011), as well as more impaired cognition (Mayeux et al., 2001; Farlow et al., 2004; Caselli et al., 2011) in patients with L-MCI and AD and cognitively healthy older adults (HC). However, the role of *APOE* genotype in E-MCI has not been assessed. Therefore, the goal of this study is to evaluate the effect of *APOE* ε4 status on amyloid deposition, neurodegeneration, and cognition in patients diagnosed with E-MCI, the earliest clinically-defined prodromal stage of AD.

MATERIALS AND METHODS

ALZHEIMER'S DISEASE NEUROIMAGING INITIATIVE (ADNI)

ADNI was launched in 2004 by the National Institute on Aging (NIA), the National Institute of Biomedical Imaging and Bioengineering (NIBIB), the Food and Drug Administration (FDA), pharmaceutical companies, and non-profit organizations, as a multi-year public-private partnership. The Principal Investigator is Michael W. Weiner, MD, VA Medical Center and UCSF. ADNI is a longitudinal study, ultimately including more than 1200 participants (aged 55–90) recruited from over 50 sites across the United States and Canada. Further information can be found at http://www.adni-info.org/ and in previous reports (Jack et al., 2010; Jagust et al., 2010; Petersen et al., 2010; Saykin et al., 2010; Trojanowski et al., 2010; Weiner et al., 2010). Appropriate Institutional Review Boards approval occurred at each ADNI site and informed consent was obtained from each participant or authorized representative.

PARTICIPANTS

Participants were selected if they were designated as E-MCI or HC (continuing participants or newly enrolled) at the initial visit of the ADNI-GO or ADNI-2 phases and had *APOE* genotype data. The sample included 209 E-MCI patients and 123 HC. Patients were diagnosed with E-MCI using criteria described in the ADNI-2 procedures manual (http://www.adni-info.org/). Briefly, patients were diagnosed with E-MCI using the following criteria:

1. Subject must have a subjective memory concern as reported by subject, study partner, or clinician.
2. Abnormal memory function documented by scoring within the education adjusted ranges on the Logical Memory II subscale (Delayed Paragraph Recall, Paragraph A only) from the Wechsler Memory Scale—Revised (the maximum score is 25):
   a. 9–11 for 16 or more years of education.
   b. 5–9 for 8–15 years of education.
   c. 3–6 for 0–7 years of education.
3. Mini-Mental State Exam score between 24 and 30 (inclusive) (Exceptions may be made for subjects with less than 8 years of education at the discretion of the project director).
4. Clinical Dementia Rating = 0.5; Memory Box score must be at least 0.5.
5. General cognition and functional performance sufficiently preserved such that a diagnosis of Alzheimer's disease cannot be made by the site physician at the time of the screening visit.

In addition, all participants met ADNI inclusion and exclusion criteria which have been described previously (Weiner et al., 2010) and can be found at http://www.adni-info.org/.

APOE genotyping for all participants was performed as previously described (Saykin et al., 2010). In the present study, we sought to evaluate the impact of the presence or absence of an *APOE* ε4 allele on imaging and non-imaging phenotypes. Therefore, all participants were divided into two groups based on *APOE* ε4 status, including participants with one or more ε4 allele (*APOE* ε4 positive (ε4+); 85 E-MCI, 30 HC) and participants without an ε4 allele (*APOE* ε4 negative (ε4−); 124 E-MCI, 93 HC).

CLINICAL AND NEUROPSYCHOLOGICAL ASSESSMENTS

All clinical and neuropsychological test performance data for included participants was downloaded from the ADNI clinical data repository on the Laboratory of Neuro Imaging (LONI) site. Specifically, we evaluated participant performance on the Mini-Mental State Exam (MMSE), Alzheimer's Disease Assessment Scale (ADAS), Montreal Cognitive Assessment (MoCA; Total and all sub-scores), Rey Auditory Verbal Learning Test (RAVLT; Total score, delayed recall score, delayed recognition score), Weschler's Logical Memory Scale—Revised (LM; Immediate and Delayed), Clock Drawing Test (CDT), Trailmaking Test A and B (TMT-A,

TMT-B), Boston Naming Test (BNT), Animal Fluency, and the American National Adult Reading Test (ANART). We also evaluated clinical measures, including a measure of dementia severity [Clinical Dementia Rating Scale (CDR), Sum of Boxes score], general functioning [Functional Assessment Questionnaire (FAQ)], depression [Geriatric Depression Scale (GDS)], and stroke/vascular incident history (Modified Hachinski Scale). Cognitive complaints were assessed using the Measure of Everyday Cognition (E-Cog) from both the patient and an informant. The total level of complaints on the E-Cog (overall and within each domain) for both the participant and the informant were assessed as percentage of items endorsed as either "2 = questionably or occasionally worse," "3 = consistently a little worse," or "4 = consistently much worse." Items endorsed as "9 = I don't know" were excluded.

STRUCTURAL MRI SCANS

All available baseline 3 Tesla structural magnetic resonance imaging (MRI) scans were downloaded from LONI for included E-MCI and HC participants. Scans were corrected prior to download as previously described (Jack et al., 2008, 2010). Most participants had a minimum of two scans from the baseline visit. All available scans were processed using voxel-based morphometry (VBM) implemented in Statistical Parametric Mapping 8 (SPM8) (Ashburner and Friston, 2000) and Freesurfer version 5.1 (Dale et al., 1999; Fischl et al., 1999), as described in previous reports (Dale et al., 1999; Fischl et al., 1999; Ashburner and Friston, 2000; Risacher et al., 2009, 2010) and briefly below:

VBM

Scans were co-registered to a T1-weighted template, segmented into grey matter (GM), white matter (WM), and CSF compartments with bias correction, unmodulated normalized to Montreal Neurologic Institute (MNI) space as $1 \times 1 \times 1$ mm voxels, and smoothed with an 8 mm Gaussian kernel. All scans underwent extensive quality control. Mean GM density was extracted from all available baseline scans for target regions of interest (ROIs) using MarsBaR (Brett et al., 2002). Since most participants had two or more baseline MRI scans, an average GM density measure was calculated for each ROI using the mean GM density values extracted from each of the available baseline scans. Eighteen participants (5 HC ε4−, 2 HC ε4+, 5 E-MCI ε4−, 6 E-MCI ε4+) were excluded from the GM density analyses for missing data or failed processing.

Automated parcellation

Freesurfer version 5.1 was used to extract volumetric and cortical thickness measures. Similar to the VBM ROI data, values from all available baseline scans were averaged to create a mean volumetric or cortical thickness value for each ROI. Seven participants (2 HC ε4−, 1 HC ε4+, 2 E-MCI ε4−, 2 E-MCI ε4+) were excluded from the cortical thickness and volumetric analyses for incomplete data or failed processing.

AMYLOID PET SCANS ([^{11}C]FLORBETAPIR)

Pre-processed [^{11}C]Florbetapir PET scans (Coregistered, Averaged, Standardized Image and Voxel Size, Uniform Resolution) were downloaded from LONI (http://adni.loni.ucla.edu/). Before download, images were averaged, aligned to a standard space, re-sampled to a standard image and voxel size, smoothed to a uniform resolution and normalized to a cerebellar GM reference region resulting in standardized uptake value ratio (SUVR) images as previously described (Jagust et al., 2010). After downloading, the images were aligned to each participant's same visit MRI scan and normalized to MNI space as $2 \times 2 \times 2$ mm voxels using parameters from the MRI segmentation. The normalized scans were evaluated for the effect of *APOE* ε4 status on a voxel-wise basis using a two-sample t-test, masked using a whole-brain mask, and covaried for age, gender, education, and handedness. Significant results were displayed at a voxel-wise threshold of $p < 0.01$ [family-wise error (FWE) correction for multiple comparisons] with a minimum cluster size (k) of 50 voxels. SPM8 was used for all processing and voxel-wise analysis. Mean regional SUVR values were also extracted for target ROIs using MarsBaR. Fourteen participants (6 HC ε4−, 5 HC ε4+, 3 E-MCI ε4−) were excluded from [^{11}C]Florbetapir analyses for missing scan data or failed processing.

CSF BIOMARKERS

Levels of amyloid-beta 1-42 (Aβ), total tau, and phosphorylated tau (p-tau) were measured from all available CSF samples as previously described (Shaw et al., 2009, 2011; Trojanowski et al., 2010). CSF data was downloaded from the LONI site and extracted for all included participants. Of the 332 included participants, 44 participants (25 E-MCI and 19 HC) were missing all CSF data. 4 additional participants (2 E-MCI, 3 HC) were missing CSF tau data and 2 additional HC participants were missing CSF p-tau data. Furthermore, participants with CSF levels outside 3 SDs above or below the mean were excluded, including 6 E-MCI participants with tau levels more than 3 SDs above the mean and 2 E-MCI participants with p-tau levels more than 3 SDs above the mean. Thus, the final samples for CSF analyses included 288 participants in the CSF Aβ analysis, 278 participants in the CSF tau analysis, and 284 participants in the CSF p-tau analysis.

STATISTICAL ANALYSES

We evaluated the effect of diagnosis and *APOE* ε4 status on demographics, cognition, cognitive complaints, amyloid deposition, atrophy, and CSF biomarkers using two-way analysis of covariance (ANCOVA) for continuous variables and a chi-square test for categorical variables implemented in SPSS 19.0 (SPSS, Inc., Chicago, IL). Specifically, the effect of diagnosis (HC vs. E-MCI), *APOE* ε4 status (ε4+ vs. ε4−), and the interaction of diagnosis and ε4 status on performance on clinical and psychometric tests, cognitive complaints, amyloid deposition (mean SUVR from target ROIs), CSF levels of Aβ, tau, and p-tau, and brain atrophy (volume, cortical thickness, and GM density from target ROIs) were assessed. All ANCOVA analyses were covaried for age, gender, education, and handedness. The analysis of neurodegenerative measures was also covaried for total intracranial volume (ICV). The frequency of having one or more *APOE* ε4 alleles was also compared between diagnostic groups (HC vs. E-MCI) using a chi-square test.

Table 1 | Demographics, neuropsychological and clinical test performance, and cognitive complaints [Mean (Standard Error)].

		HC: ε4– (*n* = 93)	HC: ε4+ (*n* = 30)	E-MCI: ε4– (*n* = 124)	E-MCI: ε4+ (*n* = 85)	*p*-values		
						DX	*APOE*	Interaction
Demographics	Age (years)	74.1 (0.72)	73.67 (1.27)	71.47 (0.62)	70.26 (0.75)	0.0007	0.3506	0.6572
	Education (years)	16.47 (0.27)	16.37 (0.48)	15.9 (0.24)	15.78 (0.28)	0.0810	0.7251	0.9756
	Gender (M, F)	49, 44	13, 17	64, 60	52, 33	0.3686	0.4394	0.3258
	Handedness (R, L)	85, 8	28, 2	109, 15	79, 6	0.5619	0.2777	0.5831
Clinical performance	CDR-Sum of Boxes	0.04 (0.06)	0.08 (0.11)	1.15 (0.05)	1.34 (0.06)	0.0000	0.0979	0.2989
	FAQ Total[a]	0.17 (0.25)	0.05 (0.45)	1.66 (0.21)	2.22 (0.26)	0.0000	0.4699	0.2637
	Modified Hachinski Total	0.59 (0.07)	0.37 (0.12)	0.77 (0.06)	0.58 (0.07)	0.0257	0.0164	0.8585
	GDS Total[b]	0.80 (0.14)	0.53 (0.25)	1.87 (0.12)	1.55 (0.15)	0.0000	0.0901	0.8687
Reading	ANART Errors[c]	10.61 (0.83)	9.05 (1.47)	11.22 (0.71)	12.35 (0.88)	0.0606	0.8320	0.1832
General cognition	MMSE Total Score	29.05 (0.14)	28.91 (0.25)	28.57 (0.12)	28.06 (0.15)	0.0002	0.0565	0.2847
	ADAS Cognitive Subtotal[d]	6.25 (0.36)	6.76 (0.63)	7.77 (0.30)	8.60 (0.37)	0.0002	0.1211	0.7147
	ADAS Total Score[e]	9.63 (0.51)	10.38 (0.90)	11.99 (0.44)	13.98 (0.53)	0.0000	0.0266	0.3168
	MoCA Total Score[f]	25.64 (0.27)	24.90 (0.47)	24.12 (0.22)	23.57 (0.28)	0.0000	0.0446	0.7835
Memory	Logical Memory - Immediate	14.78 (0.29)	13.26 (0.50)	10.84 (0.24)	10.85 (0.30)	0.0000	0.0273	0.0267
	Logical Memory - Delayed	13.89 (0.23)	12.51 (0.39)	8.76 (0.19)	8.97 (0.24)	0.0000	0.0318	0.0036
	RAVLT Total Score[d]	44.99 (0.93)	42.48 (1.65)	39.98 (0.79)	37.63 (0.97)	0.0000	0.0320	0.9459
	RAVLT Delayed Recall[d]	7.26 (0.39)	6.61 (0.70)	6.18 (0.33)	5.24 (0.41)	0.0128	0.0976	0.7601
	RAVLT Delayed Recognition[d]	12.82 (0.27)	12.20 (0.48)	11.98 (0.23)	12.01 (0.28)	0.1249	0.3687	0.3238
	MoCA Delayed Memory[g]	2.36 (0.16)	1.67 (0.29)	1.40 (0.14)	1.49 (0.17)	0.0061	0.1356	0.0509
Language and naming	Boston Naming Test Total[e]	28.24 (0.31)	28.64 (0.55)	27.08 (0.26)	27.34 (0.32)	0.0015	0.3790	0.8413
	Animal Fluency Total[d]	21.07 (0.49)	21.63 (0.87)	18.98 (0.42)	18.62 (0.51)	0.0000	0.8704	0.4444
	MoCA Naming[d]	2.90 (0.03)	3.01 (0.06)	2.83 (0.03)	2.89 (0.04)	0.0311	0.0374	0.5251
	MoCA Language[d]	2.52 (0.08)	2.57 (0.13)	2.45 (0.06)	2.34 (0.08)	0.1150	0.7619	0.3858
Visuospatial and executive function	Clock Drawing Score[d]	4.62 (0.06)	4.63 (0.11)	4.69 (0.05)	4.60 (0.07)	0.8319	0.5891	0.4899
	Clock Drawing - Copy Score[d]	4.86 (0.04)	4.93 (0.08)	4.80 (0.04)	4.84 (0.05)	0.2157	0.3119	0.7972
	Trailmaking A[d]	33.40 (1.16)	34.28 (2.05)	34.52 (0.99)	39.06 (1.21)	0.0418	0.0542	0.1943
	Trailmaking B[h]	81.07 (4.34)	79.47 (7.85)	90.52 (3.76)	107.64 (4.58)	0.0007	0.1469	0.0807
	Trailmaking B-A[h]	47.66 (3.99)	45.54 (7.21)	55.94 (3.45)	68.52 (4.2)	0.0021	0.2868	0.1347
	MoCA Visuospatial-Executive[a]	4.29 (0.09)	4.37 (0.16)	4.28 (0.08)	4.04 (0.10)	0.1440	0.4833	0.1444
	MoCA Attention[d]	5.77 (0.07)	5.55 (0.12)	5.64 (0.06)	5.47 (0.07)	0.2040	0.0123	0.7272
	MoCA Abstraction[d]	1.80 (0.06)	1.79 (0.11)	1.69 (0.05)	1.56 (0.06)	0.0276	0.3399	0.4321
	MoCA Orientation[d]	5.94 (0.04)	5.94 (0.08)	5.83 (0.04)	5.74 (0.04)	0.0040	0.3920	0.4418

(Continued)

Table 1 | Continued

		HC: ε4− (*n* = 93)	HC: ε4+ (*n* = 30)	E-MCI: ε4− (*n* = 124)	E-MCI: ε4+ (*n* = 85)	*p*-values		
						DX	*APOE*	Interaction
Patient complaints	E-Cog Patient: Total[d,k]	27.01 (2.59)	28.00 (4.52)	49.04 (2.18)	52.10 (2.67)	0.0000	0.5147	0.7396
	E-Cog Patient: Memory[d,k]	43.09 (2.92)	45.91 (5.11)	73.03 (2.46)	77.60 (3.02)	0.0000	0.2932	0.8033
	E-Cog Patient: Language[d,k]	32.59 (3.16)	33.39 (5.52)	56.31 (2.66)	55.96 (3.26)	0.0000	0.9520	0.8805
	E-Cog Patient: Visuospatial[d,k]	11.55 (3.11)	13.91 (5.43)	28.44 (2.61)	33.46 (3.20)	0.0000	0.3222	0.7216
	E-Cog Patient: Planning[d,k]	12.94 (3.33)	11.29 (5.82)	32.82 (2.80)	38.40 (3.43)	0.0000	0.6230	0.3654
	E-Cog Patient: Organization[d,k]	20.69 (3.56)	17.07 (6.22)	38.33 (2.99)	38.16 (3.67)	0.0000	0.6576	0.6858
	E-Cog Patient: Divided Attention[d,k]	36.55 (4.10)	41.95 (7.16)	59.36 (3.44)	64.13 (4.23)	0.0000	0.3011	0.9485
Informant complaints	E-Cog Informant: Total[i,k]	11.38 (2.39)	14.83 (4.18)	40.00 (2.01)	45.78 (2.47)	0.0000	0.1087	0.6866
	E-Cog Informant: Memory[i,k]	21.04 (2.98)	25.77 (5.21)	61.73 (2.51)	64.77 (3.08)	0.0000	0.2778	0.8138
	E-Cog Informant: Language[i,k]	8.71 (2.95)	15.11 (5.16)	38.32 (2.48)	44.24 (3.05)	0.0000	0.0829	0.9454
	E-Cog Informant: Visuospatial[j,k]	5.42 (2.78)	4.18 (4.86)	21.23 (2.35)	32.97 (2.87)	0.0000	0.1166	0.0528
	E-Cog Informant: Planning[i,k]	7.44 (3.25)	10.97 (5.68)	31.80 (2.73)	37.94 (3.35)	0.0000	0.2155	0.7375
	E-Cog Informant: Organization[i,k]	7.62 (3.25)	9.34 (5.68)	32.36 (2.73)	37.20 (3.35)	0.0000	0.4009	0.6891
	E-Cog Informant: Divided Attention[i,k]	18.38 (4.07)	23.69 (7.12)	56.69 (3.43)	57.89 (4.20)	0.0000	0.5051	0.6736

[a] *2 HC (1 ε4+, 1 ε4−) missing data.*

[b] *2 E-MCI (1 ε4+, 1 ε4−) missing data.*

[c] *2 HC (1 ε4+, 1 ε4−), 5 E-MCI (2 ε4+, 3 ε4−) missing data.*

[d] *1 HC (ε4+) missing data.*

[e] *1 HC (ε4+), 1 E-MCI (ε4−) missing data.*

[f] *3 HC (1 ε4+, 2 ε4−), 1 E-MCI (ε4+) missing data*

[g] *2 HC (1 ε4+, 1 ε4−), 1 E-MCI (ε4+) missing data.*

[h] *2 HC (2 ε4+), 4 E-MCI (1 ε4+, 3 ε4−) missing data.*

[i] *4 HC (1 ε4+, 3 ε4−) missing data.*

[j] *4 HC (ε4+), 1 E-MCI (ε4−) missing data.*

[k] *Patient and informant E-Cog values are expressed as a percentage of items endorsed (total and within each domain); see text for additional description.*

RESULTS

DEMOGRAPHICS, PSYCHOMETRIC PERFORMANCE, AND COGNITIVE COMPLAINTS

Significantly more E-MCI were *APOE* ε4+ than HC ($p = 0.003$), with 85 of 209 E-MCI participants (40.7%) showing one or more ε4 alleles relative to only 30 of 123 HC participants (24.4%). Demographics and psychometric performance variables for E-MCI and HC participants stratified by *APOE* ε4 status are shown in **Table 1**. The effect of diagnosis, ε4 status, and the interaction between diagnosis and ε4 status are displayed. Age was significantly different between diagnostic groups ($p < 0.05$) but not *APOE* ε4 groups. A significant interaction between diagnosis and ε4 status on LM Immediate and Delayed performance was observed, with ε4+ HC showing worse performance on both measures than ε4− HC participants but no difference by ε4 status in E-MCI participants. A trend for a significant interaction on the MoCA delayed recall sub-score ($p = 0.05$) was also observed, again with a significant effect of ε4 status in HC but not E-MCI participants. Finally, a marginally significant interaction of diagnosis and ε4 status for informant complaints in the visuospatial domain ($p = 0.05$) was also seen, with ε4 status having an effect only in E-MCI participants.

Significant effects of diagnosis on the CDR-SB, FAQ, Modified Hachinski Total, and GDS were observed ($p < 0.05$), with E-MCI participants showing a greater CDR-SB, as well as higher scores on the FAQ, Modified Hachinski, and GDS. Differences in psychometric performance by diagnosis were observed for nearly every test ($p < 0.05$), except for the RAVLT Delayed Recognition, CDT (Total and Copy Scores), and the MoCA language, executive-visuospatial function, and attention sub-scores. Significant differences in cognitive complaints from both the participant and the informant by diagnosis were also observed in all domains ($p < 0.001$). In all cases, E-MCI participants had worse cognition and more cognitive complaints than HC participants.

Vascular risk factors and/or stroke history was significantly different by *APOE* ε4 status ($p < 0.05$), with ε4+ participants showing lower Modified Hachinski Total scores. In addition, ε4 status was significantly associated with performance on a number of psychometric tests, including the ADAS Total score, MoCA Total score, RAVLT Total score, and the MoCA naming and attention sub-scores ($p < 0.05$). The effect of ε4 status was also significant at a trend level for TMT-A ($p = 0.05$). For these comparisons, ε4+ participants demonstrated worse performance than ε4−.

VOXEL-BASED COMPARISONS OF AMYLOID DEPOSITION

ε4+ E-MCI showed significantly greater amyloid deposition upon voxel-wise analysis than ε4− (**Figure 1**; voxel-wise threshold: $p < 0.01$ (FWE), $k = 50$ voxels). The most significant cluster was observed in the left orbitofrontal cortex (**Figure 1A**). Additional significant clusters were observed in the medial frontal

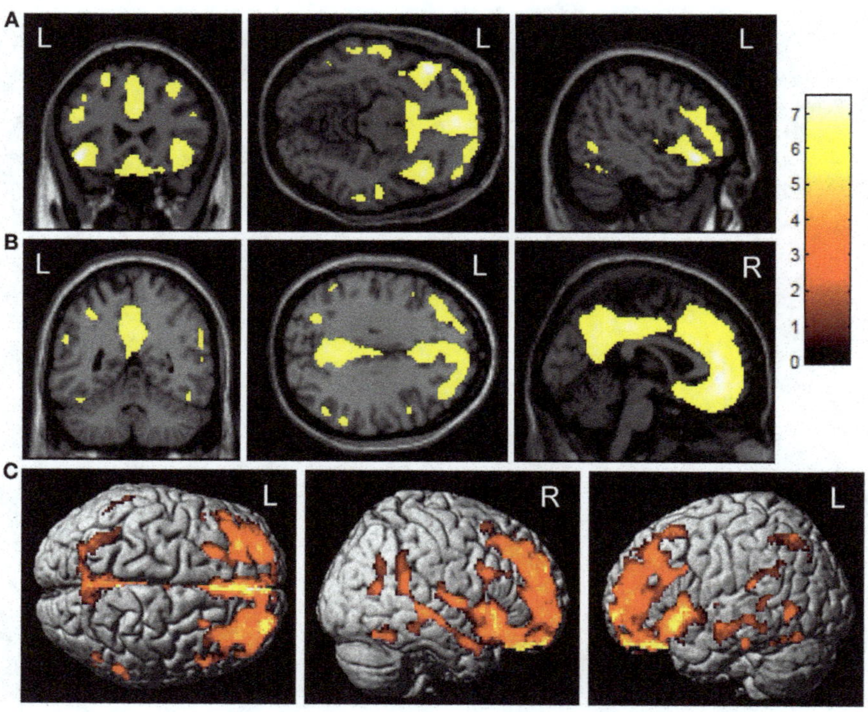

FIGURE 1 | Voxel-wise association of *APOE* ε4 status and amyloid deposition in E-MCI participants. Greater cortical amyloid deposition was observed in *APOE* ε4+ ($n = 85$) relative to *APOE* ε4− ($n = 121$) E-MCI participants. Significant clusters were observed in the medial and lateral frontal lobes **(A)**, anterior and posterior cingulate **(B)**, and lateral temporal lobes. Surface renderings show the diffuse pattern of significant clusters **(C)**. All analyses were covaried for age, gender, education, and handedness and a voxel-wise threshold of $p < 0.01$ (FWE correction for multiple comparisons) and minimum cluster size (k) of 50 voxels was considered significant.

lobe/anterior cingulate cortex, the right orbitofrontal cortex, and the posterior cingulate/precuneus (**Figure 1B**). The surface rendering also reflects the widespread pattern of significant differences with significant clusters throughout the frontal, parietal, and temporal lobes (**Figure 1C**). No significant clusters were observed in the reverse comparison (ε4− > ε4+; *data not shown*).

ROI COMPARISONS OF AMYLOID DEPOSITION

ROI results were consistent with voxel-wise findings demonstrating significantly greater global and regional amyloid deposition in ε4+ relative to ε4− E-MCI participants in the global cortex, mean frontal lobe, anterior cingulate, and precuneus (**Figure 2**). A significant effect of ε4 status ($p < 0.001$) but not diagnosis was observed in all ROI measures, with ε4+ participants showing greater amyloid than ε4− participants regardless of diagnosis (HC or E-MCI). Overall, amyloid PET results indicate that ε4+ individuals showed greater amyloid deposition than ε4− regardless of cognitive impairment in the earliest stages of decline.

ROI COMPARISONS OF NEURODEGENERATION

Hippocampal neurodegeneration (volume and GM density) was associated with diagnosis ($p < 0.001$; **Figures 3A,B**) but not *APOE* ε4 status. E-MCI participants showed more hippocampal atrophy than HC. However, a significant interaction effect of diagnosis and ε4 status on mean temporal lobe cortical thickness was observed ($p = 0.008$; **Figure 3C**), with ε4+ HC participants showing thicker mean temporal lobes than all other groups. Mean temporal lobe GM density was also significantly associated with diagnosis ($p = 0.005$) and ε4 status ($p = 0.047$; **Figure 3D**), as E-MCI patients showed smaller mean temporal lobe GM density than HC and ε4− participants showed smaller mean temporal lobe GM density than ε4+ participants.

CSF LEVELS OF Aβ, TAU, AND p-tau

CSF levels of Aβ, tau, and p-tau were significantly affected by diagnosis and *APOE* ε4 status (**Figure 4**). Levels of CSF Aβ were significantly associated with ε4 status ($p < 0.001$), with ε4+ participants showing lower levels of Aβ than ε4− participants (**Figure 4A**). CSF tau levels were significantly affected by

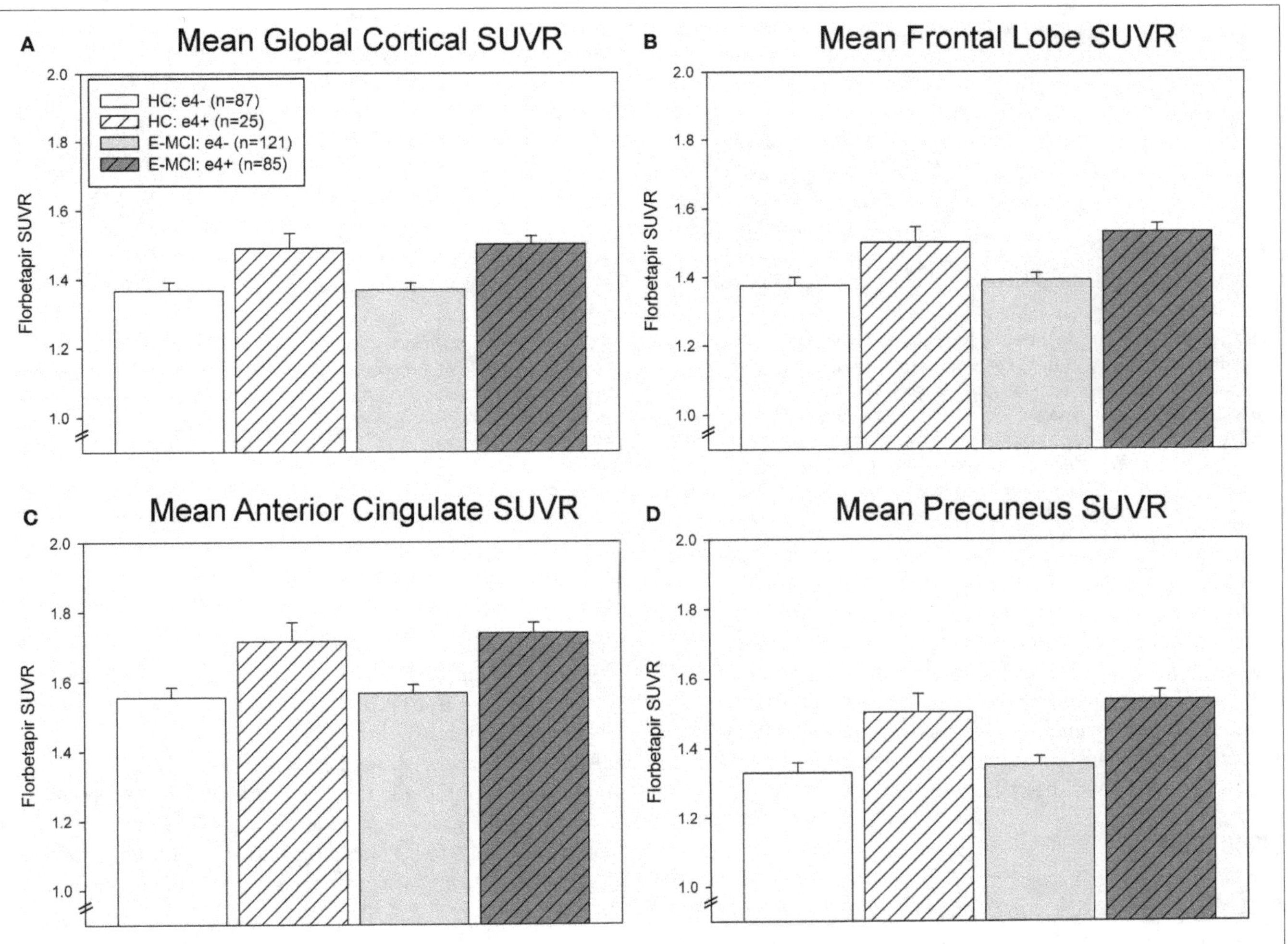

FIGURE 2 | Regional effects of *APOE* ε4 status on amyloid deposition in E-MCI and HC participants. A significant effect of *APOE* ε4 status on regional amyloid deposition was observed ($p < 0.001$), including in the global cortical mean amyloid **(A)**, mean bilateral frontal lobes **(B)**, anterior cingulate **(C)**, and precuneus **(D)**. In all evaluated regions, *APOE* ε4+ E-MCI ($n = 85$) and HC ($n = 25$) participants showed a higher mean standardized uptake value ratio (SUVR) than *APOE* ε4− E-MCI ($n = 121$) and HC ($n = 87$) participants. No significant effect of diagnostic status was observed.

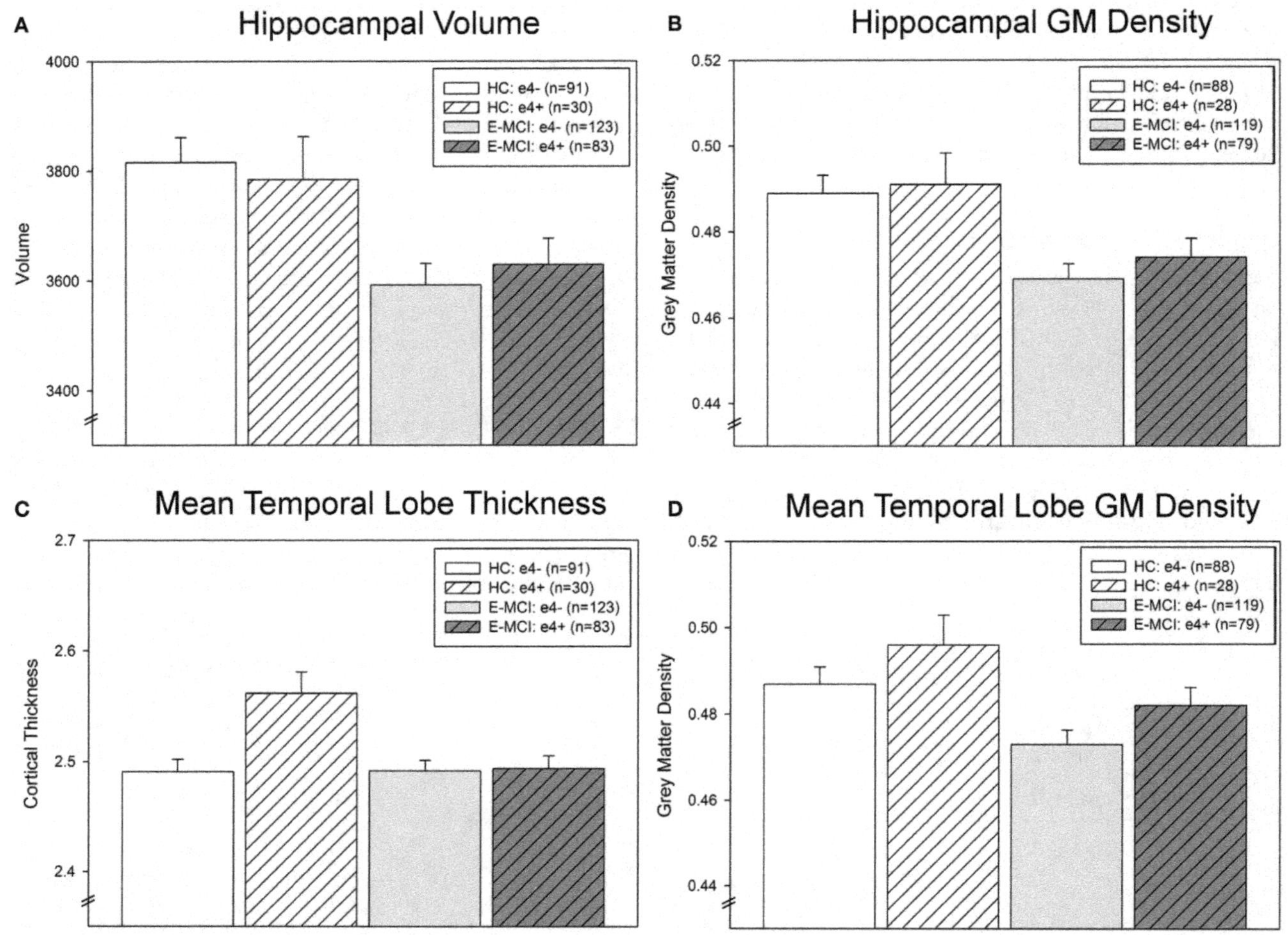

FIGURE 3 | Temporal lobe atrophy is associated with *APOE* ε4 status and diagnostic group in E-MCI and HC participants. A significant effect of diagnosis on neurodegeneration in the temporal lobe was observed ($p < 0.05$), including in hippocampal volume **(A)** and grey matter (GM) density **(B)**, mean temporal lobe cortical thickness **(C)**, and mean temporal lobe GM density **(D)**. In all evaluated regions, E-MCI participants showed more temporal lobe atrophy than HC participants. In addition, *APOE* ε4 status was significantly associated with mean temporal lobe GM density, with *APOE* ε4− participants showing smaller mean temporal lobe GM density than *APOE* ε4+ participants. Finally, a significant interaction effect of diagnosis and *APOE* ε4 status was observed in mean temporal lobe cortical thickness, with ε4− HC participants showing thicker mean temporal lobes than all other groups. All analyses were covaried for age, gender, education, handedness, and total intracranial volume (ICV). The total number of participants for each analysis is indicated on each graph (Panels **A–D**). Note: Thirteen participants were excluded from the GM density analyses, but not the cortical thickness and volumetric analyses, for failed VBM segmentation (3 HC ε4−, 2 HC ε4+, 4 E-MCI ε4−, 4 E-MCI ε4+).

both diagnosis ($p = 0.041$) and ε4 status ($p < 0.001$; **Figure 4B**). E-MCI patients had higher tau levels than HC participants and ε4+ participants had higher levels than ε4− participants. Finally, an interaction between diagnosis and ε4 status on p-tau was also observed ($p = 0.046$), primarily driven by a higher level of p-tau in ε4+ HC and E-MCI participants (**Figure 4C**).

DISCUSSION

This study provides a comprehensive evaluation of the impact of *APOE* ε4 status on cognition, cognitive complaints, amyloid deposition, neurodegeneration, and CSF Aβ, tau, and p-tau levels in E-MCI and HC. As expected, we observed a significant association of diagnosis with clinical and cognitive status. Furthermore, diagnosis was associated with neurodegeneration and CSF tau and p-tau levels but not with amyloid deposition. Cognitive performance, amyloid deposition, temporal lobe atrophy, and CSF tau and p-tau levels were significantly associated with ε4 status, with ε4+ participants showing poorer cognition, less temporal lobe atrophy, and higher CSF tau and p-tau levels. ε4+ participants also showed greater cortical amyloid deposition and lower CSF Aβ levels. Finally, an interaction between diagnosis and ε4 status was observed for memory performance, temporal lobe cortical thickness, and CSF p-tau levels. Overall, the results suggest that *APOE* ε4 status impacts AD-related pathological and clinical changes in E-MCI and HC.

The effect of *APOE* genotype on amyloid deposition has been shown previously, including in middle-aged and older cognitively healthy adults, as well as patients with L-MCI and AD (Drzezga et al., 2009; Shaw et al., 2009; Morris et al., 2010; Fleisher et al., 2011; Tosun et al., 2011). Biochemically, *APOE* genotype has

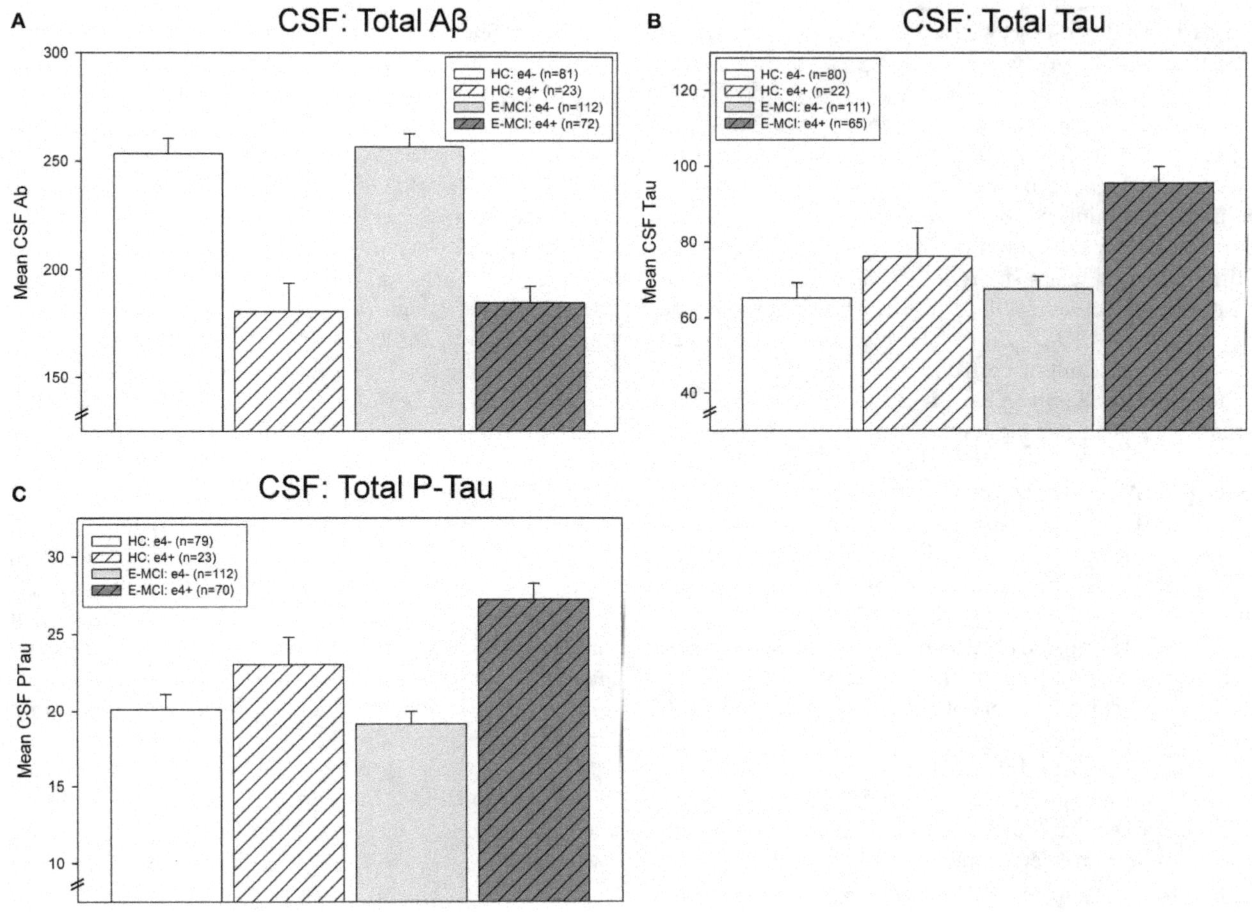

FIGURE 4 | Effects of *APOE* ε4 status and diagnosis on CSF protein levels in E-MCI and HC participants. Diagnostic group and *APOE* ε4 status significantly affected CSF levels of Aβ **(A)**, total tau **(B)**, and p-tau **(C)**. CSF Aβ was significantly associated to *APOE* ε4 status ($p < 0.001$), with *APOE* ε4+ E-MCI and HC participants showing lower levels of Aβ than *APOE* ε4− E-MCI and HC participants, regardless of diagnosis. Total tau levels were significantly affected by both diagnosis ($p < 0.05$) and *APOE* ε4 status ($p < 0.001$), with E-MCI patients showing higher total tau levels than HC participants and *APOE* ε4+ showing higher levels than *APOE* ε4− participants. Finally, an interaction between diagnostic status and *APOE* ε4 status on CSF p-tau levels was also observed ($p < 0.05$), primarily driven by a higher level of p-tau in *APOE* ε4+ HC and E-MCI participants relative to *APOE* ε4− HC and E-MCI participants. The total number of participants in each analysis is shown for each graph (Panels **A–C**). Note: See text for description of participants excluded from the CSF analysis.

been shown to affect Aβ clearance rate, with the APOE ε4 isoform showing significantly slower clearance (Deane et al., 2008; Castellano et al., 2011; Holtzman et al., 2012). The lack of diagnostic effect on amyloid deposition in this study suggests that in the earliest stages of cognitive change, *APOE* ε4 status has a stronger relationship to amyloid deposition than cognitive status.

The additional findings of a diagnostic effect on cognition, cognitive complaints, neurodegeneration, and CSF tau and p-tau levels underscore the importance of E-MCI as a diagnostic entity. Thus, this report has notable clinical implications, particularly in the potential implementation and utilization of E-MCI as a clinical diagnostic entity. Patients with E-MCI show changes in cognition and selected biomarkers, suggesting that these individuals may have a higher likelihood of clinical progression. The association of cognition and complaints to atrophic changes, rather than amyloid levels, supports E-MCI as an intermediate stage with pathology beyond amyloid accumulation.

These results further support the Jack et al. model of AD biomarkers, suggesting that changes in cognition and neurodegeneration occur after measurable amyloid accumulation (Saykin et al., 2010; Jack et al., 2011). Additionally, *APOE* ε4 genotype may alter the hypothesized sigmoidal curves, in particular amyloid accumulation. These results also indicate the importance of genetic background in determining likelihood and extent of amyloid accumulation, even in preclinical stages, which may be particularly important in clinical trial enrollment. Further, in the era of personalized medicine, the implications of *APOE* genotype disclosure to patients in a clinical setting must be carefully considered, given the impact of *APOE* on AD risk and amyloid deposition (Green et al., 2009; Roberts et al., 2011).

The observed greater temporal lobe cortical thickness and GM density in ε4+ participants, particularly in HC, is somewhat unexpected and may be related to the modest sample size of the ε4+ HC group. However, previous studies have observed increased cortical thickness, including in middle-aged *APOE* ε4 positive participants (Espeseth et al., 2008), in cognitively HC who are transitioning to become CSF Aβ biomarker positive (Fortea et al., 2011), and in asymptomatic patients positive for a *PSEN1* mutation more than 9 years prior to the clinical onset (Fortea et al., 2010). Thus, future studies including longitudinal follow-up with an expanded sample will be important in determining the significance of this finding.

The present study has a few notable limitations. First, we evaluated the effect of *APOE* ε4 status on AD biomarkers in only HC and E-MCI rather than across the disease spectrum. Although our goal was to evaluate *APOE* in the earliest stages of AD, future studies assessing the full clinical spectrum are warranted. In addition, we did not evaluate all known biomarkers of AD, including FDG PET or advanced MRI techniques (i.e., diffusion tensor imaging, resting-state functional MRI, etc.). These measures are available in subsets of the ADNI-GO/2 cohort and thus, future studies evaluating these measures would augment the findings of the present report. Thirdly, genome-wide genetic data for this cohort was recently released. Future studies assessing other variants may provide information about the role of genetics in very early stages of AD. Finally, the present study evaluates only cross-sectional measures. Future studies using longitudinal and clinical outcome data will allow assessment of the role of *APOE* in progression of HC and E-MCI.

In summary, we assessed the role of *APOE* ε4 status on clinical and cognitive measures, cognitive complaints, and imaging and CSF biomarkers in HC and E-MCI participants from the ADNI-GO/2 cohort. We determined that *APOE* ε4 status is associated with increased amyloid deposition in both HC and E-MCI, while diagnostic category is associated with measures of cognition and cognitive complaints, as well as neurodegeneration. Therefore, we conclude that *APOE* is an important mediator of amyloid pathology in the earliest stages of AD-associated clinical decline.

ACKNOWLEDGMENTS

Data collection and sharing for this project was funded by the Alzheimer's Disease Neuroimaging Initiative (ADNI) [National Institutes of Health (NIH) Grant U01 AG024904 (PI: MW Weiner)]. ADNI is funded by the National Institute on Aging (NIA), the National Institute of Biomedical Imaging and Bioengineering (NIBIB), and through generous contributions from the following: Abbott; Alzheimer's Association; Alzheimer's Drug Discovery Foundation; Amorfix Life Sciences Ltd.; AstraZeneca; Bayer HealthHCare; BioClinica, Inc.; Biogen Idec Inc.; Bristol-Myers Squibb Company; Ei6sai Inc.; Elan Pharmaceuticals Inc.; Eli Lilly and Company; F. Hoffmann-La Roche Ltd. and its affiliated company Genentech, Inc.; GE HealthHCare; Innogenetics, N.V.; IXICO Ltd.; Janssen Alzheimer Immunotherapy Research & Development, LLC.; Johnson & Johnson Pharmaceutical Research & Development LLC.; Medpace, Inc.; Merck & Co., Inc.; Meso Scale Diagnostics, LLC.; Novartis Pharmaceuticals Corporation; Pfizer Inc.; Servier; Synarc Inc.; and Takeda Pharmaceutical Company, with participation from the US FDA. The Canadian Institutes of Health Research is providing funds to support ADNI clinical sites in Canada. Private sector contributions are facilitated by the Foundation for the National Institutes of Health (www.fnih.org). The grantee organization is the Northern California Institute for Research and Education, and the study is coordinated by the Alzheimer's Disease Cooperative Study at the University of California, San Diego. ADNI data are disseminated by Laboratory for Neuro Imaging at the University of California, Los Angeles. ADNI was also supported by NIH grants P30 AG010129, K01 AG030514, and the Dana Foundation. Additional support for analyses included in the present report was provided by the following sources: NIA R01 AG19771 (to Andrew J. Saykin), NIA P30 AG10133-18S1 (to Dr. Bernardino Ghetti and Andrew J. Saykin), NLM R01 LM011360 (to Li Shen and Andrew J. Saykin), K24 AG027841 (to Robert C. Green), an Indiana CTSI Predoctoral Fellowship (TL1 RR025759 to Shannon L. Risacher), NIA U01-AG10483 [to Paul S. Aisen (PI)], NIA U01-AG024904 [to Paul S. Aisen (Coordinating Center Director)], NIA R01-AG030048 [to Paul S. Aisen (PI)], NIA R01-AG16381 [to Paul S. Aisen (Co-I)], NIH AG027859 [to William J. Jagust (PI)], NIH AG027984 [to William J. Jagust (PI)], and NIH AG 024904 [William J. Jagust (Co-I)].

REFERENCES

Albert, M. S., Dekosky, S. T., Dickson, D., Dubois, B., Feldman, H. H., Fox, N. C., et al. (2011). The diagnosis of mild cognitive impairment due to Alzheimer's disease: recommendations from the National Institute on Aging-Alzheimer's Association workgroups on diagnostic guidelines for Alzheimer's disease. *Alzheimers Dement.* 7, 270–279.

Ashburner, J., and Friston, K. J. (2000). Voxel-based morphometry–the methods. *Neuroimage* 11, 805–821.

Association, A. S. (2011). 2011 Alzheimer's disease facts and figures. *Alzheimers Dement.* 7, 208–244.

Bertram, L., Lill, C. M., and Tanzi, R. E. (2010). The genetics of Alzheimer disease: back to the future. *Neuron* 68, 270–281.

Bondi, M. W., Houston, W. S., Eyler, L. T., and Brown, G. G. (2005). fMRI evidence of compensatory mechanisms in older adults at genetic risk for Alzheimer disease. *Neurology* 64, 501–508.

Bookheimer, S. Y., Strojwas, M. H., Cohen, M. S., Saunders, A. M., Pericak-Vance, M. A., Mazziotta, J. C., et al. (2000). Patterns of brain activation in people at risk for Alzheimer's disease. *N. Engl. J. Med.* 343, 450–456.

Brett, M., Anton, J.-L., Valabregue, R., and Poline, J.-B. (2002). "Region of interest analysis using an SPM toolbox [abstract]," in *Presented at the 8th International Conference on Functional Mapping of the Human Brain, June 2–6, 2002.* (Sendai, Japan).

Caroli, A., and Frisoni, G. B. (2010). The dynamics of Alzheimer's disease biomarkers in the Alzheimer's Disease Neuroimaging Initiative cohort. *Neurobiol. Aging* 31, 1263–1274.

Caselli, R. J., Dueck, A. C., Locke, D. E., Hoffman-Snyder, C. R., Woodruff, B. K., Rapcsak, S. Z., et al. (2011). Longitudinal modeling of frontal cognition in APOE epsilon4 homozygotes, heterozygotes, and noncarriers. *Neurology* 76, 1383–1388.

Castellano, J. M., Kim, J., Stewart, F. R., Jiang, H., Demattos, R. B., Patterson, B. W., et al. (2011). Human apoE isoforms differentially regulate brain amyloid-beta peptide clearance. *Sci. Transl. Med.* 3, 89ra57.

Corder, E. H., Saunders, A. M., Strittmatter, W. J., Schmechel, D. E., Gaskell, P. C., Small, G. W., et al. (1993). Gene dose of apolipoprotein E type 4 allele and the risk of Alzheimer's disease in late onset families. *Science* 261, 921–923.

Dale, A., Fischl, B., and Sereno, M. (1999). Cortical surface-based analysis. I. Segmentation and surface reconstruction. *Neuroimage* 9, 179–194.

Deane, R., Sagare, A., Hamm, K., Parisi, M., Lane, S., Finn, M. B., et al. (2008). apoE isoform-specific disruption of amyloid beta peptide clearance from mouse brain. *J. Clin. Invest.* 118, 4002–4013.

Drzezga, A., Grimmer, T., Henriksen, G., Muhlau, M., Perneczky, R., Miederer, I., et al. (2009). Effect of APOE genotype on amyloid plaque load and gray matter volume in Alzheimer disease. *Neurology* 72, 1487–1494.

Espeseth, T., Westlye, L. T., Fjell, A. M., Walhovd, K. B., Rootwelt, H., and Reinvang, I. (2008). Accelerated age-related cortical thinning in healthy carriers of apolipoprotein E epsilon 4. *Neurobiol. Aging* 29, 329–340.

Farlow, M. R., He, Y., Tekin, S., Xu, J., Lane, R., and Charles, H. C. (2004). Impact of APOE in mild cognitive impairment. *Neurology* 63, 1898–1901.

Fischl, B., Sereno, M., and Dale, A. (1999). Cortical surface-based analysis. II: Inflation, flattening, and a surface-based coordinate system. *Neuroimage* 9, 195–207.

Fleisher, A. S., Chen, K., Liu, X., Roontiva, A., Thiyyagura, P., Ayutyanont, N., et al. (2011). Using positron emission tomography and florbetapir F18 to image cortical amyloid in patients with mild cognitive impairment or dementia due to Alzheimer disease. *Arch. Neurol.* 68, 1404–1411.

Fortea, J., Sala-Llonch, R., Bartres-Faz, D., Bosch, B., Llado, A., Bargallo, N., et al. (2010). Increased cortical thickness and caudate volume precede atrophy in PSEN1 mutation carriers. *J. Alzheimers Dis.* 22, 909–922.

Fortea, J., Sala-Llonch, R., Bartres-Faz, D., Llado, A., Sole-Padulles, C., Bosch, B., et al. (2011). Cognitively preserved subjects with transitional cerebrospinal fluid ss-amyloid 1-42 values have thicker cortex in Alzheimer's disease vulnerable areas. *Biol. Psychiatry* 70, 183–190.

Green, R. C., Roberts, J. S., Cupples, L. A., Relkin, N. R., Whitehouse, P. J., Brown, T., et al. (2009). Disclosure of APOE genotype for risk of Alzheimer's disease. *N. Engl. J. Med.* 361, 245–254.

Holtzman, D. M., Herz, J., and Bu, G. (2012). Apolipoprotein e and apolipoprotein e receptors: normal biology and roles in Alzheimer disease. *Cold Spring Harb. Perspect. Med.* 2:a006312. doi: 10.1101/cshperspect.a006312

Jack, C. R. Jr., Bernstein, M. A., Borowski, B. J., Gunter, J. L., Fox, N. C., Thompson, P. M., et al. (2010). Update on the magnetic resonance imaging core of the Alzheimer's disease neuroimaging initiative. *Alzheimers Dement.* 6, 212–220.

Jack, C. R. Jr., Bernstein, M. A., Fox, N. C., Thompson, P., Alexander, G., Harvey, D., et al. (2008). The Alzheimer's Disease Neuroimaging Initiative (ADNI): MRI methods. *J. Magn. Reson. Imaging* 27, 685–691.

Jack, C. R. Jr., Vemuri, P., Wiste, H. J., Weigand, S. D., Aisen, P. S., Trojanowski, J. Q., et al. (2011). Evidence for ordering of Alzheimer disease biomarkers. *Arch. Neurol.* 68, 1526–1535.

Jagust, W. J., Bandy, D., Chen, K., Foster, N. L., Landau, S. M., Mathis, C. A., et al. (2010). The Alzheimer's Disease Neuroimaging Initiative positron emission tomography core. *Alzheimers Dement.* 6, 221–229.

Langbaum, J. B., Chen, K., Lee, W., Reschke, C., Bandy, D., Fleisher, A. S., et al. (2009). Categorical and correlational analyses of baseline fluorodeoxyglucose positron emission tomography images from the Alzheimer's Disease Neuroimaging Initiative (ADNI). *Neuroimage* 45, 1107–1116.

Mayeux, R., Small, S. A., Tang, M., Tycko, B., and Stern, Y. (2001). Memory performance in healthy elderly without Alzheimer's disease: effects of time and apolipoprotein-E. *Neurobiol. Aging* 22, 683–689.

McKhann, G. M., Knopman, D. S., Chertkow, H., Hyman, B. T., Jack, C. R. Jr., Kawas, C. H., et al. (2011). The diagnosis of dementia due to Alzheimer's disease: recommendations from the National Institute on Aging-Alzheimer's Association workgroups on diagnostic guidelines for Alzheimer's disease. *Alzheimers Dement.* 7, 263–269.

Moffat, S. D., Szekely, C. A., Zonderman, A. B., Kabani, N. J., and Resnick, S. M. (2000). Longitudinal change in hippocampal volume as a function of apolipoprotein E genotype. *Neurology* 55, 134–136.

Morris, J. C., Roe, C. M., Xiong, C., Fagan, A. M., Goate, A. M., Holtzman, D. M., et al. (2010). APOE predicts amyloid-beta but not tau Alzheimer pathology in cognitively normal aging. *Ann. Neurol.* 67, 122–131.

Petersen, R. C., Aisen, P. S., Beckett, L. A., Donohue, M. C., Gamst, A. C., Harvey, D. J., et al. (2010). Alzheimer's Disease Neuroimaging Initiative (ADNI): clinical characterization. *Neurology* 74, 201–209.

Petersen, R. C., Smith, G. E., Waring, S. C., Ivnik, R. J., Tangalos, E. G., and Kokmen, E. (1999). Mild cognitive impairment: clinical characterization and outcome. *Arch. Neurol.* 56, 303–308.

Risacher, S. L., Saykin, A. J., West, J. D., Shen, L., Firpi, H. A., and McDonald, B. C. (2009). Baseline MRI predictors of conversion from MCI to probable AD in the ADNI cohort. *Curr. Alzheimer Res.* 6, 347–361.

Risacher, S. L., Shen, L., West, J. D., Kim, S., McDonald, B. C., Beckett, L. A., et al. (2010). Longitudinal MRI atrophy biomarkers: relationship to conversion in the ADNI cohort. *Neurobiol. Aging* 31, 1401–1418.

Roberts, J. S., Christensen, K. D., and Green, R. C. (2011). Using Alzheimer's disease as a model for genetic risk disclosure: implications for personal genomics. *Clin. Genet.* 80, 407–414.

Saykin, A. J., Shen, L., Foroud, T. M., Potkin, S. G., Swaminathan, S., Kim, S., et al. (2010). Alzheimer's Disease Neuroimaging Initiative biomarkers as quantitative phenotypes: genetics core aims, progress, and plans. *Alzheimers Dement.* 6, 265–273.

Shaw, L. M., Vanderstichele, H., Knapik-Czajka, M., Clark, C. M., Aisen, P. S., Petersen, R. C., et al. (2009). Cerebrospinal fluid biomarker signature in Alzheimer's disease neuroimaging initiative subjects. *Ann. Neurol.* 65, 403–413.

Shaw, L. M., Vanderstichele, H., Knapik-Czajka, M., Figurski, M., Coart, E., Blennow, K., et al. (2011). Qualification of the analytical and clinical performance of CSF biomarker analyses in ADNI. *Acta Neuropathol.* 121, 597–609.

Tosun, D., Schuff, N., Shaw, L. M., Trojanowski, J. Q., and Weiner, M. W. (2011). Relationship between CSF biomarkers of Alzheimer's disease and rates of regional cortical thinning in ADNI data. *J. Alzheimers Dis.* 26(Suppl. 3), 77–90.

Trojanowski, J. Q., Vandeerstichele, H., Korecka, M., Clark, C. M., Aisen, P. S., Petersen, R. C., et al. (2010). Update on the biomarker core of the Alzheimer's Disease Neuroimaging Initiative subjects. *Alzheimers Dement.* 6, 230–238.

Vemuri, P., Wiste, H. J., Weigand, S. D., Knopman, D. S., Shaw, L. M., Trojanowski, J. Q., et al. (2010). Effect of apolipoprotein E on biomarkers of amyloid load and neuronal pathology in Alzheimer disease. *Ann. Neurol.* 67, 308–316.

Weiner, M. W., Aisen, P. S., Jack, C. R. Jr., Jagust, W. J., Trojanowski, J. Q., Shaw, L., et al. (2010). The Alzheimer's disease neuroimaging initiative: progress report and future plans. *Alzheimers Dement.* 6, 202 e207-211 e207.

Wu, L., Rowley, J., Mohades, S., Leuzy, A., Dauar, M. T., Shin, M., et al. (2012). Dissociation between Brain Amyloid Deposition and Metabolism in Early Mild Cognitive Impairment. *PLoS ONE* 7:e47905. doi: 10.1371/journal.pone.0047905

Conflict of Interest Statement: Dr. Jack serves as a consultant for Janssen, Bristol-Meyer-Squibb, General Electric, Siements, and Johnson & Johnson; is involved in clinical trials sponsored by Allon and Baxter, Inc.; receives research funding from the NIH and the Alexander Family Alzheimer's Disease Research Professorship of the Mayo Foundation. Dr. Aisen serves on a scientific advisory board for NeuroPhage; serves as a consultant to Elan Corporation, Wyeth, Eisai Inc., Schering-Plough Corp., Bristol-Myers-Squibb, Eli Lilly and Company, NeuroPhage, Merck & Co., Roche, Amgen, Genentech, Inc., Abbott, Pfizer Inc., Novartis, Bayer, Astellas, Dainippon, Biomarin, Solvay, Otsuka, Daiichi, AstraZeneca, Janssen and Medivation, Inc.; and receives research support from Pfizer Inc., Eli Lilly and Company, and Baxter International Inc. Dr. Jagust has served on a scientific advisory board for Genentech, Inc.; has served as a consultant for Synarc, Janssen Alzheimer Immunotherapy, Genentech, Inc., Siemens, and TauRx. Dr. Shaw has served on a technical advisory board for Innogenetics and Saladax; serves as a consultant for Janssen; is involved in clinical trials sponsored by Eisai, Inc., and Baxter, Inc.; and receives research funding from the NIH and MJ Fox Foundation for Parkinson's research. Dr. Trojanowski may accrue revenue in the future on patents submitted by the University of Pennsylvania wherein he is co-Inventor and he received revenue from the sale of Avid to Eli Lily as co-inventor on imaging related patents submitted by the University of Pennsylvania; and receives research support from the NIH, Bristol Myer Squib, AstraZenica and several non-profits. Dr. Weiner has served on scientific advisory boards for Eli Lilly, Araclon, Institut Catala de Neurociencies Aplicades, the Gulf War Veterans Illnesses Advisory Committee, Biogen Idec, and Pfizer; has served as a consultant to Astra Zeneca, Araclon, Medivation/Pfizer, Ipsen, TauRx Therapeutics LDT, Bayer Healthcare, Biogen Idec, Exonhit Therapeutics,

Servier, Synarc, Janssen, Harvard University, and KLJ Associates; has received funding for travel from NeuroVigil, Inc., CHRU Hopital Roger Salengro, Siemens, AstraZeneca, Geneva University Hospitals, Eli Lilly, Paris University, Institut Catala de Neurociencies Aplicades, University of New Mexico School of Medicine, Ipsen, Clinical Trials on Alzheimer's Disease, the AD/PD Meeting, Paul Sabatier University, Novartis, Tohoku University, Fundacio ACE, and Travel eDreams, Inc.; has received honoraria from NeuroVigil, Inc., Institut Catala de Neurociencies Aplicades, PMDA/Japanese Ministry of Health, Labour, and Welfare, Tohoku University, and the Alzheimer's Drug Discovery Foundation; has received research support from Merck and Avid; and has stock options for Synarc and Elan. Dr. Saykin has received investigator-initiated research funding from Welch Allyn and Siemens Healthcare; has served as a consultant or advisory board member for Siemens Healthcare and Eli Lilly. Drs. Risacher, Shen, Kim, Nho, Foroud, Petersen, and Koeppe declare that the research was conducted in the absence of any commercial or financial relationships that could be construed as a potential conflict of interest.

23

Primary phagocytosis of neurons by inflamed microglia: potential roles in neurodegeneration

Jonas J. Neher*, Urte Neniskyte and Guy C. Brown

Department of Biochemistry, University of Cambridge, Cambridge, UK

Edited by:
Roger A. Barker, University of Cambridge, UK

Reviewed by:
Steve Lacroix, Laval University, Canada
V. Hugh Perry, University of Southampton, UK

****Correspondence:***
Jonas J. Neher, Department of Biochemistry, University of Cambridge, Tennis Court Road, Cambridge CB2 1QW, UK.
e-mail: jjn24@bioc.cam.ac.uk

Microglial phagocytosis of dead or dying neurons can be beneficial by preventing the release of damaging and/or pro-inflammatory intracellular components. However, there is now evidence that under certain conditions, such as inflammation, microglia can also phagocytose viable neurons, thus executing their death. Such phagocytic cell death may result from exposure of phosphatidylserine (PS) or other eat-me signals on otherwise viable neurons as a result of physiological activation or sub-toxic insult, and neuronal phagocytosis by activated microglia. In this review, we discuss the mechanisms of phagocytic cell death and its potential roles in Alzheimer's Disease, Parkinson's Disease, and Frontotemporal Dementia.

Keywords: microglia, phagocytosis, inflammation, neurodegeneration, phosphatidylserine, MFG-E8, lactadherin, reactive oxygen and nitrogen species

INTRODUCTION

Phagocytosis of host cells is generally thought to be *secondary* to the target cell dying by some means such as apoptosis (Savill et al., 2002; Ravichandran, 2003). However, phagocytosis can execute cell death of viable cells, and we shall refer to this form of cell death as "*primary* phagocytosis," with the defining characteristic that inhibition of phagocytosis prevents cell death. Examples of primary phagocytosis outside the brain include macrophage phagocytosis of "aged" erythrocytes (Föller et al., 2008; Lee et al., 2011) and activated neutrophils (Lagasse and Weissman, 1994; Jitkaew et al., 2009; Stowell et al., 2009; Bratton and Henson, 2011). In *C. elegans*, primary phagocytosis has been shown to contribute to programmed cell death of neuronal precursors during development (Hoeppner et al., 2001; Reddien et al., 2001), the elimination of cells subjected to sub-toxic insults (Neukomm et al., 2011) or simply as a result of phosphatidylserine (PS) exposure on the surface of cells (Darland-Ransom et al., 2008). In this review, we will briefly discuss the mechanisms of phagocytosis of cells, current evidence for primary phagocytosis in the central nervous system (CNS) and the resulting implications for neurodegenerative disease.

MECHANISMS OF PHAGOCYTOSIS OF HOST CELLS

The process of phagocytosis is normally initiated by the release of attractive signals from the target cell (referred to as "come-get-me" signals) leading to chemotaxis of a nearby macrophage. Upon reaching the target cell, the macrophage recognizes cell-surface signals on the target cell ("eat-me" signals), which then induce its uptake. The best characterized "eat-me" signal is the cell-surface exposure of phosphatidylserine (PS; Fadok et al., 1992; Martin et al., 1995), although display of proteins such as calreticulin has also been implicated (Gardai et al., 2005). In healthy cells, PS is found exclusively on the inner leaflet of the plasma membrane, because the aminophospholipid translocase removes PS from the outer leaflet. However, a second enzyme, the phospholipid scramblase, can cause PS exposure by randomizing phospholipid distribution between the inner and outer leaflets. PS exposure may occur as a result of: (i) apoptosis (by unknown mechanisms), (ii) necrosis (due to plasma membrane rupture), (iii) calcium elevation (which stimulates the phospholipid scramblase and inhibits the aminophospholipid translocase), (iv) ATP depletion (which inhibits the aminophospholipid translocase), (v) oxidative stress (which inhibits the aminophospholipid translocase and stimulates the scramblase), and/or (vi) fusion of intracellular vesicles with the plasma membrane (Bratton et al., 1997; Gleiss et al., 2002; Tyurina et al., 2007).

While PS display has generally been regarded as an early sign of apoptotic cell death, it is now clear that PS exposure can be reversible and independent of apoptosis (Dias-Baruffi et al., 2003; Mackenzie et al., 2005; Tyurina et al., 2007; Jitkaew et al., 2009; Neher et al., 2011), and therefore may lead to the phagocytosis of viable host cells in the presence of macrophages. For example, galectin-1 induces PS exposure on the surface of neutrophils, which is fully reversible when galectin-1 is removed and does not lead to cell death. However, when macrophages are present at the time of PS exposure these cells are phagocytosed and thus killed (Dias-Baruffi et al., 2003; Stowell et al., 2009). Whether exposure of PS by itself is sufficient for recognition and removal is not entirely clear: PS exposure may be sufficient for some cells (Fadok et al., 2001), while others may require PS oxidation or other co-stimulatory signals to induce phagocytosis (Borisenko et al., 2003, 2004). Furthermore, some healthy cells actively protect themselves from phagocytic removal by displaying signals on their surface,

---

Abbreviations: AD, Alzheimer's disease; DAP12, DNAX adaptor protein-12; FTD, Frontotemporal dementia; MerTK, Mer receptor tyrosine kinase; MFG-E8, milk fat globule EGF-like factor 8; MS, multiple sclerosis; PD, Parkinson's disease; PS, phosphatidylserine; Tim4, T-cell immunoglobulin- and mucin-domain-containing molecule-4; TLR, Toll-like receptor; TREM2, triggering receptor expressed by myeloid cells-2; VR, vitronectin receptor.

which inhibit phagocytosis ("don't-eat-me" signals, such as CD200 or CD47; see below).

A range of receptors on the macrophage can mediate recognition of PS on target cells, implying redundancy on first glance. However, not all receptors are expressed by a macrophage at any one time, but rather are dependent on its activation state, e.g., classically activated/pro-inflammatory vs. alternatively activated/anti-inflammatory macrophages. For example, resting peritoneal mouse macrophages express the PS receptors Tim4 (T-cell immunoglobulin- and mucin-domain-containing molecule-4; Kobayashi et al., 2007; Miyanishi et al., 2007), and alternatively activated human monocyte-derived macrophages express stabilin-1 (Park et al., 2009) and stabilin-2 (Park et al., 2008). In contrast, inflammatory activated (thioglycollate-elicited) peritoneal macrophages upregulate the PS-binding protein MFG-E8 (Milk fat globule EGF-like factor 8, also known as lactadherin, SED1; Hanayama et al., 2002) and the Mer receptor tyrosine kinase (MerTK), which recognizes PS or other eat-me signals through bridging molecules Gas6, protein S, galectin-3, tubby, and Tulp1 (Scott et al., 2001; Seitz et al., 2007; Shao et al., 2009; Caberoy et al., 2011). At the same time, activated (thioglycollate-elicited) macrophages downregulate expression of other phagocytic proteins such as Tim4 (Miyanishi et al., 2007). Interestingly, it therefore appears from the literature that resting macrophages express receptors that bind PS directly (i.e., Tim4, stabilin-1/2), whereas activated/pro-inflammatory macrophages utilize phagocytic pathways that recruit bridging proteins (e.g., MFG-E8, Gas6), which bind both PS on the target cell and a receptor on the macrophage [e.g., vitronectin receptor (VR), MerTK].

Microglia are resident brain macrophages, which continuously and actively survey their microenvironment (Nimmerjahn et al., 2005). Microglia represent a distinct population of tissue macrophages as they arise at least in part from primitive myeloid progenitors during early embryonic stages and are thought to be maintained by self-replication throughout life in the healthy brain (Ginhoux et al., 2010). However, under specific conditions, such as brain injury and inflammation, peripheral monocytes can be recruited to the brain. This occurs for example after stroke, but whether peripheral monocytes modify the pathology of chronic neurodegenerative diseases is disputed. In Alzheimer's disease (AD) for example, recent evidence indicates that peripheral monocytes do not invade the brain, but contribute to removal of amyloid-β (Aβ) in the perivascular environment (Mildner et al., 2011). While it is beyond the scope of this review to discuss this issue in detail, it appears that invading peripheral monocytes may mediate effects distinct from resident microglia (Prinz et al., 2011). Nevertheless, microglia share a number of similarities with peripheral macrophages, including their recognition of both exogenous "non-self" ligands (e.g., lipopolysaccharide, LPS) and endogenous "self" ligands (such as Aβ, HSP60, and HMGB1) through pattern recognition receptors (such as Toll-like receptor-2 and -4; Kawai and Akira, 2010). Recognition of these ligands results in inflammation and associated neurodegeneration due to inflammatory activation of microglia, which also renders the microglia highly phagocytic (Babcock et al., 2006; Boivin et al., 2007; Hanisch and Kettenmann, 2007; Neher et al., 2011; Neniskyte et al., 2011). Other macrophage populations in the brain, with phenotypes distinct from microglia, include those associated with the perivascular space, the circumventricular organs, the choroid plexus, and the meninges (Ransohoff and Perry, 2009).

Although data on microglia is limited, they appear to express similar phagocytic receptors and bridging proteins as peripheral macrophages. For example, primary microglia in culture express MFG-E8 (Neher et al., 2011) and MerTK (Grommes et al., 2008), possibly consistent with a partially activated microglial phenotype induced by cell-isolation procedures (Streit et al., 1999) as expression levels of these two proteins are low in homogenates of the naïve brain (Binder et al., 2008; Fuller and Van Eldik, 2008). In support of this notion, it has been reported that stimulation of microglia with the TLR4 ligand LPS increases MerTK expression in culture, and MerTK and its ligand Gas6 are also upregulated after a demyelinating insult in the brain (Binder et al., 2008). The expression of PS receptors in resting microglia has not been investigated in detail, but the mRNA levels of Tim4 appear to be low in brain homogenates (Miyanishi et al., 2007; Tanaka et al., 2009). Importantly, in the CNS, surrounding astrocytes may support microglial phagocytic function by producing bridging proteins such as MFG-E8 (Boddaert et al., 2007; Cahoy et al., 2008; Kranich et al., 2010) and protein S (Stitt et al., 1995), thus enabling efficient clearance of PS-exposing neurons.

A different phagocytic receptor, triggering receptor expressed by myeloid cells-2 (TREM2), mediates microglial clearance of debris and apoptotic neurons *in vitro* after activation by TREM2 ligands expressed on neuronal cells. Accordingly, knockdown of TREM2 impairs phagocytic function of microglia and increases the generation of pro-inflammatory cytokines *in vitro* (Takahashi et al., 2005). The function of TREM2 and its signaling partner DNAX adaptor protein-12 (DAP12) are essential for CNS immune homeostasis as loss-of-function mutations cause Nasu–Hakola disease (also known as polycystic lipomembranous osteodysplasia with sclerosing leukoencephalopathy, PLOSL), which presents with inflammation and neurodegeneration (Neumann and Takahashi, 2007). This supports the idea that microglial phagocytosis of dead and dying cells (rather than viable cells) can be protective and anti-inflammatory. The only identified TREM2 agonist is the endogenous "self" ligand HSP60, which upon binding to TREM2 strongly stimulates microglial phagocytosis (Stefano et al., 2009). Interestingly, HSP60 is also a ligand for TLR4, and TLR4 activation by HSP60 can cause microglial activation and inflammatory neurodegeneration *in vitro* (Lehnardt et al., 2008). Thus, TLR4 activation by HSP60 may contribute to the inflammation and neurodegeneration seen in Nasu–Hakola disease, where the anti-inflammatory signaling via HSP60 and TREM2 would be missing.

Wang and Neumann (2010) identified Siglec-11 as a microglial receptor, which binds polysialylated proteins on the surface of neurons (in particular neuronal cell adhesion molecule, NCAM) resulting in inhibition of inflammation and phagocytosis. Transfection of mouse microglia with human Siglec-11 reduced the spontaneous phagocytosis of neurites and neuronal cell bodies occurring in neuronal–microglial co-cultures, and this was dependent on the presence of polysialylated proteins on the surface of neurons. Thus polysialylation can act as a "don't-eat-me" signal for neurons *in vitro*.

Several other molecules can downregulate microglial activity. CD200 and CD47 are both expressed on the surface of neurons, and are known to act as "don't-eat-me-signals." The CD200 receptor (OX2) is found on microglia (Wright et al., 2000), and CD200 suppresses brain inflammation in experimental autoimmune encephalomyelitis and after facial nerve transection (Hoek et al., 2000). CD47 expression on cells and myelin sheaths inhibits phagocytosis by microglia via a CD47 receptor, SIRPα (Gitik et al., 2011).

Another signaling pathway that has been shown to modulate microglial activity is the CX3CL1 (fractalkine)/CX3CR1 pathway. CX3CL1 is expressed by neurons, while its receptor is predominantly expressed by microglia in the brain (Harrison et al., 1998). Inflammatory microglial activity can be suppressed by the neuronal chemokine CX3CL1 (also known as fractalkine) via the microglial chemokine receptor CX3CR1 as shown in neuron–microglia co-cultures (Zujovic et al., 2000) and in CX3CR1-deficient mice after systemic injection of LPS, in the MPTP model of Parkinson's Disease (PD), as well as in a transgenic model of amyotrophic lateral sclerosis (Cardona et al., 2006). Furthermore, CX3CR1 knockout restricts natural killer cell recruitment in experimental autoimmune encephalomyelitis thereby worsening disease outcome (Huang et al., 2006). However, in other circumstances fractalkine/fractalkine receptor knockout has been shown to improve neuropathology. For example, CX3CR1 deficiency resulted in improved outcome after spinal cord injury possibly due to enhanced recruitment of bone marrow derived macrophages, which also displayed reduced release of inflammatory mediators (Donnelly et al., 2011). Further, it has been reported that CX3CL1 deficient mice displayed smaller infarcts (about 30%) 24 h after middle cerebral artery occlusion (MCAo; Soriano et al., 2002), although the mechanisms of this effect were not analyzed in this study. However, a different group showed an even more pronounced reduction of infarct size (more than 50%), reduced blood brain barrier damage, leukocyte infiltration, neuronal death, and levels of IL-1β (Denes et al., 2008) between 1 and 3 days after MCAo. Importantly, a recent study analyzed the influence of the fractalkine/fractalkine receptor pathway after permanent MCAo (Cipriani et al., 2011). Similar to the two studies described above, they found reduced infarct size in both CX3CL1 and CX3CR1 knockout mice 24 h after the insult. Interestingly, *icv* infusion of recombinant CX3CL1 in rats also reduced infarct size and this effect persisted for up to 56 days. When analyzing the *in vitro* responses of wildtype and CX3CL1 knockout microglia to medium from oxygen–glucose deprived neurons, the authors found that microglial phagocytic activity was suppressed only in wildtype, but not in CX3CL1 knockout microglia. In the same experiment, the release of TNF-α was reduced in CX3CL1 knockout but not in wildtype microglia demonstrating a changed microglial response resulting from fractalkine knockout.

Fractalkine is normally displayed on the cell surface of neurons, but its release is induced by stress such as nerve injury or excitotoxicity, when it may suppress microglial inflammation but can also act as a chemokine for leukocyte infiltration as well as microglial recruitment. Additionally, soluble fractalkine may also promote microglial phagocytosis of neuronal debris by stimulating microglial production and release of MFG-E8 (Harrison et al., 1998; Cook et al., 2010; Fuhrmann et al., 2010; Noda et al., 2011) and induces upregulation of microglial integrin β_5 expression, which is one of the subunits of the receptor for MFG-E8, the VR (Leonardi-Essmann et al., 2005). Interpretation of experiments in CX3CL1 or CX3CR1 knockout animals are therefore difficult as the outcome may be due to any of the above mechanisms or combinations thereof. However, from the literature described above, it appears that suppression of leukocyte recruitment and microglial inflammation may dominate the outcome.

EVIDENCE FOR PRIMARY PHAGOCYTOSIS IN THE CNS

Activation of microglial phagocytosis is generally considered to be beneficial via removal of pathogens or potentially pro-inflammatory debris and apoptotic cells (Neumann et al., 2009). However, we and others have shown that microglia can also phagocytose viable synapses and neurons. For example, during development microglia may be involved in synaptic pruning, i.e., elimination of synapses, and mice lacking the fractalkine receptor, CX3CR1, show higher densities of spines and functional synapses during early postnatal development, which the authors attributed to temporarily reduced microglial density (Paolicelli et al., 2011). Furthermore, microglia kill developing neurons in cerebellar organotypic slices leading to an increase in the number of fully differentiated Purkinje cell clusters (Marín-Teva et al., 2004). Similarly, two phagocytosis-related proteins, CD11b and DAP12, appear to mediate developmental neuronal death in the hippocampus *in vivo* (Wakselman et al., 2008). In animals with a loss-of-function mutation in DAP12 as well as by inhibition of the complement receptor 3 subunit CD11b, neuronal death was reduced at postnatal day 1 by about 25%. Both in cerebellar slices and in the hippocampus, this effect appeared to be mediated through the release of reactive oxygen species, although it is unclear whether phagocytosis is required for this developmental death. These data are reminiscent of findings in the nematode, where knockdown of phagocytic genes was shown to result in the survival of neuronal precursor cells that would otherwise die during development (Hoeppner et al., 2001; Reddien et al., 2001) indicating a potential role for primary phagocytosis of immature neurons.

Importantly, we and others have found that stressed but viable cells can reversibly expose PS *in vitro* (Tyurina et al., 2007; Jitkaew et al., 2009; Kim et al., 2010; Neher et al., 2011) and therefore macrophages may potentially phagocytose viable cells. In particular, we have shown that microglia activated with LPS (a bacterial TLR4 agonist), lipoteichoic acid (LTA, a bacterial TLR2 agonist), or nanomolar concentrations of Aβ (an endogenous TLR2/4 agonist) phagocytose viable neurons *in vitro* (**Figure 1**). We found that microglial activation with these ligands greatly increases their phagocytic activity, and video imaging of the inflamed glial-neuronal cultures showed highly mobile microglia phagocytosing large numbers of neurons appearing morphologically healthy (Neher et al., 2011). Mechanistically, we showed that inflammatory activated microglia release reactive oxygen and nitrogen species, which induce reversible PS exposure on neurons and neuronal phagocytosis by microglia (Neher et al., 2011; Neniskyte et al.,

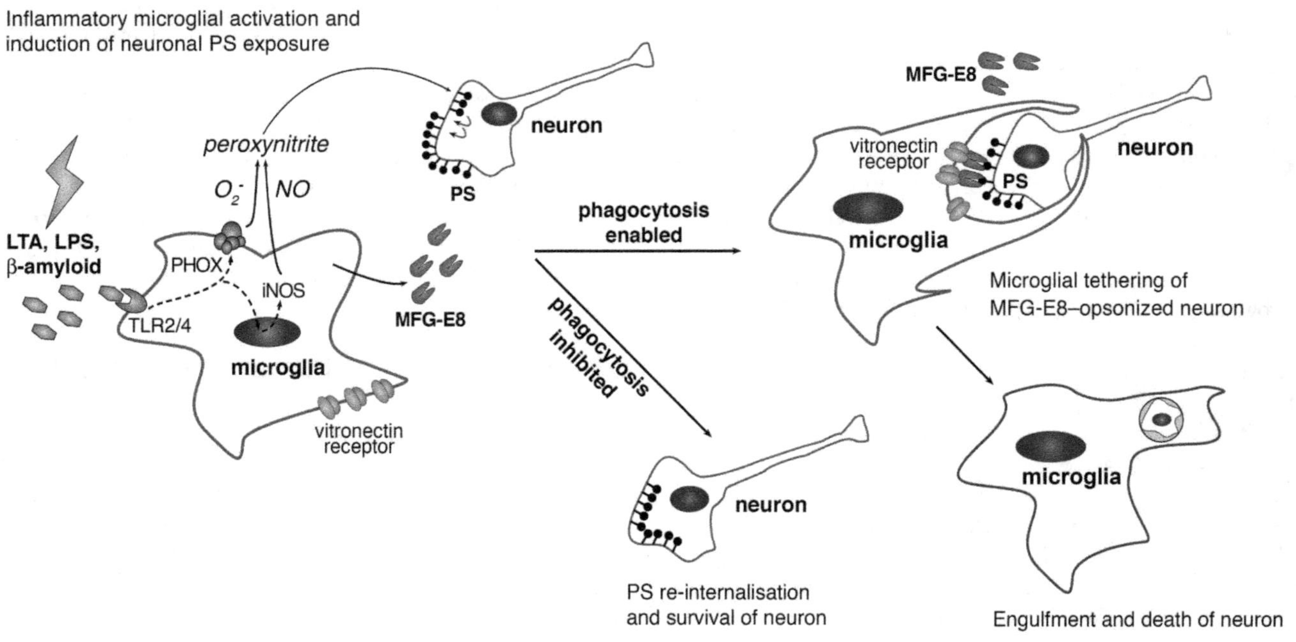

FIGURE 1 | Suggested mechanism of primary phagocytosis in inflammatory neurodegeneration. Inflammatory microglial activation with lipopolysaccharide (LPS), lipoteichoic acid (LTA), or amyloid-β (Aβ) through Toll-like receptors-2/4 induces expression of inducible nitric oxide synthase (iNOS) and assembly of the phagocytic NADPH oxidase (PHOX). iNOS and PHOX produce nitric oxide (NO) and superoxide (O_2^-), respectively, which react to form low concentrations of peroxynitrite. These sublethal levels of peroxynitrite (while not causing neuronal death) are sufficient to cause neuronal exposure of phosphatidylserine (PS), which is recognized by the bridging protein MFG-E8 (milk fat globule EGF-like factor 8). MFG-E8 also binds to the microglial vitronectin receptor (the heterodimeric $\alpha_v\beta_{3/5}$ integrin), thereby causing engulfment of the PS-exposing neuron. If phagocytosis is blocked, however, neurons are able to re-internalize PS, thus evading phagocytosis and death.

2011). Specifically, when inflammatory activated microglia were co-cultured with neurons but physically separated by a transwell membrane, neurons showed increased PS exposure but no signs of cell death. When microglia were then allowed to interact with these neurons, the neurons were phagocytosed and thus killed. However, if the activated microglia were removed from the transwell co-culture, the neuronal PS exposure was fully reversed and neurons remained viable for as long as they were cultured. This implied that inflamed microglia release soluble mediators that cause reversible PS exposure on neurons. We identified these soluble mediators to be reactive oxygen or nitrogen species, probably peroxynitrite, based on the findings that the reversible PS exposure and neuronal loss in glial-neuronal cultures is prevented by inhibitors of the NADPH oxidase (PHOX) or nitric oxide synthases (NOS), or addition of superoxide dismutase or a peroxynitrite scavenger. Furthermore, addition of 5–10 μM peroxynitrite alone caused neuronal loss in the presence of microglia, but reversible PS exposure and no neuronal loss or death in the absence of microglia (Neher et al., 2011).

We further identified a pathway consisting of neuronal PS exposure, recognition of PS by the bridging molecule MFG-E8, and MFG-E8 binding to the VR to be essential for neuronal loss. Again, blocking different components of the PS/MFG-E8/VR pathway (proteins blocking the exposed PS, antibodies to MFG-E8, VR antagonists) rescued neurons, leaving apparently healthy cells behind (Neher et al., 2011; Neniskyte et al., 2011; Fricker et al., 2012). If the neurons had been killed first and then eaten, then blocking phagocytosis would leave dead neurons. Instead, blocking phagocytosis in LPS or LTA-treated cultures prevented essentially all neuronal loss and death, leaving neurons with intact plasma and mitochondrial membrane potentials, and these neurons remained alive for as long as untreated cultures (Neher et al., 2011).

More recently we have found that LPS-induced neuronal loss is absent in glial-neuronal cultures from *Mfge8* knockout mice, but can be reconstituted by adding purified MFG-E8 to these cultures (Fricker et al., 2012). The absence or presence of MFG-E8 had no apparent effect on microglial inflammation, and this is very strong evidence that the inflammatory neuronal death is mediated by the MFG-E8 pathway of phagocytosis. Further, we have shown that LPS (5 μg and 1 μg, respectively) injection into the striatum of rats and mice *in vivo* causes strong microglial inflammation and loss of 20–30% of neurons, which is reduced by approximately 50% through co-injection of a VR inhibitor and in *Mfge8* knockout mice (Fricker et al., 2012).

Similarly, McArthur et al. (2010) recently reported that a microglial cell-line (BV2), when activated with LPS or Aβ phagocytosed viable neuron-like cells (PC12). Although a rescue of neurons by blocking phagocytosis was not shown in this study, these data further support the idea that inflammatory activated microglia may phagocytose stressed but viable neurons, thereby executing neuronal death. Altogether, this suggests the possibility that inflammatory neuronal loss in human pathologies may be prevented by inhibitors of specific phagocytic pathways.

POTENTIAL ROLES OF PRIMARY PHAGOCYTOSIS IN NEURODEGENERATIVE DISEASES

Alzheimer's disease is characterized by extracellular plaques of which the main constituent is Aβ. These plaques are associated with inflammatory activated microglia, and there is evidence that inflammation may contribute to the disease (Griffin et al., 1998; Combs, 2009). Some studies have indicated a beneficial role of microglia in the disease process, which may be due to phagocytic removal of Aβ, although it is possible that this effect is mostly mediated by invading (CCR2+) peripheral monocytes rather than resident microglia (Simard et al., 2006; El Khoury et al., 2007). However, it has recently become clear that these data may have been confounded by the fact that many studies investigating monocyte recruitment to the brain used whole-body irradiation, which may prompt invasion of peripheral monocytes. By shielding the brain, a recent study found that peripheral monocytes did not invade the brain and that amyloid clearance was mediated by perivascular myeloid cells (Mildner et al., 2011).

In humans, AD is also characterized by extensive loss of neurons and synapses by means that are not entirely clear. In contrast, in most animal models of AD neuronal loss is limited, restricted to specific brain regions and negatively correlated to plaque load. However, interestingly in these models neuronal loss occurs predominantly in the hippocampus, the area affected most severely in the human condition (Calhoun et al., 1998; Fuhrmann et al., 2010; Rupp et al., 2011).

High concentrations of Aβ (μM) can induce direct toxicity to neurons, but low concentrations (nM, which may be more relevant to AD) induce neuronal loss via inflammatory activation of glia *in vitro* (Maezawa et al., 2011). We found that nanomolar concentrations of Aβ caused microglia to phagocytose viable neurons and synapses in culture, and if we blocked this phagocytosis then all neuronal loss and death was prevented (Neniskyte et al., 2011). This suggests the possibility that microglial phagocytosis of synapses and neurons contributes to AD.

In line with this hypothesis, Aβ can induce PS exposure on neurons (Mohmmad Abdul and Butterfield, 2005), and there appears to be an increase in PS-exposed neurons in AD and mild cognitive impairment, as evidenced by PS-exposing synaptosomes isolated from patients' brains (Bader Lange et al., 2008, 2010). We have found that the PS-binding bridging protein MFG-E8 and its VR mediate inflammatory neuronal loss by primary phagocytosis *in vitro* (Neher et al., 2011; Neniskyte et al., 2011; Fricker et al., 2012). Levels of MFG-E8 are reduced in the brains of AD mice and patients with AD (Boddaert et al., 2007; Fuller and Van Eldik, 2008) possibly due to phagocytosis and degradation, while integrin β_3, a subunit of the MFG-E8 recognizing VR is strongly upregulated on reactive microglia in AD (Akiyama et al., 1991). However, it has also been reported that MFG-E8 can interact directly with Aβ (Boddaert et al., 2007), and it therefore remains to be determined whether in AD MFG-E8 mediates phagocytosis of Aβ or of PS-exposing synapses and/or neurons.

Microglia have been shown to contribute to neuronal loss in an Alzheimer's mouse model (Fuhrmann et al., 2010). Two-photon imaging of neuronal loss in the brain of living triple transgenic APP/PS1/tau AD mice revealed an involvement of microglia in neuron elimination. Microglial number and migration velocity was increased prior to loss of neurons and knockout of the microglial chemokine receptor CX3CR1, which is critical for microglial chemotaxis, prevented this neuron loss (Fuhrmann et al., 2010). However, testing whether phagocytosis of neurons in AD is primary or secondary to neuronal death by other means *in vivo* is challenging. Primary phagocytosis (unlike apoptosis or necrosis) leaves no cell corpse to diagnose the cause of death. Furthermore, most mouse models expressing mutant APP and presenilins lack significant neuronal loss unless they also include mutant tau, and we currently lack suitable phagocytosis inhibitors that cross the blood–brain barrier. However, in principle, mouse models deficient in phagocytic genes could be used to test for primary phagocytosis.

More support for an involvement of phagocytosis of cells in AD comes from recent genome wide association studies. These analyses revealed that variants in a number of phagocytosis-related genes promote late onset AD, including ApoE, ApoJ (clusterin), ABCA7, and CR1 (Jun et al., 2010; Morgan, 2011). ApoE genotype has the largest effect on AD incidence, and is known to modulate phagocytosis of apoptotic cells *in vitro* and *in vivo* (Grainger et al., 2004). Clusterin expression is upregulated by exposure to phosphatidylserine and it facilitates the uptake of cellular debris through a pathway mediated by the LDL receptor-related protein (LRP), megalin, and other yet undefined endocytic receptors (Bach et al., 2001; Bartl et al., 2001). Optimal ligand-induced signaling through LRP requires the presence of another protein related to increased AD risk, namely ABCA7. After stimulation, ABCA7 is transported to the cell membrane, localizes to the phagocytic cup and enhances the clearance of apoptotic cells *in vitro* and *in vivo* (Jehle et al., 2006). Altogether, accumulating evidence suggests that microglial phagocytosis of neurons may have a role in AD. Since impaired phagocytosis of cells can lead to inflammation, it remains to be determined whether phagocytosis may contribute to AD pathology through primary phagocytosis of viable synapses/neurons or through inflammation resulting from impaired phagocytosis of dying cells.

Parkinson's disease is characterized by motor dysfunction, resulting from progressive loss of neurons, particularly dopaminergic neurons of the pars compacta region of the substantia nigra (SN). The causes of neuronal loss may include: α-synuclein inclusions (which may be directly toxic to neurons), mitochondrial dysfunction, and glial inflammation (Tansey et al., 2007). A role for glial inflammation is suggested by the findings of: (i) inflamed glia and pro-inflammatory cytokines in the SN of patients and animal models, (ii) pro-inflammatory agents, e.g., LPS, causing loss of dopaminergic neurons in culture and *in vivo*, and (iii) anti-inflammatory drugs being protective in patients and animal models (McGeer et al., 1988; Herrera et al., 2005; Block et al., 2007; Tansey et al., 2007). We have found that LPS injection into rodent striatum causes microglial inflammation and neuronal loss reminiscent of the dopaminergic neuronal loss in LPS-induced PD. Using this model, we found that neuronal loss and death is reduced in *Mfge8* knockout mice or by co-injection of phagocytosis inhibitors (Fricker et al., 2012), suggesting that primary phagocytosis may contribute to inflammatory neuronal loss as it may occur in PD.

Substantia nigra neurons are black because they contain neuromelanin. Neuromelanin granules are found within activated microglia of the SN in PD patients, suggesting microglial phagocytosis of neurons (McGeer et al., 1988; Banati et al., 1998), even though there is little evidence of neuronal apoptosis in PD (Banati et al., 1998). Furthermore, addition of human neuromelanin causes microglial activation and dopaminergic neuronal loss in culture and *in vivo*, and this neuronal loss is prevented if a microglial phagocytosis receptor (Mac-1/CR3) is genetically deleted (Zhang et al., 2011b). Thus the neuromelanin-induced neuronal loss could be due to primary phagocytosis, however these results were interpreted in terms of a Mac-1 requirement for phagocytosis of neuromelanin (Zhang et al., 2011b). Interestingly, Aβ-induced neuronal loss is also dependent on Mac-1 (Zhang et al., 2011a), suggesting either that Mac-1 is an Aβ receptor or that neuronal loss is occurring by primary phagocytosis.

Importantly, it has been reported that in the 6-hydroxydopamine model of PD microglia become activated before any significant decrease in the number of dopaminergic neurons. Phagocytic microglia are found attached to morphologically intact neurons with normal chromatin distribution, suggesting that microglia may engulf pre-apoptotic neurons precluding the possibility of their recovery (Marinova-Mutafchieva et al., 2009), in accordance with a role for primary phagocytosis in PD.

Frontotemporal lobar degeneration (FTD) has a strong genetic component, and one of the major causes is inactivating mutations in the progranulin gene (Baker et al., 2006; Cruts et al., 2006). Progranulin deficiency leads to exaggerated microglial response after insult as well as to age-dependent accumulation of activated microglia (Ahmed et al., 2007; Yin et al., 2010a,b). Importantly, progranulin was recently found to inhibit phagocytosis of apoptotic/PS-exposed cells in culture and *in vivo*, and it was suggested that neuronal loss in FTD was due to primary phagocytosis that progranulin normally suppressed (Kao et al., 2011). Strikingly, polymorphisms in the progranulin gene are also associated with AD, PD, and amyotrophic lateral sclerosis (Brouwers et al., 2007, 2008; Sleegers et al., 2008). Therefore it is possible that premature neuronal phagocytosis as observed in the FTD model may also contribute to pathogenesis of other neurodegenerative diseases.

CONCLUSION

We have recently found that inflammatory activated microglia can execute neuronal death through phagocytosis. This primary phagocytosis is a potential mechanism for neuronal loss in neurodegenerative diseases that present with inflammation and microglial activation, and we have reviewed evidence here suggestive of such a mechanism. Primary phagocytosis may have been overlooked as a form of cell death as it is difficult to assess whether a neuron was viable prior to its phagocytosis and because the general assumption has always been that a cell must die before it is phagocytosed. The only way to determine whether phagocytosis mediates cell death is by comparing neuronal survival in the presence and absence of phagocytosis. It will be important to test the contribution of primary phagocytosis to neuronal death using models of neurodegenerative disease in mice that are deficient in phagocytic components.

ACKNOWLEDGMENTS

This work was supported by the Wellcome Trust (Grant RG50995).

REFERENCES

Ahmed, Z., Mackenzie, I. R., Hutton, M. L., and Dickson, D. W. (2007). Progranulin in frontotemporal lobar degeneration and neuroinflammation. *J. Neuroinflammation* 4, 7.

Akiyama, H., Kawamata, T., Dedhar, S., and McGeer, P. L. (1991). Immunohistochemical localization of vitronectin, its receptor and beta-3 integrin in Alzheimer brain tissue. *J. Neuroimmunol.* 32, 19–28.

Babcock, A. A., Wirenfeldt, M., Holm, T., Nielsen, H. H., Dissing-Olesen, L., Toft-Hansen, H., Millward, J. M., Landmann, R., Rivest, S., Finsen, B., and Owens, T. (2006). Toll-like receptor 2 signaling in response to brain injury: an innate bridge to neuroinflammation. *J. Neurosci.* 26, 12826–12837.

Bach, U. C., Baiersdörfer, M., Klock, G., Cattaruzza, M., Post, A., and Koch-Brandt, C. (2001). Apoptotic cell debris and phosphatidylserine-containing lipid vesicles induce apolipoprotein J (clusterin) gene expression in vital fibroblasts. *Exp. Cell Res.* 265, 11–20.

Bader Lange, M. L., Cenini, G., Piroddi, M., Abdul, H. M., Sultana, R., Galli, F., Memo, M., and Butterfield, D. A. (2008). Loss of phospholipid asymmetry and elevated brain apoptotic protein levels in subjects with amnestic mild cognitive impairment and Alzheimer disease. *Neurobiol. Dis.* 29, 456–464.

Bader Lange, M. L., St Clair, D., Markesbery, W. R., Studzinski, C. M., Murphy, M. P., and Butterfield, D. A. (2010). Age-related loss of phospholipid asymmetry in APP(NLh)/APP(NLh) x PS-1(P264L)/PS-1(P264L) human double mutant knock-in mice: relevance to Alzheimer disease. *Neurobiol. Dis.* 38, 104–115.

Baker, M., Mackenzie, I. R., Pickering-Brown, S. M., Gass, J., Rademakers, R., Lindholm, C., Snowden, J., Adamson, J., Sadovnick, A. D., Rollinson, S., Cannon, A., Dwosh, E., Neary, D., Melquist, S., Richardson, A., Dickson, D., Berger, Z., Eriksen, J., Robinson, T., Zehr, C., Dickey, C. A., Crook, R., McGowan, E., Mann, D., Boeve, B., Feldman, H., and Hutton, M. (2006). Mutations in progranulin cause tau-negative frontotemporal dementia linked to chromosome 17. *Nature* 442, 916–919.

Banati, R. B., Daniel, S. E., and Blunt, S. B. (1998). Glial pathology but absence of apoptotic nigral neurons in long-standing Parkinson's disease. *Mov. Disord.* 13, 221–227.

Bartl, M. M., Luckenbach, T., Bergner, O., Ullrich, O., and Koch-Brandt, C. (2001). Multiple receptors mediate apoJ-dependent clearance of cellular debris into nonprofessional phagocytes. *Exp. Cell Res.* 271, 130–141.

Binder, M. D., Cate, H. S., Prieto, A. L., Kemper, D., Butzkueven, H., Gresle, M. M., Cipriani, T., Jokubaitis, V. G., Carmeliet, P., and Kilpatrick, T. J. (2008). Gas6 deficiency increases oligodendrocyte loss and microglial activation in response to cuprizone-induced demyelination. *J. Neurosci.* 28, 5195–5206.

Block, M., Zecca, L., and Hong, J. (2007). Microglia-mediated neurotoxicity: uncovering the molecular mechanisms. *Nat. Rev. Neurosci.* 8, 57–69.

Boddaert, J., Kinugawa, K., Lambert, J. C., Boukhtouche, F., Zoll, J., Merval, R., Blanc-Brude, O., Mann, D., Berr, C., Vilar, J., Garabedian, B., Journiac, N., Charue, D., Silvestre, J. S., Duyckaerts, C., Amouyel, P., Mariani, J., Tedgui, A., and Mallat, Z. (2007). Evidence of a role for lactadherin in Alzheimer's disease. *Am. J. Pathol.* 170, 921–929.

Boivin, A., Pineau, I., Barrette, B., Filali, M., Vallieres, N., Rivest, S., and Lacroix, S. (2007). Toll-like receptor signaling is critical for Wallerian degeneration and functional recovery after peripheral nerve injury. *J. Neurosci.* 27, 12565–12576.

Borisenko, G. G., Iverson, S. L., Ahlberg, S., Kagan, V. E., and Fadeel, B. (2004). Milk fat globule epidermal growth factor 8 (MFG-E8) binds to oxidized phosphatidylserine: implications for macrophage clearance of apoptotic cells. *Cell Death Differ.* 11, 943–945.

Borisenko, G. G., Matsura, T., Liu, S. X., Tyurin, V. A., Jianfei, J., Serinkan, F. B., and Kagan, V. E. (2003). Macrophage recognition of externalized phosphatidylserine and phagocytosis of apoptotic Jurkat cells – existence of a threshold. *Arch. Biochem. Biophys.* 413, 41–52.

Bratton, D. L., Fadok, V. A., Richter, D. A., Kailey, J. M., Guthrie, L. A., and Henson, P. M. (1997). Appearance of phosphatidylserine on apoptotic cells requires calcium-mediated nonspecific flip-flop and is enhanced by loss of the aminophospholipid translocase. *J. Biol. Chem.* 272, 26159–26165.

Bratton, D. L., and Henson, P. M. (2011). Neutrophil clearance: when the party is over, clean-up begins. *Trends Immunol.* 32, 350–357.

Brouwers, N., Nuytemans, K., van der Zee, J., Gijselinck, I., Engelborghs, S., Theuns, J., Kumar-Singh, S., Pickut, B. A., Pals, P., Dermaut, B., Bogaerts, V., De Pooter, T., Serneels, S., Van den Broeck, M., Cuijt, I., Mattheijssens, M., Peeters, K., Sciot, R., Martin, J. J., Cras, P., Santens, P., Vandenberghe, R., De Deyn, P. P., Cruts, M., Van Broeckhoven, C., and Sleegers, K. (2007). Alzheimer and Parkinson diagnoses in progranulin null mutation carriers in an extended founder family. *Arch. Neurol.* 64, 1436–1446.

Brouwers, N., Sleegers, K., Engelborghs, S., Maurer-Stroh, S., Gijselinck, I., van der Zee, J., Pickut, B. A., Van den Broeck, M., Mattheijssens, M., Peeters, K., Schymkowitz, J., Rousseau, F., Martin, J. J., Cruts, M., De Deyn, P. P., and Van Broeckhoven, C. (2008). Genetic variability in progranulin contributes to risk for clinically diagnosed Alzheimer disease. *Neurology* 71, 656–664.

Caberoy, N. B., Alvarado, G., Bigcas, J. L., and Li, W. (2011). Galectin-3 is a new MerTK-specific eat-me signal. *J. Cell. Physiol.* 227, 401–407.

Cahoy, J., Emery, B., Kaushal, A., Foo, L., Zamanian, J., Christopherson, K., Xing, Y., Lubischer, J., Krieg, P., Krupenko, S., Thompson, W. J., and Barres, B. A. (2008). A transcriptome database for astrocytes, neurons, and oligodendrocytes: a new resource for understanding brain development and function. *J. Neurosci.* 28, 264–278.

Calhoun, M. E., Wiederhold, K. H., Abramowski, D., Phinney, A. L., Probst, A., Sturchler-Pierrat, C., Staufenbiel, M., Sommer, B., and Jucker, M. (1998). Neuron loss in APP transgenic mice. *Nature* 395, 755–756.

Cardona, A. E., Pioro, E. P., Sasse, M. E., Kostenko, V., Cardona, S. M., Dijkstra, I. M., Huang, D., Kidd, G., Dombrowski, S., Dutta, R., Lee, J. C., Cook, D. N., Jung, S., Lira, S. A., Littman, D. R., and Ransohoff, R. M. (2006). Control of microglial neurotoxicity by the fractalkine receptor. *Nat. Neurosci.* 9, 917–924.

Cipriani, R., Villa, P., Chece, G., Lauro, C., Paladini, A., Micotti, E., Perego, C., De Simoni, M. G., Fredholm, B. B., Eusebi, F., and Limatola, C. (2011). CX3CL1 is neuroprotective in permanent focal cerebral ischemia in rodents. *J. Neurosci.* 31, 16327–16335.

Combs, C. K. (2009). Inflammation and microglia actions in Alzheimer's disease. *J. Neuroimmune Pharmacol.* 4, 380–388.

Cook, A., Hippensteel, R., Shimizu, S., Nicolai, J., Fatatis, A., and Meucci, O. (2010). Interactions between chemokines: regulation of fractalkine/CX3CL1 homeostasis by SDF/CXCL12 in cortical neurons. *J. Biol. Chem.* 285, 10563–10571.

Cruts, M., Gijselinck, I., van der Zee, J., Engelborghs, S., Wils, H., Pirici, D., Rademakers, R., Vandenberghe, R., Dermaut, B., Martin, J. J., van Duijn, C., Peeters, K., Sciot, R., Santens, P., De Pooter, T., Mattheijssens, M., Van den Broeck, M., Cuijt, I., Vennekens, K., De Deyn, P. P., Kumar-Singh, S., and Van Broeckhoven, C. (2006). Null mutations in progranulin cause ubiquitin-positive frontotemporal dementia linked to chromosome 17q21. *Nature* 442, 920–924.

Darland-Ransom, M., Wang, X., Sun, C. L., Mapes, J., Gengyo-Ando, K., Mitani, S., and Xue, D. (2008). Role of *C. elegans* TAT-1 protein in maintaining plasma membrane phosphatidylserine asymmetry. *Science* 320, 528–531.

Denes, A., Ferenczi, S., Halasz, J., Kornyei, Z., and Kovacs, K. J. (2008). Role of CX3CR1 (fractalkine receptor) in brain damage and inflammation induced by focal cerebral ischemia in mouse. *J. Cereb. Blood Flow Metab.* 28, 1707–1721.

Dias-Baruffi, M., Zhu, H., Cho, M., Karmakar, S., McEver, R. P., and Cummings, R. D. (2003). Dimeric galectin-1 induces surface exposure of phosphatidylserine and phagocytic recognition of leukocytes without inducing apoptosis. *J. Biol. Chem.* 278, 41282–41293.

Donnelly, D. J., Longbrake, E. E., Shawler, T. M., Kigerl, K. A., Lai, W., Tovar, C. A., Ransohoff, R. M., and Popovich, P. G. (2011). Deficient CX3CR1 signaling promotes recovery after mouse spinal cord injury by limiting the recruitment and activation of Ly6Clo/iNOS+ macrophages. *J. Neurosci.* 31, 9910–9922.

El Khoury, J., Toft, M., Hickman, S. E., Means, T. K., Terada, K., Geula, C., and Luster, A. D. (2007). Ccr2 deficiency impairs microglial accumulation and accelerates progression of Alzheimer-like disease. *Nat. Med.* 13, 432–438.

Fadok, V. A., de Cathelineau, A, Daleke, D. L., Henson, P. M., and Bratton, D. L. (2001). Loss of phospholipid asymmetry and surface exposure of phosphatidylserine is required for phagocytosis of apoptotic cells by macrophages and fibroblasts. *J. Biol. Chem.* 276, 1071–1077.

Fadok, V. A., Voelker, D. R., Campbell, P. A., Cohen, J. J., Bratton, D. L., and Henson, P. M. (1992). Exposure of phosphatidylserine on the surface of apoptotic lymphocytes triggers specific recognition and removal by macrophages. *J. Immunol.* 148, 2207–2216.

Föller, M., Huber, S. M., and Lang, F. (2008). Erythrocyte programmed cell death. *IUBMB Life* 60, 661–668.

Fricker, M., Neher, J. J., Zhao, J. W., Thery, C., Tolkovsky, A. M., and Brown, G. C. (2012). MFG-E8 mediates primary phagocytosis of viable neurons during neuroinflammation. *J. Neurosci.* (in press).

Fuhrmann, M., Bittner, T., Jung, C. K., Burgold, S., Page, R. M., Mitteregger, G., Haass, C., LaFerla, F. M., Kretzschmar, H., and Herms, J. (2010). Microglial Cx3cr1 knockout prevents neuron loss in a mouse model of Alzheimer's disease. *Nat. Neurosci.* 13, 411–413.

Fuller, A., and Van Eldik, L. (2008). MFG-E8 regulates microglial phagocytosis of apoptotic neurons. *J. Neuroimmune Pharmacol.* 3, 246–256.

Gardai, S. J., McPhillips, K. A., Frasch, S. C., Janssen, W. J., Starefeldt, A., Murphy-Ullrich, J. E., Bratton, D. L., Oldenborg, P. A., Michalak, M., and Henson, P. M. (2005). Cell-surface calreticulin initiates clearance of viable or apoptotic cells through trans-activation of LRP on the phagocyte. *Cell* 123, 321–334.

Ginhoux, F., Greter, M., Leboeuf, M., Nandi, S., See, P., Gokhan, S., Mehler, M. F., Conway, S. J., Ng, L. G., Stanley, E. R., Samokhvalov, I. M., and Merad, M. (2010). Fate mapping analysis reveals that adult microglia derive from primitive macrophages. *Science* 330, 841–845.

Gitik, M., Liraz-Zaltsman, S., Oldenborg, P. A., Reichert, F., and Rotshenker, S. (2011). Myelin down-regulates myelin phagocytosis by microglia and macrophages through interactions between CD47 on myelin and SIRPα (signal regulatory protein-α) on phagocytes. *J. Neuroinflammation* 8, 24.

Gleiss, B., Gogvadze, V., Orrenius, S., and Fadeel, B. (2002). Fas-triggered phosphatidylserine exposure is modulated by intracellular ATP. *FEBS Lett.* 519, 153–158.

Grainger, D. J., Reckless, J., and McKilligin, E. (2004). Apolipoprotein E modulates clearance of apoptotic bodies in vitro and in vivo, resulting in a systemic proinflammatory state in apolipoprotein E-deficient mice. *J. Immunol.* 173, 6366–6375.

Griffin, W. S., Sheng, J. G., Royston, M. C., Gentleman, S. M., McKenzie, J. E., Graham, D. I., Roberts, G. W., and Mrak, R. E. (1998). Glial-neuronal interactions in Alzheimer's disease: the potential role of a 'cytokine cycle' in disease progression. *Brain Pathol.* 8, 65–72.

Grommes, C., Lee, C. Y., Wilkinson, B. L., Jiang, Q., Koenigsknecht-Talboo, J. L., Varnum, B., and Landreth, G. E. (2008). Regulation of microglial phagocytosis and inflammatory gene expression by Gas6 acting on the Axl/Mer family of tyrosine kinases. *J. Neuroimmune Pharmacol.* 3, 130–140.

Hanayama, R., Tanaka, M., Miwa, K., Shinohara, A., Iwamatsu, A., and Nagata, S. (2002). Identification of a factor that links apoptotic cells to phagocytes. *Nature* 417, 182–187.

Hanisch, U., and Kettenmann, H. (2007). Microglia: active sensor and versatile effector cells in the normal and pathologic brain. *Nat. Neurosci.* 10, 1387–1394.

Harrison, J. K., Jiang, Y., Chen, S., Xia, Y., Maciejewski, D., McNamara, R. K., Streit, W. J., Salafranca, M. N., Adhikari, S., Thompson, D. A., Botti, P., Bacon, K. B., and Feng, L. (1998). Role for neuronally derived fractalkine in mediating interactions between neurons and CX3CR1-expressing microglia. *Proc. Natl. Acad. Sci. U.S.A.* 95, 10896–10901.

Herrera, A. J., Tomás-Camardiel, M., Venero, J. L., Cano, J., and Machado, A. (2005). Inflammatory process as a determinant factor for the degeneration of substantia nigra dopaminergic neurons. *J. Neural Transm.* 112, 111–119.

Hoek, R. M., Ruuls, S. R., Murphy, C. A., Wright, G. J., Goddard, R., Zurawski, S. M., Blom, B., Homola, M. E., Streit, W. J., Brown, M. H., Barclay, A. N., and Sedgwick, J. D. (2000). Down-regulation of the macrophage lineage through interaction with OX2 (CD200). *Science* 290, 1768–1771.

Hoeppner, D. J., Hengartner, M. O., and Schnabel, R. (2001). Engulfment genes cooperate with ced-3 to promote cell death in *Caenorhabditis elegans. Nature* 412, 202–206.

Huang, D., Shi, F. D., Jung, S., Pien, G. C., Wang, J., Salazar-Mather, T. P., He, T. T., Weaver, J. T., Ljunggren, H. G., Biron, C. A., Littman, D. R., and Ransohoff, R. M. (2006). The neuronal chemokine CX3CL1/fractalkine selectively recruits NK cells that modify experimental autoimmune encephalomyelitis within the central nervous system. *FASEB J.* 20, 896–905.

Jehle, A. W., Gardai, S. J., Li, S., Linsel-Nitschke, P., Morimoto, K., Janssen, W. J., Vandivier, R. W., Wang, N., Greenberg, S., Dale, B. M., Qin, C., Henson, P. M., and Tall, A. R. (2006). ATP-binding cassette transporter A7 enhances phagocytosis of apoptotic cells and associated ERK signaling in macrophages. *J. Cell Biol.* 174, 547–556.

Jitkaew, S., Witasp, E., Zhang, S., Kagan, V. E., and Fadeel, B. (2009). Induction of caspase- and reactive oxygen species-independent phosphatidylserine externalization in primary human neutrophils: role in macrophage recognition and engulfment. *J. Leukoc. Biol.* 85, 427–437.

Jun, G., Naj, A. C., Beecham, G. W., Wang, L. S., Buros, J., Gallins, P. J., Buxbaum, J. D., Ertekin-Taner, N., Fallin, M. D., Friedland, R., Inzelberg, R., Kramer, P., Rogaeva, E., St George-Hyslop, P., Alzheimer's Disease Genetics Consortium, Cantwell, L. B., Dombroski, B. A., Saykin, A. J., Reiman, E. M., Bennett, D. A., Morris, J. C., Lunetta, K. L., Martin, E. R., Montine, T. J., Goate, A. M., Blacker, D., Tsuang, D. W., Beekly, D., Cupples, L. A., Hakonarson, H., Kukull, W., Foroud, T. M., Haines, J., Mayeux, R., Farrer, L. A., Pericak-Vance, M. A., and Schellenberg, G. D. (2010). Meta-analysis confirms CR1, CLU, and PICALM as Alzheimer disease risk loci and reveals interactions with APOE genotypes. *Arch. Neurol.* 67, 1473–1484.

Kao, A. W., Eisenhut, R. J., Martens, L. H., Nakamura, A., Huang, A., Bagley, J. A., Zhou, P., de Luis, A., Neukomm, L. J., Cabello, J., Farese, R. V. Jr., and Kenyon, C. (2011). A neurodegenerative disease mutation that accelerates the clearance of apoptotic cells. *Proc. Natl. Acad. Sci. U.S.A.* 108, 4441–4446.

Kawai, T., and Akira, S. (2010). The role of pattern-recognition receptors in innate immunity: update on Toll-like receptors. *Nat. Immunol.* 11, 373–384.

Kim, Y. E., Chen, J., Chan, J. R., and Langen, R. (2010). Engineering a polarity-sensitive biosensor for time-lapse imaging of apoptotic processes and degeneration. *Nat. Methods* 7, 67–73.

Kobayashi, N., Karisola, P., Peña-Cruz, V., Dorfman, D. M., Jinushi, M., Umetsu, S. E., Butte, M. J., Nagumo, H., Chernova, I., Zhu, B., Sharpe, A. H., Ito, S., Dranoff, G., Kaplan, G. G., Casasnovas, J. M., Umetsu, D. T., Dekruyff, R. H., and Freeman, G. J. (2007). TIM-1 and TIM-4 glycoproteins bind phosphatidylserine and mediate uptake of apoptotic cells. *Immunity* 27, 927–940.

Kranich, J., Krautler, N. J., Falsig, J., Ballmer, B., Li, S., Hutter, G., Schwarz, P., Moos, R., Julius, C., Miele, G., and Aguzzi, A. (2010). Engulfment of cerebral apoptotic bodies controls the course of prion disease in a mouse strain-dependent manner. *J. Exp. Med.* 207, 2271–2281.

Lagasse, E., and Weissman, I. L. (1994). bcl-2 inhibits apoptosis of neutrophils but not their engulfment by macrophages. *J. Exp. Med.* 179, 1047–1052.

Lee, S. J., Park, S. Y., Jung, M. Y., Bae, S. M., and Kim, I. S. (2011). Mechanism for phosphatidylserine-dependent erythrophagocytosis in mouse liver. *Blood* 117, 5215–5223.

Lehnardt, S., Schott, E., Trimbuch, T., Laubisch, D., Krueger, C., Wulczyn, G., Nitsch, R., and Weber, J. (2008). A vicious cycle involving release of heat shock protein 60 from injured cells and activation of toll-like receptor 4 mediates neurodegeneration in the CNS. *J. Neurosci.* 28, 2320–2331.

Leonardi-Essmann, F., Emig, M., Kitamura, Y., Spanagel, R., and Gebicke-Haerter, P. (2005). Fractalkine-upregulated milk-fat globule EGF factor-8 protein in cultured rat microglia. *J. Neuroimmunol.* 160, 92–101.

Mackenzie, A. B., Young, M. T., Adinolfi, E., and Surprenant, A. (2005). Pseudoapoptosis induced by brief activation of ATP-gated P2 × 7 receptors. *J. Biol. Chem.* 280, 33968–33976.

Maezawa, I., Zimin, P. I., Wulff, H., and Jin, L. W. (2011). Amyloid-beta protein oligomer at low nanomolar concentrations activates microglia and induces microglial neurotoxicity. *J. Biol. Chem.* 286, 3693–3706.

Marinova-Mutafchieva, L., Sadeghian, M., Broom, L., Davis, J. B., Medhurst, A. D., and Dexter, D. T. (2009). Relationship between microglial activation and dopaminergic neuronal loss in the substantia nigra: a time course study in a 6-hydroxydopamine model of Parkinson's disease. *J. Neurochem.* 110, 966–975.

Marín-Teva, J., Dusart, I., Colin, C., Gervais, A., van Rooijen, N., and Mallat, M. (2004). Microglia promote the death of developing Purkinje cells. *Neuron* 41, 535–547.

Martin, S. J., Reutelingsperger, C. P., McGahon, A. J., Rader, J. A., van Schie, R. C., LaFace, D. M., and Green, D. R. (1995). Early redistribution of plasma membrane phosphatidylserine is a general feature of apoptosis regardless of the initiating stimulus: inhibition by overexpression of Bcl-2 and Abl. *J. Exp. Med.* 182, 1545–1556.

McArthur, S., Cristante, E., Paterno, M., Christian, H., Roncaroli, F., Gillies, G. E., and Solito, E. (2010). Annexin A1: a central player in the anti-inflammatory and neuroprotective role of microglia. *J. Immunol.* 185, 6317–6328.

McGeer, P. L., Itagaki, S., Boyes, B. E., and McGeer, E. G. (1988). Reactive microglia are positive for HLA-DR in the substantia nigra of Parkinson's and Alzheimer's disease brains. *Neurology* 38, 1285–1291.

Mildner, A., Schlevogt, B., Kierdorf, K., Bottcher, C., Erny, D., Kummer, M. P., Quinn, M., Bruck, W., Bechmann, I., Heneka, M. T., Priller, J., and Prinz, M. (2011). Distinct and non-redundant roles of microglia and myeloid subsets in mouse models of Alzheimer's disease. *J. Neurosci.* 31, 11159–11171.

Miyanishi, M., Tada, K., Koike, M., Uchiyama, Y., Kitamura, T., and Nagata, S. (2007). Identification of Tim4 as a phosphatidylserine receptor. *Nature* 450, 435–439.

Mohmmad Abdul, H., and Butterfield, D. A. (2005). Protection against amyloid beta-peptide (1-42)-induced loss of phospholipid asymmetry in synaptosomal membranes by tricyclodecan-9-xanthogenate (D609) and ferulic acid ethyl ester: implications for Alzheimer's disease. *Biochim. Biophys. Acta* 1741, 140–148.

Morgan, K. (2011). The three new pathways leading to Alzheimer's disease. *Neuropathol. Appl. Neurobiol.* 37, 353–357.

Neher, J. J., Neniskyte, U., Zhao, J. W., Bal-Price, A., Tolkovsky, A. M., and Brown, G. C. (2011). Inhibition of microglial phagocytosis is sufficient to prevent inflammatory neuronal death. *J. Immunol.* 186, 4973–4983.

Neniskyte, U., Neher, J. J., and Brown, G. C. (2011). Neuronal death induced by nanomolar amyloid beta is mediated by primary phagocytosis of neurons by microglia. *J. Biol. Chem.* 286, 39904–39913.

Neukomm, L. J., Frei, A. P., Cabello, J., Kinchen, J. M., Zaidel-Bar, R., Ma, Z., Haney, L. B., Hardin, J., Ravichandran, K. S., Moreno, S., and Hengartner, M. O. (2011). Loss of the RhoGAP SRGP-1 promotes the clearance of dead and injured cells in *Caenorhabditis elegans. Nat. Cell Biol.* 13, 79–86.

Neumann, H., Kotter, M. R., and Franklin, R. J. (2009). Debris clearance by microglia: an essential link between degeneration and regeneration. *Brain* 132, 288–295.

Neumann, H., and Takahashi, K. (2007). Essential role of the microglial triggering receptor expressed on myeloid cells-2 (TREM2) for central nervous tissue immune homeostasis. *J. Neuroimmunol.* 184, 92–99.

Nimmerjahn, A., Kirchhoff, F., and Helmchen, F. (2005). Resting microglial cells are highly dynamic surveillants of brain parenchyma in vivo. *Science* 308, 1314–1318.

Noda, M., Doi, Y., Liang, J., Kawanokuchi, J., Sonobe, Y., Takeuchi, H., Mizuno, T., and Suzumura, A. (2011). Fractalkine attenuates excito-neurotoxicity via microglial clearance of damaged neurons and antioxidant enzyme heme oxygenase-1 expression. *J. Biol. Chem.* 286, 2308–2319.

Paolicelli, R. C., Bolasco, G., Pagani, F., Maggi, L., Scianni, M., Panzanelli, P., Giustetto, M., Ferreira, T. A., Guiducci, E., Dumas, L., Ragozzino, D., and Gross, C. T. (2011). Synaptic pruning by microglia is necessary for normal brain development. *Science* 333, 1456–1458.

Park, S. Y., Jung, M. Y., Lee, S. J., Kang, K. B., Gratchev, A., Riabov, V., Kzhyshkowska, J., and Kim, I. S. (2009). Stabilin-1 mediates phosphatidylserine-dependent clearance of cell corpses in alternatively activated macrophages. *J. Cell. Sci.* 122, 3365–3373.

Park, S. Y., Kim, S. Y., Jung, M. Y., Bae, D. J., and Kim, I. S. (2008). Epidermal growth factor-like domain repeat of stabilin-2 recognizes phosphatidylserine during cell corpse clearance. *Mol. Cell. Biol.* 28, 5288–5298.

Prinz, M., Priller, J., Sisodia, S. S., and Ransohoff, R. M. (2011). Heterogeneity of CNS myeloid cells and their roles in neurodegeneration. *Nat. Neurosci.* 13, 1227–1235.

Ransohoff, R. M., and Perry, V. H. (2009). Microglial physiology: unique stimuli, specialized responses. *Annu. Rev. Immunol.* 27, 119–145.

Ravichandran, K. S. (2003). "Recruitment signals" from apoptotic cells: invitation to a quiet meal. *Cell* 113, 817–820.

Reddien, P., Cameron, S., and Horvitz, H. (2001). Phagocytosis promotes programmed cell death in *C. elegans. Nature* 412, 198–202.

Rupp, N. J., Wegenast-Braun, B. M., Radde, R., Calhoun, M. E., and Jucker, M. (2011). Early onset amyloid lesions lead to severe neuritic abnormalities and local, but not global neuron loss in APPPS1 transgenic mice. *Neurobiol. Aging* 32, 2324 e2321–e2326.

Savill, J., Dransfield, I., Gregory, C., and Haslett, C. (2002). A blast from the past: clearance of apoptotic cells regulates immune responses. *Nat. Rev. Immunol.* 2, 965–975.

Scott, R. S., McMahon, E. J., Pop, S. M., Reap, E. A., Caricchio, R., Cohen, P. L., Earp, H. S., and Matsushima, G. K. (2001). Phagocytosis and clearance of apoptotic cells is mediated by MER. *Nature* 411, 207–211.

Seitz, H. M., Camenisch, T. D., Lemke, G., Earp, H. S., and Matsushima, G. K. (2007). Macrophages and dendritic cells use different Axl/Mertk/Tyro3 receptors in clearance of apoptotic cells. *J. Immunol.* 178, 5635–5642.

Shao, W. H., Zhen, Y., Eisenberg, R. A., and Cohen, P. L. (2009). The Mer receptor tyrosine kinase is expressed on discrete macrophage subpopulations and mainly uses Gas6 as its ligand for uptake of apoptotic cells. *Clin. Immunol.* 133, 138–144.

Simard, A. R., Soulet, D., Gowing, G., Julien, J. P., and Rivest, S. (2006). Bone marrow-derived microglia play a critical role in restricting senile plaque formation in Alzheimer's disease. *Neuron* 49, 489–502.

Sleegers, K., Brouwers, N., Maurer-Stroh, S., van Es, M. A., Van Damme, P., van Vught, P. W., van der Zee, J., Serneels, S., De Pooter, T., Van den Broeck, M., Cruts, M., Schymkowitz, J., De Jonghe, P., Rousseau, F., van den Berg, L. H., Robberecht, W., and Van Broeckhoven, C. (2008). Progranulin genetic variability contributes to amyotrophic lateral sclerosis. *Neurology* 71, 253–259.

Soriano, S. G., Amaravadi, L. S., Wang, Y. F., Zhou, H., Yu, G. X., Tonra, J. R., Fairchild-Huntress, V., Fang, Q., Dunmore, J. H., Huszar, D., and Pan, Y. (2002). Mice deficient in fractalkine are less susceptible to cerebral ischemia-reperfusion injury. *J. Neuroimmunol.* 125, 59–65.

Stefano, L., Racchetti, G., Bianco, F., Passini, N., Gupta, R. S., Panina Bordignon, P., and Meldolesi, J. (2009). The surface-exposed chaperone, Hsp60, is an agonist of the microglial TREM2 receptor. *J. Neurochem.* 110, 284–294.

Stitt, T. N., Conn, G., Gore, M., Lai, C., Bruno, J., Radziejewski, C., Mattsson, K., Fisher, J., Gies, D. R., and Jones, P. F. (1995). The anticoagulation factor protein S and its relative, Gas6, are ligands for the Tyro 3/Axl family of receptor tyrosine kinases. *Cell* 80, 661–670.

Stowell, S. R., Karmakar, S., Arthur, C. M., Ju, T., Rodrigues, L. C., Riul, T. B., Dias-Baruffi, M., Miner, J., McEver, R. P., and Cummings, R. D. (2009). Galectin-1 induces reversible phosphatidylserine exposure at the plasma membrane. *Mol. Biol. Cell* 20, 1408–1418.

Streit, W. J., Walter, S. A., and Pennell, N. A. (1999). Reactive microgliosis. *Prog. Neurobiol.* 57, 563–581.

Takahashi, K., Rochford, C. D., and Neumann, H. (2005). Clearance of apoptotic neurons without inflammation by microglial triggering receptor expressed on myeloid cells-2. *J. Exp. Med.* 201, 647–657.

Tanaka, T., Ueno, M., and Yamashita, T. (2009). Engulfment of axon debris by microglia requires p38 MAPK activity. *J. Biol. Chem.* 284, 21626–21636.

Tansey, M. G., McCoy, M. K., and Frank-Cannon, T. C. (2007). Neuroinflammatory mechanisms in Parkinson's disease: potential environmental triggers, pathways, and targets for early therapeutic intervention. *Exp. Neurol.* 208, 1–25.

Tyurina, Y., Basova, L., Konduru, N., Tyurin, V., Potapovich, A., Cai, P., Bayir, H., Stoyanovsky, D., Pitt, B., Shvedova, A., Fadeel, B., and Kagan, V. E. (2007). Nitrosative stress inhibits the aminophospholipid translocase resulting in phosphatidylserine externalization and macrophage engulfment: implications for the resolution of inflammation. *J. Biol. Chem.* 282, 8498–8509.

Wakselman, S., Béchade, C., Roumier, A., Bernard, D., Triller, A., and Bessis, A. (2008). Developmental neuronal death in hippocampus requires the microglial CD11b integrin and DAP12 immunoreceptor. *J. Neurosci.* 28, 8138–8143.

Wang, Y., and Neumann, H. (2010). Alleviation of neurotoxicity by microglial human Siglec-11. *J. Neurosci.* 30, 3482–3488.

Wright, G. J., Puklavec, M. J., Willis, A. C., Hoek, R. M., Sedgwick, J. D., Brown, M. H., and Barclay, A. N. (2000). Lymphoid/neuronal cell surface OX2 glycoprotein recognizes a novel receptor on macrophages implicated in the control of their function. *Immunity* 13, 233–242.

Yin, F., Banerjee, R., Thomas, B., Zhou, P., Qian, L., Jia, T., Ma, X., Ma, Y., Iadecola, C., Beal, M. F., Nathan, C., and Ding, A. (2010a). Exaggerated inflammation, impaired host defense, and neuropathology in progranulin-deficient mice. *J. Exp. Med.* 207, 117–128.

Yin, F., Dumont, M., Banerjee, R., Ma, Y., Li, H., Lin, M. T., Beal, M. F., Nathan, C., Thomas, B., and Ding, A. (2010b). Behavioral deficits and progressive neuropathology in progranulin-deficient mice: a mouse model of frontotemporal dementia. *FASEB J.* 24, 4639–4647.

Zhang, D., Hu, X., Qian, L., Chen, S. H., Zhou, H., Wilson, B., Miller, D. S., and Hong, J. S. (2011a). Microglial MAC1 receptor and PI3K are essential in mediating β-amyloid peptide-induced microglial activation and subsequent neurotoxicity. *J. Neuroinflammation* 8, 3.

Zhang, W., Phillips, K., Wielgus, A. R., Liu, J., Albertini, A., Zucca, F. A., Faust, R., Qian, S. Y., Miller, D. S., Chignell, C. F., Wilson, B., Jackson-Lewis, V., Przedborski, S., Joset, D., Loike, J., Hong, J. S., Sulzer, D., and Zecca, L. (2011b). Neuromelanin activates microglia and induces degeneration of dopaminergic neurons: implications for progression of Parkinson's disease. *Neurotox. Res.* 19, 63–72.

Zujovic, V., Benavides, J., Vigé, X., Carter, C., and Taupin, V. (2000). Fractalkine modulates TNF-alpha secretion and neurotoxicity induced by microglial activation. *Glia* 29, 305–315.

24

VBM with viscous fluid registration of gray matter segments in SPM

Joao M. S. Pereira[1,2]*, Julio Acosta-Cabronero[2], George Pengas[2], Li Xiong[3], Peter J. Nestor[4] and Guy B. Williams[2]

[1] Laboratory of Biostatistics and Medical Informatics, IBILI - Faculty of Medicine, University of Coimbra, Coimbra, Portugal
[2] Department of Clinical Neurosciences, School of Clinical Medicine, University of Cambridge, Cambridge, UK
[3] Neurology Department, Zhongnan Hospital of Wuhan University, Wuhan, China
[4] German Center for Neurodegenerative Diseases (DZNE), Magdeburg, Germany

Edited by:
Manuel Menéndez-González, Hospital Álvarez-Buylla, Spain

Reviewed by:
Katsutoshi Furukawa, Tohoku University, Japan
Yunfei Huang, Albany Medical College, USA

***Correspondence:**
Joao M. S. Pereira, Laboratory of Biostatistics and Medical Informatics, IBILI - Faculty of Medicine, University of Coimbra, Azinhaga de Santa Comba – Celas, 3000-548 Coimbra, Portugal
e-mail: joao.mspereira@gmail.com

Improved registration of gray matter segments in SPM has been achieved with the DARTEL algorithm. Previous work from our group suggested, however, that such improvements may not translate to studies of clinical groups. To address the registration issue in atrophic brains, this paper relaxed the condition of diffeomorphism, central to DARTEL, and made use of a viscous fluid registration model with limited regularization constraints to register the modulated gray matter probability maps to an intra-population template. Quantitative analysis of the registration results after the additional viscous fluid step showed no worsening of co-localization of fiducials compared to DARTEL or unified segmentation methods, and the resulting voxel based morphometry (VBM) analyses were able to better identify atrophic regions and to produce results with fewer apparent false positives. DARTEL showed great sensitivity to atrophy, but the resulting VBM maps presented broad, amorphous regions of significance that are hard to interpret. We propose that the condition of diffeomorphism is not necessary for basic VBM studies in atrophic populations, but also that it has disadvantages that must be taken into consideration before a study. The presented viscous fluid registration method is proposed for VBM studies to enhance sensitivity and localizing power.

Keywords: MRI, VBM, SPM, DARTEL, registration, dementia

INTRODUCTION

Imaging biomarkers are of considerable interest in dementia research. Aside from the qualities of the biomarker itself, the method with which it is analysed is crucial to consider as insensitive or unstable methods could mean that real information is lost (false negatives) or that spurious changes (false positives) are reported. Voxel-based image analysis has become a cornerstone of assessing structural imaging biomarkers, yet such methods are typically validated in simulations and the healthy population. The DARTEL algorithm (Diffeomorphic Anatomical Registration Through Exponentiated Lie Algebra) has been presented as an improvement for the registration of gray matter probability maps used in voxel based morphometry (VBM) (Ashburner, 2007) in the software package SPM (http://www.fil.ion.ucl.ac.uk/spm/). One of the key advantages of DARTEL is its explicit search for an inverse consistent, diffeomorphic transformation. This leads to very smooth, large deformation fields that follow elegant mathematical descriptors and that can be easily inverted. Although such characteristics can be useful for applications where it is important to consistently use reverse deformation fields, that is not the case with standard VBM studies of dementia, where most often scans are simply registered to standard space and nothing more is done with the deformation fields (aside from their use for modulation for volume change) (Ridgway et al., 2008). Moreover, a previously published study (Pereira et al., 2010) demonstrated variability in the registration accuracy both by region and disease categorization, raising questions about the spatially variant sensitivity of the resulting VBM significance maps. Even though DARTEL shows improved performance when using preprocessed scans (bias corrected and skull stripped), the associated VBM results showed apparent false positives when compared to the standard SPM5 results using the same scans (Pereira et al., 2010). The motivation for the present study was to explore a simpler, standard registration algorithm without diffeomorphism, in order to assess whether DARTEL's stringent mathematical approach, is in effect inappropriately regularized for use in neurodegenerative disease research. The approach taken in the present study makes use of a long established high degrees of freedom registration algorithm as an alternative: a viscous fluid registration (Christensen et al., 1996). The novelty in the current study compared to past fluid registration studies, however, is its use as an additional registration step, on top of the standard registration in SPM. The hypothesis is that by relaxing the severe regularization constraints intrinsic to DARTEL, the viscous fluid algorithm will be able to account for more anatomical variability, while also preserving structural detail post-registration. This is especially applicable to atrophic brains, which may require both finer (more local) and more extreme deformations than the ones permitted by DARTEL. The resulting VBMs will be more sensitive and more anatomically meaningful than either VBM with

DARTEL or standard VBM. As the viscous fluid methods are able to account for finer deformations than the limited degrees of freedom discrete cosine transform (DCT) used in unified segmentation (Ashburner and Friston, 2005), this study considered the utility of applying the former as an additional step to include after SPM's registration. This was implemented as a hierarchical registration model in which a low degrees of freedom algorithm (DCT in unified segmentation) is applied first in order to account for gross differences between the target and the subject, and then a high degree of freedom method (viscous fluid) is applied to address the finer details. The concept of working on top of already registered gray matter probability maps is justified by the fact that DCT registration is unable to account for all anatomical differences between the subject and the template (Ashburner and Friston, 1999). In short, rather than using a complicated, mathematically rich approach like DARTEL in order to achieve smooth deformation fields that might be of little benefit to a real clinical study, better results might be achieved by adding an extra step after the unified segmentation.

The method presented in this study was tested using real datasets from neurodegenerative studies because these are precisely the datasets where such algorithms find application as VBM studies. This is of paramount importance because other registration approaches, notably DARTEL, have been validated in abstract mathematical frameworks or on healthy volunteer data (Ashburner, 2007; Yassa and Stark, 2009) and then accepted as clinical tools without thorough testing in clinical settings. The clinical plausibility of the resulting statistical maps of VBM, as compared with known patterns of atrophy from other assessments, is a significant consideration if these methods are to be robust for clinical studies. In the current study, the results were assessed in comparison to prior knowledge of disease atrophy patterns and manual hippocampal volumetry in patient groups. Finally, fiducial markers were placed in a subset of subjects so as to directly compare the method to the standard unified segmentation and DARTEL methods.

MATERIALS AND METHODS

All algorithms presented in this section were written in Matlab7, and run on a Dual Xeon 3.2 GHz Intel X86 64 bit processor with 4GB RAM running GNU Debian Linux version 3.1, except where otherwise stated. The code of the fluid registration algorithm presented in this paper can be found in http://www.uc.pt/en/fmuc/ibili/Archives/Articles/JPereira/MiMe.

VISCOUS FLUID ALGORITHM

A viscous fluid algorithm was implemented in order to register the gray matter probability maps generated by SPM8 (http://www.fil.ion.ucl.ac.uk/spm/software/spm8/). Viscous fluid registration assumes a subject's brain *S* to behave as a viscous fluid when being registered to a target space *T*, with each point of the subject scan being deformed by the action of an external driving force field **F**. This force field is cancelled out at equilibrium by the internal forces of the fluid body, as described by the Navier-Stokes equation:

$$\mu\nabla^2\mathbf{v}(\mathbf{x},\ t) + (\mu + \lambda)\nabla(\nabla \cdot \mathbf{v}(\mathbf{x},\ t)) + \mathbf{F}(\mathbf{x}, \mathbf{u}(\mathbf{x}, t)) = 0 \quad (1)$$

with:

$$\mathbf{v}(\mathbf{x}, t) = \frac{d\mathbf{u}(\mathbf{x}, t)}{dt} \quad (2)$$

In Equation 1, $\mathbf{F}(\mathbf{x}, \mathbf{u}(\mathbf{x}, t))$ is the external force acting on the body deformed by the displacement field $\mathbf{u}(\mathbf{x}, t)$ at location $\mathbf{x}$ at time t, ∇ is the gradient operator, ∇^2 is the Laplacian operator, and μ and λ are the viscosity constants. From this point on, dependencies will be dropped for the sake of simplicity [e.g., $\mathbf{v}(\mathbf{x}, t)$ will be written as $\mathbf{v}$]. For the external forces calculation, a simple difference metric was used, based on the difference between the target and the deformed subject, multiplied by the gradient of the latter (Christensen et al., 1996).

As a linear differential equation, and using finite differences to discretize it (Press et al., 1992), Equation 1 can be written as:

$$\mathbf{Lv} = \mathrm{F} \quad (3)$$

where **L** is a linear operator, **v** is the velocity field and **F** is the external force field. This system can be either explicitly solved or a solution can be estimated using approximations to the linear operator **L**.

The explicit solution requires the use of the successive over-relaxation (SOR) method (Press et al., 1992; Wollny and Kruggel, 2002), which may be too time consuming. One possibility is to speed it up by using adaptive updates (SOR with adaptative updates, SORA) (Wollny and Kruggel, 2002). Another option is to approximate the linear operator **L** with an adequate convolution kernel **K**. As a consequence, the velocity response to each individual force vector can be estimated by its convolution with **K**. It is known that **K** can be a Gaussian filter (Thirion, 1998). This is a simplistic solution that has been shown to cause a decrease in registration quality (Gramkow and Bro-Nielsen, 1997). Another approximation, based on the eigenfunctions of **L**, can be used to yield more accurate results through a "viscous kernel" (Bro-Nielsen and Gramkow, 1996; Gramkow and Bro-Nielsen, 1997). We assessed all three approaches in this paper.

An Eulerian frame of reference describes the non-linear warp field variables through fixed positions **x** associated with time dependent displacement vectors $\mathbf{u}(\mathbf{x}, t)$ such that the deformed position at time t is described as $\mathbf{x}-\mathbf{u}(\mathbf{x}, t)$ (Christensen et al., 1996). The material derivative *d/dt* provides the instantaneous rate of change a point **x** of the grid observes at time *t*. A particle of the viscous body flowing through position **x** at that time will have a velocity **v** described by:

$$\mathbf{v} = \frac{d\mathbf{u}}{dt} = \frac{\partial \mathbf{u}}{\partial t} + \sum_{i=1}^{3} v_i \frac{\partial \mathbf{u}}{\partial x_i} \Leftrightarrow \frac{\partial \mathbf{u}}{\partial t} = \mathbf{R} = \mathbf{v} - \sum_{i=1}^{3} v_i \frac{\partial \mathbf{u}}{\partial x_i} \quad (4)$$

where $\mathbf{v} = (v_1, v_2, v_3)$ and $\mathbf{x} = (x_1, x_2, x_3)$.

The sum element in Equation 4 accounts for the deformation applied on the body and is zero when the body and the reference grid match. As a consequence, the partial derivative of the deformation **u** with respect to time yields a perturbation field **R** that is used to update the warping. The deformation field **u** is updated for iteration $k + 1$ of the registration algorithm by $\mathbf{R}$ such that:

$$\mathbf{u}^{(k+1)} = \mathbf{u}^{(k)} + \Delta\mathbf{u}^{(k)} = \mathbf{u}^{(k)} + \mathbf{R}^{(k)} \cdot \Delta T^{(k)} \quad (5)$$

where $\Delta T^{(k)}$ is an iteration dependent time step, thus performing an explicit Euler integration of the perturbation vectors, which in themselves form a velocity field. The choice of time step will depend on the maximum value of the perturbation field, $\|\mathbf{R}^{(k)}\|_{\max}$. In the current work, $\Delta T^{(k)}$ was chosen such that a maximum displacement value m was enforced for each iteration (D'Agostino et al., 2003):

$$\Delta T^{(k)} = \frac{m}{\| \mathbf{R}^{(k)} \|_{\max}} \quad (6)$$

B. TOPOLOGY PRESERVATION

The determinant of the Jacobian of the deformation field must at all times be positive in order to ensure that topology is preserved (Christensen et al., 1996). This is ensured by regridding the deformation field every time this determinant crosses a certain threshold. Details of how this is done can be found in the supplementary material.

VISCOUS FLUID ASSESSMENT

The viscous fluid registration method was used to register gray matter probability maps in the context of VBM analyses of clinical cohorts. The first set of analyses was performed using groups of healthy controls ($n = 18$), Alzheimer's disease (AD) ($n = 19$), semantic dementia (SD) ($n = 10$) and behavioral variant frontotemporal dementia subjects (bvFTD) ($n = 8$). Subjects in each of the disease groups were diagnosed according to standard criteria (McKhann et al., 1984; Neary et al., 1998). These subjects made up Set A. This diverse set of atrophy profiles—AD, SD, and bvFTD—allowed for a thorough assessment of the proposed viscous fluid method in contrast to DARTEL and a standard SPM method. Demographic information about these groups can be found in the supplementary material (**Table S1**). Hippocampal volumes had been measured on the AD and control cohorts of Set A for a previous study (Pengas et al., 2010), and are presented in **Table 1**.

In order to not confine the assessment to a set of scans sharing the same acquisition parameters, another set of scans (designated Set B) was also used. Set B comprised controls ($n = 21$), AD subjects ($n = 16$), SD subjects ($n = 10$), and $n = 17$ patients diagnosed with mild cognitive impairment (MCI). The demographic details of these groups are listed in the supplementary material (**Table S2**). Hippocampal volumes were measured for all cohorts of Set B and are presented in **Table 2**. Details of how these volumes were obtained can be found in the supplementary material.

Set A was acquired with a 1.5 T GE Signa MRI scanner (GE Medical Systems, Milwaukee, WI). Volumetric T_1-weighted images were coronally acquired using SPGR (pixel dimensions $0.86 \times 0.86\,\text{mm}^2$, slice thickness 1.5 or 1.8 mm). Set B was acquired on a Siemens Trio 3T system (Siemens Medical Systems, Erlangen, Germany) using a 3D MPRAGE pulse sequence for the acquisition of volumetric T_1-weighted images with 144 slices, 192×192 matrix dimensions and $1.25\,\text{mm}^3$ voxel size. Scans were preprocessed according to a previously described pipeline (Acosta-Cabronero et al., 2008) (see supplementary material).

All scans were registered and segmented using the unified segmentation model provided in SPM8 (Ashburner and Friston, 2005). Probability maps of GM, WM, and CSF were also obtained in native space from all subjects for automated total intracranial volume (TIV) estimation (Pengas et al., 2008).

Subjects were also processed with the DARTEL algorithm, designated $\text{DARTEL}_{\text{pre}}$ when used with preprocessed scans, using default parameters and modulated gray matter probability maps. The output probability maps of the DARTEL algorithm were used in all subsequent analyses without any further processing.

VISCOUS FLUID REGISTRATION

Heuristic tests suggested that the eigenfunction-based kernel approximation was faster than SORA, while providing better results than the gaussian kernel approximation. As such, this was the method of choice in this paper. The others methods, however, presented similar results, which will not be discussed herein. All gray matter probability maps, normalized and resliced to an isotropic resolution of $2\,\text{mm}^3$ were registered with the viscous fluid method using the eigenfunction-based approximation to the linear operator to solve the differential equation. This viscous fluid method will be named "Fluid" from this point on.

For all sets of scans, a fixed random gray matter probability map from the control cohort was used as the target to which

Table 1 | Hippocampal volumes for subjects used in the AD VBM study of Set A, normalized to the mean total intracraneal volume (TIV) of the control cohort.

	Right hippocampus volume (mm³)	Left hippocampus volume (mm³)
Controls	1667 ± 301.0	1574 ± 214.4
AD	1399 ± 294.3 (−16.1%)	1270 ± 369.0 (−19.3%)

Values presented are mean ± standard deviation. Average percentage volume reduction relative to controls is shown in brackets. Values for the AD subjects are significantly lower than controls ($p < 0.05$, one-tail t-test). TIV was not statistically different between cohorts (not shown).

Table 2 | Hippocampal volumes for Controls, as well as for AD and MCI subjects in Set B, normalized to the mean TIV of the control cohort.

	Right hippocampus volume (mm³)	Left hippocampus volume (mm³)
Controls	1286 ± 157.5	1206 ± 209.6
AD	986 ± 192.9 (−23.4%)	886 ± 166.2 (−26.6%)
MCI	1037 ± 124.4 (−19.4%)	1008 ± 101.3 (−16.4%)

Values presented are mean ± standard deviation. Average percentage volume reduction is shown in brackets. Values are significantly lower than controls in all patient cohorts ($p < 0.05$ one-tail t-test). TIV was not statistically different between cohorts (not shown).

all other probability maps were registered. Given that these gray matter probability maps are already registered to a template, no further linear registration was performed.

VBM ANALYSES

A two-group *t*-test comparison was made between each diseased cohort and the relevant control group (i.e., with the same acquisition parameters). The control target was also included in the control group for the statistical analyses.

A relative threshold mask of 0.2 was used for all studies, except where otherwise stated. Scans were smoothed with an 8 mm full width half maximum (FWHM) Gaussian kernel. All analyses were also performed with 6 and 10 mm FWHM kernels, but as results were very similar to those obtained with the 8 mm kernel these are not shown or discussed. All tests were performed with total intracraneal volume (TIV) as a nuisance covariate.

The analyses of the scans of Set A included both gray matter probability maps from raw (not preprocessed) volumes and preprocessed volumes. Set B was only analysed using preprocessed scans. All probability maps were modulated by the Jacobian determinant of the non-linear viscous transformation. The modulation step was required for consistency with the original probability maps; moreover, the fine deformation fields result in determinant values that contain important information about local volume changes in the brain. All analyses had a statistical threshold of $p_{\text{FWE corrected}} = 0.05$, unless the resulting glass brains were blank (or showed only noise), in which case the threshold of $p_{\text{uncorrected}} = 0.001$ was used. The extent threshold k was set at 0 for all analyses. No correction was made for the differing initial voxel dimensions in Set A as this was a systematic error introduced in all studies and can be discounted when comparing the results (Pereira et al., 2008). Results of DARTEL, $\text{DARTEL}_{\text{pre}}$, Fluid and $\text{Fluid}_{\text{pre}}$ were analysed in their own template space.

REGISTRATION ASSESSMENT

Registration quality was assessed by comparing the results of the viscous fluid re-registration analyses with those of SPM8's unified segmentation and DARTEL.

A quantitative analysis of the registration performance was also performed using a subgroup of Set A that had fiducial points placed on the original scans as part of a previous study (Pereira et al., 2010). A set of 20 locations were chosen for fiducial marker placement. The consistency of location for each fiducial marker cluster was analysed with three metrics–the degree of dispersion error after warping in the direction of greatest location uncertainty (λ_1), and the extent to which dispersion was distributed along a given plane (R_1). The first metric (λ_1) is similar to a standard deviation of the registration error on a specific location—ideally, it should be zero. The second metric (R_1) is a ratio between the amount of registration misalignment in the main error direction and the total sum of errors in all directions—it complements the amount of error by providing information on the anisotropy of that error, i.e., if the misalignment has a preferential direction (anisotropic) or if it is randomly distributed in space (isotropic). The resulting λ_1 and R_1 values of the fiducial clusters from Fluid and $\text{Fluid}_{\text{pre}}$ were then compared with the corresponding results from SPM, SPM_{pre}, DARTEL, and $\text{DARTEL}_{\text{pre}}$. Further details of this method and results can be found in the supplementary material.

RESULTS

VBM RESULTS

The VBM results for Set A are presented in **Figures 1–3**, and the results for Set B are in **Figures 4–6**.

It was observed that VBMs performed with the Fluid registration algorithms showed greater sensitivity than both SPM and DARTEL. This effect was especially evident for mild atrophy scenarios, namely for the AD cohorts. In these cases, hippocampal atrophy—known to be present from the manually measured hippocampi—in Fluid was more extensive than with SPM and (especially) SPM_{pre}, without the apparent cost of localization reduction visible in the DARTEL results. In fact, the DARTEL algorithm fared better in terms of eliminating apparent extraneous results in mild atrophy cases, but at the apparent cost of eliminating true positives, a problem previously described in detail (Pereira, 2010) and seen here in **Figure 1**, where the detection of hippocampal atrophy, in DARTEL without preprocessing, was less pronounced than with the other methods.

Compared to DARTEL, the results obtained with the Fluid algorithms retained greater anatomical detail, comparable to the detail obtained with both SPM methods. DARTEL destroys the anatomical detail of the results, especially in severely atrophic regions that appear as amorphous areas, as seen in the SD analyses shown in **Figures 2, 6**.

ASSESSMENT OF FIDUCIAL POINTS

A detailed analysis of the fiducial study has been included in the supplementary material. The λ_1 values dispersion values for Fluid (both with and without preprocessed scans) remained comparable to those of all other methods for most cases. The Fluid results were very consistent with the other methods. Also as observed previously using SPM and DARTEL (Pereira et al., 2010), there was an interaction between brain pathology and registration difficulties shown across all metrics, with severe focal atrophy still presenting the greatest challenge.

DISCUSSION

The use of viscous fluid registration algorithms to re-register gray matter probability maps demonstrates potential for VBM analyses. Overall, the VBM results from the analysis of each cohort were consistent with prior knowledge of atrophy profiles. Fluid registration enhanced the sensitivity of VBM while retaining anatomical detail. There was evidence for improvement over both standard SPM and DARTEL in several analyses.

REGISTRATION ASSESSMENT

The quantitative assessment of Fluid registration when compared to both SPM and DARTEL (further details and results can be found in the supplementary material) showed that all methods were broadly comparable. Despite the good match between target and subject, the registration algorithms seemed to be limited by the inherent variability between subjects that eludes warping. The registration performance values were quite variable across brain regions, and a disease grouping interaction for all methods was visible. The quantitative analysis of fiducial metrics closely

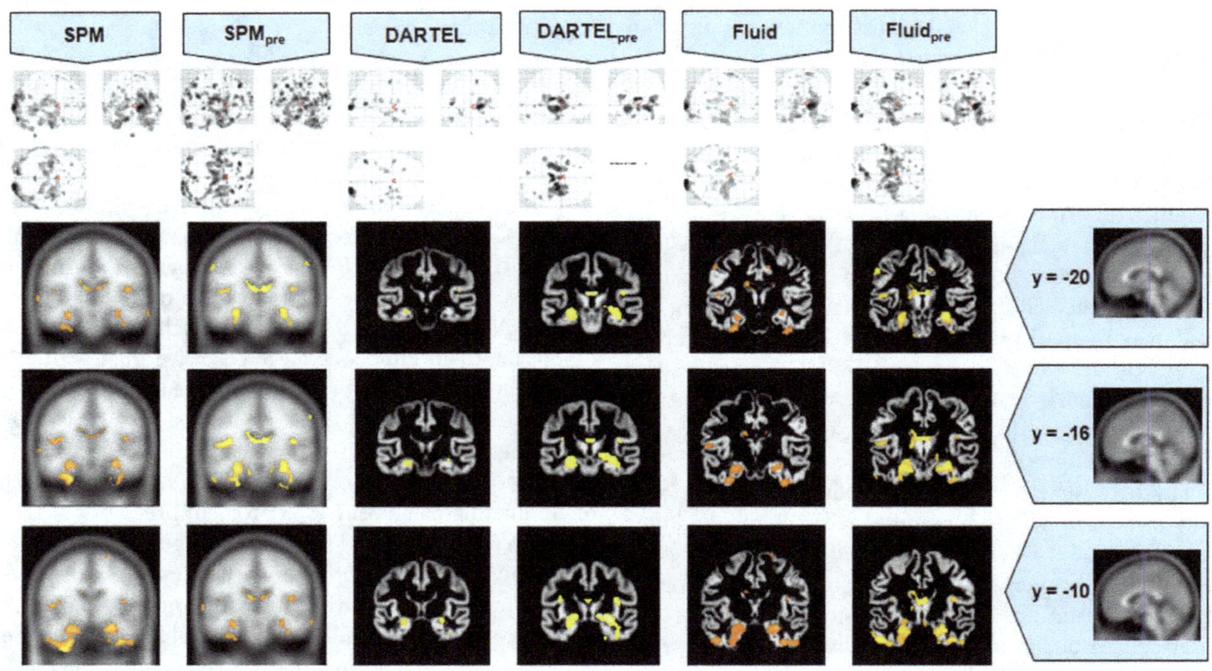

FIGURE 1 | VBM results for the AD cohort of Set A, with $p_{uncorrected}$ = 0.001. The projection of the results on three coronal slices are presented, at y = −20, −16, and 0 mm, emphasizing the hippocampal region, expected to be atrophic in this pathology and visible in all methods. The entorhinal cortex, however, also likely atrophic, is lost in both DARTEL results. The MNI template was used for SPM and SPM_{pre}, and the bespoke target was used for both DARTEL results, as well as for both Fluid results. Due to the use of bespoke template spaces, the presented coronal slices are not strictly comparable across different methods.

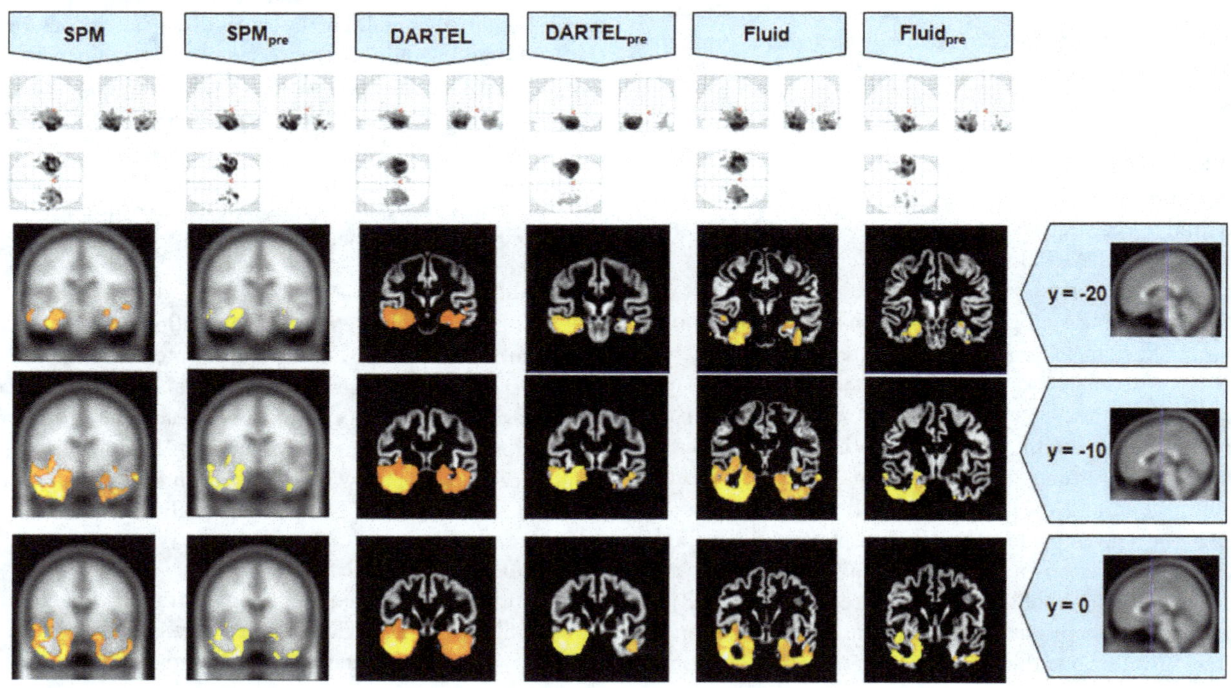

FIGURE 2 | VBM results for the SD cohort of Set A, with $p_{FWEcorrected}$ = 0.05. The projection of the results on three coronal slices are presented, at y = −20, −10, and 0 mm, emphasizing the temporal lobes, expected to be atrophic in this pathology. The lack of anatomical detail in DARTEL is notable, especially around the mesial temporal lobe. This detail is regained with the Fluid methods, with an increase in sensitivity compared to the SPM methods. The MNI template was used for SPM and SPM_{pre}, and the bespoke target was used for both DARTEL results, as well as for both Fluid results. Due to the use of bespoke template spaces, the presented coronal slices are not strictly comparable across different methods.

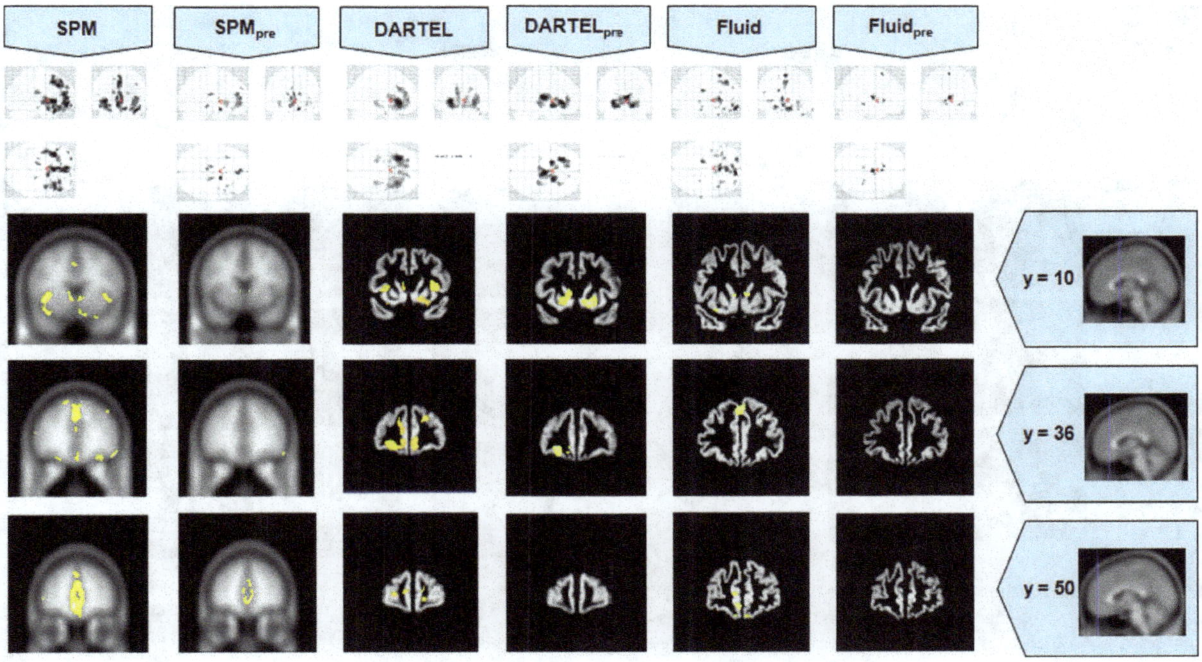

FIGURE 3 | VBM results for the bvFTD cohort of Set A, with $p_{FWEcorrected} = 0.05$. The projection of the results on three coronal slices are presented, at y = 10, 36, and 50 mm, emphasizing the frontal lobe, expected to be atrophic in this pathology. This was the only case where the use of Fluid methods did not provide tangible benefits; DARTEL was also not more informative than the SPM methods. The MNI template was used for SPM and SPM_{pre}, and the bespoke target was used for both DARTEL results, as well as for both Fluid results. Due to the use of bespoke template spaces, the presented coronal slices are not strictly comparable across different methods.

resembled the results for SPM5's unified segmentation that were reported previously (Pereira et al., 2010). This is not unexpected, as the viscous fluid registration was based on SPM8's registered probability maps (similar to SPM5's) and the algorithm was also limited to 15 iterations[1].

Importantly, the observation that the dispersion values of the fiducial markers were not significantly worsened by the Fluid methods suggesting that these registration algorithms are preserving the anatomical validity of the registration—in theory, there is a danger that geometric overfitting could lead to a loss of anatomical validity (i.e., that better fitting comes at the expense of moving anatomical structures). The quantitative results indicate that this did not occur.

VBM ANALYSES

All methods were able to identify the key abnormalities known from prior knowledge: hippocampal atrophy in AD and MCI groups (Galton et al., 2001; Du et al., 2004; Pennanen et al., 2004; Du et al., 2007); rostral temporal lobe atrophy in SD (Chan et al., 2001; Rosen et al., 2002; Williams et al., 2005; Nestor et al., 2006); and frontal atrophy in bvFTD (Rosen et al., 2002; Williams et al., 2005; Cardenas et al., 2007; Pereira et al., 2009). The preprocessed viscous registration results were, however, more concentrated on these areas of known atrophy in several of the analyses. This might suggest a reduction in false positives though it is important to highlight that, in the absence of ground-truth measurements for unexpected locations, this might also reflect lack of sensitivity to true, albeit unanticipated, abnormalities. On the other hand there was evidence to suggest that adding the viscous registration step offered superior results in detecting true positives and preserving anatomical detail, particularly in contrast to DARTEL. For instance, the AD analysis found fairly restricted hippocampal abnormalities in the temporal lobe using DARTEL. In contrast, the fluid registration method showed blobs extending into the adjacent temporal lobe (**Figure 1**). This result is far more consistent with previous manual volumetric studies of the entorhinal region (Du et al., 2004; Pennanen et al., 2004) and with knowledge of the spread of neuropathology in very early AD (Braak and Braak, 1991). It should be noted that SPM without DARTEL also detected change in this region. Regarding anatomical precision, the SD analysis also suggested superior performance with viscous registration over DARTEL. As seen in **Figures 2, 6**, DARTEL identified the rostral temporal abnormality but the blobs were essentially amorphous. In contrast, the viscous method produced results that adhered to the gray matter and were maximal in the rostral inferior surface, again consistent with prior knowledge from manual volumetrics (Chan et al., 2001; Galton et al., 2001; Davies et al., 2004). The difficulties shown by DARTEL when analysing atrophic brains have also been made evident in a recent paper (Ashburner and Friston, 2011), where it is clear that the algorithm underperforms when large deformations are required.

[1] A more liberal convergence criterion was also tested, up to a maximum of 25 iterations, but the resulting VBM glass brains started to show false positives around the cerebellum. These results suggested that the chosen number of iterations was adequate.

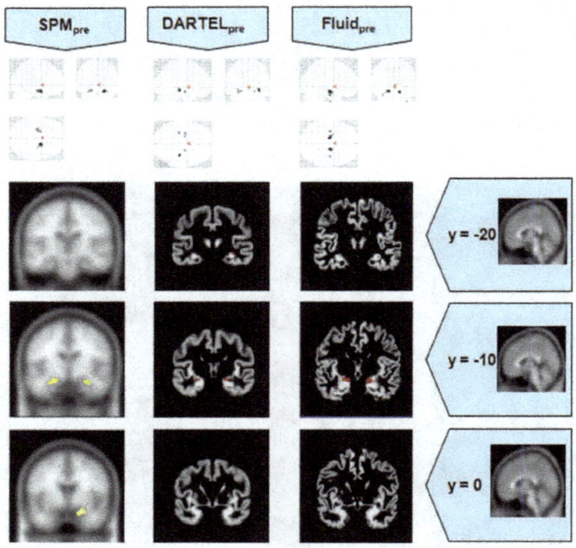

FIGURE 4 | VBM results for the MCI cohort of Set B, with $p_{FWEcorrected}$ = 0.05. The projection of the results on three coronal slices are presented, at y = −20, −10, and 0 mm, emphasizing the hippocampal region, expected to be atrophic in this pathology. Whereas DARTEL detects the atrophy, the Fluid methods are also able to detect it with further anatomical detail. The loss of sensitivity with DARTEL is clear. The MNI template was used for SPM and SPM_{pre}, and the bespoke target was used for the DARTEL result, as well as for the Fluid result. Due to the use of bespoke template spaces, the presented coronal slices are not strictly comparable across different methods. A different colour scale was use for $Fluid_{pre}$ to highlight the detected areas.

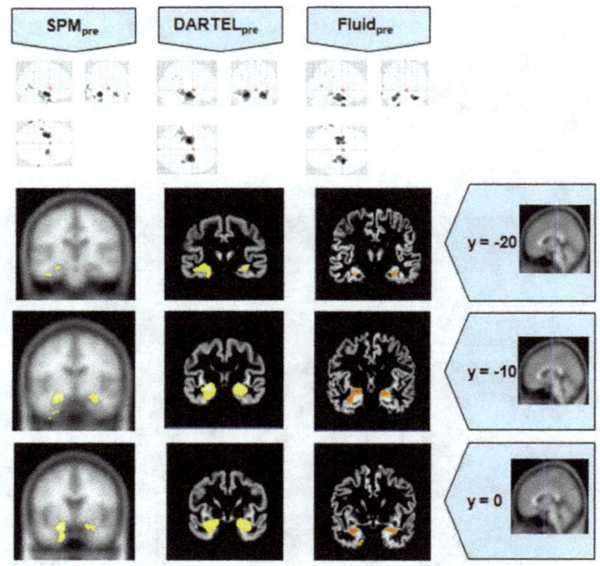

FIGURE 5 | VBM results for the AD cohort of Set B, with $p_{FWEcorrected}$ = 0.05. The projection of the results on three coronal slices are presented, at y = −20, −10, and 0 mm, emphasizing the hippocampal region, expected to be atrophic in this pathology. As before, whereas DARTEL detects the atrophy, the Fluid methods are also able to detect it with further anatomical detail. The MNI template was used for SPM and SPM_{pre}, and the bespoke target was used for the DARTEL result, as well as for the Fluid result. Due to the use of bespoke template spaces, the presented coronal slices are not strictly comparable across different methods. A different color scale was use for $Fluid_{pre}$ to highlight the detected areas.

The loss of anatomical detail due to averaging of subjects with DARTEL is shown in **Figure 7**. Even though DARTEL iteratively builds the template in order to reduce differences between subjects and to create a sharp average, the effects of blurring were still present. The viscous fluid algorithms, in contrast, generate gray matter probability maps that are locally deformed in order to conform to precise anatomical reference structures, whereas the DARTEL probability map results are degraded, leading to loss of localization power and to VBM results that are smoother and seemingly amorphous (**Figures 2**, **6**). Moreover, DARTEL has more regularization constraints than the viscous registration method presented in this paper that prevent it from creating the very local warps that a viscous fluid method can generate. This creates smooth diffeomorphic deformation fields but leads to limited local warping capabilities.

It must be acknowledged, nevertheless, that the use of a single subject template has some potential disadvantages, namely biasing the registration result for more similar brains. The nature of the gray matter probability maps, however, bypasses some of those limitations as the registered subjects already share a space very similar to the template. To address this concern, the Fluid algorithms were also tested by using as registration target the average of all subjects in each analysis, but results were essentially the same as the ones presented. Even if the templates were similar, the Fluid methods are more lightly regularized and are able to produce fields that can flow more freely than with DARTEL. It must be also noted that the use of a bespoke template in DARTEL, based on the iterative average of the registered gray matter probability maps, is prone to errors if at least one of the probability maps is poorly segmented. Heuristic tests have shown that such an approach may lead to false positives and to the propagation of segmentation errors. This issue will be addressed in future work.

It also important to highlight that while fluid registration yielded results that were more consistent with prior knowledge and/or manual volumetry (AD and MCI) and greater preservation of anatomical detail (SD), the bvFTD analyses did not show a benefit for this technique. All three approaches showed changes in the frontal lobe as would be expected from prior knowledge, though they were least extensive with fluid registration. The frontal lobes are large, and this results suggests that in the face of a large spatial extent of atrophy, the registration step is less important. Interestingly, in this group, it was not DARTEL but rather the default SPM analysis that yielded the most significant and extensive frontal abnormalities.

Finally, in common with many previous clinical VBM studies, this work made use of low numbers of subjects per cohort in order to simulate the real world application as closely as possible. We speculate that low numbers of subjects hinder the quality of a bespoke template—this would explain why DARTEL underperformed so often in the scenarios presented in this article. Moreover, a future application of the work presented in this paper is to make single subject VBM-like analyses possible in a clinical

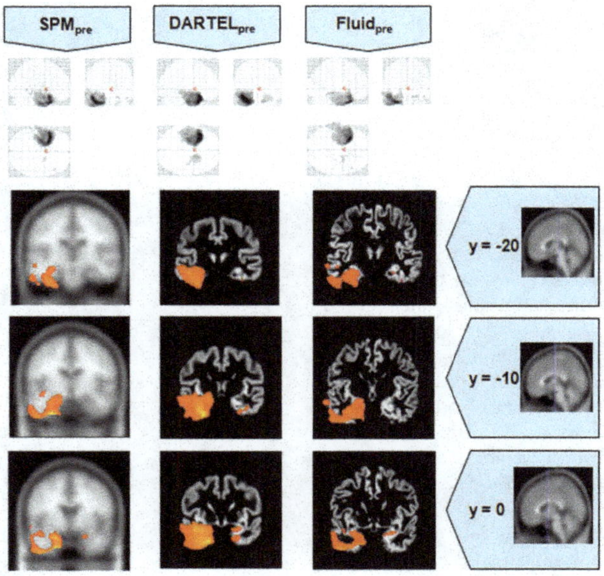

FIGURE 6 | VBM results for the SD cohort of Set B, with $p_{FWEcorrected} = 0.05$. The projection of the results on three coronal slices are presented, at y = −20, −10, and 0 mm, emphasizing the temporal lobes, expected to be atrophic in this pathology. The gain in sensitivity with the Fluid methods compared to the SPM approaches is clear; the gain in anatomical detail compared to DARTEL is again notable. The MNI template was used for SPM and SPM_{pre}, and the bespoke target was used for the DARTEL result, as well as for the Fluid result. Due to the use of bespoke template spaces, the presented coronal slices are not strictly comparable across different methods.

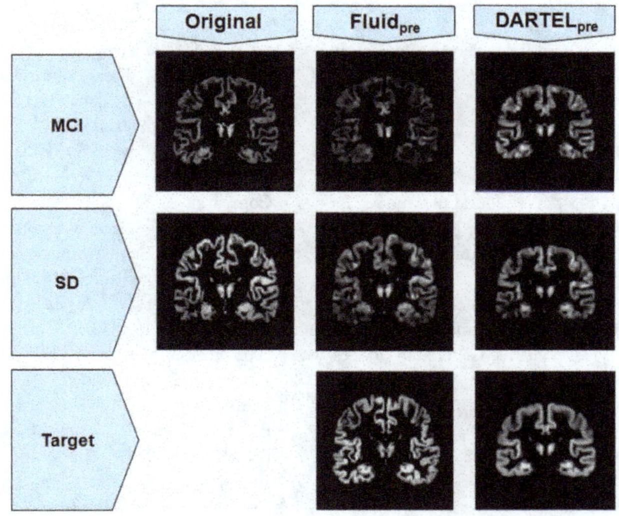

FIGURE 7 | Gray matter segments before and after registration to a target, for both MCI and SD cohorts from Set B, using both $Fluid_{pre}$ and $DARTEL_{pre}$. Notice the smoothness of $DARTEL_{pre}$'s target (for the *SD* population only, as an example) compared to the target used in $Fluid_{pre}$.

context. Understanding the practical limitations of the available methods when using low numbers of subjects is therefore fundamental to this aim.

CONCLUSIONS

The use of a viscous fluid registration algorithm to re-register the gray matter probability maps produced by the unified segmentation proved to be a useful tool, especially in terms of the qualitative assessment of VBM results. This Fluid registration method was able to provide detailed results with probability maps generated from both unpreprocessed and (especially) preprocessed scans; this was true for both a very focal atrophic cohort such as SD and in milder, more diffuse, atrophy such as AD and MCI. When compared to alternatives, especially DARTEL, which also uses a comparable methodology, the VBM outputs were more contiguous and anatomically localized with the Fluid methods. Additionally, these results suggest that most high-degree of freedom registration algorithm, with very little regularization, may be useful to re-register the probability maps in order to improve VBM results.

ACKNOWLEDGMENTS

Joao M. S. Pereira would like to acknowledge the support of his funding body, Fundação para a Ciência e a Tecnologia, Portugal. George Pengas and Julio Acosta-Cabronero were funded by the Alzheimer's Research Trust (UK). The work also received support from an MRC grant to Peter J. Nestor and from the NIHR Cambridge Biomedical Research Centre.

REFERENCES

Acosta-Cabronero, J., Williams, G. B., Pereira, J. M. S., Pengas, G., and Nestor, P. J. (2008). The impact of skull-stripping and radio-frequency bias correction on grey-matter segmentation for voxel-based morphometry. *Neuroimage* 39, 1654–1665. doi: 10.1016/j.neuroimage.2007.10.051

Ashburner, J. (2007). A fast diffeomorphic image registration algorithm. *Neuroimage* 38, 95–113. doi: 10.1016/j.neuroimage.2007.07.007

Ashburner, J., and Friston, K. J. (2011). Diffeomorphic registration using geodesic shooting and Gauss-Newton optimisation. *Neuroimage* 55, 954–967. doi: 10.1016/j.neuroimage.2010.12.049

Ashburner, J., and Friston, K. J. (1999). Nonlinear spatial normalisation using basis functions. *Hum. Brain Mapp.* 7, 254–266.

Ashburner, J., and Friston, K. J. (2005). Unified segmentation. *Neuroimage* 15, 839–851. doi: 10.1016/j.neuroimage.2005.02.018

Braak, H., and Braak, E. (1991). Neuropathological stageing of Alzheimer-related changes. *Acta Neuropathol.* 82, 239–259. doi: 10.1007/BF00308809

Bro-Nielsen, M., and Gramkow, C. (1996). "Fast fluid registration of medical images," in *Proceedings Visualization in Biomedical Computing (VBC'96)*, Vol. 1131, (Hamburg: Springer Lecture Notes in Computer Science), 267–276.

Cardenas, V. A., Boxer, A. L., Chao, L. L., Gorno-Tempini, M. L., Miller, B. L., Weiner, M. W., et al. (2007). Deformation-based morphometry reveals brain atrophy in frontotemporal dementia. *Arch. Neurol.* 64, 873–877. doi: 10.1001/archneur.64.6.873

Chan, D., Fox, N. C., Scahill, R. I., Crum, W. R., Whitwell, J. L., Leschziner, G., et al. (2001). Patterns of temporal lobe atrophy in semantic dementia and Alzheimer's disease. *Ann. Neurol.* 49, 433–442. doi: 10.1002/ana.92

Christensen, G. E., Rabbitt, R. D., and Miller, M. I. (1996). Deformable templates using large deformation kinematics. *IEEE Trans. Image Process.* 5, 1435–1447. doi: 10.1109/83.536892

D'Agostino, E., Maes, F., Vandermeulen, D., and Suetens, P. (2003). A viscous fluid model for multimodal non-rigid image registration using mutual information. *Med. Image Anal.* 7, 565–575. doi: 10.1016/S1361-8415(03)00039-2

Davies, R. R., Graham, K. S., Xuereb, J. H., Williams, G. B., and Hodges, J. R. (2004). The human perirhinal cortex and semantic memory. *Eur. J. Neurosci.* 20, 2441–2446. doi: 10.1111/j.1460-9568.2004.03710.x

Du, A.-T., Schuff, N., Kramer, J. H., Rosen, H. J., Gorno-Tempini, M. L., Rankin, K., et al. (2007). Different regional patterns of cortical thinning in Alzheimer's disease and frontotemporal dementia. *Brain* 130, 1159–1166. doi: 10.1093/brain/awm016

Du, A. T., Schuff, N., Kramer, J. H., Ganzer, S., Zhu, X. P., Jagust, W. J., et al. (2004). Higher atrophy rate of entorhinal cortex than hippocampus in AD. *Neurology* 62, 422–427. doi: 10.1212/01.WNL.0000106462.72282.90

Galton, C. J., Patterson, K., Graham, K., Lambon-Ralph, M. A., Williams, G., Antoun, N., et al. (2001). Differing patterns of temporal atrophy in Alzheimer's disease and semantic dementia. *Neurology* 57, 216–225. doi: 10.1212/WNL.57.2.216

Gramkow, C., and Bro-Nielsen, M. (1997). "Comparison of three filters in the solution of the navier-stokes equation in registration," in *Scandinavian Conference on Image Analysis*, (Lappenranta), 795–802.

McKhann, G., Drachman, D., Folstein, M., Katzman, R., Price, D., and Stadlan, E. M. (1984). Clinical diagnosis of Alzheimer's disease: report of the NINCDS-ADRDA Work Group under the auspices of Department of Health and Human Services Task Force on Alzheimer's Disease. *Neurology* 34, 939–944. doi: 10.1212/WNL.34.7.939

Neary, D., Snowden, J. S., Gustafson, L., Passant, U., Stuss, D., Black, S., et al. (1998). Frontotemporal lobar degeneration: a consensus on clinical diagnostic criteria. *Neurology* 51, 1546–1554. doi: 10.1212/WNL.51.6.1546

Nestor, P. J., Fryer, T. D., and Hodges, J. (2006). Declarative memory impairments in Alzheimer's disease and semantic dementia. *Neuroimage* 30, 1010–1020. doi: 10.1016/j.neuroimage.2005.10.008

Pengas, G., Hodges, J. R., Watson, P., and Nestor, P. J. (2010). Focal posterior cingulate atrophy in incipient Alzheimer's disease. *Neurobiol. Aging* 31, 25–33. doi: 10.1016/j.neurobiolaging.2008.03.014

Pengas, G., Pereira, J. M. S., Williams, G. B., and Nestor, P. J. (2008). Comparative reliability of total intracranial volume estimation methods and the influence of atrophy in a longitudinal semantic dementia cohort. *J. Neuroimag.* 19, 37–46. doi: 10.1111/j.1552-6569.2008.00246.x

Pennanen, C., Kivipelto, M., Tuomainen, S., Hartikainen, P., Hanninen, T., Laakso, M. P., et al. (2004). Hippocampus and entorhinal cortex in mild cognitive impairment and early AD. *Neurobiol. Aging* 25, 303–310. doi: 10.1016/S0197-4580(03)00084-8

Pereira, J. M., Nestor, P. J., and Williams, G. B. (2008). Impact of inconsistent resolution on VBM studies. *Neuroimage* 40, 1711–1717. doi: 10.1016/j.neuroimage.2008.01.031

Pereira, J. M. S. (2010). *Characterisation, Optimisation and Application of Voxel Based Morphometry in MRI Studies of Dementia.* Ph.D. thesis. Cambridge: University of Cambridge.

Pereira, J. M. S., Williams, G. B., Acosta-Cabronero, J., Pengas, G., Spillantini, M. G., Xuereb, J. H., et al. (2009). Atrophy patterns in histologic vs clinical groupings of frontotemporal lobar degeneration. *Neurology* 72, 1653–1660. doi: 10.1212/WNL.0b013e3181a55fa2

Pereira, J. M. S., Xiong, L., Acosta-Cabronero, J., Pengas, G., Williams, G. B., and Nestor, P. J. (2010). Registration accuracy for VBM studies varies according to region and degenerative disease grouping. *Neuroimage* 49, 2205–2215. doi: 10.1016/j.neuroimage.2009.10.068

Press, W. H., Teukolsky, S. A., Vetterling, W. T., and Flannery, B. P. (1992). "Numerical recipes," in *C: the Art of Scientific Computing, 2nd Edn.* Cambridge: Cambridge University Press.

Ridgway, G. R., Henley, S. M. D., Rohrer, J. D., Scahill, R. I., Warren, J. D., and Fox, N. C. (2008). Ten simple rules for reporting voxel-based morphometry studies. *Neuroimage* 40, 1429–1435. doi: 10.1016/j.neuroimage.2008.01.003

Rosen, H., Gorno-Tempini, M., Goldman, W., Perry, R., Schuff, N., Weiner, M., et al. (2002). Patterns of brain atrophy in frontotemporal dementia and semantic dementia. *Neurology* 58, 198–208. doi: 10.1212/WNL.58.2.198

Thirion, J.-P. (1998). Image matching as a diffusion process: an analogy with Maxwell's Demons. *Med. Image Anal.* 2, 243–260. doi: 10.1016/S1361-8415(98)80022-4

Williams, G. B., Nestor, P. J., and Hodges, J. R. (2005). Neural correlates of semantic and behavioural deficits in frontotemporal dementia. *Neuroimage* 24, 1042–1051. doi: 10.1016/j.neuroimage.2004.10.023

Wollny, G., and Kruggel, F. (2002). Computational cost of nonrigid registration algorithms based on fluid dynamics. *IEEE Trans. Med. Imag.* 21, 946–952. doi: 10.1109/TMI.2002.803113

Yassa, M. A., and Stark, C. E. L. (2009). A quantitative evaluation of cross-participant registration techniques for MRI studies of the medial temporal lobe. *Neuroimage* 44, 319–327. doi: 10.1016/j.neuroimage.2008.09.016

25

The role of the innate immune system in ALS

Sudarshan Phani[1,2], Diane Berengere Re[1,2] and Serge Przedborski[1,2]*

[1] Department of Pathology and Cell Biology, Columbia University, New York, NY, USA
[2] Center for Motor Neuron Disease, Department of Neurology, Columbia University, New York, NY, USA

Edited by:
Roger A. Barker, University of Cambridge and Addenbrooke' Hospital, UK

Reviewed by:
Raja S. Settivari, The Dow Chemical Company, USA
Kevin Talbot, Oxford University, UK

***Correspondence:**
Serge Przedborski, Department of Pathology, Cell Biology and Neurology, Center for Motor Neuron Disease, Columbia University, 630 West 168th Street, P&S 5-420 NY, USA.
e-mail: sp30@columbia.edu

Amyotrophic lateral sclerosis (ALS) is a fatal, adult-onset neurodegenerative disease that is characterized by the death of upper and lower motor neurons. Recent studies have made it clear that although motor neurons are the primary targets of the degenerative process, other cell types play key roles in the death of motor neurons. Most notably, cells of the immune system, including astrocytes and microglia have come under increasing scrutiny, after multiple lines of evidence have shown these cells to be deleterious to motor neurons. Both *in vitro* and *in vivo* experiments have shown that astrocytes and microglia containing mutated SOD1 are harmful to motor neurons. Several studies on ALS and other neurodegenerative diseases have revealed that reactive astrocytes and microglia are capable of releasing pro-inflammatory factors such as cytokines and chemokines, which are harmful to neighboring neurons. In addition, it is believed that diseased astrocytes can specifically kill motor neurons through the release of toxic factors. Furthermore, in an animal model of the disease, it has been shown that the reduction of SOD1 in microglia may be able to slow the progression of ALS symptoms. Although the exact pathways of motor neuron death in ALS have yet to be elucidated, studies have suggested that they die through aBax-dependent signaling pathway. Mounting evidence suggests that neuroinflammation plays an important role in the degeneration of motor neurons. Based on these findings, anti-inflammatory compounds are currently being tested for their potential to reduce disease severity; however, these studies are only in the preliminary stages. While we understand that astrocytes and microglia play a role in the death of motor neurons in ALS, much work needs to be done to fully understand ALS pathology and the role the immune system plays in disease onset and progression.

Keywords: amyotrophic lateral sclerosis, astrocyte, microglia, motor neuron, innate immune system

INTRODUCTION

Amyotrophic Lateral Sclerosis (ALS) is a fatal adult-onset neurodegenerative disorder that is characterized clinically by muscle weakness and wasting. Pathologically, it is identified by the degeneration of upper and lower motor neurons (Boillee et al., 2006a). Generally, death results from respiratory failure due to paralysis of the respiratory muscles. The incidence of ALS is reported to be between 1.5 and 3 per 100,000 in Europe and North America (Wijesekera and Leigh, 2009; Hardiman et al., 2011). ALS onset peaks between the ages of 50–75 and declines thereafter. These factors suggest that ALS may not be a disease of aging, but rather that age may be one of a multitude of contributing factors (Hardiman et al., 2011). Thus far, there are no effective treatments and no cure for ALS.

Amyotrophic lateral sclerosis is essentially a sporadic disorder, with greater than 90% of the cases originating from an unknown cause. However, approximately 10% of the cases are considered familial (FALS) and are generally inherited as a dominant disorder (Ince et al., 2011) due to mutations in a number of seemingly disparate genes. These include, but are not limited to, mutations in genes such as TAR DNA binding protein (TDP)-43 and Fused in Sarcoma (FUS) (Sreedharan et al., 2008; Kwiatkowski et al., 2009; Vance et al., 2009). Despite major enthusiasm by the research community about the recent discoveries of mutations in FUS and TDP-43, the best characterized form of FALS still remains that which is linked to mutations in the copper-zinc superoxide dismutase gene (SOD1) and which accounts for 10–20% of all FALS cases (Andersen, 2001). Myriad mutations in SOD1 all seem to give rise to an ALS phenotype via a toxic gain-of-function mechanism, which is clinically almost indistinguishable from sporadic cases. Histopathologically, however, recent studies have found TDP-43 to be a reliable marker for differentiating sALS from SOD1-related fALS. These studies have shown that all of the cases of sporadic ALS and SOD1-negative fALS had neural and glial inclusions which were immunoreactive for both ubiquitin and TDP-43, whereas fALS cases with mutations in SOD1 were universally absent of TDP-43 immunoreactivity (MacKenzie et al., 2007; Tan et al., 2007).

More recently, studies have identified an expanded GGGGCC hexanucleotide repeat in a non-coding region of C9ORF72. This expansion has been shown to be linked to chromosome 9p-linked FTD and ALS. Interestingly, this same repeat expansion was also identified in the majority of families with a combined FTD/ALS phenotype and TDP-43 pathology. Extended studies have identified the C9ORF72 expansion as the most common genetic abnormality in fALS (23.5%; DeJesus-Hernandez et al., 2011).

A number of studies have pointed to oxidative stress, protein aggregation, or mitochondrial dysfunction as mechanisms of mutant SOD1 toxicity. In addition, SOD1 toxicity has been shown to be linked to changes in the immune system, which has also been shown to contribute to the motor neuron pathology seen in ALS; however, the exact nature of the pathogenic mechanisms provoking motor neuron degeneration in mutant SOD1-linked ALS remains elusive (Ince et al., 2011). Interestingly, the repeat expansion in C9ORF72 results in the formation of nuclear RNA foci not seen in SOD1-linked pathology, suggesting multiple disease mechanisms (DeJesus-Hernandez et al., 2011).

While the discovery of the C9ORF72 repeat expansion has opened new avenues of ALS research, the abundance and well-studied nature of SOD1-mutant animals make them the *de facto* models of choice to study ALS pathology for the time being. Although imperfect, these models allow for a great deal of insight into potential mechanisms involved in ALS pathology, with the hope that the mechanisms elucidated through the use of these models may also provide understanding of sALS and non-SOD1-mediated fALS.

INFLAMMATION AND NEURODEGENERATION

Although ALS is a disease primarily affecting upper and lower motor neurons, it is increasingly recognized that the entire pathogenic process of ALS is not restricted to a set of cell-autonomous deleterious mechanisms taking place within motor neurons. Instead, it is now believed that non-cell autonomous mechanisms, such as neuroinflammation may also contribute to the disease process.

Germane to this issue is the fact that the immune system has been found to be altered in sporadic ALS. Studies have shown immunological differences in the blood of ALS patients compared to healthy controls. These include increased levels of CD4+ cells, and reduced CD8+ T-lymphocytes (Mantovani et al., 2009). Interestingly, blood samples analyzed from patients at an earlier and less severe stage of the disease also show altered expression of immune cells, such as significant reductions in CD4+CD25+ T-regulatory (T-reg) cells as well as CD14+ monocytes (Mantovani et al., 2009). Additionally, T-reg cells have been shown to play significant roles as neuroprotectants responsible for modulating the neuroinflammatory response in mouse models of neurodegeneration (Kipnis et al., 2004). It is therefore possible to hypothesize that the reduction of T-reg cells in the blood of sporadic ALS patients might represent a recruitment of these cells from the periphery into the CNS in order to activate resident innate immune cells such as microglia, as well as anti-inflammatory cytokines such as interleukin-10 and transforming growth factor-β in an effort to protect the area most affected by the early effects of ALS degeneration (Kipnis et al., 2004; Mantovani et al., 2009).

Markers for resident innate immune cells have also been found to be altered in the brains of ALS patients as well as in animal models of ALS. For instance, immunostaining for glial fibrillary acid protein (GFAP), a common marker for astrocytes, is markedly increased in all forms of ALS in the precentral gyrus of human samples (Kawamata et al., 1992). In addition, staining for leukocyte common antigen (LCA), lymphocyte function associate molecule-1 (LFA-1), and complement receptors CR3 (CD11b) and CR4 (CD11c) are increased, supporting the idea that microglia and macrophages are activated in the areas of ALS degeneration, such as the motor cortex, brainstem, and corticospinal tract (Kawamata et al., 1992; Papadimitriou et al., 2010). Remarkably, it is believed that the early site of pathological changes in ALS is the neuromuscular junction, and while this particular site of the lower motor neuron pathway has been extensively studied, very little information exists about the immune response at that level. Nonetheless, the data reviewed above provide compelling evidence that a robust neuroinflammatory response is part of the neuropathological changes that characterize ALS. However, none of the aforementioned studies address the actual role, if any, of neuroinflammation in ALS. Investigations in other neurodegenerative disorders have shown that neuroinflammation may exert dual effects, that it can be protective or harmful. In order to distinguish between these two possibilities, efforts have generally concentrated on studying animal models of ALS.

The blood brain barrier renders the brain as immune-privileged, therefore, the brain contains resident astrocytes and microglia that perform the duties of immune surveillance and act as an innate response system. Reactive astrocytes are most commonly recruited to the site of an injury, such as a spinal cord injury or ischemic events. Their main functions are to compact inflammatory cells, and to re-establish the blood brain barrier (Okada et al., 2006) they may also be involved in clearing CNS debris, such as amyloid plaques (Papadimitriou et al., 2010). Aside from astrocytes, the CNS immune system also consists of ramified resting microglial cells, whose processes play an active role in maintaining the homeostasis of the neural environment. Once activated by the presence of antigens and during times of distress, such as is the case during neurodegeneration, microglia, like other immune cells, become activated taking on an ameboid morphology. Once activated, microglia can secrete a myriad of neurotrophic factors and cytokines (Napoli and Neumann, 2009), and engage in the clearance of pathogens and debris through phagocytosis. However, unregulated activation of microglial activation may be harmful to neurons through the release of potentially harmful neurotoxins including quinolinic acid, reactive oxygen and nitrogen species (ROS; RNS), and pro-inflammatory cytokines. Although a large number of studies have shown that microglia and, to a lesser extent, astrocytes are activated in the affected areas of the CNS in ALS, thus far little attention has been paid to the determination of the actual phenotype of these cells. For instance, since activated resident immune cells can display either a pro-inflammatory or anti-inflammatory phenotype, sometimes referred to as M1 or M2, it will be critical to determine which phenotype they exhibit as a whole, and if possible as individual cells. It is also important to determine whether such profiles differ among the various affected structures of the CNS and stages of the disease. Aside from these outstanding questions, it is also critical to elucidate whether these inflammatory cells play a role in the pathogenesis of ALS. The use of animal models is greatly aiding in the attempts to answer the questions raised by the findings described above.

The most commonly studied animal models of ALS are rats and mice expressing mutant SOD1 (mSOD1). Although, as indicated above, SOD 1 mutations only account for a small percentage of human cases, animal models using mSOD1 are used with the hope that the mechanisms leading the disease are shared across cases, and knowledge gained from these models can be used to understand the development of the disease in humans. Notably, evidence for increases in astrocytes and microglia have also been found in transgenic mice expressing different forms of mutant SOD1 (mSOD1), supporting human pathology studies (Fischer et al., 2004). Specifically, GFAP and CD11b staining showed evidence for significant increases in reactive astrocytes and microglia in the motor regions of transgenic mice containing mSOD1 (Fischer et al., 2004). Although both astrocytosis and microgliosis have been observed in rodent models, the timing of events seems to be unclear. Some studies using mSOD1 mice have suggested astrocytosis to be an early stage event, with microgliosis as a late stage reaction (Yang et al., 2011). However, others have suggested that microglial response occurs at a much earlier stage of the disease (Sanagi et al., 2010). Nevertheless, it does appear that microglial activation starts after motor neuron degeneration, and initially tries to protect motor neurons from degeneration (Fischer et al., 2004; Henkel et al., 2009).

IMMUNE CELL MEDIATED NON-CELL AUTONOMY IN ALS

Motor neuron death and degeneration has been implicated in causing the debilitating symptoms characteristic of ALS, however, mounting evidence indicates that motor neuron death is, at least in part, non-cell autonomous. *In vivo* studies have shown that mSOD1 expressed only in motor neurons of transgenic mice is either not sufficient to cause neurodegeneration or causes only a mild ALS-like phenotype (Jaarsma et al., 2008). Support for non-cell autonomy comes from studies showing that when mSOD1 expression was reduced in microglia and macrophages in transgenic mice (Boillee et al., 2006b; Wang et al., 2009), motor neuron degeneration was decreased. Aside from microglia, evidence has shown that astrocytes may also play a role in motor neuron death. Early studies using transgenic mice expressing mSOD1 in astrocytes suggested the need for motor neurons to be impaired for a degenerative phenotype (Gong et al., 2000), however more recent studies have concluded that astrocytes expressing mSOD1 released toxic factor(s) which were sufficient to cause motor neuron degeneration in an *in vitro* model of ALS (Nagai et al., 2007).

THE ROLE OF ASTROCYTES IN ALS NON-CELL AUTONOMY

Astrocytes are one of the main cell types responsible for the clearance of potentially excitotoxic glutamate from the synaptic space, and as mentioned earlier, play a distinct role when they become activated by the immune system. Quite interestingly, glutamate handling has been reported to be modified in both sporadic and familial ALS (Boillee et al., 2006a). Studies have found that brain and spinal cord samples from ALS patients showed altered glutamate transport (Rothstein et al., 1992) resulting from changes in the glutamate transporter EAAT2 (Maragakis et al., 2004). Evidence suggests that EAAT2 is significantly decreased in the motor cortex and spinal cords of ALS patients (Fray et al., 1998), as well as in the spinal cords of mSOD1 transgenic mice (Bruijn et al., 1997) and rats (Howland et al., 2002). It should come as no coincidence then, that astrocytes were quickly targeted for their role in the ALS disease processes.

More interestingly in terms of inflammation, samples analyzed from the brains and spinal cords of ALS patients were found to contain greater numbers of activated or reactive astrocytes, a clear sign of an immune response (Sta et al., 2011). Of note, and useful for research purposes, increased reactive astrocyte expression has been found both in ALS patients and in animal models of ALS (Sta et al., 2011).

Although the main function of astrocytes in the synaptic space is the maintenance of a homeostatic environment for neurons though activities such as the clearance of neurotransmitters, reactive astrocytes gain properties that resting astrocytes do not exhibit. It has been shown that during and after injury, astrocytes have the ability to ameliorate symptoms by physically isolating the injured area through the formation of a glial scar, as well as release neurotrophins and growth factors such as IGF-1 which have been deemed beneficial to injured cells (Dong and Benveniste, 2001). Astrocytes have also been found to release NGF and induce additional sprouting both *in vitro* and *in vivo*, a key step in neuronal recovery (Chalmers et al., 1996; Wu et al., 1998).

Even though astrocytes do have the potential to be beneficial to neurons, the majority of evidence suggests that astrocytes actually contribute to neuronal degeneration during disease, with ALS being no exception. Interestingly, NGF release, which has generally been regarded as a positive attribute of reactive astrocytes, has been shown to directly lead to motor neuron apoptosis through the p75 pathway (Pehar et al., 2004). Notably, mSOD1-containing astrocytes have been found to be even more toxic to their environments than reactive astrocytes alone. Studies have found that reducing mSOD1 expressing astrocyte levels in an *in vivo* model of ALS decreased motor neuron degeneration and correspondingly increased the life span of the affected animals (Lepore et al., 2008; Barbeito et al., 2010). Although the exact mechanisms for astrocyte-mediated motor neuron toxicity is not known, several lines of evidence have pointed to the activation and release of toxic or harmful products such as pro-inflammatory cytokine oxidative stressors. These include, but are not limited to prostaglandins, leukotrienes, and RNS (Hensley et al., 2006a,b). In addition, *in vitro* models of ALS have shown that astrocytes containing mSOD1 release toxic factors that are preferentially toxic to motor neurons. Furthermore, it was noted that even wild-type motor neurons die in the presence of mSOD1-containing astrocytes. Moreover, wild-type motor neurons die when grown in media conditioned by mSOD1 containing astrocytes. These *in vitro* studies have suggested the pro-apoptotic Bax pathway as another mechanism through which astrocytes mediate motor neuron cell death (Nagai et al., 2007).

THE ROLE OF MICROGLIA IN ALS

Microglial cells perform the duties of immune surveillance in the CNS, and once activated, such as is the case during neurodegeneration, these cells secrete cytokines and neurotrophins in order to help restore homeostasis to the neuronal environment (Napoli and Neumann, 2009). However, just as astrocytes may play a deleterious role in ALS, microglia have also been found to exacerbate neuronal injury. *In vivo* studies have shown that microglial cells increase their expression and release of pro-inflammatory cytokines, such as TNF-α and IL-1β in a mouse model of ALS. Additionally, activated microglia have been shown to promote the generation of reactive oxidative species, causing more harm than good to motor neurons (Henkel et al., 2009).

In the case of ALS, a number of studies have looked at mSOD1 expression in microglia, and its effect on ALS disease progression and motor neuron degeneration. Recent studies have found that diminishing mSOD1 levels in microglia in a mouse model of ALS did not alter the age of onset of paralysis, however it was able to significantly slow the disease progression (Boillee et al., 2006b). Yet, the lack of effects on onset must be regarded with caution, as one cannot exclude that the reduction in mSOD1 in microglia was only at the time when some actual motor neuron degeneration has already occurred. Indeed, the technology used in this study to reduce mSOD1 expression was driven by the microglial specific promoter CD11b which only acquires significant driving forces in response to pathological stimuli such as motor neuron degeneration. Accordingly, it would not be surprising that the disease phenotype in these mice has only been modified after the onset of motor neuron degeneration. It has also been found that mSOD1 containing microglia produce and release greater levels of pro-inflammatory cytokines and free radicals than their wild-type counterparts (Henkel et al., 2009). While the presence of mSOD1 in microglia has been shown to be deleterious, new evidence has begun to pinpoint the mechanisms that may control ALS-related microglial toxicity. Specifically, increases in the pro-inflammatory cytokines and prostaglandin E_2 have been reported to be present in ALS patients (Papadimitriou et al., 2010). Additionally, *in vitro* data suggested that conditioned media obtained from activated microglia is sufficient to cause neuronal degeneration through the concurrent stimulation of TNF-α and NMDA receptors. These pathways are thought to up-regulate inducible nitric oxide synthase activity, thus causing oxidative stress which leads to cell death. Of note is the fact that activation of either the TNF-α or NMDA receptor alone was not found to cause cell death, and the blockade of either of these receptor pathways was found to alleviate cell death caused by microglial-conditioned media, suggesting that both of these receptors need to be activated for MN death to occur (Moisse and Strong, 2006).

Although there is compelling evidence supporting the notion that microglial activation could be sufficient to kill motor neurons in ALS, *in vivo* studies have cast doubt on this theory by showing that repopulating microglial-deficient mice with mSOD-containing microglia failed to cause motor neuron death. These studies have yet to be repeated (Boillee et al., 2006a,b). In addition, studies done in mSOD1 mice absent in TNF-α, a potent inflammatory signaling molecule, did not show any decrease in motor neuron death (Gowing et al., 2006). These data are perhaps suggestive of alternate inflammatory pathways, and may implicate inflammatory mechanisms as coincidental, but not causative.

When viewed together, mounting *in vitro* and *in vivo* evidence have given credence to the toxic effects of astrocytes and microglia on motor neurons and have suggested multiple mechanisms that may be involved. In addition to these, it must be noted that mSOD1 containing motor neurons are particularly vulnerable to Fas ligand and NO-triggered cell death (Moisse and Strong, 2006). Therefore, it is thought that the combined effects of mSOD1 in motor neurons as well as in neighboring astrocytes and microglia are what ultimately result in cell death and degeneration in ALS. While the discovery of the expansion repeat in C9ORF72 is too recent to know its relationship with the inflammatory system, it would be conceivable that the immune system response to such a widespread mutation would be equal to or greater than what has already been observed in other forms of ALS.

ANTI-INFLAMMATORY THERAPEUTICS IN ALS

With inflammation potentially playing a significant role in ALS pathogenesis and progression, it is logical to attempt anti-inflammatory drugs for use as therapeutics in combating ALS. Using SOD1 mice, a number of groups have attempted to administer COX2 inhibitors such as cyclosporine, thalidomide, and lenalidomide to COX2-deficient mice in order to attenuate the negative effects of inflammation. Interestingly, the use of these drugs in mSOD1 animal models was sufficient to prolong lifespan (Karlsson et al., 2004; Kiaei et al., 2006). Cyclosporine is currently in clinical trials. Initial double-blind, placebo-controlled clinical trials suggest that men may benefit from cyclosporine administration when given within 18 months of initial diagnosis (Appel et al., 1988). Based on these results, the group of Karlsson et al. are currently running Phase II clinical trials.

Another approach to anti-inflammatory therapy was the use of the drug Copaxone, which has most often been used to treat patients diagnosed with multiple sclerosis. The active ingredient, glatiramer acetate, was used both in animal models as well as clinical trials. While there was initial excitement for the drug, which increased survival in mSOD1 mouse models of ALS (Angelov et al., 2003), these results could not be replicated (Turner and Talbot, 2008). Clinical trials with glatiramer acetate were also unsuccessful (Meininger et al., 2009), suggesting the mouse strain or the delivery mechanism in the original study may have played a greater role than initially indicated.

Perhaps the most well-known of the anti-inflammatory compounds used against ALS is minocycline, a second-generation tetracycline which has been shown to have anti-inflammatory properties (Yrjanheikki et al., 1999). The use of minocycline was shown to delay motor neuron degeneration as well as increase survival in several different mSOD1 mouse models of ALS (Kriz et al., 2002; Zhu et al., 2002). These studies found that minocycline may have had a direct impact on motor neurons by decreasing apoptosis through a reduction in cytochrome *c* release (Zhu et al., 2002; Moisse and Strong, 2006). Furthermore, it may have decreased the level of microglial activation and proliferation in mSOD1 mouse models of ALS (Kriz et al., 2002; Moisse and Strong, 2006). Given these promising results, minocycline was moved into clinical trials, and thus far, no observable difference was found between placebo and drug cohorts in phase III trials (Barbeito et al., 2010).

It should be noted however, that the use of anti-inflammatory drugs in animal models does not lead to direct knowledge of drug dosing and further study may be needed in order to find correct dosing levels, and potentially more importantly, dosing schedules. The use of animal models allows researchers to administer therapeutics before, during, after, or any combination therein relative to symptom onset. Unfortunately, patients being treated for neurodegenerative disorders do not have the luxury of being pre-treated for ALS symptoms before they arise, thus vastly complicating any therapeutic regimen.

CONCLUSION

Recent lines of evidence have given strong support to the role of astrocytes and microglia in ALS disease pathology. Tissue samples from ALS patients have been found to contain increased inflammatory by-products, and animal models of ALS have corroborated these increases. There is some debate as to whether inflammation in ALS could potentially be protective, however most studies have found the activation of microglia and astrocytes to be more harmful than beneficial. These harmful effects may come through the up-regulation and increased release of pro-inflammatory cytokines and reactive oxidative species, as well as through decreased uptake of excitotoxic neurotransmitters such as glutamate from the synaptic space. One major unanswered question, however, is whether an external event causes neuroinflammatory activation leading to ALS, or whether an external event leads to ALS causing neuroinflammation. In either case, both ALS pathology and neuroinflammation seem to act concurrently to exacerbate the symptoms of neurodegeneration. Future therapies to combat motor neuron death may involve a combination of approaches which recognize the role of multiple mechanisms and cell types in the progression of ALS.

REFERENCES

Andersen, P. M. (2001). Genetics of sporadic ALS. *Amyotroph. Lateral Scler. Other Motor Neuron Disord.* 2(Suppl. 1), S37–S41.

Angelov, D. N., Waibel, S., Guntinas-Lichius, O., Lenzen, M., Neiss, W. F., Tomov, T. L., Yoles, E., Kipnis, J., Schori, H., Reuter, A., Ludolph, A., and Schwartz, M. (2003). Therapeutic vaccine for acute and chronic motor neuron diseases: implications for amyotrophic lateral sclerosis. *Proc. Natl. Acad. Sci. U.S.A.* 100, 4790–4795.

Appel, S. H., Stewart, S. S., Appel, V., Harati, Y., Mietlowski, W., Weiss, W., and Belendiuk, G. W. (1988). A double-blind study of the effectiveness of cyclosporine in amyotrophic lateral sclerosis. *Arch. Neurol.* 45, 381–386.

Barbeito, A. G., Mesci, P., and Boillee, S. (2010). Motor neuron-immune interactions: the vicious circle of ALS. *J. Neural Transm.* 117, 981–1000.

Boillee, S., Vande Velde, C., and Cleveland, D. W. (2006a). ALS: a disease of motor neurons and their nonneuronal neighbors. *Neuron* 52, 39–59.

Boillee, S., Yamanaka, K., Lobsiger, C. S., Copeland, N. G., Jenkins, N. A., Kassiotis, G., Kollias, G., and Cleveland, D. W. (2006b). Onset and progression in inherited ALS determined by motor neurons and microglia. *Science* 312, 1389–1392.

Bruijn, L. I., Becher, M. W., Lee, M. K., Anderson, K. L., Jenkins, N. A., Copeland, N. G., Sisodia, S. S., Rothstein, J. D., Borchelt, D. R., Price, D. L., and Cleveland, D. W. (1997). ALS-linked SOD1 mutant G85R mediates damage to astrocytes and promotes rapidly progressive disease with SOD1-containing inclusions. *Neuron* 18, 327–338.

Chalmers, G. R., Peterson, D. A., and Gage, F. H. (1996). Sprouting adult CNS cholinergic axons express NILE and associate with astrocytic surfaces expressing neural cell adhesion molecule. *J. Comp. Neurol.* 371, 287–299.

DeJesus-Hernandez, M., MacKenzie, I. R., Boeve, B. F., Boxer, A. L., Baker, M., Rutherford, N. J., Nicholson, A. M., Finch, N. A., Flynn, H., Adamson, J., Kouri, N., Wojtas, A., Sengdy, P., Hsiung, G. Y., Karydas, A., Seeley, W. W., Josephs, K. A., Coppola, G., Geschwind, D. H., Wszolek, Z. K., Feldman, H., Knopman, D. S., Petersen, R. C., Miller, B. L., Dickson, D. W., Boylan, K. B., Graff-Radford, N. R., and Rademakers, R. (2011). Expanded GGGGCC hexanucleotide repeat in noncoding region of C9ORF72 causes chromosome 9p-linked FTD and ALS. *Neuron* 72, 245–256.

Dong, Y., and Benveniste, E. N. (2001). Immune function of astrocytes. *Glia* 36, 180–190.

Fischer, L. R., Culver, D. G., Tennant, P., Davis, A. A., Wang, M., Castellano-Sanchez, A., Khan, J., Polak, M. A., and Glass, J. D. (2004). Amyotrophic lateral sclerosis is a distal axonopathy: evidence in mice and man. *Exp. Neurol.* 185, 232–240.

Fray, A. E., Ince, P. G., Banner, S. J., Milton, I. D., Usher, P. A., Cookson, M. R., and Shaw, P. J. (1998). The expression of the glial glutamate transporter protein EAAT2 in motor neuron disease: an immunohistochemical study. *Eur. J. Neurosci.* 10, 2481–2489.

Gong, Y. H., Parsadanian, A. S., Andreeva, A., Snider, W. D., and Elliott, J. L. (2000). Restricted expression of G86R Cu/Zn superoxide dismutase in astrocytes results in astrocytosis but does not cause motoneuron degeneration. *J. Neurosci.* 20, 660–665.

Gowing, G., Dequen, F., Soucy, G., and Julien, J. P. (2006). Absence of tumor necrosis factor-alpha does not affect motor neuron disease caused by superoxide dismutase 1 mutations. *J. Neurosci.* 26, 11397–11402.

Hardiman, O., Van Den Berg, L. H., and Kiernan, M. C. (2011). Clinical diagnosis and management of amyotrophic lateral sclerosis. *Nat. Rev. Neurol.* 7, 639–649.

Henkel, J. S., Beers, D. R., Zhao, W., and Appel, S. H. (2009). Microglia in ALS: the good, the bad, and the resting. *J. Neuroimmune Pharmacol.* 4, 389–398.

Hensley, K., Abdel-Moaty, H., Hunter, J., Mhatre, M., Mou, S., Nguyen, K., Potapova, T., Pye, Q. N., Qi, M., Rice, H., Stewart, C., Stroukoff, K., and West, M. (2006a). Primary glia expressing the G93A-SOD1 mutation present a neuroinflammatory phenotype and provide a cellular system for studies of glial inflammation. *J. Neuroinflammation* 3, 2.

Hensley, K., Mhatre, M., Mou, S., Pye, Q. N., Stewart, C., West, M., and Williamson, K. S. (2006b). On the relation of oxidative stress to neuroinflammation: lessons learned from the G93A-SOD1 mouse model of amyotrophic lateral sclerosis. *Antioxid. Redox Signal.* 8, 2075–2087.

Howland, D. S., Liu, J., She, Y., Goad, B., Maragakis, N. J., Kim, B., Erickson, J., Kulik, J., Devito, L., Psaltis, G., Degennaro, L. J., Cleveland, D. W., and Rothstein, J. D. (2002). Focal loss of the glutamate transporter EAAT2 in a transgenic rat model of SOD1 mutant-mediated amyotrophic lateral sclerosis (ALS). *Proc. Natl. Acad. Sci. U.S.A.* 99, 1604–1609.

Ince, P. G., Highley, J. R., Kirby, J., Wharton, S. B., Takahashi, H., Strong, M. J., and Shaw, P. J. (2011). Molecular pathology and genetic advances in amyotrophic lateral sclerosis: an emerging molecular pathway and the significance of glial pathology. *Acta Neuropathol.* 122, 657–671.

Jaarsma, D., Teuling, E., Haasdijk, E. D., De Zeeuw, C. I., and Hoogenraad, C. C. (2008). Neuron-specific expression of mutant superoxide dismutase is sufficient to induce amyotrophic lateral sclerosis in transgenic mice. *J. Neurosci.* 28, 2075–2088.

Karlsson, J., Fong, K. S., Hansson, M. J., Elmer, E., Csiszar, K., and Keep, M. F. (2004). Life span extension and reduced neuronal death after weekly intraventricular cyclosporin injections in the G93A transgenic mouse model of amyotrophic lateral sclerosis. *J. Neurosurg.* 101, 128–137.

Kawamata, T., Akiyama, H., Yamada, T., and McGeer, P. L. (1992). Immunologic reactions in amyotrophic lateral sclerosis brain and spinal cord tissue. *Am. J. Pathol.* 140, 691–707.

Kiaei, M., Petri, S., Kipiani, K., Gardian, G., Choi, D. K., Chen, J., Calingasan, N. Y., Schafer, P., Muller, G. W., Stewart, C., Hensley, K., and Beal, M. F. (2006). Thalidomide and lenalidomide extend survival in a transgenic mouse model of amyotrophic lateral sclerosis. *J. Neurosci.* 26, 2467–2473.

Kipnis, J., Avidan, H., Caspi, R. R., and Schwartz, M. (2004). Dual effect of CD4+CD25+ regulatory T cells in neurodegeneration: a dialogue with microglia. *Proc. Natl. Acad. Sci. U.S.A.* 101(Suppl. 2), 14663–14669.

Kriz, J., Nguyen, M. D., and Julien, J. P. (2002). Minocycline slows disease progression in a mouse model of amyotrophic lateral sclerosis. *Neurobiol. Dis.* 10, 268–278.

Kwiatkowski, T. J. Jr., Bosco, D. A., Leclerc, A. L., Tamrazian, E., Vanderburg, C. R., Russ, C., Davis, A., Gilchrist, J., Kasarskis, E. J., Munsat, T., Valdmanis, P., Rouleau, G. A., Hosler, B. A., Cortelli, P., De Jong, P. J., Yoshinaga, Y., Haines, J. L., Pericak-Vance, M. A., Yan, J., Ticozzi, N., Siddique, T., McKenna-Yasek, D., Sapp, P. C., Horvitz, H. R., Landers, J. E., and Brown, R. H. Jr. (2009). Mutations in the FUS/TLS gene on chromosome 16 cause familial amyotrophic lateral sclerosis. *Science* 323, 1205–1208.

Lepore, A. C., Rauck, B., Dejea, C., Pardo, A. C., Rao, M. S., Rothstein, J. D., and Maragakis, N. J. (2008). Focal transplantation-based astrocyte replacement is neuroprotective in a model of motor neuron disease. *Nat. Neurosci.* 11, 1294–1301.

MacKenzie, I. R., Bigio, E. H., Ince, P. G., Geser, F., Neumann, M., Cairns, N. J., Kwong, L. K., Forman, M. S., Ravits, J., Stewart, H., Eisen, A., McClusky, L., Kretzschmar, H. A., Monoranu, C. M., Highley, J. R., Kirby, J., Siddique, T., Shaw, P. J., Lee, V. M., and Trojanowski, J. Q. (2007). Pathological TDP-43 distinguishes sporadic amyotrophic lateral sclerosis from amyotrophic lateral sclerosis with SOD1 mutations. *Ann. Neurol.* 61, 427–434.

Mantovani, S., Garbelli, S., Pasini, A., Alimonti, D., Perotti, C., Melazzini, M., Bendotti, C., and Mora, G. (2009). Immune system alterations in sporadic amyotrophic lateral sclerosis patients suggest an ongoing neuroinflammatory process. *J. Neuroimmunol.* 210, 73–79.

Maragakis, N. J., Dietrich, J., Wong, V., Xue, H., Mayer-Proschel, M., Rao, M. S., and Rothstein, J. D. (2004). Glutamate transporter expression and function in human glial progenitors. *Glia* 45, 133–143.

Meininger, V., Drory, V. E., Leigh, P. N., Ludolph, A., Robberecht, W., and Silani, V. (2009). Glatiramer acetate has no impact on disease progression in ALS at 40 mg/day: a double- blind, randomized, multicentre, placebo-controlled trial. *Amyotroph. Lateral Scler.* 10, 378–383.

Moisse, K., and Strong, M. J. (2006). Innate immunity in amyotrophic lateral sclerosis. *Biochim. Biophys. Acta* 1762, 1083–1093.

Nagai, M., Re, D. B., Nagata, T., Chalazonitis, A., Jessell, T. M., Wichterle, H., and Przedborski, S. (2007). Astrocytes expressing ALS-linked mutated SOD1 release factors selectively toxic to motor neurons. *Nat. Neurosci.* 10, 615–622.

Napoli, I., and Neumann, H. (2009). Microglial clearance function in health and disease. *Neuroscience* 158, 1030–1038.

Okada, S., Nakamura, M., Katoh, H., Miyao, T., Shimazaki, T., Ishii, K., Yamane, J., Yoshimura, A., Iwamoto, Y., Toyama, Y., and Okano, H. (2006). Conditional ablation of Stat3 or Socs3 discloses a dual role for reactive astrocytes after spinal cord injury. *Nat. Med.* 12, 829–834.

Papadimitriou, D., Le Verche, V., Jacquier, A., Ikiz, B., Przedborski, S., and Re, D. B. (2010). Inflammation in ALS and SMA: sorting out the good from the evil. *Neurobiol. Dis.* 37, 493–502.

Pehar, M., Cassina, P., Vargas, M. R., Castellanos, R., Viera, L., Beckman, J. S., Estevez, A. G., and Barbeito, L. (2004). Astrocytic production of nerve growth factor in motor neuron apoptosis: implications for amyotrophic lateral sclerosis. *J. Neurochem.* 89, 464–473.

Rothstein, J. D., Martin, L. J., and Kuncl, R. W. (1992). Decreased glutamate transport by the brain and spinal cord in amyotrophic lateral sclerosis. *N. Engl. J. Med.* 326, 1464–1468.

Sanagi, T., Yuasa, S., Nakamura, Y., Suzuki, E., Aoki, M., Warita, H., Itoyama, Y., Uchino, S., Kohsaka, S., and Ohsawa, K. (2010). Appearance of phagocytic microglia adjacent to motoneurons in spinal cord tissue from a presymptomatic transgenic rat model of amyotrophic lateral sclerosis. *J. Neurosci. Res.* 88, 2736–2746.

Sreedharan, J., Blair, I. P., Tripathi, V. B., Hu, X., Vance, C., Rogelj, B., Ackerley, S., Durnall, J. C., Williams, K. L., Buratti, E., Baralle, F., De Belleroche, J., Mitchell, J. D., Leigh, P. N., Al-Chalabi, A., Miller, C. C., Nicholson, G., and Shaw, C. E. (2008). TDP-43 mutations in familial and sporadic amyotrophic lateral sclerosis. *Science* 319, 1668–1672.

Sta, M., Sylva-Steenland, R. M., Casula, M., De Jong, J. M., Troost, D., Aronica, E., and Baas, F. (2011). Innate and adaptive immunity in amyotrophic lateral sclerosis: evidence of complement activation. *Neurobiol. Dis.* 42, 211–220.

Tan, C. F., Eguchi, H., Tagawa, A., Onodera, O., Iwasaki, T., Tsujino, A., Nishizawa, M., Kakita, A., and Takahashi, H. (2007). TDP-43 immunoreactivity in neuronal inclusions in familial amyotrophic lateral sclerosis with or without SOD1 gene mutation. *Acta Neuropathol.* 113, 535–542.

Turner, B. J., and Talbot, K. (2008). Transgenics, toxicity and therapeutics in rodent models of mutant SOD1-mediated familial ALS. *Prog. Neurobiol.* 85, 94–134.

Vance, C., Rogelj, B., Hortobagyi, T., De Vos, K. J., Nishimura, A. L., Sreedharan, J., Hu, X., Smith, B., Ruddy, D., Wright, P., Ganesalingam, J., Williams, K. L., Tripathi, V., Al-Saraj, S., Al-Chalabi, A., Leigh, P. N., Blair, I. P., Nicholson, G., De Belleroche, J., Gallo, J. M., Miller, C. C., and Shaw, C. E. (2009). Mutations in FUS, an RNA processing protein, cause familial amyotrophic lateral sclerosis type 6. *Science* 323, 1208–1211.

Wang, L., Sharma, K., Grisotti, G., and Roos, R. P. (2009). The effect of mutant SOD1 dismutase activity on non-cell autonomous degeneration in familial amyotrophic lateral sclerosis. *Neurobiol. Dis.* 35, 234–240.

Wijesekera, L. C., and Leigh, P. N. (2009). Amyotrophic lateral sclerosis. *Orphanet. J. Rare Dis.* 4, 3.

Wu, V. W., Nishiyama, N., and Schwartz, J. P. (1998). A culture model of reactive astrocytes: increased nerve growth factor synthesis and reexpression of cytokine responsiveness. *J. Neurochem.* 71, 749–756.

Yang, W. W., Sidman, R. L., Taksir, T. V., Treleaven, C. M., Fidler, J. A., Cheng, S. H., Dodge, J. C., and Shihabuddin, L. S. (2011). Relationship between neuropathology and disease progression in the SOD1(G93A) ALS mouse. *Exp. Neurol.* 227, 287–295.

Yrjanheikki, J., Tikka, T., Keinanen, R., Goldsteins, G., Chan, P. H., and Koistinaho, J. (1999). A tetracycline derivative, minocycline, reduces inflammation and protects against focal cerebral ischemia with a wide therapeutic window. *Proc. Natl. Acad. Sci. U.S.A.* 96, 13496–13500.

Zhu, S., Stavrovskaya, I. G., Drozda, M., Kim, B. Y., Ona, V., Li, M., Sarang, S., Liu, A. S., Hartley, D. M., Wu, D. C., Gullans, S., Ferrante, R. J., Przedborski, S., Kristal, B. S., and Friedlander, R. M. (2002). Minocycline inhibits cytochrome *c* release and delays progression of amyotrophic lateral sclerosis in mice. *Nature* 417, 74–78.

26

Environmental enrichment may protect against hippocampal atrophy in the chronic stages of traumatic brain injury

Lesley S. Miller[1], Brenda Colella[2], David Mikulis[3,4], Jerome Maller[5] and Robin E. A. Green[2,6]*

[1] Applied Psychology and Human Development, Ontario Institute for Studies in Education, University of Toronto, Toronto, ON, Canada
[2] Cognitive Neurorehabilitation Sciences Lab, Research Department, Toronto Rehab-University Health Network, Toronto, ON, Canada
[3] fMRI Laboratory, Division of Applied and Interventional Research, Toronto Western Research Institute, University Health Network, Toronto, ON, Canada
[4] Faculty of Medicine, Department of Medical Imaging, University of Toronto, Toronto, ON, Canada
[5] Brain Stimulation and Neuroimaging Laboratory, Monash Alfred Psychiatry Research Centre, Alfred Hospital, Melbourne, VIC, Australia
[6] Graduate Department of Rehabilitation Science, University of Toronto, Toronto, ON, Canada

Edited by:
Alvaro Pascual-Leone, Beth Israel Deaconess Medical Center/Harvard Medical School, USA

Reviewed by:
Bogdan Draganski, University Lausanne, Switzerland
Stefano Sandrone, Institute of Neuroinformatics, Switzerland

***Correspondence:**
Robin E. A. Green, Cognitive Neurorehabilitation Sciences Lab, Research Department, Toronto Rehab-University Health Network, 550 University Ave., Toronto, ON M5A 2G2, Canada
e-mail: robin.green@uhn.ca

Objective: To examine the relationship between environmental enrichment (EE) and hippocampal atrophy in the chronic stages of moderate to severe traumatic brain injury (TBI).

Design: Retrospective analysis of prospectively collected data; observational, within-subjects.

Participants: Patients ($N = 25$) with moderate to severe TBI.

Measures: Primary predictors: (1) An aggregate of self-report rating of EE (comprising hours of cognitive, physical, and social activities) at 5 months post-injury; (2) pre-injury years of education as a proxy for pre-morbid EE (or cognitive reserve). Primary outcome: bilateral hippocampal volume change from 5 to 28 months post-injury.

Results: As predicted, self-reported EE was significantly negatively correlated with bilateral hippocampal atrophy ($p < 0.05$), with greater EE associated with less atrophy from 5 to 28 months. Contrary to prediction, years of education (a proxy for cognitive reserve) was not significantly associated with atrophy.

Conclusion: Post-injury EE may serve as a buffer against hippocampal atrophy in the chronic stages of moderate-severe TBI. Clinical application of EE should be considered for optimal maintenance of neurological functioning in the chronic stages of moderate-severe TBI.

Keywords: traumatic brain injury, environmental enrichment, subacute atrophy, adult, moderate to severe

INTRODUCTION

Conventionally, moderate-severe traumatic brain injury (TBI) has been viewed as a non-progressive brain disorder with a predictable trajectory of recovery leading to a stable course thereafter (Lezak et al., 2004). However, growing research findings show progressive gray matter atrophy and loss of white matter integrity in the post-acute and chronic phases of injury (Trivedi et al., 2007; Greenberg et al., 2008; Ng et al., 2008; Farbota et al., 2012; Adnan et al., in press). Further, some individuals with TBI also show progressive cognitive and functional declines in the ensuing months and years following injury (Corkin et al., 1989; Millis et al., 2001; Himanen et al., 2006; Till et al., 2008), supporting the notion that TBI is not a stable condition (Ng et al., 2008; Till et al., 2008)

A brain structure of key importance in TBI is the hippocampus. Memory impairment is one of the most common complaints following TBI, in part due to the acute effects of hippocampal injury, which include excitotoxic and hypoxic insult (Rosenfeld et al., 2012). On top of these acute injuries, post-acute atrophy of the hippocampus has now been demonstrated in several TBI studies (Bigler et al., 1997; Ng et al., 2008). Tate and Bigler (2000) have suggested that post-acutely, hippocampal cell loss may be the result of transneuronal degeneration secondary to hippocampal deafferentation and/or deefferentation. Indeed, the unique pattern of neuronal projections within the hippocampus (Duvernoy et al., 2005), which is comprised of six architecturally distinct regions linked via unidirectional projections (Amaral and Witter, 1995), has been referred to as an Achilles' heel of sorts, whereby damage to one region of the hippocampus can lead to downstream damage to other regions via loss of activity-dependent survival factors (McCarthy, 2003). Thus, disuse-mediated loss, either secondary to disconnection or to a dearth of behavioral stimulation, may be an important factor in observed hippocampal volume loss in the post-acute stages of injury.

Disuse-mediated loss—or "use it or lose it"—is a concept that has received extensive attention in the older adult literature. It has been argued for decades that greater day-to-day cognitive stimulation is associated with less cognitive decline and delayed onset of dementia. The "negative neuroplasticity" framework of

Mahncke et al. (2006), advanced to explain functional losses in normal aging, offers a disuse-mediated framework that can also be applied to atrophy in the chronic stages of TBI (Evans et al., 2008). In their framework, the authors posit that cognitive, perceptual, emotional, physical, psychosocial, and vocational changes associated with aging limit engagement in the busy schedules and complexity of activities of earlier life, leading to a cycle of behavioral inactivation and avoidance—or learned disuse (Taub et al., 2006), and resulting in reduced activation of brain networks (Blake et al., 2006). Although behavioral losses are more sudden in brain injury, moderate-severe TBI patients, too, are commonly unable to engage in the complex activities of work, school and social activities as a result of TBI-induced decrements in cognitive, physical, perceptual and emotional functioning. These patients are especially at risk of reduced behavioral (and thereby neural) stimulation in the sub-acute and chronic stages of injury (after discharge from in-patient rehabilitation facilities), where there is often reduced environmental stimulation and/or reduced supports to foster engagement in the environment (Evans et al., 2008; Frasca et al., 2013).

Related to the above, the concept of environmental enrichment (EE) refers to exposure to and engagement with complex and stimulating environments, and there is extensive evidence that EE can beneficially influence the size, morphology and function of the brain, through synaptic modification and synaptogenesis, the shape and size of dendritic spines (or spine remodeling), axon collateral sprouting, hippocampal (dentate gyrus) neurogenesis and survival of neurons, and brain network connectivity; and such changes have been associated with improvements in functional performance (Rosenzweig and Bennett, 1996; Diamond, 2001; Mohammed et al., 2002; Draganski et al., 2006; Kasai et al., 2010; Kolb et al., 2010; Berlucchi, 2011). Indeed, seminal reviews of the literature conclude that brains that have received increased stimulation, via enhanced mental and physical activity, are better able to mount neuroprotective responses against neurodegenerative processes, traumatic insults and other forms of adult-onset neural dysfunction (Nithianantharajah and Hannan, 2009).

Taken together, the above literature (Mohammed et al., 2002; Kolb et al., 2010; Berlucchi, 2011) suggests that environmental influences, such as intensified cognitive stimulation, might buffer against chronic stage atrophy in moderate-severe TBI. The primary objective of the present study, therefore, was to examine the relationship between post-injury EE, and hippocampal atrophy in the chronic stages of injury. To our knowledge, no studies have yet examined this relationship. We hypothesized that greater EE (i.e., frequency of cognitive, physical, and social engagement) measured in the early post-acute stages of injury (i.e., 5 months post-injury) would be associated with less long-term bilateral hippocampal atrophy over the ensuing years (measured from 5 to 28 months post-injury).

The secondary objective concerned pre-injury EE factors, namely exposure to higher levels of education in development and early adulthood, which has been associated with better cognitive recovery following TBI (Kesler et al., 2003). Given evidence of (1) a positive association between education and cognitive and functional recovery following TBI (Green et al., 2008) and stroke (Elkins et al., 2006), (2) a positive association between education and dendritic branching in healthy adult humans (Jacobs et al., 1993), and (3) a positive correlation between years of education and cognitive functioning in normal aging (Corral et al., 2006; Fritsch et al., 2007), it was hypothesized that greater years of education would be associated with less bilateral hippocampal atrophy, measured from 5 to 28 months post-injury.

METHODS

PARTICIPANTS

The 25 clinical participants in this study (see **Table 1**) were part of a larger research study being conducted at the Toronto Rehabilitation Institute, a large publicly-funded inpatient neurorehabilitation hospital. The focus of the larger study was to investigate the natural history and mechanisms of recovery following moderate-severe TBI. Informed consent was obtained from all participants in the study, and procedures for the present study were approved by the Research Ethics Board of the Toronto Rehabilitation Institute and the Office of Research Ethics at the University of Toronto. Participants underwent prospective assessments at approximately 5, 12, and 28 months post-injury. As the current design was a retrospective analysis of data collected in the course of the larger study data were *only* available at the 5, 12, and 28 month time points.

Inclusion criteria for the larger study comprised: (1) acute care medical diagnosis of TBI; (2) posttraumatic amnesia (PTA) of 1 h or more and/or Glasgow Coma Scale (GCS) score of 12 or less either at emergency or at the scene of the accident and/or positive CT or MRI findings; (3) age between 17 and 80 years old; (4) able to follow simple commands in English based upon Speech Language Pathologist intake assessment; and, (5) competent to provide informed consent for study or availability of a legal decision maker.

Exclusion criteria for the larger study included: (1) orthopaedic injuries affecting both upper extremities; (2) diseases primarily or frequently affecting the central nervous system, including dementia of Alzheimer's type, Parkinson's disease, multiple sclerosis, Huntington's disease, lupus, or stroke; (3) a history of psychotic disorder; (4) non-emergence from posttraumatic amnesia by 6 weeks post-injury, as measured by the Galveston Orientation Amnesia Test (Levin et al., 1979); (5) TBI secondary to another neurological event, such as a fall due to stroke; and, (6) failure on a symptom validity test (Test of Memory Malingering) (Tombaugh, 1996) at any of the assessments. The demographic and injury characteristics of the clinical sample are shown in **Table 1**. The additional inclusion criteria for the current study were: relevant behavioral and MRI outcome measures at 5 months post-injury plus MRI data at 28 months post-injury.

There were 30 individuals from the larger study with all relevant outcome measures at 5 months post-injury who had reached or surpassed the 28 month post-injury time-point at the time of data analysis. Of those, 25 underwent the 28-month post-injury MRI and were, therefore, eligible for inclusion in the present study, indicating a retention rate of 83%.

Of the sample included in the present study, none showed evidence of severe anxiety or depression, and less than 30% reported experiencing mild or moderate depression or anxiety during the

Table 1 | Demographic information and hippocampal volume loss.

Subject ID	Age/sex	Education	GCS	PTA	IQ (WTAR)	% Change in bilateral hippocampal volume from 5–28 months post-injury
368	68/M	8	Unknown	5	ESL	−19.79
380	48/M	12	3	4	89	−14.45
358	59/F	17	4	5	107	−14.27
376	29/M	16	3	4	124	−11.06
364	54/M	20	7	5	120	−8.82
369	25/M	12	Unknown	5	LD	−7.91
362	60/M	15	Unknown	5	111	−7.05
337	17/M	12	4	1	83	−6.85
363	46/M	17	3	5	Dysarthria	−6.01
389	48/M	11	6	6	105	−5.49
353	27/F	18	3	5	117	−5.35
352	59/M	12	3	6	104	−4.79
339	37/M	12	3	6	89	−4.46
333	44/F	16	6	4	120	−4.06
379	31/M	16	8	6	108	−3.31
349	50/F	17	10	3	120	−3.29
338	57/F	12	13	6	98	−3.27
359	18/F	12	6	5	LD	−2.55
329	19/M	9	Unknown	4	103	−0.97
346	28/F	14	7	5	106	0.27
374	66/M	12	6	5	Aphasia	0.83
331	30/M	16	6	6	97	2.77
327	41/M	11	3	4	99	2.98
330	40/F	13	3	0	116	3.34
335	25/M	16	7	4	124	5.43
	($M = 41$yrs; $SD = 16$)	($M = 14$yrs; $SD = 3$)	($M = 5$; $SD = 3$)	($M = 4.6$days; $SD = 1.5$)	($M = 109$; $SD = 11.4$)	($M = -4.7\%$; $SD = 6.0$)

first year post-injury based on the Beck Depression Inventory (Beck, 1987) and Beck Anxiety Inventory (Beck, 1990).

MATERIALS

Lifestyle activities questionnaire

Assessment of post-injury EE was based on participants' self-reported frequency of engagement in a variety of activities involving cognitive, physical, and social demands. Given the absence of reliable or valid published measures of EE in humans at the time of data analysis, EE activities were listed on a self-report questionnaire designed for the purpose of the present study, entitled the Lifestyle Activities Questionnaire (LAQ). Cognitive, physical, and social activities on the LAQ were obtained from a theoretically-derived and empirically-tested inventory developed by Salthouse et al. (2002), which was constructed by specifying 22 common activities that a sample of 1200 adults, ranging from the age of 18–97 years, rated in terms of their cognitive demand (where 1 = low demand, corresponding to sleeping, and 5 = high demand, corresponding to working on a tax form). An activity added to the LAQ that was not on Salthouse's inventory was the frequency of engagement in sports or physical activity at the gym. Participants were asked to rate the frequency with which they engaged in each of the listed activities on an ordinal scale ranging from 1 to 5.

The scale comprised descriptors that ranged from (1) *didn't do at all* to (5) *several hours, every day of the week*. For statistical analysis, each number of the scale was weighted based on estimated associated hours. "Didn't do at all and less than once a week" was assigned a weight of zero; "once or twice a week" was assigned a weight of 1 (i.e., for 1 h/week); "several times a week" was assigned a weight of 3 (3 h/week); "an hour or so most days" was assigned a weight of 7; and "several hours a day" was assigned a weight of 20 (20 h/week). Transformation of ordinal scores into weighted scale scores corresponding to estimated hours/week provided a meaningful and more ecological marker of EE. However, for patient responses, the scale was kept as ordinal (i.e., 1–5), because self-reported ratings were deemed by clinical experts consulted to be more easily understood by patients and less likely to result in missing or inaccurate data. We suggest that this approach enabled us to provide richer data than previous methods of aggregating EE activities, in which individuals were classified as "active" if they endorsed doing even one mentally-challenging activity for 1 h per week or more, for example (Bosma et al., 2002; Richards et al., 2003).

Items were sub-classified into cognitive, social or physical activity types to allow for a comparison of the respective influences of each on hippocampal volume loss. For all items, consensus was reached by two trained clinicians regarding assignment to a cognitive, social or physical aggregate. Nineteen items were classified as cognitive activities, 8 items were classified as social activities, and 2 items were classified as physical activities. For each subject, the weighted score for each item type (i.e., social, cognitive, physical) was summed to create a sub-aggregate score for each component of EE; the grand sum was the total score for the larger EE aggregate.

MRI acquisition protocol

MRI scans were acquired on a General Electric (GE) Signa-Echospeed 1.5 Tesla HD scanner (SIGNA EXCITE, GE Healthcare, Milwaukee WI), using an eight channel head coil. Sequences included sagittal T1 (TR/TE = 300/13 ms), slice thickness = 5 mm, space 2.5 mm, matrix 256 × 128 axial gradient recalled echo TR/TE = 450/20, flip angle = 20°, slice thickness = 3 mm no gap, matrix 256 × 192 axial fluid-attenuated-inversion-recovery TR/TE = 9000/45 ms, TI (inversion time) = 2200 ms, slice thickness = 5 mm no gap, matrix 256 × 192 axial fast spin echo proton density (PD)/T2 TR/TE 5500/30, 90 ms, slice thickness = 3 mm no gap, matrix 256 × 192. All above mentioned sequences were obtained with a 22 cm field of view. The high-resolution isotropic T1 weighted, three-dimensional IR prepped radio-frequency spoiled-gradient recalled-echo images TI/TR/TE = 12/300/5, TI, FA = 20, slice thickness = 1 mm no gap, matrix = 256 × 256 were acquired in the axial plane utilizing a 25 cm field of view. The entire scanning session lasted ~55 min.

Image processing and analysis

The MR images were transferred to a workstation for image processing. The scans were received in the Digital Imaging and Communications in Medicine file format and were subsequently converted into (Medical Imaging Network Common Data Form) file format that was created at McConnell Brain Imaging Centre of the Montreal Neurological Institute. Following this procedure, the files were anonymized.

A number of image processing steps were performed in order to make the MRI data usable for image analysis. First, an intensity non-uniformity correction was performed, followed by linear registration of the images into stereotaxic coordinates based on the Talairach atlas. The linear registration to Talairach coordinates was accomplished through 3D cross-correlation between a given volume and an average MR brain image previously converted into the Talairach coordinate system allowing for direct anatomical comparisons between subjects. Finally, a second non-uniformity correction was performed after the registration, which helped to remove any residual non-uniformity artifacts.

The hippocampi were manually outlined using Analyze 7.0 (Brain Imaging Resource, Mayo Clinic, MN) by an experienced tracer (JM) from coronally orientated MR images in the anterior-posterior direction. Calculations of volumes were computed automatically by multiplying the number of voxels traced in each slice, by their depth (i.e., slice thickness). As described by Watson et al. (1992, 1997), the anterior tip of the hippocampus until the slice before the opening of the crux of the fornix was measured as the hippocampal head and body and included the subiculum, CA1-(4) areas, and dentate gyrus. The hippocampus tail was measured from the slice immediately posterior to that which represented the last slice according to the Watson protocol (Watson et al., 1992, 1997) (see Maller et al., 2007 for a more detailed description of this procedure).

All raw hippocampal volumes were expressed in mm^3. For the purpose of the present study, hippocampal volume change between 5 months (T1) post-injury and 28 months (T2) post-injury was measured using the following formula:

$$\text{Hippocampal volume change} = \frac{(\text{Vol T2} - \text{Vol T1})}{(\text{Vol T2} + \text{Vol T1})/2} * 100$$

DESIGN AND PROCEDURES

The study employed a retrospective, within subjects, longitudinal design. For clinical participants, LAQs were collected and initial MRI scans were acquired at a mean of 5.3 months ($SD = 1.2$; range = 4.3–10.3 months) post-injury; follow-up MRI scans were acquired at 28.48 months ($SD = 5.5$; range = 24–42 months) post-injury.

The primary dependent measure for the study was bilateral hippocampal volume. The primary independent measures were (1) EE as measured by the total score of the LAQ at 5 months post-injury and (2) years of education prior to the injury. We also examined the relative contributions of the cognitive, social and physical EE sub-aggregate scores.

The primary control variables were injury severity (measured by the Glasgow Coma Scale, duration of PTA, and duration of acute care length of stay), estimated premorbid intelligence (based on the mean score on the Wechsler Test of Adult Reading administered [Wechsler, 2001] at 12 and 28 months post-injury), socioeconomic status, and age at injury.

RESULTS

Using Pearson product moment correlation, primary control variables were correlated with hippocampal atrophy and with the measure of overall EE. Each variable was correlated separately due to limited power secondary to sample size. Any variables with significant correlation were included in subsequent analyses. No significant correlations were observed between any of the primary control variables and EE or hippocampal atrophy, with the exception of age, which correlated significantly with the EE aggregate ($r = -0.45$, $p < 0.05$, $N = 25$) whereby increasing age was associated with less overall EE. As well, there was a trend for higher age at injury to be associated with greater bilateral hippocampal atrophy ($r = 0.39$, $p = 0.06$, $N = 25$). These findings, combined with previous research findings of greater deleterious effects of injury on aging brains (Popa-Wagner et al., 2007; Onyszchuk et al., 2008; Petcu et al., 2008), necessitated controlling for age at injury in the present study analyses.

Partial correlation was used to test the primary hypothesis of the study, namely the relationship between the EE aggregate and bilateral hippocampal atrophy, while controlling for age at injury. A significant negative correlation was observed ($r = -0.42$, $p < 0.05$, $df = 21$) whereby greater general activity level at 5 months post-injury was associated with less bilateral hippocampal atrophy from 5 to 28 months post-injury.

Partial correlation between years of education and hippocampal atrophy, controlling for age at injury was used to examine the secondary hypothesis. Contrary to prediction, no significant relationship was observed ($r = -0.05, p = 0.82, df = 22$).

Lastly, we also explored preliminarily the respective contribution to hippocampal atrophy of the cognitive, social and physical sub-aggregates. Here, a hierarchical linear regression was conducted, which revealed significant negative correlations between bilateral hippocampal atrophy and cognitive activity ($r = -0.53, p < 0.01$), and between bilateral hippocampal atrophy and social activity ($r = -0.47, p < 0.05$) but no significant correlation between bilateral hippocampal atrophy and physical activity.

DISCUSSION

Consistent with our prediction, there was a significant negative association between EE (i.e., engagement in cognitive, physical, and social activities) at 5 months post-injury and bilateral hippocampal atrophy from 5 to 28 months post-injury. Although the observational design of the present study precludes conclusions regarding causality, our findings are consistent with previous associations found between EE and enhanced hippocampal structure, and they are potentially explained by increased production, survival and integration of newly generated dentate gyrus neurons (Kempermann et al., 2002; Olson et al., 2006; Tanti et al., 2013); findings in animals—where EE has been correlated with neurogenesis in TBI and moreover correlated with better recovery (Kovesdi et al., 2011; Matter et al., 2011)—bolster such an interpretation. At a behavioral level, the current findings are consistent with use-it-or-lose-it frameworks, and support the extrapolation of the Mahncke et al. (2006) framework—where reduced schedules of activities and avoidance of cognitively-challenging activities were purported to lead to under-stimulation of critical neural networks and loss of associated functions—to chronic TBI (Evans et al., 2008). The findings are also consistent with Robertson and Murre's (1999) computational model of brain plasticity and guided recovery of function, whereby damaged, but potentially viable circuits may be repaired via cognitive activity, cognitive arousal, and Hebbian learning mechanisms. As well, these findings converge with findings from the cognitive-training literature, which shows evidence that engagement in cognitively-demanding tasks is associated with increased cerebral volume in brain areas that are functionally-related to the demands of the task (Draganski et al., 2006).

Unexpectedly, the results of the present study showed no significant relationship between hippocampal atrophy and pre-injury cognitive reserve, as measured by level of education. This finding was surprising given the extensive evidence of a positive association between level of education and cognitive functioning in normal aging (Corral et al., 2006; Fritsch et al., 2007), stroke recovery (Elkins et al., 2006), and TBI recovery (Kesler et al., 2003). Therefore, the study findings do not offer evidence that this proxy for pre-injury EE protects against the structural progression of subacute hippocampal atrophy following TBI. One interpretation of this null finding is that a fixed degree of neural reserve at the time of brain injury does not confer neuroprotection against progressive pathology (e.g., disconnection, [Tate and Bigler, 2000]; neuroinflammation [Bigler, 2013; Johnson et al., 2013]) as would be logically predicted by conventional theories of brain reserve (Satz, 1993; Stern, 2002) and by negative associations found between premorbid cognitive reserve and progression of pathology in Alzheimers disease (Stern, 2006), multiple sclerosis (Amato et al., 2013) and stroke (Willis and Hakim, 2013). In particular, our findings suggest that in order for EE to positively modulate brain disorders via neuroprotective and/or compensatory mechanisms, EE exposure must occur after the disorder has commenced, and during the period of progression of neuropathology (Nithianantharajah and Hannan, 2009). Such an explanation is consistent with EE influences on neurogenesis, as discussed above (Kovesdi et al., 2011; Matter et al., 2011). As neurogenesis is an active process, it may be that temporally congruent factors, namely current EE, but not past education, play a more significant role (Lee et al., 2009; Surget et al., 2011). Unfortunately, our retrospective analysis did not allow us to quantitate the dentate gyrus, the site of neurogenesis.

EE in humans is viewed conventionally as being comprised of three primary elements: cognitive, physical, and social stimulation (Scarmeas and Stern, 2003; Studenski et al., 2006). Of the three conventional elements of EE, our preliminary findings indicated that cognitive activity accounted for the most outcome variance in bilateral hippocampal atrophy. The question whether it is cognitive, social or physical enrichment that confers the greatest neuroplastic advantage is under active debate; our findings are consistent with those comparison studies in animals that found greater survival and integration of new hippocampal neurons after cognitive stimulation than exercise (Kempermann et al., 2002, 2010; Olson et al., 2006; Curlik and Shors, 2011; Shors et al., 2012; Tanti et al., 2013).

A limitation of the present study was the small sample size and relatively small (albeit typical) representation of female subjects, which limits the generalizability of the study findings and precluded examination of gender as a control variable.

It is important to note that in our preliminary and exploratory analysis of the relative contributions of the sub-aggregates (cognitive vs. social vs. physical stimulation), the greater number of cognitive items on the LAQ may have conferred greater analytic stability to the cognitive outcome measure, with the very small number of physical items (2) providing limited stability. Therefore, further research into the relationship between cognitive vs. other types of stimulation and atrophy in the chronic stages of TBI is needed.

Many studies of EE in humans are observational and correlational in design, including the present study. Future EE research would benefit from inclusion of elements that would permit conclusions regarding causality and directionality of relationships, as offered by Salthouse et al. (2002). They suggested that random assignment to experimental and control groups would minimize influences of relevant pre-existing individual differences, such as initial level of cognitive ability and amount of education. Further, rigorous control of enrichment groups, in terms of type and amount of EE, is needed as well as long-term objective monitoring of the amount and frequency of EE activities. Though, given that objective monitoring of lifestyle activities is often unfeasible, experience sampling might offer greater accuracy than retrospective self-report (Csikszentmihalyi and Larson, 1987). Further general challenges in the measurement and manipulation of EE in humans pertain to inter-individual differences in motivation, interest and engagement: what is cognitively challenging, stimulating, and enjoyable to one may be overly difficult and thus stressful for another, or excessively easy and thus insufficiently stimulating to confer neural benefits to another. These limitations affect the strength of conclusions in our own study and warrant future experimental studies with the controls described above.

With regard to models of rehabilitation, the present study arguably provides preliminary empirical support for the contextualized model of cognitive rehabilitation proposed by Ylvisaker et al. (2002), in which therapeutic activities embedded in the patient's real life outside of the clinical setting may lead to greater recovery following brain injury. Cognitive rehabilitation researchers have recommended that rehabilitation strategies should be embedded in real-life contexts in order to maximize far transfer of learned skills and to impact real-life functioning (Murre and Robertson, 1999; Mateer and Sira, 2006). Consistent with these recommendations and with the Ylvisaker et al. (2002) contextualized model of rehabilitation, the majority of activities examined in the present study were embedded in real-life contexts, thus increasing the practical utility of the present study findings. Future prospective research should compare augmentation or intensification of those activities that are a part of patients' day to day life, with EE conferred by more conventional interventions such as computerized cognitively stimulating activities. Longitudinal measures of EE are also needed. Here, we inferred that EE at 5 months post-injury is a proxy for ongoing EE.

Regarding future research avenues, preliminary findings indicate that the default mode network (DMN; Raichle et al., 2001) in humans is implicated in TBI, with functional connectivity decrements within the DMN predicting sustained attention deficits (Bonnelle et al., 2011; Sandrone and Bacigaluppi, 2012). Future studies could investigate the benefits of EE factors purported to impact connectivity within the DMN, such as meditation practice (Taylor et al., 2013), an area of burgeoning interest in the literature on recovery from TBI.

CONCLUSIONS

The present study is the first to examine EE factors and their relationship with hippocampal atrophy in the chronic stages of moderate-severe TBI. EE that followed TBI and was temporally proximal to injury had a negative association with hippocampal atrophy, while years of education, a proxy for pre-injury EE (or cognitive reserve) was not significantly associated. Validation of the present findings through replication with larger samples of TBI patients is needed, ideally in a study in which the type and duration of EE is experimentally manipulated. EE is intimately associated with modification of existing synapses, synaptogenesis as well as neurogenesis. Its role in neurorehabilitation appears critical. The findings of this correlational study can be used to generate testable hypotheses regarding the directional impact of EE, as well as the active ingredients of EE for buffering against cerebral atrophy, and its functional consequences. Such questions have significant implications for the development of effective rehabilitation methods for people suffering the long-term consequences of moderate-severe TBI.

ACKNOWLEDGMENTS

The study was supported by funding from the Ontario Neurotrauma foundation, Canadian Institutes for Health Research, Canada Research Chair and Physicians' Services Incorporated foundation.

REFERENCES

Adnan, A., Crawley, A., Mikulis, D., Moscovitch, M., Colella, B., and Green, R. E. A. (in press). Moderate-severe traumatic brain injury causes delayed loss of white matter integrity: evidence of fornix deterioration in the chronic stage of injury. *Brain Injury*.

Amaral, D. G., and Witter, M. P. (1995). "Hippocampal formation," in *The Rat Nervous System*, ed G. Paxinos (New York, NY: Academic Press), 443–493.

Amato, M. P., Razzolini, L., Goretti, B., Stromillo, M. L., Rossi, F., Giorgio, A., et al. (2013). Cognitive reserve and cortical atrophy in multiple sclerosis: a longitudinal study. *Neurology* 80, 1728–1733. doi: 10.1212/WNL.0b013e3182918c6f

Beck, A. T. (1987). *Beck Depression Inventory*. San Antonio, TX: The Psychological Corporation.

Beck, A. T. (1990). *Beck Anxiety Inventory*. San Antonio, TX: Psychological Corporation.

Berlucchi, G. (2011). Brain plasticity and cognitive neurorehabilitation. *Neuropsychol. Rehabil.* 21, 560–578. doi: 10.1080/09602011.2011.573255

Bigler, E. D. (2013). Neuroinflammatin and the dynamic lesion. *Brain* 136, 9–11. doi: 10.1093/brain/aws342

Bigler, E. D., Blatter, D. D., Anderson, C. V., Johnson, S. C., Gale, S. D., Hopkins, R. O., et al. (1997). Hippocampal volume in normal aging and traumatic brain injury. *AJNR Am. J. Neuroradiol.* 18, 11–23.

Blake, D. T., Heiser, M. A., Caywood, M., and Merzenich, M. M. (2006). Experience-dependent adult cortical plasticity requires cognitive association between sensation and reward. *Neuron* 52, 371–381. doi: 10.1016/j.neuron.2006.08.009

Bonnelle, V., Leech, R., Kinnunen, K. M., Ham, T. E., Beckmann, C. F., De Boissezon, X., et al. (2011). Default mode network connectivity predicts sustained attention deficits after traumatic brain injury. *J. Neurosci.* 31, 13442–13451. doi: 10.1523/JNEUROSCI.1163-11.2011

Bosma, H., Van Boxtel, M. P., Ponds, R. W., Jelicic, M., Houx, P., Metsemakers, J., et al. (2002). Engaged lifestyle and cognitive function in middle and old-aged, non-demented persons: a reciprocal association? *Z. Gerontol. Geriatr.* 35, 575–581. doi: 10.1007/s00391-002-0080-y

Corkin, S., Rosen, T. J., Sullivan, E. V., and Clegg, R. A. (1989). Penetrating head injury in young adulthood exacerbates cognitive decline in later years. *J. Neurosci.* 9, 3876–3883.

Corral, M., Rodriguez, M., Amenedo, E., Sanchez, J. L., and Diaz, F. (2006). Cognitive reserve, age, and neuropsychological performance in healthy participants. *Dev. Neuropsychol.* 29, 479–491. doi: 10.1207/s15326942dn2903_6

Csikszentmihalyi, M., and Larson, R. (1987). Validity and reliability of the experience-sampling method. *J. Nerv. Ment. Dis.* 175, 526–536. doi: 10.1097/00005053-198709000-00004

Curlik, D. M., and Shors, T. J. (2011). Learning increases the survival of newborn neurons provided that learning is difficult to achieve and successful. *J. Cogn. Neurosci.* 23, 2159–2170. doi: 10.1162/jocn.2010.21597

Diamond, M. C. (2001). Response of the brain to enrichment. *An. Acad. Bras. Cienc.* 73, 211–220.

Draganski, B., Gaser, C., Kempermann, G., Kuhn, H. G., Winkler, J., Buchel, C., et al. (2006). Temporal and spatial dynamics of brain structure changes during extensive learning. *J. Neurosci.* 26, 6314–6317. doi: 10.1523/JNEUROSCI.4628-05.2006

Duvernoy, H. M., Cattin, F., and Naidich, T. (2005). *Human Hippocampus: Functional Anatomy, Vascularization and Serial Sections with MRI.* Heidelberg: Springer-Verlag.

Elkins, J. S., Longstreth, W. T. Jr., Manolio, T. A., Newman, A. B.,

Bhadelia, R. A., et al. (2006). Education and the cognitive decline associated with MRI-defined brain infarct. *Neurology* 67, 435–440. doi: 10.1212/01.wnl.0000228246.89109.98

Evans, J. J., Bateman, A., Turner, G., and Green, R. E. A. (2008). Understanding brain injury resources and evidence base. *Neuropsychol. Rehabil. Res. Dig.* 18, 372–384. doi: 10.1080/09602010801909153

Farbota, K. D., Bendlin, B. B., Alexander, A. L., Rowley, H. A., Dempsey, R. J., and Johnson, S. C. (2012). Longitudinal diffusion tensor imaging and neuropsychological correlates in traumatic brain injury patients. *Front. Hum. Neurosci.* 6:160. doi: 10.3389/fnhum.2012.00160

Frasca, D., Tomaszczyk, J., McFadyen, B. J., and Green, R. E. A. (2013). Traumatic brain injury and post-acute decline: what role does environmental enrichment play? A scoping review. *Front. Hum. Neurosci.* 7:31. doi: 10.3389/fnhum.2013.00031

Fritsch, T., McClendon, M. J., Smyth, K. A., Lerner, A. J., Friedland, R. P., and Larsen, J. D. (2007). Cognitive functioning in healthy aging: the role of reserve and lifestyle factors early in life. *Gerontologist* 47, 307–322. doi: 10.1093/geront/47.3.307

Green, R. E. A., Colella, B., Herbert, D. A., Bayley, M., Kang, H. S., Till, C., et al. (2008). Prediction of return to productivity after severe traumatic brain injury: investigations of optimal neuropsychological tests and timing of assessment. *Arch. Phys. Med. Rehabil.* 89, S51–S60.

Greenberg, G., Mikulis, D. J., Ng, K., Desouza, D., and Green, R. E. (2008). Use of diffusion tensor imaging to examine subacute white matter injury progression in moderate to severe traumatic brain injury. *Arch. Phys. Med. Rehabil.* 89, 45–50. doi: 10.1016/j.apmr.2008.09.552

Himanen, L., Portin, R., Isoniemi, H., Helenius, H., Kurki, T., and Tenovuo, O. (2006). Longitudinal cognitive changes in traumatic brain injury: a 30-year follow-up study. *Neurology* 66 187–192. doi: 10.1212/01.wnl.0000194264.60150.d3

Jacobs, B., Schall, M., and Scheibel, A. B. (1993). A quantitative dendritic analysis of Wernicke's area in humans. II. Gender, hemispheric, and environmental factors. *J. Comp. Neurol.* 327, 97–111. doi: 10.1002/cne.903270108

Johnson, V. E., Stewart, J. E., Begbie, F. D., Trojanowski, J. Q., Smith, D. H., and Stewart, W. (2013). Inflammation and white matter degeneration persist for years after a single traumatic brain injury. *Brain* 136(Pt 1), 28–42. doi: 10.1093/brain/aws322

Kasai, H., Fukuda, M., Watanabe, S., Hayashi-Takagi, A., and Noguchi, J. (2010). Structural dynamics of dendritic spines in memory and cognition. *Trends Neurosci.* 33 121–129.

Kempermann, G., Fabel, K., Ehninger, D., Babu, H., Leal-Galicia, P., Garthe, A., et al. (2010). Why and how physical activity promotes experience-induced brain plasticity. *Front. Neurosci.* 4:189. doi: 10.3389/fnins.2010.00189

Kempermann, G., Gast, D., and Gage, F. H. (2002). Neuroplasticity in old age: sustained fivefold induction of hippocampal neurogenesis by long-term environmental enrichment. *Ann. Neurol.* 52, 135–143. doi: 10.1002/ana.10262

Kesler, S. R., Adams, H. F., Blasey, C. M., and Bigler, E. D. (2003). Premorbid intellectual functioning, education, and brain size in traumatic brain injury: an investigation of the cognitive reserve hypothesis. *Appl. Neuropsychol.* 10, 153–162. doi: 10.1207/S15324826AN1003_04

Kolb, B., Teskey, G. C., and Gibb, R. (2010). Factors influencing cerebral plasticity in the normal and injured brain. *Front. Hum. Neurosci.* 4:204. doi: 10.3389/fnhum.2010.00204

Kovesdi, E., Gyorgy, A. B., Kwon, S. C., Wingo, D. L., Kamnaksh. A., Long, J. B., et al. (2011). The effect of enriched environment on the outcome of traumatic brain injury; a behavioral, proteomics, and histological study. *Front. Neurosci.* 5:42. doi: 10.3389/fnins.2011.00042

Lee, T., Jarome, T., Li, S. J., Kim, J. J., and Helmstetter, F. J. (2009). Chronic stress selectively reduces hippocampal volume in rats: a longitudinal magnetic resonance imaging study. *Neuroreport* 20, 1554–1558. doi: 10.1097/WNR.0b013e328332bb09

Levin, H. S., O'donnell, M. A., and Grossman, R. G. (1979). The Galveston orientation and amnesia test: a practical scale to assess cognition after head injury. *J. Nerv. Ment. Dis.* 167, 675–684. doi: 10.1097/00005053-197911000-00004

Lezak, M. D., Howieson, D. B., and Loring, D. W. (2004). *Neuropsychological Assessment.* New York, NY: Oxford University Press.

Mahncke, H. W., Bronstone, A., and Merzenich, M. M. (2006). Brain plasticity and functional losses in the aged: scientific bases for a novel intervention. *Prog. Brain Res.* 157, 81–109.

Maller, J. J., Daskalakis, Z. J., and Fitzgerald, P. B. (2007). Hippocampal volumetrics in depression: the importance of the posterior tail. *Hippocampus* 17, 1023–1027.

Mateer, C. A., and Sira, C. S. (2006). Cognitive and emotional consequences of TBI: intervention strategies for vocational rehabilitation. *Neurorehabilitation* 21, 315–326.

Matter, A. M., Folweiler, K. A., Curatolo, L. M., and Kline, A. E. (2011). Temporal effects of environmental enrichment–mediated functional improvement after experimental traumatic brain injury in rats. *Neurorehabil. Neural Repair* 25, 558–564. doi: 10.1177/1545968310397206

McCarthy, M. M. (2003). Stretching the truth. Why hippocampal neurons are so vulnerable following traumatic brain injury. *Exp. Neurol.* 184, 40–43. doi: 10.1016/j.expneurol.2003.08.020

Millis, S. R., Rosenthal, M., Novack, T. A., Sherer, M., Nick, T. G., Kreutzer, J. S., et al. (2001). Long-term neuropsychological outcome after traumatic brain injury. *J. Head Trauma Rehabil.* 16, 343–355. doi: 10.1097/00001199-200108000-00005

Mohammed, A. H., Zhu, S. W., Darmopil, S., Hjerling-Leffler, J., Ernfors, P., Winblad, B., et al. (2002). Environmental enrichment and the brain. *Prog. Brain Res.* 138, 109–133. doi: 10.1016/S0079-6123(02)38074-9

Murre, R., and Robertson, I. (1999). Rehabilitation of brain damage: brain plasticity and principles of guided recovery. *Psychol. Bull.* 125, 544–575. doi: 10.1037/0033-2909.125.5.544

Ng, K., Mikulis, D. J., Glazer, J., Kabani, N., Till, C., Greenberg, G., et al. (2008). Magnetic resonance imaging evidence of progression of subacute brain atrophy in moderate to severe traumatic brain injury. *Arch. Phys. Med. Rehabil.* 89, S35–S44. doi: 10.1016/j.apmr.2008.07.006

Nithianantharajah, J., and Hannan, A. J. (2009). The neurobiology of brain and cognitive reserve: mental and physical activity as modulators of brain disorders. *Prog. Neurobiol.* 89, 369–382. doi: 10.1016/j.pneurobio.2009.10.001

Olson, A. K., Eadie, B. D., Ernst, C., and Christie, B. R. (2006). Environmental enrichment and voluntary exercise massively increase neurogenesis in the adult hippocampus via dissociable pathways. *Hippocampus* 16, 250–260. doi: 10.1002/hipo.20157

Onyszchuk, G., He, Y. Y., Berman, N. E., and Brooks, W. M. (2008). Detrimental effects of aging on outcome from traumatic brain injury: a behavioral, magnetic resonance imaging, and histological study in mice. *J. Neurotrauma* 25, 153–171. doi: 10.1089/neu.2007.0430

Petcu, E. B., Sfredel, V., Platt, D., Herndon, J. G., Kessler, C., and Popa-Wagner, A. (2008). Cellular and molecular events underlying the dysregulated response of the aged brain to stroke: a mini-review. *Gerontology* 54, 6–17. doi: 10.1159/000112845

Popa-Wagner, A., Carmichael, S. T., Kokaia, Z., Kessler, C., and Walker, L. C. (2007). The response of the aged brain to stroke: too much, too soon? *Curr. Neurovasc. Res.* 4, 216–227.

Raichle, M. E., MacLeod, A. M., Snyder, A. Z., Powers, W. J., Gusnard, D. A., and Shulman, G. L. (2001). A default mode of brain function. *Proc. Natl. Acad. Sci. U.S.A.* 98, 676–682. doi: 10.1073/pnas.98.2.676

Richards, M., Hardy, R., and Wadsworth, M. E. (2003). Does active leisure protect cognition? Evidence from a national birth cohort. *Soc. Sci. Med.* 56, 785–792.

Robertson, I. H., and Murre, J. M. (1999). Rehabilitation of brain damage: brain plasticity and principles of guided recovery. *Psychol. Bull.* 125, 544–575. doi: 10.1037/0033-2909.125.5.544

Rosenzweig, M. R., and Bennett, E. L. (1996). Psychobiology of plasticity: effects of training and experience on brain and behavior. *Behav. Brain Res.* 78, 57–65. doi: 10.1016/0166-4328(95)00216-2

Rosenfeld, J. V., Maas, A. I., Bragge, P., Morganti-Kossmann, M. C., Manley, G. T., and Gruen, R. L. (2012). Early management of severe traumatic brain injury. *Lancet* 380, 1088–1098. doi: 10.1016/S0140-6736(12)60864-2

Salthouse, T. A., Berish, D. E., and Miles, J. D. (2002). The role of cognitive stimulation on the relations between age and cognitive functioning. *Psychol. Aging* 17, 548–557. doi: 10.1037/0882-7974.17.4.548

Sandrone, S., and Bacigaluppi, M. (2012). Learning from default mode network: the predictive value of resting state in traumatic brain injury. *J. Neurosci.* 32, 1915–1917. doi: 10.1523/JNEUROSCI.5637-11.2012

Satz, P. (1993). Brain reserve capacity on symptom onset after brain injury: a formulation and review of evidence for threshold theory. *Neuropsychology* 7, 273–295. doi: 10.1037/0894-4105.7.3.273

Scarmeas, N., and Stern, Y. (2003). Cognitive reserve and lifestyle. *J. Clin. Exp. Neuropsychol.* 25, 625–633. doi: 10.1076/jcen.25.5.625.14576

Shors, T. J., Anderson, M. L., Curlik, D. M., and Nokia, M. S. (2012). Use it or lose it: How neurogenesis keeps the brain fit for learning. *Behav. Brain Res.* 227, 450–458. doi: 10.1016/j.bbr.2011.04.023

Stern, Y. (2002). What is cognitive reserve? Theory and research application of the reserve concept. *J. Int. Neuropsychol. Soc.* 8, 448–460. doi: 10.1017/S1355617702813248

Stern, Y. (2006). Cognitive reserve and Alzheimer disease. *Alzheimer Dis. Assoc. Disord.* 20, 112–117.

Studenski, S., Carlson, M. C., Fillit, H., Greenough, W. T., Kramer, A., and Rebok, G. W. (2006). "From bedside to bench: does mental and physical activity promote cognitive vitality in late life?" in *Proceeding of the Conference on Science Aging Knowledge Environment 2006* (Philadelphia, PA), pe21.

Surget, A., Tanti, A., Leonardo, E. D., Laugeray, A., Rainer, Q., Touma, C., et al. (2011). Antidepressants recruit new neurons to improve stress response regulation. *Mol. Psychiatry* 16, 1177–1188. doi: 10.1038/mp.2011.48

Tanti, A., Westphal, W. P., Girault, V., Brizard, B., Devers, S., Leguisquet, A. M., et al. (2013). Region-dependent and stage-specific effects of stress, environmental enrichment and antidepressant treatment on hippocampal neurogenesis. *Hippocampus* 23, 797–811. doi: 10.1002/hipo.22134

Tate, and Bigler, E. D. (2000). Fornix and hippocampal atrophy in traumatic brain injury. *Learn. Mem.* 7, 442–446. doi: 10.1101/lm.33000

Taub, E., Uswatte, G., Mark, V. W., and Morris, D. M. (2006). The learned nonuse phenomenon: implications for rehabilitation. *Eura. Medicophys.* 42, 241–256.

Taylor, V. A., Daneault, V., Grant, J., Scavone, G., Breton, E., Roffe-Vidal, S., et al. (2013). Impact of meditation training on the default mode network during a restful state. *Soc. Cogn. Affect. Neurosci.* 8, 4–14. doi: 10.1093/scan/nsr087

Till, C., Colella, B., Verwegen, J., and Green, R. E. (2008). Postrecovery cognitive decline in adults with traumatic brain injury. *Arch. Phys. Med. Rehabil.* 89(12 Suppl.), S25–S34. doi: 10.1016/j.apmr.2008.07.004

Tombaugh, T. N. (1996). *Test of Memory Malingering (TOMM).* New York, NY: Multi-Health Systems, Inc.

Trivedi, M. A., Ward, M. A., Hess, T. M., Gale, S. D., Dempsey, R. J., Rowley, H. A., et al. (2007). Longitudinal changes in global brain volume between 79 and 409 days after traumatic brain injury: relationship with duration of coma. *J. Neurotrauma* 24, 766–771. doi: 10.1089/neu.2006.0205

Watson, C., Andermann, F., Gloor, P., Jones-Gotman, M., Peters, T., Evans, A., et al. (1992). Anatomic basis of amygdaloid and hippocampal volume measurement by magnetic resonance imaging. *Neurology* 42, 1743–1750. doi: 10.1212/WNL.42.9.1743

Watson, C., Cendes, F., Fuerst, D., Dubeau, F., Williamson, B., Evans, A., et al. (1997). Specificity of volumetric magnetic resonance imaging in detecting hippocampal sclerosis. *Arch. Neurol.* 54, 67–73. doi: 10.1001/archneur.1997.00550130049015

Wechsler, D. (2001). *Wechsler Test of Adult Reading (WTAR).* San Antonio, TX: The Psychological Corporation.

Willis, K. J., and Hakim, A. M. (2013). Stroke prevention and cognitive reserve: emerging approaches to modifying risk and delaying onset of dementia. *Front. Neurol.* 4:13. doi: 10.3389/fneur.2013.00013

Ylvisaker, M., Hanks, R., and Johnson-Greene, D. (2002). Perspectives on rehabilitation of individuals with cognitive impairment after brain injury: rationale for reconsideration of theoretical paradigms. *J. Head Trauma Rehabil.* 17, 191–209.

27

Is abeta a sufficient biomarker for monitoring anti-abeta clinical studies?

Jens Moreth, Chrystelle Mavoungou and Katharina Schindowski*

Faculty for Biotechnology, Institute of Applied Biotechnology, Biberach University of Applied Science, Biberach/Riss, Germany

Edited by:
Manuel Menéndez-González, Hospital Álvarez-Buylla, Spain

Reviewed by:
Eugenia Rota, Ospedale Guglielmo da Saliceto di Piacenza, Italy
Xue Hua, University of California, Los Angeles, USA
Sandra A. Acosta, University of South Florida, USA

***Correspondence:**
Katharina Schindowski, Faculty for Biotechnology, Institute of Applied Biotechnology, Biberach University of Applied Science, Karlstrasse 11, D-88400 Biberach/Riss, Germany
e-mail: zimmermann@hochschule-bc.de

Amyloid-beta (Aβ) in Alzheimer's disease (AD) appeared to be a promising target for disease-modifying therapeutic strategies like passive immunotherapy with anti-Aβ monoclonal antibodies (mAbs). Biochemical markers in cerebrospinal fluid (CSF) include alterations of Aβ that allow the diagnosis of AD. Biomarker strategies, such as the levels of Aβ in CSF and plasma, currently play an important role in early clinical trials for AD. Indeed, these strategies have a relevant impact on the outcome of such studies, since the biomarkers are used to monitor the bioactivity of anti-Aβ mAbs. The clinical trials of Solanezumab were mainly based on the readout of Aβ levels in CSF and plasma, whereas those of Bapineuzumab were based on cognition; however, little is known about the mechanisms altering these biomarker levels, and no biomarker has yet been proven to be a successful predictor for AD therapy. In addition, the Aβ biomarkers allow for the determination of free and bound anti-Aβ mAb in order to monitor the available amount of bioactive drug and could give hints to the mechanism of action. In this review, we discuss clinical Aβ biomarker data and the latest regulatory strategies.

Keywords: passive immunization, dementia, therapeutic monoclonal antibodies, regulatory strategy, CSF, plasma increase, mode of action, pharmacogenetics and pharmacogenomics

Aβ-AGGREGATES AND THEIR IMPLICATIONS ON IMMUNIZATION

With about 70% of all cases, Alzheimer's disease (AD) is the most-common form of dementia (Alzheimer's Disease International, 2009) and countries in demographic transition will experience the greatest growth. AD is defined as a multifactorial disease with the pathogenic cerebral deposition of the aggregated proteins Amyloid-β (Aβ) and hyper-phosphorylated tau (phospho-tau). Despite the well-accepted pathogenic role of Aβ (Selkoe, 2001), the underlying pathogenic mechanism is still elusive (Broersen et al., 2010). Aβ-aggregates—majorly derived from $A\beta_{40}$ and $A\beta_{42}$—are generated from amyloid precursor protein by sequential proteolysis (Haass and Selkoe, 2007) followed by self-association from monomeric to soluble oligomeric and protofibrillar Aβ. Protofibrillar Aβ further aggregates into insoluble Aβ-fibrils and deposits in the brain as amyloid plaques. Since the number of these plaques does not correlate well with the severity of dementia (Terry, 2006)—as opposed to soluble Aβ-aggregates (McDonald et al., 2010)—the amyloid hypothesis has been reformulated, positioning soluble Aβ aggregates as hallmark in AD pathology (Walsh and Selkoe, 2007; Broersen et al., 2010). A plethora of different Aβ-species with overlapping size and morphology have been described (Broersen et al., 2010; Benilova et al., 2012): Aβ-dimers (Shankar et al., 2008; O'Nuallain et al., 2010), low-molecular weight oligomers comprising dimeric to tetrameric Aβ (Walsh et al., 2005), pentamers and hexamers (Ahmed et al., 2010), dodecameric Aβ56* (Lesne et al., 2006; Reed et al., 2011), globulomers (Barghorn et al., 2005), Aβ-oligomers (Kayed et al., 2003), Alzheimer-derived diffusible ligands (ADDLs; Lambert et al., 1998), protofibrils (Walsh et al., 1999), and amylospheroids (Hoshi et al., 2003). Although, the size and molecular weight of these Aβ-species have predominantly been used for differentiation, the peptide source, either synthetic or endogenous, and the applied methods for characterization—e.g., SDS-PAGE, TEM, AFM, Ultracentrifugation—hamper a direct comparison (Moreth et al., 2013). Despite the pathological relevance of endogenous Aβ-species, low protein concentrations and protein heterogeneity elude a precise characterization of the molecular identity. The synthetic Aβ-aggregate is applicable to a more-precise characterization, but still retains limited relevance, since the variety of reported Aβ-aggregates has yet to be proven to be present in AD brain. Furthermore, the identification of Aβ-aggregates is hampered owing to their meta-stability and the ability for inter-conversion in different aggregation pathways (Moreth et al., 2013), which was also mentioned by Bitan et al. (2005). This is of great importance for immunization, since the fate of the pre-aggregated Aβ is elusive after injection.

OCCURRENCE OF Aβ SPECIES IN PLASMA AND CSF

From a set of upcoming biomarkers (Fagan and Perrin, 2012), the most-established biomarkers for AD diagnosis in cerebrospinal

Abbreviations: aa, amino acid; Aβ, amyloid-beta; AβO, Aβ oligomers; AD, Alzheimer's disease; ADAS-Cog, Alzheimer's Disease Assessment Scale-cognitive subscale; ADDLs, Alzheimer derived diffusible ligands; ADNI, Alzheimer's disease neuroimaging initiative; AFM, atomic force microscopy; ApoE4, ApolipoproteinE4; CSF, cerebrospinal fluid; DAD, disability assessment for dementia; EMA, European Medicine Agency; FDA, food and drug administration; J&J, Johnson&Johnson; LRP, low density lipoprotein receptor-related protein; MRI, magnetic resonance imaging; PET, positron emission tomography; phospho-tau, hyperphosphorylated tau; PK, pharmacokinetic; SDS-PAGE, sodium dodecyl sulfate polyacrylamide gel electrophoresis; TEM, transmission electron microscopy.

fluid (CSF) are still the determination of Aβ_{42}, total-Tau and phospho-Tau$_{181}$ (Di Carlo et al., 2012). Only a combination of these three CSF biomarkers increases the validity of the diagnosis with a combined sensitivity of 95% (Blennow et al., 2010). In AD, CSF-Aβ_{42} is significantly decreased, which is believed to be due to decreased clearance of aggregated Aβ_{42} from the brain. The Aβ_{40} levels seem to be constant and therefore the increased Aβ_{42}/Aβ_{40} ratio has been suggested to improve early AD-diagnosis. However, this is still controversial and for plasma-derived Aβ reports are even more contradictory (Zetterberg, 2008; Zetterberg et al., 2010). To mention the prefibrillar Aβ-aggregates as the prime toxic agents in AD, one might address these as potential biomarkers. However, there is still a lack of a robust method for the detection of larger Aβ-aggregates *in vivo* (e.g., ADDL, Aβ-oligomers). Some recent reports showed methods for Aβ-aggregate detection based on ELISA, IP western blotting and Aβ-aggregate capture assays. All of these methods are based on conformation-specific antibodies, which do not detect monomeric or fibrillar, but rather the prefibrillar aggregates (Funke et al., 2009), even though the most relevant Aβ-aggregate for AD diagnosis is still elusive. Furthermore, based on the described meta-stability of Aβ-aggregates (Moreth et al., 2013), it might be misleading to focus on a single aggregate species if the whole spectrum of aggregates from the dimer up to protofibrillar Aβ are present in the brain and of importance in AD-progression.

PLASMA AND CSF Aβ AS BIOMARKERS TO MONITOR PASSIVE ANTI-Aβ IMMUNOTHERAPY CLINICAL STUDIES

Aβ has a complex pharmacokinetic profile, as it is permanently produced in brain as well as in the periphery, and transported back and forth between both pharmacokinetic compartments (Zlokovic et al., 1993; Ghersi-Egea et al., 1996; Shibata et al., 2000). Soluble Aβ is either degraded by proteases (Iwata et al., 2005), transported via the blood-brain barrier by receptors like LRP (Sagare et al., 2007), RAGE (Deane et al., 2003), and P-glycoprotein (Ito et al., 2006), or aggregates to multimers and plaques. Likewise, plaque Aβ is in steady-state equilibrium with soluble Aβ (Kawarabayashi et al., 2001). Finally, Aβ is rapidly eliminated by hepatic and renal degradation (Ghiso et al., 2004). PET scanning with the Pittsburgh compound (PiB) detects fibrillar Aβ. CSF Aβ_{42} and PET measures of fibrillar Aβ are significantly inversely correlated with each other, likely to reflect Aβ deposition in the brain (Fagan et al., 2006).

Proteins in plasma, like antibodies that capture soluble Aβ, are capable of sequestering soluble forms of Aβ from their bound and circulating forms. Total Aβ plasma levels will therefore increase while free Aβ levels reduce due to the longer half-life of protein-complexed Aβ [see **Figure 1A**; (Park et al., 2012)]. The elimination of the Aβ-protein complex is according to the complex's half-life, which is rather long in the case of FcRn-recycled monoclonal antibodies (mAbs). Complexed Aβ is predictably not transported across the blood brain barrier, does not form multimers, and influences the equilibrium between soluble Aβ and plaque Aβ that appears to result in improved clearance of cerebral Aβ, e.g., CSF Aβ. The Aβ-binding proteins should have an affinity to Aβ high enough to compete with endogenous Aβ-binding proteins and transporters. Free Aβ drops rapidly after Aβ is sequestered, but due to its rapid synthesis in various tissues, it is restored to basal endogenous levels rather quickly (Barten et al., 2005).

Peripherally-administered mAbs that sequester soluble Aβ result in an increase of plasma Aβ (DeMattos et al., 2002) that is correlated to its affinity; some mAbs are even capable of reducing CSF Aβ (Mavoungou and Schindowski, 2013). Several studies used these biomarkers as clinical strategy (**Table 1**). Solanezumab caused a sharp, sustained, and dose-dependent increase of plasma Aβ_{1-40} and Aβ_{1-42} (Farlow et al., 2012). CSF Aβ_{1-40} and Aβ_{1-42} increased in the mild to moderate AD patients with 0.1% of plasma levels of Solanezumab found in the CSF. The rise in level of total Aβ in plasma and CSF is assumed to be related to target engagement (Strobel and Bowman Rogers, 2012). Free CSF Aβ was determined by protein G sepharose immunoprecipitation to deplete immunoglobins and subsequent ELISA (Farlow et al., 2012). Therefore, this method was used for CSF samples only, since immunoglobulin plasma concentrations are too high for this method. In a rather small cohort of patients, free CSF Aβ_{1-40} decreased with treatment, while free Aβ_{1-42} did not. It is suspected that the higher amount of free CSF Aβ_{1-42} is related to the dissolution of plaques that were mainly composed of Aβ_{42}. However, PiB scans of another subcohort showed no significant change between the groups, although treated patients with mild AD had a trend toward less amyloid, this lacked statistical significance (Matthews and Bader, 2012).

The clinical biomarker data from Bapineuzumab are more difficult to interpret, due to the fact that Bapineuzumab binds both soluble and plaque Aβ, and the methodological strategy is rather unclear. Aβ_{1-40} and Aβ_{x-42} were detected by a sandwich ELISA using 4G8 for capture and a C-terminal mAb for detection (**Figure 1B**). 4G8 does not interfere with Bapineuzumab binding (Johnson-Wood et al., 1997; Clarke and Shearman, 2000). Interestingly, Aβ_{1-42} was determined with an ELISA using 3D6 as capture. 3D6 is the parental molecule of Bapineuzumab and therefore these two mAbs compete with each other when binding Aβ. Consequently, Bapineuzumab-Aβ complexes in CSF will predictably not be detected in this assay, though according to PK data Bapineuzumab occurs in CSF with 0.3% incidence of plasma levels (Blennow et al., 2012). Hence, the clinical data reveal no changes in CSF Aβ_{1-42} levels with Bapineuzumab treatment, while Solanezumab treatment revealed an increase in Aβ_{1-42} detected with the C-terminal mAb 21F12 and the N-terminal 3D6. Moreover, to avoid signal suppression due to steric hindrance, the authors of the Solanezumab study spiked an excess of Solanezumab in the assay buffer (Farlow et al., 2012). Furthermore, Bapineuzumab treatment decreased CSF phospho-tau (Salloway et al., 2012; Sperling et al., 2012). Like Solanezumab, Bapineuzumab was not active on patient's cognition and activities of daily living unless subsequent post-test of subcohorts were considered for re-analysis (Salloway et al., 2009; Lilly, 2012; Matthews and Bader, 2012). In summary, both antibodies engaged their target, but they hardly improved clinical signs (Strobel and Bowman Rogers, 2012). Bapineuzumab's clinical development was discontinued for AD in 2012 (Johnson & Johnson, 2012), AAB-003/PF-0523681 an engineered 3D6

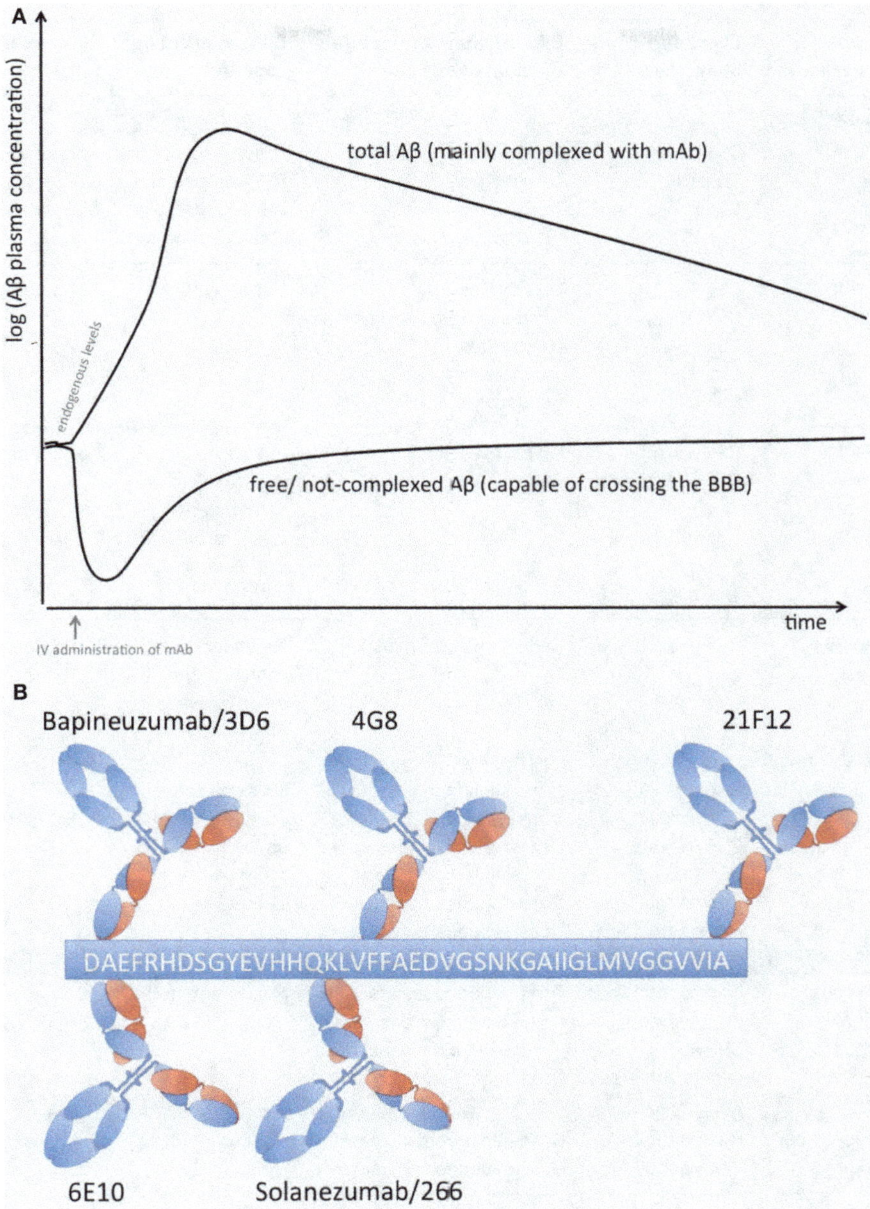

FIGURE 1 | (A) Plasma Aβ levels after treatment with an Aβ sequestering compound. Anti-Aβ mAbs capture soluble Aβ and form Aβ-mAb complexes, which have a much longer half-life than free Aβ alone. Therefore, total Aβ (i.e., free and bound) plasma levels rise while free Aβ levels drop rapidly but return rather quickly to normal levels due to its rapid synthesis in many tissues. **(B)** Binding sites on $A\beta_{1-42}$ of therapeutic and diagnostic mAbs. Adapted from Johnson-Wood et al. (1997); Clarke and Shearman (2000).

replaced Bapineuzumab in the sponsor's pipeline (Pfizer, 2013). Dose-dependent plasma total Aβ increases were reported from GSK933776 and Crenezumab with decreased free plasma Aβ levels (GlaxoSmithKline, 2011; Adolfsson et al., 2012).

THE IMPORTANCE OF AN APPROPRIATE BIOMARKER STRATEGY FOR AD

In an ideal world with a successful anti-AD therapy, the detection of AD biomarkers should indicate appropriate patient selection likely to derive therapeutic benefit. The EMA tried first to get closer to this ideal world, at least from the regulatory side, and introduced research diagnostic criteria that added specificity to the prevailing concept of mild cognitive impairment (Dubois et al., 2007). This set the stage for new types of trials (Strobel and Bowman Rogers, 2012). The criteria are closer to the disease, combining a mild but measurable memory impairment with a biomarker change. The EMA considered firstly that a pathological signature based on CSF $A\beta_{42}$ and phospho-tau was acceptable for identifying prodromal-stage patients who are at risk of developing AD (European Medicines Agency, 2011b), secondly, using

Table 1 | Clinical effects of anti-Aβ mAbs on CSF and plasma Aβ, adapted from Mavoungou and Schindowski (2013).

Study/cohort	Subcohort size for biomarker evaluation	Evaluated biomarker	Clinical effect of treatment on biomarker	Clinical effect on cognition	PK data of mAb	References
BAPINEUZUMAB (HUMANIZED 3D6)						
201 Phase II	Placebo: $n = 14$ BAPI: $n = 20$	CSF $A\beta_{x-42}$ Total CSF tau CSF phospho-tau	No changes No changes Trend to reduction ($p = 0.056$)	In small cohort 6% less loss of ADAS-Cog scores after 18 months	Approximately 0.3% CSF-plasma ratio	Salloway et al., 2009
Phase II: pooled 201 and 202	Placebo: $n = 19$ BAPI: $n = 26–27$	CSF $A\beta_{1-40}$ CSF $A\beta_{x-42}$ CSF $A\beta_{1-42}$ Total CSF tau CSF phospho-tau	No changes Decrease from baseline No changes No changes Reduction ($p = 0.03$)	Not determined	Not determined	Blennow et al., 2012
Phase III: 301 (*ApoE4* carrier)	Placebo: $n = 77$ 0.5 mg/kg: $n = 47$ 1.0 mg/kg: $n = 54$	CSF phospho-tau CSF phospho-tau	No changes at 0.5 mg/kg Reduction at 1.0 mg/kg	In a subcohort of mild cases at 1.0 mg/kg ~30% less loss of DAD scores after 18 months	Not determined	Salloway et al., 2012
Phase III: 302 (*ApoE4* non-carrier)	Placebo: $n = 85$ 0.5 mg/kg: $n = 127$	CSF phospho-tau	Reduction at 0.5 mg/kg	No effect on cognition after 18 months, even not for mild cases	Not determined	Sperling et al., 2012
SOLANEZUMAB (HUMANIZED m266)						
Phase II	Placebo: $n = 8$; SOLA: $n = 10–11$ per dose group	CSF total $A\beta_{40}$ CSF total $A\beta_{42}$ CSF free $A\beta_{40}$ CSF free $A\beta_{42}$ Plasma total $A\beta_{40}$ Plasma total $A\beta_{42}$	Increase at high dose Increase at high dose Decrease at high dose Increase at high dose Dose-dependent increase Dose-dependent decrease	No significant cognitive benefit on the ADAS-cog score over after 12-weeks	0.1% CSF-plasma ratio	Farlow et al., 2012
GSK933776 (DISCONTINUED FOR AD)						
Phase I	Placebo: $n = 14$; GSK933776: $n = 3–6$ per dose group	Plasma total Aβ Plasma free Aβ CSF $A\beta_{1-38}$ tau/phospho-tau	Dose-dependent increase Dose-dependent decrease Increase at the highest dose No changes	Not determined	>0.2% CSF-plasma ratio	GlaxoSmithKline, 2011
CRENEZUMAB (MABT5102A)						
Phase I	MABT: $n = 25–31$ per regime group	Plasma total $A\beta_{40}$ Plasma total $A\beta_{40}$	Dose-dependent increase Dose-dependent increase	Not determined	Not determined	Adolfsson et al., 2012

hippocampal volume (European Medicines Agency, 2011a), and thirdly, using amyloid PET as a biomarker to enrich pre-dementia trials (European Medicines Agency, 2011c). Likewise, the FDA revised its criteria as well. Nevertheless, evidence is needed that a surrogate marker predicts a subsequent clinical outcome. Qualifying disease- and disorder-specific biomarkers for AD can still be considered "exploratory" from a regulatory point of view, therefore making an accurate validation and qualification questionable. Nevertheless, biomarkers, in particular those appropriate to guide selection of patients for clinical trials as well as those used as surrogate endpoint for drug efficacy, have reached the status of "probable valid biomarker" within the scope of investigation drugs along with an effective clinical trial strategy. In conclusion, the results show that CSF biomarkers are better predictors of progression to AD than plasma Aβ isoforms (Hansson et al., 2010).

Florbetapir, which binds Aβ plaques like PiB, was fast-track reviewed by the FDA and is currently the first granted and therefore qualified imaging agent for clinical use (Food and Drug Administration, 2012a). Following the results of the evaluation, even though a positive scan indicates moderate to frequent plaques, a positive Florbetapir scan is not AD specific, indicating that it is not appropriate to establish an accurate diagnosis of AD (Food and Drug Administration, 2012b). In fact, nobody currently knows why cognitively normal people accumulate Aβ in their brains, and what that might mean for their future brain health. The AD Neuroimaging Initiative (ADNI) belongs to one of the instruments to gain more information on the disease by means of PET and MRI linked to genetic disposition, cognitive impairment as well as CSF and plasma biomarkers. The use of such information obviously is crucial to set future clinical designs for AD (Food and Drug Administration, 2012a) but also as prophylactic examination for physicians in case of genetic predisposition for AD. On the other hand, exploring a set of imaging and biochemical biomarkers helps to develop regulatory guidelines to change diagnostic criteria, their validation and finally to support the potential use of biomarkers in different stages of drug development.

While the expressed view is that CSF biomarkers indicate the pathologic processes underlying AD, it is also important to keep in mind that specific genotypes like *ApoE4* and presenilin mutations affect the degree of pathological change. Therefore, using pharmacogenetics will enrich clinical drug development. From the presented data it seems that use of CSF markers is an unavoidable step for a correct and early diagnosis. However, the data reported show only the positive results, with no negative comments or discussion on potential pitfalls. Uncritical support without showing areas of uncertainty or controversy could be misleading, in helping to improve the design of subsequent randomized controlled clinical trials. The hazard ratio in longitudinal studies shows an extremely large confidence interval, which is not that supportive for the utility of monitoring. The specifications of the confidence interval for such a multifactorial disease like AD might be nowadays too tight in the light of the recent findings about the disease. That means it is understandable that the confidence interval cannot be met for most of the cases. A combination of biomarkers to boost the sensitivity and reliability for tracking AD progression at different stage and widening the current specification limits with respect to confidential interval would better match with the variability of the results.

CONCLUSION

To summarize, Aβ-aggregates reveal a remarkable metastability and the ability for reorganization within different aggregate equilibria. One might assume that the whole spectrum of prefibrillar Aβ-aggregates is of relevance in AD. Thus, targeting one specific species of Aβ with immunotherapy and using Aβ as preclinical and clinical biomarker is based on tentative, though countless data that apparently do not reflect the clinical reality. Therefore, the clinical biomarker data from the phase II and III studies of the most-advanced anti-Aβ mAbs are not appropriate to predict the cognitive outcome, even though the results show that CSF Aβ appears to be more relevant than plasma Aβ. This stresses the urgent need to understand the molecular basis of AD and to find adequate surrogate biomarkers. From a regulatory point of view, the approval of a highly-innovative active substance for the treatment for AD still remains a challenge. Although biomarker strategies have been taken more and more into account, the current study designs for AD superficially address the silent pathogenesis of the disease. The EMA and FDA are looking forward to qualifying new surrogate endpoints that encompass appropriate biomarker concepts in support of a robust biomarker strategy, which would enable the discovery of medicinal products that are active in interfering with AD pathogenesis.

AUTHORS CONTRIBUTIONS

Jens Moreth supported with novel data on Aβ conformation and aggregation, Chrystelle Mavoungou supported with insight from regulatory affairs and Katharina Schindowski supported with insight on Aβ immunotherapy und neuroimmunology. All authors drafted the manuscript. All authors read and approved the final manuscript.

ACKNOWLEDGMENTS

The authors thank Owen Scudamore for language editing and help with the manuscript.

REFERENCES

Adolfsson, O., Pihlgren, M., Toni, N., Varisco, Y., Buccarello, A. L., Antoniello, K., et al. (2012). An effector-reduced anti-β-amyloid (Aβ) antibody with unique Aβ binding properties promotes neuroprotection and glial engulfment of Aβ. *J. Neurosci.* 32, 9677–9689. doi: 10.1523/JNEUROSCI.4742-11.2012

Ahmed, M., Davis, J., Aucoin, D., Sato, T., Ahuja, S., Aimoto, S., et al. (2010). Structural conversion of neurotoxic amyloid-beta(1-42) oligomers to fibrils. *Nat. Struct. Mol. Biol.* 17, 561–567. doi: 10.1038/nsmb.1799

Alzheimer's Disease International. (2009). *World Alzheimer Report 2009*. Available online at: http://www.alz.co.uk/research/world-report

Barghorn, S., Nimmrich, V., Striebinger, A., Krantz, C., Keller, P., Janson, B., et al. (2005). Globular amyloid beta-peptide oligomer a homogenous and stable neuropathological protein in Alzheimer's disease. *J. Neurochem.* 95, 834–847. doi: 10.1111/j.1471-4159.2005.03407.x

Barten, D. M., Guss, V. L., Corsa, J. A., Loo, A., Hansel, S. B., Zheng, M., et al. (2005). Dynamics of beta-amyloid reductions in brain, cerebrospinal fluid, and plasma of beta-amyloid precursor protein transgenic mice treated with a gamma-secretase inhibitor. *J. Pharmacol. Exp. Ther.* 312, 635–643. doi: 10.1124/jpet.104.075408

Benilova, I., Karran, E., and De Strooper, B. (2012). The toxic Abeta oligomer and Alzheimer's disease: an emperor in need of clothes. *Nat. Neurosci.* 15, 349–357. doi: 10.1038/nn.3028

Bitan, G., Fradinger, E. A., Spring, S. M., and Teplow, D. B. (2005). Neurotoxic protein oligomers what you see is not always what you get. *Amyloid* 12, 88–95. doi: 10.1080/13506120500106958

Blennow, K., Hampel, H., Weiner, M., and Zetterberg, H. (2010). Cerebrospinal fluid and plasma biomarkers in Alzheimer disease. *Nat. Rev. Neurol.* 6, 131–144. doi: 10.1038/nrneurol.2010.4

Blennow, K., Zetterberg, H., Rinne, J. O., Salloway, S., Wei, J., Black, R., et al. (2012). Effect of immunotherapy with bapineuzumab on cerebrospinal fluid biomarker levels in patients with mild to moderate Alzheimer Disease. *Arch. Neurol.* 69, 1002–1010. doi: 10.1001/archneurol.2012.90

Broersen, K., Rousseau, F., and Schymkowitz, J. (2010). The culprit behind amyloid beta peptide related neurotoxicity in Alzheimer's disease: oligomer size or conformation. *Alzheimers Res. Ther.* 2, 12. doi: 10.1186/alzrt36

Clarke, E. E., and Shearman, M. S. (2000). Quantitation of amyloid-beta peptides in biological milieu using a novel homogeneous time-resolved fluorescence (HTRF) assay. *J. Neurosci. Methods* 102, 61–68. doi: 10.1016/S0165-0270(00)00280-6

Deane, R., Du Yan, S., Submamaryan, R. K., LaRue, B., Jovanovic, S., Hogg, E., et al. (2003). RAGE mediates amyloid-beta peptide transport across the blood-brain barrier and accumulation in brain. *Nat. Med.* 9, 907–913. doi: 10.1038/nm890

DeMattos, R. B., Bales, K. R., Cummins, D. J., Paul, S. M., and Holtzman, D. M. (2002). Brain to plasma amyloid-β efflux: a measure of brain amyloid burden in a mouse model of Alzheimer's disease. *Science* 295, 2264–2267. doi: 10.1126/science.1067568

Di Carlo, M., Giacomazza, D., and San Biagio, P. L. (2012). Alzheimer's disease: biological aspects, therapeutic perspectives and diagnostic tools. *J. Phys. Condens. Matter* 24:244102. doi: 10.1088/0953-8984/24/24/244102

Dubois, B., Feldman, H., Jacova, C., Dekosky, S., Barberger-Gateau,

P., Cummings, J., et al. (2007). Research criteria for the diagnosis of Alzheimer's disease: revising the NINCDS-ADRDA criteria. *Lancet* 6, 734–746. doi: 10.1016/S1474-4422(07)70178-3

European Medicines Agency. (2011a). *European Medicines Agency Releases Qualification Opinion on Diagnosis of Pre-Dementia Alzheimer's for Public Consultation*. Available online at: http://www.ema.europa.eu/ema/index.jsp?curl=pages/news_and_events/news/2011/10/news_detail_001359.jspandmid=WC0b01ac058004d5c1. (Accessed January 30, 2013).

European Medicines Agency. (2011b). *First Clinical Biomarker Qualification Released for Public Consultation*. Available online at: http://www.ema.europa.eu/ema/index.jsp?curl=pages/news_and_events/news/2011/02/news_detail_001207.jspandmid=WC0b01ac058004d5c1. (Accessed March 3, 2013).

European Medicines Agency. (2011c). *Qualification Opinion of Alzheimer's Disease Novel Methodologies/Biomarkers for the use of CSF AB 1-42 and t-tau Signature and/or PET-Amyloid Imaging (Positive/Negative) as a Biomarkers for Enrichment, for use in Regulatory Clinical Trials in Mild*. Available online at: http://www.ema.europa.eu/docs/en_GB/document_library/Regulatory_and_procedural_guideline/2011/12/WC500118365.pdf. (Accessed January 30, 2013).

Fagan, A. M., Mintun, M. A., Mach, R. H., Lee, S.-Y., Dence, C. S., Shah, A. R., et al. (2006). Inverse relation between *in vivo* amyloid imaging load and cerebrospinal fluid Abeta42 in humans. *Ann. Neurol.* 59, 512–519. doi: 10.1002/ana.20730

Fagan, A. M., and Perrin, R. J. (2012). Upcoming candidate cerebrospinal fluid biomarkers of Alzheimer's disease. *Biomark. Med.* 6, 455–476. doi: 10.2217/bmm.12.42

Farlow, M., Arnold, S. E., Van Dyck, C. H., Aisen, P. S., Snider, B. J., Porsteinsson, A. P., et al. (2012). Safety and biomarker effects of solanezumab in patients with Alzheimer's disease. *Alzheimer's Dement.* 8, 261–271. doi: 10.1016/j.jalz.2011.09.224

Food and Drug Administration. (2012a). *FDA Approves Imaging Drug Amyvid*. Available online at: http://www.fda.gov/NewsEvents/Newsroom/PressAnnouncements/ucm299678.htm. (Accessed January 30, 2013).

Food and Drug Administration. (2012b). *FY 2012 Innovative Drug Approvals*. Available online at: http://www.fda.gov/downloads/aboutfda/reportsmanualsforms/reports/ucm330859.pdf. (Accessed March 27, 2013).

Funke, S. A., Birkmann, E., and Willbold, D. (2009). Detection of Amyloid-beta aggregates in body fluids: a suitable method for early diagnosis of Alzheimer's disease. *Curr. Alzheimer Res.* 6, 285–289. doi: 10.2174/156720509788486536

Ghersi-Egea, J. F., Gorevic, P. D., Ghiso, J., Frangione, B., Patlak, C. S., and Fenstermacher, J. D. (1996). Fate of cerebrospinal fluid-borne amyloid beta-peptide: rapid clearance into blood and appreciable accumulation by cerebral arteries. *J. Neurochem.* 67, 880–883. doi: 10.1046/j.1471-4159.1996.67020880.x

Ghiso, J., Shayo, M., Calero, M., Ng, D., Tomidokoro, Y., Gandy, S., et al. (2004). Systemic catabolism of Alzheimer's Abeta40 and Abeta42. *J. Biol. Chem.* 279, 45897–45908. doi: 10.1074/jbc.M407668200

GlaxoSmithKline. (2011). *A Randomised, Single-Blind, Placebo-Controlled Study to Investigate the Safety, Tolerability, Immunogenicity, Pharmacokinetics and Pharmacodynamics of Intravenous Infusion of GSK933776 in Patients with Alzheimer's Disease*. Available online at: http://www.gsk-clinicalstudyregister.com/result_comp_list.jsp?phase=AllandstudyType=Allandpopulation=AllandmarketingNoandcompound=GSK933776. (Accessed June 1, 2012).

Haass, C., and Selkoe, D. J. (2007). Soluble protein oligomers in neurodegeneration: lessons from the Alzheimer's amyloid β-peptide. *Nat. Rev. Mol. Cell Biol.* 8, 101–112. doi: 10.1038/nrm2101

Hansson, O., Zetterberg, H., Vanmechelen, E., Vanderstichele, H., Andreasson, U., Londos, E., et al. (2010). Evaluation of plasma Abeta40 and Abeta42 as predictors of conversion to Alzheimer' s disease in patients with mild cognitive impairment. *Neurobiol. Aging* 31, 357–367. doi: 10.1016/j.neurobiolaging.2008.03.027

Hoshi, M., Sato, M., Matsumoto, S., Noguchi, A., Yasutake, K., Yoshida, N., et al. (2003). Spherical aggregates of beta-amyloid (amylospheroid) show high neurotoxicity and activate tau protein kinase I/glycogen synthase kinase-3beta. *Proc. Natl. Acad. Sci. U.S.A.* 100, 6370–6375. doi: 10.1073/pnas.1237107100

Ito, S., Ohtsuki, S., and Terasaki, T. (2006). Functional characterization of the brain-to-blood efflux clearance of human amyloid-beta peptide (1-40) across the rat blood-brain barrier. *Neurosci. Res.* 56, 246–252. doi: 10.1016/j.neures.2006.07.006

Iwata, N., Higuchi, M., and Saido, T. C. (2005). Metabolism of amyloid-h peptide and Alzheimer' s disease. *Brain* 108, 403–430.

Johnson & Johnson. (2012). *Johnson & Johnson Announces Discontinuation Of Phase 3 Development of Bapineuzumab Intravenous (IV) In Mild-To-Moderate Alzheimer's Disease. 2012*. Available online at: http://www.jnj.com/connect/news/product/johnson-and-johnson-announces-discontinuation-of-phase-3-development-of-bapineuzumab-intravenous-iv-in-mild-to-moderate-alzheimers-disease

Johnson-Wood, K., Lee, M., Motter, R., Hu, K., Gordon, G., Barbour, R., et al. (1997). Amyloid precursor protein processing and Aβ42 deposition in a transgenic mouse model of Alzheimer disease. *Proc. Natl. Acad. Sci. U.S.A.* 94:1550. doi: 10.1073/pnas.94.4.1550

Kawarabayashi, T., Younkin, L. H., Saido, T. C., Shoji, M., Ashe, K. H., and Younkin, S. G. (2001). Age-dependent changes in brain, CSF, and plasma amyloid (beta) protein in the Tg2576 transgenic mouse model of Alzheimer's disease. *J. Neurosci.* 21, 372–381.

Kayed, R., Head, E., Thompson, J. L., McIntire, T. M., Milton, S. C., Cotman, C. W., et al. (2003). Common structure of soluble amyloid oligomers implies common mechanism of pathogenesis. *Science* 300, 486–489. doi: 10.1126/science.1079469

Lambert, M. P., Barlow, A. K., Chromy, B. A., Edwards, C., Freed, R., Liosatos, M., et al. (1998). Diffusible, nonfibrillar ligands derived from Abeta1-42 are potent central nervous system neurotoxins. *Proc. Natl. Acad. Sci. U.S.A.* 95, 6448–6453. doi: 10.1073/pnas.95.11.6448

Lesne, S., Koh, M. T., Kotilinek, L., Kayed, R., Glabe, C. G., Yang, A., et al. (2006). A specific amyloid-beta protein assembly in the brain impairs memory. *Nature* 440, 352–357. doi: 10.1038/nature04533

Lilly, E. (2012). *Lilly Announces Detailed Results of the Phase 3 Solanezumab Expedition Studies Following a Presentation of the Independent Analyses by the Alzheimer's Disease Cooperative Study (ADCS)*. Available online at: http://newsroom.lilly.com/releasedetail.cfm?ReleaseID=702211

Matthews, G., and Bader, V. (2012). *Indipendent Analysis of Solanezumab Provides Evidence that Compound may remove Amyloid from Brain in Alzheimer's Disease. Clinical Trials on Alzheimer's Disease* (Press Release). Available online at: http://www.ctad.fr/07-download/Congres2012/PressRelease/Sola-Release_29Oct2012.pdf. (Accessed November 5, 2012).

Mavoungou, C., and Schindowski, K. (2013). "Immunotherapy with anti-Amyloid-beta antibodies in Alzheimer's disease: a critical review on the molecules in the pipelines with regulatory considerations," in *Frontiers in Clinical Drug Research - Alzheimer Disorders*, Vol. 1, ed A. U. Rahman (Oak Park: Bentham Science Publishers), 3–85.

McDonald, J. M., Savva, G. M., Brayne, C., Welzel, A. T., Forster, G., Shankar, G. M., et al. (2010). The presence of sodium dodecyl sulphate-stable abeta dimers is strongly associated with alzheimer-type dementia. *Brain J. Neurol.* 133, 1328–1341.

Moreth, J., Kroker, K. S., Schwanzar, D., Schnack, C., Von Arnim, C. A. F., Hengerer, B., et al. (2013). Globular and protofibrillar Aβ aggregates impair neurotransmission by different mechanisms. *Biochemistry* 52, 1466–1476. doi: 10.1021/bi3016444

O'Nuallain, B., Freir, D. B., Nicoll, A. J., Risse, E., Ferguson, N., Herron, C. E., et al. (2010). Amyloid beta-protein dimers rapidly form stable synaptotoxic protofibrils. *J. Neurosci.* 30, 14411–14419. doi: 10.1523/JNEUROSCI.3537-10.2010

Park, J. E., Dorner-Ciossek, C., Hoerer, S., Kussmaul, L., Lenter, M., Zimmermann, K., et al. (2012). A-Beta binding polypeptides. *U.S. Patent 8337845 B2 filed*, 2012.

Pfizer. (2013). *Pfizer Pipeline our Medicines in Development*. Available online at: http://www.pfizer.com/research/product_pipeline/product_pipeline.jsp. (Accessed March 27, 2013).

Reed, M. N., Hofmeister, J. J., Jungbauer, L., Welzel, A. T., Yu, C., Sherman, M. A., et al. (2011). Cognitive effects of cell-derived and synthetically derived Abeta oligomers. *Neurobiol. Aging* 32, 1784–1794. doi: 10.1016/j.neurobiolaging.2009.11.007

Sagare, A., Deane, R., Bell, R. D., Johnson, B., Hamm, K., Pendu, R., et al. (2007). Clearance of amyloid-beta by circulating lipoprotein receptors. *Nat. Med.* 13, 1029–1031. doi: 10.1038/nm1635

Salloway, S., Sperling, R., Gilman, S., Fox, N. C., Blennow, K., Raskind, M., et al. (2009). A phase 2 multiple ascending dose trial of bapineuzumab in mild to moderate Alzheimer disease. *Neurology* 73, 2061–2070. doi: 10.1212/WNL.0b013e3181c67808

Salloway, S., Sperling, R., Honig, L., Porsteinsson, A., Sabbagh, M., Liu, E., et al. (2012). A randomized, double-blind, placebo-controlled clinical trial of intravenous bapineuzumab in patients with Alzheimer's disease who are apolipoprotein E ε4 non-carriers. *Eur. J. Neurol.* 19, SC312.

Selkoe, D. J. (2001). Alzheimer's disease: genes, proteins, and therapy. *Physiol. Rev.* 81, 741–766.

Shankar, G. M., Li, S., Mehta, T. H., Garcia-Munoz, A., Shepardson, N. E., Smith, I., et al. (2008). Amyloid-beta protein dimers isolated directly from Alzheimer's brains impair synaptic plasticity and memory. *Nat. Med.* 14, 837–842. doi: 10.1038/nm1782

Shibata, M., Yamada, S., Kumar, S. R., Calero, M., Bading, J., Frangione, B., et al. (2000). Clearance of Alzheimer's amyloid-ss(1-40) peptide from brain by LDL receptor-related protein-1 at the blood-brain barrier. *J. Clin. Invest.* 106, 1489–1499. doi: 10.1172/JCI10498

Sperling, R., Salloway, S., Raskind, M., Ferris, S., Liu, E., Yuen, E., et al. (2012). A randomized, double-blind, placebo-controlled clinical trial of intravenous bapineuzumab in patients with Alzheimer's disease who are apolipoprotein E ε4 carriers. *Eur. J. Neurol.* 19, SC3012.

Strobel, G., and Bowman Rogers, M. (2012). *CTAD (2012) in Monte Carlo: Getting Preclinical Trials Ship Shape. Alzheimer Research Forum.* Available online at: http://www.alzforum.org/new/pdf/CTAD2012.pdf. (Accessed January 14, 2013).

Terry, R. D. (2006). Alzheimer's disease and the aging brain. *J. Geriatric Psychiatry Neurol.* 19, 125–128. doi: 10.1177/0891988706291079

Walsh, D. M., Hartley, D. M., Kusumoto, Y., Fezoui, Y., Condron, M. M., Lomakin, A., et al. (1999). Amyloid beta-protein fibrillogenesis. Structure and biological activity of protofibrillar intermediates. *J. Biol. Chem.* 274, 25945–25952. doi: 10.1074/jbc.274.36.25945

Walsh, D. M., and Selkoe, D. J. (2007). A beta oligomers - a decade of discovery. *J. Neurochem.* 101, 1172–1184. doi: 10.1111/j.1471-4159.2006.04426.x

Walsh, D. M., Townsend, M., Podlisny, M. B., Shankar, G. M., Fadeeva, J. V., El Agnaf, O., et al. (2005). Certain inhibitors of synthetic amyloid beta-peptide (Abeta) fibrillogenesis block oligomerization of natural Abeta and thereby rescue long-term potentiation. *J. Neurosci.* 25, 2455–2462. doi: 10.1523/JNEUROSCI.4391-04.2005

Zetterberg, H. (2008). Is plasma amyloid-beta a reliable biomarker for Alzheimer's disease. *Recent Pat. CNS Drug Discov.* 3, 109–111. doi: 10.2174/157488908784534595

Zetterberg, H., Blennow, K., and Hanse, E. (2010). Amyloid beta and APP as biomarkers for Alzheimer's disease. *Exp. Gerontol.* 45, 23–29. doi: 10.1016/j.exger.2009.08.002

Zlokovic, B. V., Ghiso, J., Mackic, J. B., McComb, J. G., Weiss, M. H., and Frangione, B. (1993). Blood-brain barrier transport of circulating Alzheimer's amyloid beta. *Biochem. Biophys. Res. Commun.* 197, 1034–1040. doi: 10.1006/bbrc.1993.2582

28

PREDICT-HD study

Kevin M. Biglan[1], Ying Zhang[2], Jeffrey D. Long[3], Michael Geschwind[4], Gail A. Kang[4], Annie Killoran[1], Wenjing Lu[2], Elizabeth McCusker[5], James A. Mills[3], Lynn A. Raymond[6], Claudia Testa[7], Joanne Wojcieszek[8], Jane S. Paulsen[3]*, and the PREDICT-HD Investigators of the Huntington Study Group

[1] *Department of Neurology, University of Rochester, Rochester, NY, USA*
[2] *Department Biostatistics, University of Iowa, Iowa City, IA, USA*
[3] *Department of Psychiatry, University of Iowa, Iowa City, IA, USA*
[4] *Department of Neurology, University of California San Francisco, San Francisco, CA, USA*
[5] *Department of Neurology, Westmead Hospital, Sydney, NSW, Australia*
[6] *Division of Psychiatry, University of British Columbia, Vancouver, BC, Canada*
[7] *VCU Parkinson's and Movement Disorders Center Virginia Commonwealth University, Richmond, VA, USA*
[8] *Department of Neurology, Indiana University, Indianapolis, IN, USA*

Edited by:
Manuel Menéndez-González, Hospital Álvarez-Buylla, Spain

Reviewed by:
Hiroshi Morita, Sinshu University, Japan
Katsutoshi Furukawa, Tohoku University, Japan
Diego Ruano, University of Sevilla, Spain
Andrea Ciarmiello, S. Andrea Hospital ASL5 Spezzino, Italy

*Correspondence:
Jane S. Paulsen, Department of Psychiatry, Roy J. and Lucille A. Carver College of Medicine Research, The University of Iowa, 1-305 Medical Education Building, Iowa City, IA 52242-1000, USA.
e-mail: jane-paulsen@uiowa.edu

Participants with the gene expansion for Huntington disease (HD) but not yet diagnosed were evaluated annually. Unidimensional diagnosis (UD) was a motor diagnosis defined as a diagnostic confidence level (DCL) of 4 (unequivocal motor signs, $\geq$99% confidence) on the standardized motor exam of the Unified Huntington Disease Rating Scale (UHDRS). Multidimensional diagnosis (MD) was defined as answering yes on Question 80 (Q80) of the UHDRS, $\geq$99% confidence of manifest HD based on the *entire* UHDRS. Motor, cognitive, and behavioral measures of phenotype at first diagnosis were compared by t-tests between participants diagnosed via motor exam (UD) and those diagnosed via multidimensional input (MD). Cluster analysis identified clusters based on UHDRS domains.186 participants received a diagnosis of HD during a maximum of 6.4 years of follow-up. In 108 (58.1%) the diagnosis by MD and UD occurred simultaneously, while in 69 (37.1%) the diagnosis by MD occurred prior to UD. Participants who were diagnosed by MD prior to UD were less impaired on motor (12.2 ± 6.7 vs. 22.4 ± 9.3, $p < 0.0001$), and cognitive (290.7 ± 56.2 vs. 258.0 ± 53.7, $p = 0.0002$), but not behavioral measures (16.3 ± 21.2 vs. 18.6 ± 22.1, $p = 0.49$) when compared with those diagnosed simultaneously. Cluster analysis identified three clusters that represented primarily cognitively impaired, behaviorally impaired, and cognitively preserved phenotypes. A multidimensional method results in an earlier diagnosis with less motor and cognitive impairment than a motor diagnosis. Findings have implications for designing preventive trials and providing clinical care in prodromal HD.

Keywords: Huntington's disease, trinucleotide repeat diseases, cohort studies, natural history studies, outcome research

INTRODUCTION

Huntington disease (HD) is an adult-onset, autosomal dominant, progressive, and fatal neurodegenerative disease characterized by the clinical triad of a movement disorder, cognitive decline, and behavioral disturbances caused by a cytosine-adenine-guanine (CAG) repeat in the 5′-translated region of the gene on the short arm of chromosome 4 (Duyao et al., 1993). The precise point of disease diagnosis is poorly characterized, with clinical abnormalities emerging gradually over many years during a "pre-manifest" or prodromal phase (Huntington Study Group, 2006; Paulsen et al., 2006).

A challenge of therapeutic research is in the identification of treatments that impact the manifestation of disease in individuals at varying stages of disease progression. For the neurodegenerative diseases, much effort has been devoted to early identification and staging using clinical outcome measures or biomarkers. For instance, there are widespread efforts to detect "mild cognitive impairment" prior to dementia so that therapeutics might be considered before extensive cell death has occurred. Even in HD, in which a cohort can be identified years prior to diagnosis, challenges remain in designing trials aimed at delaying illness progression. The Neurobiological Predictors of Huntington's Disease (PREDICT-HD) study is a longitudinal prospective evaluation in individuals at risk for HD with known gene status.

Abbreviations: AD, Alzheimer disease; CAG, cytosine-adenine-guanine; DCL, diagnostic confidence level; HD, Huntington disease; PREDICT-HD, Neurobiological Predictors of Huntington's Disease; Q80, Question 80; SDM, symbol digit modalities; TFC, Total Functional Capacity; UHDRS, Unified Huntington Disease Rating Scale.

The PREDICT-HD study should help identify outcomes for use in trials aimed at delaying the manifestation of illness in prodromal HD. However, in order to show that an intervention can delay disease, there needs to be consensus on how to best define the clinical diagnosis of HD. The traditional method of HD diagnosis rests on the motor manifestation of disease though the cognitive and psychiatric aspects of HD have been recognized for decades. Efforts toward more refined disease staging may be improved with a more comprehensive consideration of HD. Therefore, we compared two methods of diagnosis in the PREDICT-HD cohort: a multidimensional diagnosis (MD) and a unidimensional diagnosis (UD) or motor diagnosis.

MATERIALS AND METHODS

All aspects of the study were approved by the Institutional Review Board at each participating institution. Participants signed consents for participation and to release their de-identified data for analyses.

OVERVIEW OF PREDICT-HD

The PREDICT-HD study is designed to prospectively characterize refined clinical, neurobiological, and neurobehavioral markers of HD prior to the point of traditional motor diagnosis in a population known to carry the HD CAG expansion (Paulsen et al., 2006). Participants at risk for HD were recruited from 32 sites in the United States, Canada, Australia, and Europe beginning in 2001. All participants were required to have voluntarily undergone genetic testing for the HD CAG expansion independent from the study. Participants were evaluated annually with standardized assessments of motor, cognition, behavior, function, and clinical diagnosis.

Only individuals with the HD CAG expansion and without manifest disease (prodromal HD) as defined by the absence of unequivocal motor signs (diagnostic confidence level of less than 4 on question 17 of the UHDRS, **Table 1A**) on their initial examination were included in the current analysis. Control subjects were those participants who had tested negative for the HD CAG expansion and had participated in at least two visits. For purposes of this analysis, the last visit in controls was used for comparison with cases.

Table 1 | The Unified Huntington Disease Rating Scale diagnostic confidence level and Q80 diagnostic criteria.

A. Diagnostic confidence level
To what degree are you confident that this person meets the operational definition of the unequivocal presence of an otherwise unexplained extrapyramidal movement disorder (e.g., chorea, dystonia, bradykinesia, rigidity) in a subject at risk for HD?
0 = normal (no abnormalities) 1 = non-specific motor abnormalities (less than 50% confidence) 2 = motor abnormalities that may be signs of HD (50–89% confidence) 3 = motor abnormalities that are likely signs of HD (90–98% confidence) **4 = motor abnormalities that are unequivocal signs of HD (≥99% confidence)**
B. Q80 diagnostic criteria
Based on the entire UHDRS (Motor, Cognitive, Behavioral, and Functional components) do you believe with a confidence level ≥99% that this participant has manifest HD? (0 = No, 1 = Yes)

CLINICAL ASSESSMENTS

Huntington disease clinical diagnosis

Motor Diagnosis: The Huntington Disease Rating Scale (UHDRS) diagnostic confidence level (DCL) is the standard measure used for clinical diagnosis in at-risk individuals and is based solely on the motor evaluation. It is a categorical scale (**Table 1A**) with a range from 0 (normal) to 4 (unequivocal signs of HD, ≥99% confidence ≥ on the part of the examiner). The DCL has previously shown fair inter-rater reliability (weighted kappa = 0.67, SE = 0.09) (Hogarth et al., 2005). Participants had a clinical diagnosis of HD at the time of the first rating of a DCL = 4.

Multidimensional Diagnosis: Question 80 (Q80) of the UHDRS asks raters to take into account all aspects of the UHDRS (motor, cognitive, behavioral, and functional) and to make a decision (yes or no) whether a subject has a diagnosis of HD with a confidence level 99% (**Table 1B**). The first occurrence of Q80 = yes was the multidimensional diagnostic criteria used for the current analyses.

The primary analysis compared participants who were diagnosed by MD prior to receiving a diagnosis by UD with participants who received a diagnosis of MD and UD simultaneously. A small proportion of individuals received a diagnosis by UD prior to MD and these participants were not included in the analysis.

UNIFIED HUNTINGTON DISEASE RATING SCALE OUTCOMES

The current analyses focused solely on the UHDRS assessments, since UD is rated on the motor UHDRS only and MD specifically asks raters to make a determination based on the entirety of the Hungtington Study Group (1996). The motor UHDRS assessed for the presence and severity of motor features (Hungtington Study Group, 1996). The motor UHDRS is a standardized assessment consisting of 31 items rated on a scale from 0 to 4 with a score of 0 indicating no abnormalities and 4 indicating the most severe impairment. The maximum possible total score is 124. Previously motor scores have been shown to distinguish controls from prodromal HD cases and subtle motor abnormalities were associated with closer estimated diagnosis of disease (Biglan et al., 2009). In manifest HD, oculomotor, rigidity, chorea, dystonia, and bradykinesia domains have been identified and were used to clarify if specific motor features were associated with specific clusters at time of clinical diagnosis (Marder et al., 2000).

The cognitive section of the UHDRS includes verbal fluency, symbol digit modalities test, and Stroop word, color, and interference tests (Hungtington Study Group, 1996; Biglan et al., 2009). Each of these cognitive tests has been shown to distinguish gene mutation carriers from controls in prodromal HD (Paulsen et al., 2008; Stout et al., 2011). Total cognitive scores are calculated by summing the five individual scores in the UHDRS cognitive domain.

The behavioral section of the UHDRS consists of 11 items evaluating various behavioral signs and symptoms. Individuals are ranked on both severity and frequency on a 0 to 4 scale with 0 being not present and 4 being severe and frequent (Hungtington Study Group, 1996). Total behavioral scores are calculated by summing the severity and frequency items and ranges from 0 (no behavioral symptoms) to 88 (most severe behavioral symptoms).

The functional section of the UHDRS includes the Functional Assessment Scale, Independence Scale, and the Total Functional Capacity (TFC) (Hungtington Study Group, 1996). The TFC is a standard assessment of overall function in HD and has a demonstrated reliability for indexing progression in various diagnosed HD populations (Marder et al., 2000; Huntington Study Group, 2001). The TFC rates individuals' function on the following domains: occupation, handling finances, domestic chores, and activities of daily living. The TFC ranges from 13 (normal function) to 0 (complete loss of function). In prodromal HD, there is a strong tendency for participants to have the maximum score, as most have normal function; thus the TFC was treated as a dichotomous variable (TFC < 13) to indicate whether an individual has some kind of impairment in functionality for daily living (Paulsen et al., 2010). For assessment of employment status UHDRS item #43 (ability to work at accustomed employment) and item #44 (ability to work at any employment) were used.

STATISTICAL ANALYSIS

Kaplan-Meier curves were generated to describe the probability of being diagnosis-free over time and to evaluate the temporal relationship between incident diagnoses using the different diagnostic criteria.

UHDRS total motor, total cognitive, and total behavioral scores at the time of incident diagnosis were compared between the different diagnostic groups using *t*-tests.

Chi-square tests were used to compare differences in the frequency of diagnosis by the same vs. different raters between the different diagnostic groups.

To evaluate the factors associated with diagnosis in those participants who received a diagnosis of MD prior to UD, K-mean clustering with the pseudo-F statistic criterion was performed to identify categories of participants (clusters) at the time of diagnosis. The UHDRS total motor score, total cognitive score, and total behavior score at diagnosis were used in the cluster analysis. In order to ascertain if raters utilized participants' functional status in the diagnostic decision, TFC, and employment status were compared across the clusters. To determine if specific motor features were associated with different clusters, the sum of each motor domain was compared across clusters. The ANOVA, Fisher Exact Tests, or Kruskall-Wallis Test were performed as appropriate to determine the difference between the clusters and the control group and *post-hoc* pairwise comparisons using *t*-tests or chi-square tests, corrected for multiple comparisons (alpha < 0.01) to determine the statistical ordering among the groups.

RESULTS

Since 2001, a total of 1054 individuals have been enrolled in the PREDICT-HD study. Of these participants, 821 (78%) carried the CAG expansion and were considered prodromal (DCL < 4) at baseline. A total of 233 (22%) of the participants enrolled did not carry the CAG expansion (controls); of these, 194 had at least two follow-up visits.

Over a mean follow-up of 3.1 years (SD $= 1.4$ years and range $= 6.4$ years) a total of 186 CAG expanded participants (23% of total CAG expanded) received a first diagnosis of manifest HD by either diagnostic criteria (MD or UD). Of these diagnosed individuals, 108 (58.1%) received a diagnosis by UD and MD simultaneously, 69 (37.1%) by MD prior to UD, and 9 (4.8%) by UD prior to MD. **Figure 1** shows the Kaplan-Meier estimates of the diagnosis-free probability curves over 6 years of follow-up for diagnosis based on the UD and MD criteria.

Of those diagnosed, 148 (79.6%) had the same rater, whereas 38 (20.4%) had different raters for UD and MD. DCL $= 4$ and Q80 diagnoses were more likely to occur simultaneously when the rater was the same (89.8%). Q80 diagnosis also preceded DCL $=$ 4 diagnosis more often when the rater was the same (73.9%) (**Table 2**).

Table 3 demonstrates the clinical features at the time of diagnosis by the different criteria. Participants who were diagnosed by MD prior to UD were less impaired on UHDRS total motor scores (12.2 ± 6.7 vs. 22.4 ± 9.3, $p < 0.0001$) and on total cognitive scores (290.7 ± 56.2 vs. 258.0 ± 53.7, $p = 0.0002$) compared with individuals who received the diagnoses simultaneously.

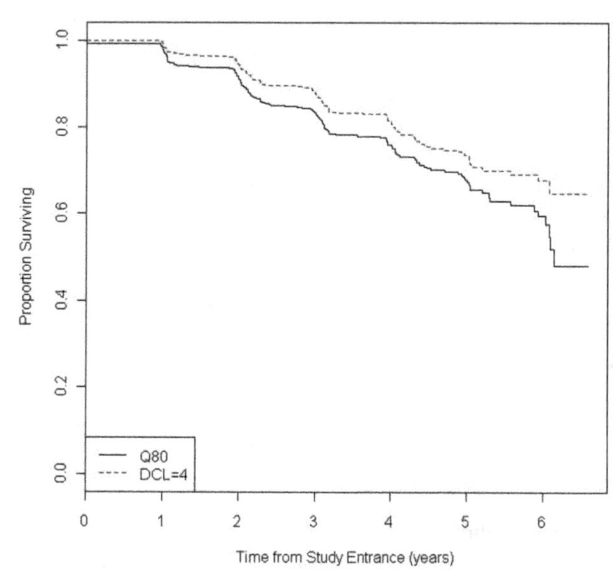

FIGURE 1 | Kaplan-Meier estimate of the probability of being diagnosis-free during follow-up by type of diagnosis (UHDRS Q80 = yes and UHDRS DCL = 4).

Table 2 | Diagnostic agreement between by same vs. different raters*,†.

Diagnosis	Same rater	Different rater	Total
Simultaneous Q80/DCL = 4	97 (89.8%)	11 (10.2%)	108
Q80 before DCL = 4	51 (73.9%)	18 (26.1%)	69
Total	148 (83.6%)	29 (16.4%)	177

**p = 0.005 for the comparison of clinical diagnosis by rater category.*

†Does not include the 9 participants where DCL = 4 occurred before Q80.

There was no statistical difference on UHDRS behavioral scores (16.3 ± 21.2 vs. 18.6 ± 22.1, $p = 0.49$) between the two groups.

A cluster analysis using K-mean clustering in the participants that received MD prior to UD was performed and a three cluster solution was identified based on the pseudo-F statistic criterion. **Table 4** shows the mean total motor, cognitive, and behavioral scores by clusters and controls. Cluster 1 identifies a predominantly cognitively impaired phenotype because it had the lowest UHDRS cognitive mean, but the second highest behavior mean and the highest total motor mean (Cluster 1 might also be labeled as predominantly cognitive/motor). Cluster 2 identifies a predominantly behaviorally impaired phenotype as it had the highest behavior mean, but had the second highest cognitive mean and the lowest total motor mean among the gene-expanded participants. Cluster 3 represents a cognitively preserved group because the cluster had the highest cognitive mean (even higher than controls), the lowest behavior mean, and the second highest total motor mean among gene-expanded participants. All clusters had significantly worse motor scores compared with controls. A more detailed assessment of motor features using the motor sub-domains (**Table 4**) suggests that cluster 3 (cognitively preserved) had the most chorea while cluster 1 (cognitively impaired) performed the worst on the bradykinesia domain. A cluster analysis of the participants that received simultaneous diagnoses identified a three-cluster solution that was qualitatively similar (i.e., cognitive, behavioral, and preserved phenotypes), except that participants performed worse on motor and cognitive measures than the same clusters in participants with MD prior to UD (results not shown). All three clusters were more likely than controls to have greater functional impairment as measured

Table 3 | Clinical features at time of diagnosis.

Variables	Q80 before DCL = 4 ($n = 69$)	Simultaneous Q80/DCL = 4 ($n = 108$)	Controls† ($n = 194$)	p-value*
Gender (%F)	65.7	66.7	66.0	0.89
Age (mean ± SD)	46.3 ± 9.2	46.7 ± 10.3	46.7 ± 11.1	0.81
CAG (mean ± SD)	43.1 ± 3.1	43.5 ± 3.1	20.1 ± 3.5	0.43
UHDRS motor (mean ± SD)	12.2 ± 6.7	22.4 ± 9.3	2.8 ± 3.1	<0.001
UHDRS cognition (mean ± SD)	290.5 ± 56.5	258.0 ± 53.7	341.4 ± 47.4	<0.001
UHDRS behavior (mean ± SD)	16.3 ± 21.2	18.6 ± 22.1	5.7 ± 9.3	0.49
UHDRS TFC (%<13)	31.9	48.1	7.0	0.03

**p-values are for the comparison between Q80 diagnosis before DCL = 4 and simultaneous diagnosis.*
†The values of controls were taken at the last visit.

Table 4 | Group comparisons between clusters.

Variables	Control ($n = 194$)	Cluster 1 ($n = 21$)	Cluster 2 ($n = 32$)	Cluster 3 ($n = 15$)	ANOVA p-value	Pair-wise comparisons (alpha 0.01)
Age (mean ± SD)	46.75 ± 11.13	45.70 ± 9.32	47.26 ± 9.97	44.70 ± 7.70	0.85	–
CAG (mean ± SD)	20.12 ± 3.45	43.58 ± 2.59	43.22 ± 3.66	42.73 ± 2.09	<0.001	Control < C1, C2, C3
UHDRS						
Total motor (mean ± SD)	2.75 ± 3.08	16.52 ± 5.60	9.56 ± 6.03	11.86 ± 6.78	<0.001	Control < C2, C3 < C1
Motor domains						
Oculo (mean ± SD)	0.65 ± 1.23	4.52 ± 2.36	2.34 ± 2.89	3.57 ± 3.06	<0.001	Control < C2 < C1; Control < C3
Brady (mean ± SD)	1.44 ± 1.91	6.67 ± 3.12	4.03 ± 3.10	3.79 ± 2.81	<0.001	Control < C2, C3 < C1
Rigidity (mean ± SD)	0.31 ± 0.68	0.67 ± 1.15	0.53 ± 0.72	0.92 ± 1.07	0.004	Control < C3
Dystonia (mean ± SD)	0.06 ± 0.34	1.05 ± 1.56	0.38 ± 0.87	0.43 ± 0.76	<0.001	Control < C2 < C1; C3 < C1
Chorea (mean ± SD)	0.29 ± 0.69	3.62 ± 2.52	2.28 ± 2.05	3.14 ± 2.28	<0.001	Control < C1, C3; C2 < C1
Cognition (mean ± SD)	341.4 ± 47.4	224.0 ± 25.7	303.8 ± 19.4	361.8 ± 22.6	<0.001	C1 < C2 < Control, C3
Behavior (mean ± SD)	5.69 ± 9.29	12.65 ± 18.63	20.25 ± 21.28	7.47 ± 10.05	<0.001	Control, C3 < C2

Cluster 1, predominantly cognitive; Cluster 2, predominantly behavioral; Cluster 3, cognitively preserved.

by TFC. Whereas participants in cluster 3 were more likely to be employable compared to the other clusters, this did not meet the threshold for significance and all clusters were less likely to be employable compared with controls (see Supplementary **Table e-1**).

There was no statistical difference between the clusters in the proportion of raters that were the same vs. raters who were different (see Supplementary **Table e-2**).

DISCUSSION

In participants with prodromal HD enrolled in the PREDICT-HD study, a multidimensional diagnosis occurs earlier and with less motor and cognitive impairment than a diagnosis based on the motor examination. Given the results of our analysis, a diagnosis that considers cognitive and behavioral features in addition to motor features has face validity. Therefore, compared to the traditional motor diagnosis, a multidimensional diagnosis may be a preferable outcome for use in future trials aimed at delaying the manifestation of HD.

The current analysis also identified different phenotypes in HD at the time of diagnosis: predominantly cognitively impaired (with motor impairments), predominantly behaviorally impaired, and cognitively preserved. These phenotypic clusters had motor impairments greater than controls at diagnosis despite marked differences among the clusters in cognitive and behavioral performance. Thus, while the traditional motor diagnosis selects for the identification of a predominantly motor phenotype, a multidimensional diagnosis may identify predominantly non-motor presentations.

It is unclear why certain participants were given a multidimensional diagnosis in the absence of significant impairment in cognition or behavior in cluster 3 (cognitively preserved). This was not related to worse functional performance in this group. It may be that worse chorea in this group influenced raters to make a diagnosis even when the overall motor impairment was not deemed sufficient to make a motor diagnosis; or this could reflect differences in how raters diagnose HD. In the future it may be useful to ask raters what factors influenced their diagnostic decision. It may also be beneficial to establish objective methods for diagnosis, such as the establishment of certain cut-off scores on the UHDRS.

Despite these findings, even individuals receiving a multidimensional diagnosis are being identified relatively late after the accumulation of significant clinical signs. PREDICT-HD and other studies suggest that striatal atrophy and clinical features may develop decades prior to diagnosis (Aylward et al., 2000; Thieben et al., 2002; Paulsen et al., 2008). Recently, Sperling et al. published recommendations from the National Institute for Aging and the Alzheimer's Association Working Group for the research diagnosis of preclinical Alzheimer disease (AD) (Sperling et al., 2011). They proposed a staged diagnosis for preclinical AD with the earliest stage being associated with biomarkers of AD pathophysiology (A-beta on PET or in CSF), followed by biomarker evidence of neuronal injury (atrophy on MRI) and finally the presence of subtle clinical signs that did not meet criteria for mild cognitive impairment (Albert et al., 2011). Using a similar strategy in prodromal HD, many CAG expanded individuals at the time of enrollment in PREDICT-HD already had evidence of subtle motor, cognitive, and behavioral features and would have fallen into the last preclinical stage using the AD model (Solomon et al., 2007; Beglinger et al., 2008; Biglan et al., 2009; Duff et al., 2010; Stout et al., 2011).

While HD does not yet have the same breadth of valid and specific biomarkers as the AD research community, the identification of a similar staged categorization of prodromal HD could be considered using neuroimaging biomarkers. Thus in stage 1, CAG expanded individuals would have no evidence of neuronal injury using volumetric MRI imaging or clinical signs of HD on examination; in stage 2, there would be evidence of neuronal injury as suggested by striatal atrophy on volumetric MRI but no clinical signs of HD; finally in stage 3, individuals would have subtle clinical signs but would not yet meet criteria for diagnosis. Ultimately, clinical trials aimed at delaying manifestation in prodromal HD could evaluate the impact of interventions on the progression through the proposed stages, changes in volumetric imaging variables, changes in clinical measures and finally the impact on a multidimensional diagnosis of HD.

The current analysis has many limitations and caveats. Foremost is the use of different raters for the motor and multidimensional diagnoses. This introduced bias with a higher likelihood of discrepant diagnoses when the raters were different. However, different raters were relatively Uncommon (see **Table 2**), and there was no difference in rater type amongst the three phenotypic clusters identified. Future studies using multidimensional diagnosis should either have the rater making the diagnostic rating complete all the appropriate assessments or, if multiple individuals are doing the assessments, the multidimensional diagnosis should be based on consensus after reviewing all the data.

Another limitation was that raters were not specifically trained on how to answer Q80. Differences in the timing of diagnosis and the observed clinical phenotypes may relate to differences in how raters make the assessment of a multidimensional diagnosis. Some raters may be comfortable with diagnosing HD based on the combination of subtle motor, cognitive, and behavioral signs, whereas others may put more weight solely on the motor exam. Future studies utilizing a multidimensional diagnosis will have to standardize this decision process.

The significance of a clinical diagnosis is unclear. Striatal atrophy and subtle clinical features develop decades before traditional diagnosis. In addition, while subjects at diagnosis were more functionally impaired compared with controls, most individuals continued to work full-time and have minimal functional impairment by the measures used in this study even at the time of diagnosis. It remains to be seen whether regulatory bodies will consider a delay in diagnosis as sufficient to show that an intervention is effective or whether it will be necessary to show a slowing in functional decline. If the latter proves to be true, more refined measures of function in prodromal HD will be necessary.

Finally, it is important to emphasize that the proposed diagnostic criteria is for research purposes only and not necessarily for the clinical diagnosis of patients. The decision to render a clinical diagnosis in individuals at risk for HD is a complicated one based on clinical features of disease, patient preferences, and a detailed understanding of relevant psychosocial factors. The potential clinical and emotional impact on patients and their families of diagnosing individuals earlier and with less motor impairment remains unknown.

A multidimensional diagnosis occurs earlier and with less motor and cognitive impairment than the traditional motor diagnosis and identifies clinical phenotypes that may have predominant non-motor features. A staging system in prodromal HD, similar to that proposed in AD, may be of value. A better understanding of diagnostic decision making may allow for better standardization of diagnosis, and the development of clear criteria for research and clinical diagnoses that may be utilized as an outcome measure in future trials aimed at delaying diagnosis in prodromal HD.

ACKNOWLEDGMENTS

We thank the PREDICT-HD sites, the study participants, and the National Research Roster for Huntington Disease Patients and Families. We would also like to thank the following PREDICT-HD Contributors for their support with this research study.

Steering Committee: Jane Paulsen, Ph.D., Principal Investigator, Eric A. Epping, MD, Ph.D., Hans Johnson, Ph.D., Megan Smith, Ph.D., Janet Williams, Ph.D., RN, FAAN, Leigh Beglinger, Ph.D., Jeffrey D. Long, Ph.D., James A. Mills, MS (University of Iowa, Iowa City, IA); Elizabeth Aylward, Ph.D. (Seattle Children's Research Institute, WA); Kevin Biglan, MD (University of Rochester, Rochester, NY); Blair Leavitt, MD (University of British Columbia, Vancouver, BC, Canada); Marcy MacDonald, Ph.D. (Massachusetts General Hospital); Martha Nance, MD (Hennepin County Medical Center, Minneapolis, MN); and Cheryl Erwin, JD, Ph.D. (University of Texas Medical School at Houston).

Scientific Sections

Bio Markers: Blair Leavitt, MDCM, FRCPC (Chair) and Michael Hayden, Ph.D. (University of British Columbia); Stefano DiDonato, MD (Neurological Institute "C. Besta," Italy); Ken Evans, Ph.D. (Ontario Cancer Biomarker Network); Wayne Matson, Ph.D. (VA Medical Center, Bedford, MA); Asa Peterson, MD, Ph.D. (Lund University, Sweden), Sarah Tabrizi, MD, Ph.D. (National Hospital for Neurology and Neurology and Neurosurgery, London); Beth Borowsky, Ph.D. (CHDI); Andrew Juhl, BS, James A. Mills, MS, Kai Wang, Ph.D. (University of Iowa); and David Weir, BSc (University of British Columbia). **Brain:** Jean Paul Vonsattell, Ph.D. (Chair), and Carol Moskowitz, ANP, MS (Columbia University Medical Center); Anne Leserman, MSW, LISW, Lynn Schaul, BA, and Stacie Vik, BA (University of Iowa). **Cognitive:** Deborah Harrington, Ph.D. (Chair), Gabriel Castillo, BS, Jessica Morison, BS, and Jason Reed, BS (University of California, San Diego), Michael Diaz, Ph.D., Ian Dobbins, Ph.D., Tamara Hershey, Ph.D., Erin Foster, OTD, and Deborah Moore, BA (Washington University Cognitive Science Battery Development); Holly Westervelt, Ph.D. (Chair, Quality Control and Training, Alpert Medical School of Brown University), Jennifer Davis, Ph.D., and Geoff Tremont, Ph.D., MS (Scientific Consultants, Alpert Medical School of Brown University); Megan Smith, Ph.D. (Chair, Administration), David J. Moser, Ph.D., Leigh J. Beglinger, Ph.D., Kelly Rowe, Gloria Wenman, and Danielle Theriault, BS (University of Iowa); Carissa Gehl, Ph.D. (VA Medical Center, Iowa City, IA); Kirsty Matheson (University of Aberdeen); Karen Siedlecki, Ph.D. (Fordham University); Marleen Van Walsem (EHDN); Susan Bonner, BA, Greg Elias, BA, Mary Gover, Rachel Bernier, and Melanie Faust, BS (Rhode Island Hospital); Beth Borowski, Ph.D. (CHDI); Noelle Carlozzi (University of Michigan); Kevin Duff, Ph.D. (University of Utah); Nellie Georgiou-Karistianis (St. Vincent's Hospital, The University of Melbourne, Australia); Julie Stout, Ph.D. (Monash University, Melbourne, Australia); Herwig Lange (Air-Rahazentrum); and Kate Papp (University of Connecticut). **Functional**: Janet Williams, Ph.D. (Chair), Leigh J. Beglinger, Ph.D., Anne Leserman, MSW, LISW, Eunyoe Ro, MA, Lee Anna Clark, Nancy Downing, RN, Ph.D., Joan Laing, Ph.D., Kristine Rees, BA, Michelle Harreld, BS, and Stacie Vik, BA (University of Iowa); Rebecca Ready, Ph.D. (University of Massachusetts); Anthony Vaccarino, Ph.D. (Ontario Cancer Biomarker Network); Sarah Farias, Ph.D. (University of California, Davis); Noelle Carlozzi, Ph.D. (University of Michigan); and Carissa Gehl, Ph.D. (VA Medical Center, Iowa City, IA). **Genetics:** Marcy MacDonald, Ph.D. (Co-Chair), Jim Gusella, Ph.D., and Rick Myers, Ph.D. (Massachusetts General Hospital); Michael Hayden, Ph.D. (University of British Columbia); Tom Wassink, MD (Co-Chair) Eric A. Epping, MD, Ph.D., Andrew Juhl, BA, James Mills, MS, and Kai Wang, Ph.D. (University of Iowa); Zosia Miedzybrodzka, MD, Ph.D. (University of Aberdeen); and Christopher Ross, MD, Ph.D. (Johns Hopkins University). **Imaging:** *Administrative:* Ron Pierson, Ph.D. (Chair), Kathy Jones, BS, Jacquie Marietta, BS, William McDowell, AA, Greg Harris, BS, Eun Young Kim, MS, Hans Johnson, Ph.D., and Thomas Wassink, MD (University of Iowa); John Ashburner, Ph.D. (Functional Imaging Lab, London); Steve Potkin, MD (University of California, Irvine); and Arthur Toga, Ph.D. (University of California, Los Angeles). *Striatal:* Elizabeth Aylward, Ph.D. (Chair, Seattle Children's Research Institute). *Surface Analysis:* Peg Nopoulos, MD (Chair), and Eric Axelson, BSE (University of Iowa). *Shape Analysis:* Christopher A. Ross (Chair), MD, Ph.D., Michael Miller, Ph.D., and Sarah Reading, MD (Johns Hopkins University); Mirza Faisal Beg, Ph.D. (Simon Fraser University). *DTI:* Vincent A. Magnotta, Ph.D. (Chair, University of Iowa); Karl Helmer, Ph.D. (Massachusetts General Hospital); Kelvin Lim, MD (University of Ulm, Germany); Mark Lowe, Ph.D. (Cleveland Clinic); Sasumu Mori, Ph.D. (Johns Hopkins University); Allen Song, Ph.D. (Duke University); and Jessica Turner, Ph.D. (University of California, Irvine). *fMRI:* Steve Rao, Ph.D. (Chair), Erik Beall, Ph.D., Katherine Koenig, Ph.D., Michael Phillips, MD, Christine Reece, BS, and Jan Zimbelman, Ph.D., PT (Cleveland Clinic); April Bryant, Andrew Juhl, BS, Kathy Jones, and Gloria Wenman (University of Iowa). **Motor:** Kevin Biglan, MD (Chair) (University of Rochester); Karen Marder, MD (Columbia University); Jody Corey-Bloom, MD, Ph.D. (University of California, San Diego); Michael Geschwind,

MD, Ph.D. (University of California, San Francisco); Ralf Reilmann, MD and Zerka Unds (Muenster, Germany); and Andrew Juhl, BS (University of Iowa). **Psychiatric:** Eric A. Epping, MD, Ph.D. (Chair), Nancy Downing, RN, Ph.D., Jess Fiedorowicz, MD, Robert Robinson, MD, Megan Smith, Ph.D., Leigh Beglinger, Ph.D., James Mills, MS, Kristine Rees, BA, Michelle Harreld, BS, Adam Ruggle, Stacie Vik, BA, Janet Williams, Ph.D., Dawei Liu, Ph.D., David Moser, Ph.D., and Kelly Rowe (University of Iowa); Karen Anderson, MD (University of Maryland); David Craufurd, MD (University of Manchester); Mark Groves, MD (Columbia University); Anthony Vaccarino, Ph.D. and Ken Evans, Ph.D. (Ontario Cancer Biomarker Network); Hugh Rickards, MD (Queen Elizabeth Psychiatric Hospital); Eric van Duijn, MD (Leiden University Medical Center, Netherlands); Phyllis Chua (The University of Melbourne, Royal Melbourne Hospital); and Kimberly Quaid, Ph.D. (Indiana University).

Core Sections
Statistics: Jeffrey D. Long, Ph.D., Ji-In Kim, Ph.D., James A. Mills, MS, Ying Zhang, Ph.D., Dawei Liu, Ph.D., Wenjing Lu, and Spencer Lourens (University of Iowa).

Recruitment/Retention: Martha Nance, MD (Chair, University of Minnesota); Anne Leserman, MSW, LISW, Nicholas Doucette, BA, Mycah Kimble, BA, Patricia Ryan, MSW, LISW, MA, Kelli Thumma, BA, Elijah Waterman, BA, and Jeremy Hinkel, BA (University of Iowa). **Ethics:** Cheryl Erwin, JD, Ph.D., (Chair, McGovern Center for Health, Humanities and the Human Spirit); Eric A. Epping, MD, Ph.D. Janet Williams, Ph.D., Nicholas Doucette, BA, Anne Leserman, MSW, LISW, James Mills, MS, Lynn Schaul, BA, and Stacie Vik, BA (University of Iowa); Martha Nance, MD (University of Minnesota); and Lisa Hughes, MEd (University of Texas Medical School at Houston). **IT/Management:** Hans Johnson, Ph.D. (Chair), R.J. Connell, BS, Karen Pease, BS, Ben Rogers, BA, BSCS, Jim Smith, AS, Shuhua Wu, MCS, Roland Zschiegner, Erin Carney, Bill McKirgan, Mark Scully, and Ryan Wyse (University of Iowa); Jeremy Bockholt (AMBIGroup).

Program Management
Administrative: Chris Werling-Witkoske (Chair), Greg Ennis, MA, Stacie Vik, BA, Karla Anderson, BS, Kristine Bjork, BA, Sean Thompson, BA, Leann Davis, Machelle Henneberry, Ann Dudler, Jamy Schumacher, and Craig Stout (University of Iowa). **Financial:** Steve Blanchard, MSHA, Kelsey Montross, BA, and Phil Danzer (University of Iowa).

STUDY FUNDING

This research is supported by the National Institutes for Health, National Institute of Neurological Disorders and Stroke (NS40068) and CHDI Foundation, Inc.

REFERENCES

Albert, M. S., Dekosky, S. T., Dickson, D., Dubois, B., Feldman, H. H., Fox, N. C., et al. (2011). The diagnosis of mild cognitive impairment due to Alzheimer's disease: recommendations from the National Institute on Aging-Alzheimer's Association workgroups on diagnostic guidelines for Alzheimer's disease. *Alzheimers Dement.* 7, 270–279.

Aylward, E. H., Codori, A. M., Rosenblatt, A., Sherr, M., Brandt, J., Stine, O. C., et al. (2000). Rate of caudate atrophy in presymptomatic and symptomatic stages of Huntington's disease. *Mov. Disord.* 15, 552–560.

Beglinger, L. J., Paulsen, J. S., Watson, D. B., Wang, C., Duff, K., Langbehn, D. R., et al. (2008). Obsessive and compulsive symptoms in prediagnosed Huntington's disease. *J. Clin. Psychiatry* 69, 1758–1765.

Biglan, K. M., Ross, C. A., Langbehn, D. R., Aylward, E. H., Stout, J. C., Queller, S., et al. (2009). Motor abnormalities in premanifest persons with Huntington's disease: the PREDICT-HD study. *Mov. Disord.* 24, 1763–1772.

Duff, K., Paulsen, J. S., Beglinger, L. J., Langbehn, D. R., Wang, C., Stout, J. C., et al. (2010). "Frontal" behaviors before the diagnosis of Huntington's disease and their relationship to markers of disease progression: evidence of early lack of awareness. *J. Neuropsychiatry Clin. Neurosci.* 22, 196–207.

Duyao, M., Ambrose, C., Myers, R., Novelletto, A., Persichetti, F., Frontali, M., et al. (1993). Trinucleotide repeat length instability and age of onset in Huntington's disease. *Nat. Genet.* 4, 387–392.

Hogarth, P., Kayson, E., Kieburtz, K., Marder, K., Oakes, D., Rosas, D., et al. (2005). Interrater agreement in the assessment of motor manifestations of Huntington's disease. *Mov. Disord.* 20, 293–297.

Hungtington Study Group. (1996). Unified Huntington's Disease Rating Scale: reliability and consistency. *Mov. Disord.* 11, 136–142.

Huntington Study Group. (2001). A randomized, placebo-controlled trial of coenzyme Q10 and remacemide in Huntington's disease. *Neurology* 57, 397–404.

Huntington Study Group PHAROS Investigators. (2006). At risk for Huntington disease: the PHAROS (Prospective Huntington At Risk Observational Study) cohort enrolled. *Arch. Neurol.* 63, 991–996.

Marder, K., Zhao, H., Myers, R. H., Cudkowicz, M., Kayson, E., Kieburtz, K., et al. (2000). Rate of functional decline in Huntington's disease. Huntington Study Group. *Neurology* 54, 452–458.

Paulsen, J. S., Hayden, M., Stout, J. C., Langbehn, D. R., Aylward, E., Ross, C. A., et al. (2006). Preparing for preventive clinical trials: the Predict-HD study. *Arch. Neurol.* 63, 883–890.

Paulsen, J. S., Langbehn, D. R., Stout, J. C., Aylward, E., Ross, C. A., Nance, M., et al. (2008). Detection of Huntington's disease decades before diagnosis: the Predict-HD study. *J. Neurol. Neurosurg. Psychiatry* 79, 874–880.

Paulsen, J. S., Wang, C., Duff, K., Barker, R., Nance, M., Beglinger, L., et al. (2010). Challenges assessing clinical endpoints in early Huntington disease. *Mov. Disord.* 25, 2595–2603.

Solomon, A. C., Stout, J. C., Johnson, S. A., Langbehn, D. R., Aylward, E. H., Brandt, J., et al. (2007). Verbal episodic memory declines prior to diagnosis in Huntington's disease. *Neuropsychologia* 45, 1767–1776.

Sperling, R. A., Aisen, P. S., Beckett, L. A., Bennett, D. A., Craft, S., Fagan, A. M., et al. (2011). Toward defining the preclinical stages of Alzheimer's disease: recommendations from the National Institute on Aging-Alzheimer's Association workgroups on diagnostic guidelines for Alzheimer's disease. *Alzheimers Dement.* 7, 280–292.

Stout, J. C., Paulsen, J. S., Queller, S., Solomon, A. C., Whitlock, K. B., Campbell, J. C., et al. (2011). Neurocognitive signs in prodromal Huntington disease. *Neuropsychology* 25, 1–14.

Thieben, M. J., Duggins, A. J., Good, C. D., Gomes, L., Mahant, N., Richards, F., et al. (2002). The distribution of structural neuropathology in pre-clinical Huntington's disease. *Brain* 125, 1815–1828.

Conflict of Interest Statement: Dr. Biglan receives grant funding from the MJFF, NINDS, NPF, HDSA, Lundbeck, Google Inc., Marvell Inc., Excellus-Blue Cross Consultant for Theravance, and Lundbeck; he also has contracts with Presbyterian Home for Central NY and the Parkinson Support Group for Central NY, and Susquehanna Nursing Home and Rehabilitation Center. Dr. Geschwind does consulting for Medacoro Consultant, Clinical Advisors, and Gerson Lehman Group and is on the Editorial Board of Dementia Cognition. Dr. Raymond's research is supported by operating grants from the Canadian Institutes of Research, the Cure Huntington Disease Initiative Foundation, Inc., and the Michael J Fox Foundation. Dr. Testa received research support from the Huntington Society of Canada (principal investigator), as well as the Tremor Research Group, HighQ Foundation, and Huntington Study Group (site principal investigator subcontracts). The Tremor Research Group subcontract sponsor is GlaxoSmithKline. Huntington Study Group subcontract sponsors are NIH/NINDS or Medivation. She was a co-investigator on NIH/NCRR 2R24RR018827-05A1. Dr. Wojcieszek receives clinical trial funding from Medivation, Novartis, Scheering Plough, and TEVA; she is also part of the TEVA speaker's bureau. All other authors report no disclosures or potential conflicts of interest.

Permissions

All chapters in this book were first published in CUBFND, by Frontiers; hereby published with permission under the Creative Commons Attribution License or equivalent. Every chapter published in this book has been scrutinized by our experts. Their significance has been extensively debated. The topics covered herein carry significant findings which will fuel the growth of the discipline. They may even be implemented as practical applications or may be referred to as a beginning point for another development.

The contributors of this book come from diverse backgrounds, making this book a truly international effort. This book will bring forth new frontiers with its revolutionizing research information and detailed analysis of the nascent developments around the world.

We would like to thank all the contributing authors for lending their expertise to make the book truly unique. They have played a crucial role in the development of this book. Without their invaluable contributions this book wouldn't have been possible. They have made vital efforts to compile up to date information on the varied aspects of this subject to make this book a valuable addition to the collection of many professionals and students.

This book was conceptualized with the vision of imparting up-to-date information and advanced data in this field. To ensure the same, a matchless editorial board was set up. Every individual on the board went through rigorous rounds of assessment to prove their worth. After which they invested a large part of their time researching and compiling the most relevant data for our readers.

The editorial board has been involved in producing this book since its inception. They have spent rigorous hours researching and exploring the diverse topics which have resulted in the successful publishing of this book. They have passed on their knowledge of decades through this book. To expedite this challenging task, the publisher supported the team at every step. A small team of assistant editors was also appointed to further simplify the editing procedure and attain best results for the readers.

Apart from the editorial board, the designing team has also invested a significant amount of their time in understanding the subject and creating the most relevant covers. They scrutinized every image to scout for the most suitable representation of the subject and create an appropriate cover for the book.

The publishing team has been an ardent support to the editorial, designing and production team. Their endless efforts to recruit the best for this project, has resulted in the accomplishment of this book. They are a veteran in the field of academics and their pool of knowledge is as vast as their experience in printing. Their expertise and guidance has proved useful at every step. Their uncompromising quality standards have made this book an exceptional effort. Their encouragement from time to time has been an inspiration for everyone.

The publisher and the editorial board hope that this book will prove to be a valuable piece of knowledge for researchers, students, practitioners and scholars across the globe.

List of Contributors

Wolfgang J. Streit and Qing-Shan Xue
Department of Neuroscience, University of Florida College of Medicine and McKnight Brain Institute, Gainesville, FL, USA

Brenda Colella, Mark Bayley and Joanna Glazer
Cognitive Neurorehabilitation Sciences Laboratory, Research Department, Toronto Rehabilitation Institute, Toronto, ON, Canada

Robin E. A. Green
Cognitive Neurorehabilitation Sciences Laboratory, Research Department, Toronto Rehabilitation Institute, Toronto, ON, Canada
Department of Psychiatry, Faculty of Medicine, University of Toronto, Toronto, ON, Canada

JeromeJ.Maller
Brain Stimulation and Neuroimaging Laboratory, Monash Alfred Psychiatry Research Centre, Alfred Hospital, Melbourne, VIC, Australia

David J. Mikulis
fMRI Laboratory, Division of Applied and Interventional Research, Toronto Western Research Institute, Toronto, ON, Canada
Department of Medical Imaging, Faculty of Medicine, University of Toronto, Toronto, ON, Canada

Roger ABarker
Department of Clinical Neuroscience, Cambridge Centre for Brain Repair, University of Cambridge, Cambridge, UK

Francesca Cicchetti
Centre de Recherch edu CHUL(CHUQ),Axe Neurosciences, Québec, QC, Canada
Département de Psychiatrie et Neurosciences, Université Laval, Québec, QC, Canada

Michelle L. Keightley
Bloorview Research Institute, Holl and Bloorview Kids Rehabilitation Hospital, Toronto, ON, Canada
Department of Occupational Science and Occupational Therapy, University of Toronto, Toronto, ON, Canada
Graduate Department of Rehabilitation Science, University of Toronto, ON, Canada
Department of Psychology, University of Toronto, ON, Canada
Cognitive Neurorehabilitation Sciences, Toronto Rehabilitation Institute, Toronto, ON, Canada

Katia J. Sinopoli
Bloorview Research Institute, Holl and Bloorview Kids Rehabilitation Hospital, Toronto, ON, Canada
Department of Psychology and Division of Neurology, Sickids Hospital for Sick Children, Toronto, ON, Canada

David J. Mikulis
Division of Brain, Imaging and Behaviour-Systems Neuroscience, Toronto Western Research Institute, University Health Network, Toronto, ON, Canada

Karen D. Davis
Division of Brain, Imaging and Behaviour-Systems Neuroscience, Toronto Western Research Institute, University Health Network, Toronto, ON, Canada
Department of Surgery and Institute of Medical Science, University of Toronto, Toronto, ON, Canada

Richard Wennberg, Maria C. Tartaglia and Charles H. Tator
Krembil Neuroscience Centre, Toronto Western Hospital, University Health Network and University of Toronto, Toronto, ON, Canada

Jen-KaiChen
Neuropsychology/CognitiveNeuroscience Unit, Montreal Neurological Institute, Montreal, QC, Canada

John Q.Trojanowski
Department of Pathology and Laboratory Medicine, Center for Neurodegenerative Disease Research, Alzheimer's Disease Core Center, Institute on Aging, University of Pennsylvania, Philadelphia, PA, USA

David J. Irwin
Department of Pathology and Laboratory Medicine, Center for Neurodegenerative Disease Research, Alzheimer's Disease Core Center, Institute on Aging, University of Pennsylvania, Philadelphia, PA, USAw
Department of Neurology, Center for Front ot emporal Dementia, Perelman School of Medicine, University of Pennsylvania, Philadelphia, PA, USA

Murray Grossman
Department of Neurology, Center for Front ot emporal Dementia, Perelman School of Medicine, University of Pennsylvania, Philadelphia, PA, USA

Diana Frasca and Robin E. Green
Graduate Department of Rehabilitation Science, University of Toronto, Toronto, ON, Canada
Cognitive Neurorehabilitation Sciences Laboratory, Toronto Rehabilitation Institute, Toronto, ON, Canada

Jennifer Tomaszczyk
Cognitive Neurorehabilitation Sciences Laboratory, Toronto Rehabilitation Institute, Toronto, ON, Canada

Bradford J. McFadyen
Département de Réadaptation, Université Laval, Québec City, QC, Canada
Centre Inter disciplinaire Recherche en Réad aptation et Intégration Sociale, Québec City, QC, Canada

YueHuang and Glenda M. Halliday
Neuroscience Research Australia, Sydney, NSW, Australia
University of New South Wales, Sydney, NSW, Australia

Maria Carmela Tartaglia
Division of Neurology, Krembil Neuroscience Centre, University Health Network, University of Toronto, Toronto, ON, Canada
Tanz Centre for Research in Neurodegenerative Disease, University of Toronto, Toronto, ON, Canada
Canadian Sports Concussion Project, Toronto, ON, Canada

Lili-NazHazrati
Tanz Centre for Research in Neurodegenerative Disease, University of Toronto, Toronto, ON, Canada
Canadian Sports Concussion Project, Toronto, ON, Canada
Department of Laboratory Medicine and Pathobiology, University of Toronto, Toronto, ON, Canada

Karen D. Davis
Canadian Sports Concussion Project, Toronto, ON, Canada
Division of Neurosurgery, University Health Network, University of Toronto, Toronto, ON, Canada
Division of Brain, Imaging and Behaviour-Systems Neuroscience, Toronto Western Research Institute, University Health Network, Toronto, ON, Canada
Department of Surgery, University of Toronto, Toronto, ON, Canada
Institute of Medical Science, University of Toronto, Toronto, ON, Canada

Robin E.A. Green
Canadian Sports Concussion Project, Toronto, ON, Canada Toronto Rehabilitation Institute, Toronto, ON, Canada

Richard Wennberg
Division of Neurology, Krembil Neuroscience Centre, University Health Network, University of Toronto, Toronto, ON, Canada
Canadian Sports Concussion Project, Toronto, ON, Canada

David Mikulis
Canadian Sports Concussion Project, Toronto, ON, Canada
Division of Neuroradiology, Joint Department of Medical Imaging, Toronto Western Hospital, The University of Toronto, Toronto, ON, Canada

Leo J. Ezerins
Canadian Sports Concussion Project, Toronto, ON, Canada
Executive Director, Canadian Football League Alumni Association, Toronto, ON, Canada

Michelle Keightley
Canadian Sports Concussion Project, Toronto, ON, Canada
Toronto Rehabilitation Institute, Toronto, ON, Canada
Bloorview Research Institute, Holl and Bloorview Kids Rehabilitation Hospital, Toronto, ON, Canada
Department of Occupational Science and Occupational Therapy, University of Toronto, Toronto, ON, Canada
Graduate Department of Rehabilitation Science, University of Toronto, Toronto, ON, Canada
Department of Psychology, University of Toronto, Toronto, ON, Canada

Charles Tator
Canadian Sports Concussion Project, Toronto, ON, Canada
Division of Neurosurgery, Krembil Neuroscience Centre, Toronto Western Hospital, University of Toronto, Toronto, ON, Canada

Egle Solito
Centre for Translational Medicine and Therapeutics, William Harvey Research Institute, Bartsand The London, Queen Mary's School of Medicine and Dentistry, London, UK

Magdalena Sastre
Centre for Neuroscience, Division of Experimental Medicine, Imperial College London, London, Uk
PhediasDiamandis
Department of Laboratory Medicine and Pathobiology, University of Toronto, Toronto, ON, Canada

Lili-Naz Hazrati and Janice C. Wong
Department of Laboratory Medicine and Pathobiology, University of Toronto, Toronto, ON, Canada
Tanz Centre for Research in Neurodegenerative Diseases, University of Toronto, Toronto, ON, Canada

Maria C. Tartaglia
Tanz Centre for Research in Neurodegenerative Diseases, University of Toronto, Toronto, ON, Canada
Division of Neurology, Krembil Neuroscience Centre, University Health Network, University of Toronto, Toronto, ON, Canada

Richard Wennberg
Division of Neurology, Krembil Neuroscience Centre, University Health Network, University of Toronto, Toronto, ON, Canada

Karen D. Davis
Division of Neurosurgery, Krembil Neuroscience Centre, University Health Network, University of Toronto, Toronto, ON, Canada
Division of Brain, Imaging, and Behaviour-Systems Neuroscience, Toronto Western Research Institute, University Health Network, Toronto, ON, Canada
Department of Surgery, University of Toronto, Toronto, ON, Canada
Institute of Medical Science, University of Toronto, Toronto, ON, Canada

Charles H. Tator
Division of Neurosurgery, Krembil Neuroscience Centre, University Health Network, University of Toronto, Toronto, ON, Canada
Institute of Medical Science, University of Toronto, Toronto, ON, Canada

Robin E.Green
Research,Cognitive Neurorehabilitation Sciences Lab, Toronto Rehabilitation Institute, University of Toronto, Toronto, ON, Canada

Leo Ezerins
Executive Director, Canadian Football League Alumni Association, Members of the Canadian Sports Concussion Projectat the Krembil Neuroscience Centre, Toronto Western Hospital and University of Toronto, Toronto, ON, Canada

Joscelyn Agron, Isael Santos, Warren Barker and Maria T. Greig
Wien Center for Alzheimer's Disease and Memory Disorders, Mount Sinai Medical Center, Miami Beach, FL,USA

David A. Loewenstein
Wien Center for Alzheimer's Disease and Memory Disorders, Mount Sinai Medical Center, Miami Beach, FL,USA
Department of Psychiatry and Behavioral Sciences, Miller School of Medicine, University of Miami, Miami, USA

Qian Shen
Wien Center for Alzheimer's Disease and Memory Disorders, Mount Sinai Medical Center, Miami Beach, FL, USA
Department of Biomedical Engineering, University of Miami, Coral Gables, FL, USA

Daniel Varon
Wien Center for Alzheimer's Disease and Memory Disorders, Mount Sinai Medical Center, Miami Beach, FL, USA
Department of Neurology, Florida International University College of Medicine, Miami, FL, USA

Rosie Curiel
Department of Psychiatry and Behavioral Sciences, Miller School of Medicine, University of Miami, Miami, USA

Ranjan Duara
Wien Center for Alzheimer's Disease and Memory Disorders, Mount Sinai Medical Center, Miami Beach, FL,USA
Departments of Medicine and Neurology, Miller School of Medicine, University of Miami, Miami, FL, USA
Department of Psychiatry and Behavioral Sciences, Miller School of Medicine, University of Miami, Miami, USA
Department of Neurology, Florida International University College of Medicine, Miami, FL, USA
Departments of Molecular Medicine and Neurology, University of South Florida, Tampa, FL, USA
Johnnie B. Byrd, Sr.Alzheimer's Center and Research Institute, Tampa, FL, USA

Huntington Potter
Departments of Molecular Medicine and Neurology, University of South Florida, Tampa, FL, USA

Junghoon Kim and John Whyte
Moss Rehabilitation Research Institute, Elkins Park, PA, USA

Brian Avants and James C. Gee
Department of Radiology, University of Pennsylvania, Philadelphia, PA, USA

Hitoshi Sohma
Department of Educational Development, Center for Medical Education, Sapporo Medical University, Sapporo, Japan
Department of Biomedical Engineering, School of Medicine, Sapporo Medical University, Sapporo, Japan

Shin-ichiImai, Norio Takei, Kayo Matsuki and Yasuo Kokai
Department of Biomedical Engineering, School of Medicine, Sapporo Medical University, Sapporo, Japan

Hirohito Honda
Mikuri Immunology Laboratory, Inc., Osaka, Japan

Kyoichi Matsumoto
Sanyo Chemical Industries, Ltd., Kyoto, Japan

Kumiko Utsumi
Department of Neuropsychiatry, Sunagawa City Medical Center, Sunagawa, Japan

Eri Hashimoto and Toshikazu Saito
Department of Neuropsychiatry, School of Medicine, Sapporo Medical University, Sapporo, Japan

Erin D. Bigler
Department of Psychology, Brigham Young University, Provo, UT, USA
Neuroscience Center, Brigham Young University, Provo, UT, USA
Department of Psychiatry, University of Utah, Salt Lake City, UT, USA
The Brain Institute of Utah, University of Utah, Salt Lake City, UT, USA

Manuel Menéndez-González
Unidad de Neurología, Hospital Álvarez-Buylla, Mieres, Spain
Departamento de Morfologíay BiologíaCelular, UniversidaddeOviedo, Oviedo, Spain Instituto de Neurociencias, Universidad de Oviedo, Oviedo, Spain

Alfonso López-Muñiz
Departamento de Morfologíay BiologíaCelular, UniversidaddeOviedo, Oviedo, Spain
Instituto de Neurociencias, Universidad de Oviedo, Oviedo, Spain

José A. Vega
Departamento de Morfologíay Biología Celular, Universidadde Oviedo, Oviedo, Spain

José M. Salas-Pacheco
Instituto de Investigación Científica, Universidad Juárez del Estado de Durango, Durango, México

Oscar Arias-Carrión
Unidad de Trastornos del Movimiento y Sueño (TMS), Hospital General Dr.Manuel Gea González/UNAM, México DF, Mexico
Unidad de Trastornos del Movimiento y Sueño (TMS), Hospital General Ajusco Medio, México DF, Mexico

Patrick L. McGeer and Edith G. McGeer
Kinsmen Laboratory of Neurological Research, University of British Columbia, Vancouver, BC, Canada

Bradford C. Dickerson
Frontotemporal Dementia Unit, Massachusetts General Hospital and Harvard Medical School, Boston, MA, USA
Department of Neurology, Massachusetts General Hospital and Harvard Medical School, Boston, MA, USA
Massachusetts Alzheimer's Disease Research Center, Massachusetts General Hospital and Harvard Medical School, Boston, MA, USA
Athinoula A. Martinos Center for Biomedical Imaging, Massachusetts General Hospital and Harvard Medical School, Boston, MA, USA

David A. Wolk
Department of Neurology, University of Pennsylvania, Philadelphia, PA, USA
Alzheimer's Disease Core Center, University of Pennsylvania, Philadelphia, PA, USA
Penn Memory Center, University of Pennsylvania, Philadelphia, PA, USA

Marios Politis, Paul Su and Paola Piccini
Division of Experimental Medicine, Faculty of Medicine, Centre for Neuroscience, Hammersmith Hospital, Imperial College London, London, UK

Olof Lindberg, Eric Westman and Lars-Olof Wahlund
Department of Neurobiology, Care Sciences and Society, Karolinska Institutet, Stockholm, Sweden

Sari Karlsson
Aging Research Centre, Karolinska Institutet, Stockholm, Sweden

Per Östberg
Division of Speech and Language Pathology, Department of Clinical Science, Intervention and Technology, Karolinska Institutet, Stockholm, Sweden

Leif A. Svensson
Department of Medical Physics, Karolinska University Hospital, Stockholm, Sweden

Andrew Simmons
Institute of Psychiatry, King's College London, London, UK
NIHR Biomedical Research Centre for Mental Health, London, UK

Christine T. Ekdahl
Inflammation and Stem Cell Therapy Group, Division of Clinical Neurophysiology, Wallenberg Neuroscience Center, Department of Clinical Sciences, Lund University and Skåne University Hospital, Lund, Sweden

Kimberly D. Farbota
Geriatric Research and Education Clinical Center, William S. Middleton Memorial Veterans Hospital, Madison, WI, USA

University of Wisconsin Neuroscience Training Program, Madison, WI, USA

Barbara B. Bendlin and Sterling C. Johnson
Geriatric Research and Education Clinical Center, William S. Middleton Memorial Veterans Hospital, Madison, WI, USA
Department of Medicine, University of Wisconsin School of Medicine and Public Health, Madison, WI, USA

Andrew L. Alexander
Department of Medical Physics, University of Wisconsin School of Medicine and Public Health, Madison, WI, USA

Howard A. Rowley
Department of Radiology, University of Wisconsin School of Medicine and Public Health, Madison, WI, USA

Robert J. Dempsey
Department of Neurological Surgery, University of Wisconsin School of Medicine and Public Health, Madison, WI, USA

Shannon L. Risacher and Kwangsik Nho
Department of Radiology and Imaging Sciences, Center for Neuroimaging, Indiana University School of Medicine, Indianapolis, IN, USA

SungeunKim and Li Shen
Department of Radiology and Imaging Sciences, Center for Neuroimaging, Indiana University School of Medicine, Indianapolis, IN, USA
Center for Computational Biology and Bioinformatics, Indiana University School of Medicine, Indianapolis, IN, USA

Tatiana Foroud
Department of Medical and Molecular Genetics, Indiana University School of Medicine, Indianapolis, IN, USA

Andrew J. Saykin
Department of Radiology and Imaging Sciences, Center for Neuroimaging, Indiana University School of Medicine, Indianapolis, IN, USA
Center for Computational Biology and Bioinformatics, Indiana University School of Medicine, Indianapolis, IN, USA
Department of Medical and Molecular Genetics, Indiana University School of Medicine, Indianapolis, IN, USA

Robert C. Green
Division of Genetics, Department of Medicine, Brighamand Women's Hospital and Harvard Medical School, Boston, MA, USA

Ronald C. Petersen
Department of Neurology, Mayo Clinic, Rochester, MN, USA

Clifford R. JackJr.
Department of Radiology, Mayo Clinic, Rochester, MN, USA

Paul S. Aisen
Department of Neurology, University of California, San Diego, San Diego, CA, USA

Robert A. Koeppe
Department of Radiology, University of Michigan, Ann Arbor, MI, USA

William J. Jagust
Department of Neurology, University of California, Berkeley, Berkeley, CA, USA

Leslie M. Shaw and John Q. Trojanowski
Department of Pathology and Laboratory Medicine, University of Pennsylvania School of Medicine, Philadelphia, PA, USA

Michael W. Weiner
Departments of Radiology, Medicine, and Psychiatry, University of California, San Francisco, San Francisco, CA, USA
Department of Veterans Affairs Medical Center, San Francisco, CA,USA

Jonas J. Neher, Urte Neniskyte and Guy C. Brown
Department of Biochemistry, University of Cambridge, Cambridge, UK

Joao M. S. Pereira
Laboratory of Biostatistics and Medical Informatics, IBILI-Faculty of Medicine, University of Coimbra, Coimbra, Portugal
Department of Clinical Neurosciences, School of Clinical Medicine, University of Cambridge, Cambridge, UK

Julio Acosta-Cabronero, George Pengas and Guy B. Williams
Department of Clinical Neurosciences, School of Clinical Medicine, University of Cambridge, Cambridge, UK

Li Xiong
Neurology Department, Zhongnan Hospital of Wuhan University, Wuhan, China

Peter J. Nestor
German Center for Neurodegenerative Diseases (DZNE), Magdeburg, Germany

Sudarshan Phani, Diane Berengere Re and Serge Przedborski
Department of Pathology and Cell Biology, Columbia University, New York, NY, USA
Center for Motor Neuron Disease, Department of Neurology, Columbia University, New York, NY, USA

Lesley S. Miller
Applied Psychology and Human Development, Ontario Institute for Studiesin Education, University of Toronto, Toronto, ON, Canada

Brenda Colella
Cognitive Neurorehabilitation Sciences Lab, Research Department, Toronto Rehab-University Health Network, Toronto, ON, Canada

David Mikulis
fMRI Laboratory, Division of Appliedand Interventional Research, Toronto Western Research Institute, University Health Network, Toronto, ON, Canada
Faculty of Medicine, Department of Medical Imaging, University of Toronto, Toronto, ON, Canada

Jerome Maller
Brain Stimulation and Neuroimaging Laboratory, Monash Alfred Psychiatry Research Centre, Alfred Hospital, Melbourne, VIC, Australia

Robin E. A. Green
Cognitive Neurorehabilitation Sciences Lab, Research Department, Toronto Rehab-University Health Network, Toronto, ON, Canada
Graduate Department of Rehabilitation Science, University of Toronto, Toronto, ON, Canada

Jens Moreth, Chrystelle Mavoungou and Katharina Schindowski
Faculty for Biotechnology, Institute of Applied Biotechnology, Biberach University of Applied Science, Biberach/Riss, Germany

Kevin M. Biglan and Annie Killoran
Department of Neurology, University of Rochester, Rochester, NY, USA

Ying Zhang and Wenjing Lu
Department Biostatistics, University of Iowa, Iowa City, IA, USA

Jeffrey D. Long, James A. Mills and JaneS.Paulsen
Department of Psychiatry, University of Iowa, Iowa City, IA, USA

Michael Geschwind and Gail A. Kang
Department of Neurology, University of California San Francisco, San Francisco, CA, USA

Elizabeth McCusker
Department of Neurology, Westmead Hospital, Sydney, NSW, Australia

Lynn A. Raymond
Division of Psychiatry, University of British Columbia, Vancouver, BC, Canada

Claudia Testa
VCU Parkinson' sand Movement Disorders Center Virginia Common wealth University, Richmond, VA, USA

Joanne Wojcieszek
Department of Neurology, Indiana University, Indianapolis, IN, USA

Index

A

Adult-born Neurons, 170-176

Alzheimer's Disease, 1, 5-7, 13, 17, 35-39, 68, 71, 73, 75-77, 79, 83-87, 89, 100, 106, 110, 112-116, 123-125, 129-131, 150-151, 155, 169, 172, 202-205, 216, 237, 241-243, 250

Amygdala, 22, 26, 57, 90-94, 130, 137

Anxiety, 101, 230-231, 234

Apolipoprotein E (apoe), 110-112, 193-194

Apoptosis, 15, 18, 42, 50-51, 54, 58, 63, 69, 82-83, 111, 118, 176, 178, 205, 209-212, 225, 228

Atrophy, 8-9, 11-16, 19-20, 31, 40, 51-52, 54-55, 57-58, 68, 73, 75, 88, 90-94, 96-102, 127-137, 148-149, 151, 153, 179, 193, 195, 199-200, 203, 229-230, 233-236, 248, 250

Axons, 3, 14, 22, 26, 74, 76, 119, 170, 173, 179-180, 186-187, 227

B

Brain Development, 7, 117, 119, 121, 177, 212

C

Cardiovascular Risk, 97, 102

Cerebrospinal Fluid, 11, 21, 24, 28, 30, 35-38, 74, 76, 98, 115, 120, 128, 135-136, 143, 145, 151, 193-194, 203, 237, 241-242

Chronic Traumatic Encephalopathy, 22, 71, 73, 87-88, 95

Corpus Callosum, 8-9, 13, 22, 24-26, 74, 76, 90-93, 107-108, 119, 122-124, 127, 131, 164, 179-180, 183-192

Cortical Thinning, 25, 127, 169, 203

D

Dementia With Lewy Bodies, 92, 110, 112, 114-116, 135

Depression, 16, 55, 72-73, 89, 92, 97, 101-102, 115-116, 124, 126, 129-130, 175, 195, 230-231, 234-235

Dopamine Neurons, 62-63, 67

Dorsolateral Prefrontal Cortex, 153, 162-163, 165, 169

E

Encephalomalacia, 9, 105

Entorhinal Cortex, 90, 93, 96-98, 101, 133, 162-163, 165, 169, 218, 222

Environmental Enrichment, 14-16, 39-41, 49-52, 55-60, 176, 229-230, 235

F

Forgetfulness, 163, 168

Frontotemporal Dementia, 28-29, 35-38, 73, 116, 135, 143, 155, 160, 162-163, 169, 205, 211, 213, 216, 222

Frontotemporal Lobar Degeneration, 28, 31, 35, 37, 71, 126, 155, 162, 210

G

Gyral Crowns, 92-93

H

Hippocampi, 8-9, 11, 13-14, 22, 25, 74, 90, 217

Huntington's Disease, 17-18, 20-21, 152, 154, 158, 160, 230, 244, 250

I

Immunohistochemistry, 6, 17, 30, 88, 139

Impaired Neuronal Protection, 1

Insula, 73, 145, 162-163, 166

L

Lactadherin, 205-206, 210

Lateral Sclerosis, 19-20, 28-29, 36, 38, 72-73, 75, 85, 87, 89-90, 207, 210, 213, 223, 227-228

M

Macrophages, 1-2, 5-6, 17, 77-78, 81, 83, 138-139, 141, 158, 171, 176-177, 205-207, 211-213, 224-225

Magnetic Resonance Imaging, 16, 22, 28, 33, 55, 60, 102, 104, 109, 111, 119, 137, 144, 161, 193, 236-237

Medial Temporal Lobe, 74, 96, 102, 124, 132, 134, 136-137, 169

Microglia, 1-7, 17-21, 62, 68-69, 77-86, 138-142, 152-161, 170-178, 205-213, 223-228

Microglial Cells, 1-7, 17-18, 21, 79-80, 85-86, 139-141, 161, 177, 212, 224-225

Microglial Senescence, 1, 3-4, 18

Mild Cognitive Impairment, 7, 79, 96, 100, 102, 123-124, 130, 132, 136, 143, 150-151, 155, 169, 193, 202, 210, 216, 239, 248, 250

Mitochondrial Dysfunction, 61, 64, 224

Moderate To Severe, 15-16, 22, 24-26, 39, 52, 56, 75-76, 104-105, 109, 128-129, 131, 229, 235

Motorneuron Disease, 19

Multiple Sclerosis, 139, 152, 156-161, 205, 226

Myelination, 25, 119-120, 160

N

Neurodegeneration, 1-2, 4-5, 7, 18-19, 22, 58, 62, 74, 79-80, 91, 104, 106, 117, 125, 135, 140, 143-145, 147-150, 156, 158, 161, 176, 199-202, 205-206, 208, 212, 224-225, 227

Neurogenic Niche, 170-173

Neuroimaging, 8, 15, 23, 26, 30-31, 33-34, 38, 71, 75-76, 105-108, 117-123, 125, 127, 129, 131-133, 135-137, 143-144, 150-151, 190, 192-194, 202-203, 229, 237, 240, 248

Neuronal Death, 5, 14-15, 61, 63, 79, 81, 85, 121, 124, 152, 158, 172, 207-210, 212-213, 227

Neuroprotection, 1-3, 5, 69, 80-81, 85, 160, 175, 177
Neuropsychiatric Disorders, 117-118
Neurotoxicity, 82-83, 86, 111, 113, 212-213, 241-242

P

Paget's Disease, 29
Parkinson's Disease, 5, 17-18, 20-21, 61, 67-70, 72-73, 85, 87-89, 95, 102, 110, 135, 152-153, 158, 160-161, 205, 207, 209-210, 213, 230
Passive Immunization, 237
Pathogenic Mutations, 29, 33
Phagocytosis, 2-4, 6, 20, 78-82, 85, 122, 139, 141-142, 159, 172, 177-178, 205-213, 224
Pharmacogenetics, 237, 241
Pharmacology, 15, 17, 19
Phosphatidylserine, 205, 208-213
Plasma Biomarker, 110, 115
Positron Emission Tomography (pet), 144, 152, 193
Post-acute Decline, 39-40, 51, 235
Primary Progressive Aphasia, 28-29, 36, 73
Proteinopathy, 71, 74, 76, 95

S

Semantic Dementia, 36, 135-136, 162-163, 216, 221-222
Sparse Canonical Correlation Analysis, 104
Subependyma, 170-173, 177
Subgranular Zone, 170, 173
Subiculum, 11, 90, 93, 101, 133, 163
Substantia Nigra, 18, 21, 43, 59, 61-62, 64, 68, 83, 88, 90-93, 141, 153-154, 159-160, 209-212
Synapse Dysfunction, 61
Synaptic Pruning, 170, 174, 207

T

Tauopathies, 28, 34, 36-38, 74-75, 87-88
Transition Home, 39, 53, 55
Traumatic Brain Injury, 8, 10, 15-16, 22, 26-27, 37, 39, 55-60, 73, 75-76, 104, 108-109, 117, 119, 124-131, 179, 190-192, 229, 234-236

U

Ubiquitination, 61-65, 83
Ulcerative Colitis, 62, 67-68

V

Volumetric Measures, 96-97, 107, 135

www.ingramcontent.com/pod-product-compliance
Lightning Source LLC
LaVergne TN
LVHW080925210926
848485LV00004B/732
* 9 7 8 1 6 3 9 8 9 0 0 1 9 *